Tuskegee's Truths

Tuskegee's

STUDIES IN SOCIAL MEDICINE

Allan M. Brandt & Larry R. Churchill, editors

Truths

RETHINKING THE TUSKEGEE SYPHILIS STUDY

EDITED BY

SUSAN M. REVERBY

University of North Carolina Press

Chapel Hill and London

© 2000 The University of North Carolina Press
All rights reserved
Set in Minion, Meta, and Franklin Gothic types
by Keystone Typesetting, Inc.
Manufactured in the United States of America
The paper in this book meets the guidelines for permanence
and durability of the Committee on Production Guidelines for
Book Longevity of the Council on Library Resources.
Library of Congress Cataloging-in-Publication Data
Tuskegee's truths: rethinking the Tuskegee syphilis study /
edited by Susan M. Reverby; foreword by James H. Jones.
    p.   cm.
Includes bibliographical references and index.
ISBN 0-8078-2539-5 (alk. paper)
ISBN 0-8078-4852-2 (pbk.: alk. paper)
1. Tuskegee Syphilis Study. 2. Human experimentation in
medicine—Alabama—Macon County—History. 3. Afro-American
men—Diseases—Alabama—Macon County—History. 4. Syphilis—
Research—Alabama—Macon County—History. I. Reverby, Susan.
R853.H8 T87   2000
174'.28'0976149—dc21   99-056379

04   03   02   01   00   5   4   3   2   1

For Darlene and Cynthia

and in memory of Rachel

CONTENTS

A section of illustrations follows page 181.

FOREWORD

JAMES H. JONES

As a historian working on the Tuskegee syphilis experiment in the early 1970s, I had to make choices in my book about what I would emphasize. What would carry the narrative tale, what would become the backdrop? I knew as I wrote *Bad Blood* that there were other questions to explore, that other people's sensibilities would broaden the scope of the inquiry. That is precisely what has happened.

The present volume, judiciously edited by Susan Reverby, provides its readers with a chance to see where this inquiry has gone. Beginning with a careful selection from several different archives of the letters between the Public Health Service and Tuskegee Institute, as well as other primary documents, it provides a glimpse into the mindset and decisions that made the study possible. Many of the other articles address differing ways to analyze the study. Some of these pieces do not always take an approach I would share; others even come to conclusions I abhor. But they do allow readers to see how the study has been understood and how differing values and beliefs shape historical understandings.

When I went to work on the Tuskegee Study in August of 1972, I was fresh out of graduate school. Several years earlier, I had worked on an unrelated topic in Record Group 90 of the PHS Records at the National Archives. These records pertained to the PHS's division of venereal diseases. Everything in the Record Group spoke either to the treatment or the prophylaxis of venereal disease, with one exception: four letter boxes of materials containing the records of an untreated syphilis program in Macon County, Alabama, in and around the county seat of Tuskegee. I remember spending two or three hours perusing these materials and being horrified by what I read. Still, I had seen other examples in my archival research of nontherapeutic medical research studies and I had no way of knowing that the Tuskegee Study was still active. I was, after all, in an archive.

When the Associated Press's Jean Heller broke the story of Tuskegee in July 1972, I had just completed my doctorate at Indiana University and was about to begin postdoctoral study in the history of medicine and medical ethics at Harvard University. I had been granted a fellowship to work on the social hygiene move-

James H. Jones holds the Alumni Distinguished Professor Chair and is professor of history at the University of Arkansas and the author of Bad Blood: The Tuskegee Syphilis Experiment. *Printed by permission of James H. Jones.*

ment. Haunted by what I had read in those four boxes three years earlier, I decided to switch to the Tuskegee Study. The result, nine years later, was my book, *Bad Blood: The Tuskegee Syphilis Experiment, A Tragedy of Race and Medicine*.

In *Bad Blood*, I set several tasks for myself. At the broadest level, I wanted to discover what had happened and to shape the story into a coherent narrative that would reach a broad audience. But I also knew that there were important analytic points that needed to be made. First and foremost, I wanted to examine the role of race in medicine. Specifically, I sought to learn how racial attitudes affected the perception of disease that white physicians brought to their African American patients, and, having done so, I wanted to learn how those attitudes altered the ways in which white physicians responded to disease in the black community. At this point, scholars had taught us a great deal about race and politics, race and social structure, and race and the economy. But we knew very little about the relationship between race and medicine. The Tuskegee Syphilis Study, I was convinced, was a critical case that could help to fill this lacuna.

Other concerns also informed my analysis. The Tuskegee Study lasted for forty years, making it the longest nontherapeutic experiment in history. Given this longevity, I was convinced that the study could teach us a great deal about the evolution of normative ethics within the medical profession, as well as the nature of decision making in bureaucracies. Moreover, I assumed that the physicians who conducted the study did not see themselves as evil agents who meant to do harm. I believed that the study could shed light on how good people could err for what many of them thought were the best of reasons. By pursuing Tuskegee, then, I hoped to learn about moral ambiguity, slippery slopes, and, in the end, moral catastrophe.

Tuskegee's Truths provides a way to see how the study can be approached from many disciplines. Historians may bemoan the incursions made by others into their turf. But historical experiences have always been fair game. It is often in this disciplinary poaching that we gain new insights into the meanings that scholars or writers can make of a historical experience. By including a wide range of materials, from poetry, to plays, to medical accounts, Susan Reverby has tapped into the various ways the Tuskegee Study continues to have contemporary resonance.

What has impressed me the most about the Tuskegee Study is its staying power as a subject of public concern. We know that knowledge about the study circulates continually among many members of the African American community. The presidential apology, the film *Miss Evers' Boys*, the revelations of other kinds of research that trampled on the rights of subjects, and the continued teaching of the scholarship on the study all help to introduce differing understandings to broader and broader members of the public and research communities.

What worries me the most is when the Tuskegee Study is forgotten. When I get calls from medical researchers who tell me they are just learning about the study, I am the most troubled. This study needs to stay on our moral horizons forever. As a historian, I can only hope that the horror I felt more than two decades ago as I read page after page in the National Archives continues to be a beacon of warning. Susan Reverby's edited volume should be a step toward making sure this happens.

PREFACE

ALLAN M. BRANDT & LARRY R. CHURCHILL

The Tuskegee Syphilis Study holds a central place in our understanding of twentieth-century medicine, science, race, and research. This study of "untreated syphilis in the Negro male," begun by the United States Public Health Service in 1932, has galvanized attention, interest, and debate since it was widely reported in the national media in 1972. At that time, the study was stopped, but the debate about what happened at Tuskegee and what it means has continued virtually unabated into our own time. Researchers and writers, ethicists and activists have repeatedly turned their attention to the Tuskegee Study in the last quarter-century. In this respect, the study has become more than an important and tragic episode in the ongoing history of human subjects research. As the writings collected here by Susan Reverby so clearly indicate, the study reels with significance for the most central questions of contemporary medicine and society.

Social medicine adheres to a basic premise that the organization and practices of medical science will inevitably reveal powerful social forces active in the contemporary society. This is, no doubt, particularly true of human subjects research, where the desire for knowledge is pitted against the potential risks and harms to human beings. Investigating how this complex calculus is determined and rationalized—how the balance is struck between the rights of subjects and the demands of science—forces a fuller examination of the historically specific social, political, and economic contexts in which research occurs. In the case of the Tuskegee Study, in which some 400 poor, mostly illiterate African American sharecroppers became the unwitting objects of investigation, the seeds of ethical disaster were planted in the selection of such vulnerable subjects, so easily exploited by the combined power of government and science.

There are, of course, many examples of ethically egregious research in the twentieth century, from Nazi experimentation to the now well-documented human radiation experiments in the United States. But as this book so powerfully shows, Tuskegee has continued to generate concerted attention and has served as a repeated referent for many subsequent debates. The study has impressively become a template by which other experiments are measured and evaluated. Perhaps this is because the underlying social conditions that gave rise to the Tuskegee Study remain so fundamentally problematic in contemporary American medicine and science. The Tuskegee Study's design itself was predicated on an epidemiological finding: the wide disparity in patterns of disease between African Americans and whites. Such disparities persist and in some cases have actually expanded in recent years. Tuskegee was also predicated on the problem of unequal access to health services. Equity of access to medical care and treatment remains a central dilemma in American society. The Tuskegee Study also reflected fundamental obstacles to the participation of African Americans as physicians, nurses, and researchers. The diversity of these professions remains limited. Finally, the Tuskegee Study represents deeply held views about the relationship of race, sexuality, and disease; these views reflected racist assumptions in the early twentieth century and continue to shape debates about race and difference in our own time as well. For these reasons—and others—the Tuskegee Study continues to generate vigorous attention and concern. Even President Clinton's recent official apology is unlikely to bring an end to the debates about Tuskegee.

Tuskegee remains emblematic of ongoing debates that are far from resolution, creating a strong justification for continued inquiry into the Tuskegee Study itself. Examining these debates—and the eclectic writings they have produced—will not only deepen our understanding of the Tuskegee Study. These writings also offer an important lens for viewing ethics and morals in the course of twentieth-century medicine. Until we master those social injustices and conflicts which inspired this tragic study, our motivation for returning to Tuskegee will remain.

ACKNOWLEDGMENTS

This book began as a challenge to me from historian Darlene Clark Hine to write about Nurse Rivers after we both saw the Atlanta staging of David Feldshuh's play *Miss Evers' Boys*, a fictionalized telling of the Tuskegee Syphilis Study story. What I thought was going to be just a short paper on Rivers' involvement in the study just kept on growing as my visits to Tuskegee for research hooked me on the community and its history. I have taught the study in my classes and spoken about it in a wide range of forums, including professional meetings, a convention of the Public Health Service Commissioned Officers, a meeting of the Boston Visiting Nurse Association, and a talk-radio show aimed at Chicago's black community. In doing this, the necessity to provide more information and explore multiple viewpoints became obvious. This collection is my effort to make a wide variety of materials available to anyone who wants to know more and to think about what it means. It would not have happened without Darlene Clark Hine's faith in me as a scholar and stand-up woman. I cannot begin to thank her for this support.

Many other people made this book possible and provided support in large and small ways. Evelynn M. Hammonds traded stories and insights regularly. Dixie Dysart gave me a home in Alabama, taught me to appreciate southern cooking, sent me clippings, and introduced me to the joys of playing bar trivia with selected members of the Auburn University history department. Cynthia Wilson and Daniel Williams, the archivists of the Washingtonian Collection at Tuskegee University, were generous with their sage advice and finding skills. Cynthia Wilson cares passionately about Tuskegee, was a wonderful guide to its mores and history, and in this long process became a good friend. James H. Jones, the author of *Bad Blood*, was unstinting in his willingness to share information and to push me to make hard decisions. In this process we got to spend time together in Tuskegee, in the White House for the federal apology, and at an Astros' game. Not a bad deal. Allan M. Brandt, also a historian of the study, willingly agreed to include this complicated project in his series.

I am very grateful to Wellesley College for providing funds from the faculty grants program that made my travel possible, a sabbatical leave a reality, and the extensive permissions costs payable. In addition, funds from two of the "folding chairs" I held at Wellesley made research easier. My departmental colleagues— Rosanna Hertz, Elena Creef, Geeta Patel, Lidwien Kapteijns—listened forever. Students in my classes were great guides to the questions that needed to be asked. Wellesley College graduates worked on the multiple details of this book with me.

Kristel Maney and Jennifer Murray were invaluable assistants, as Maggie Felts and Sally Coombs had been earlier in the process.

I wish to thank Skip Gates and the staff and fellows of the Du Bois Institute for Afro-American Research, where I spent a sabbatical year getting much of this organized. I also had support from a grant from the American Association of University Women and the National Endowment for the Humanities for another book on Tuskegee I am still writing, but which jump-started this collection. Sian Hunter, my editor at the University of North Carolina Press, waited patiently for the book. She and her staff guided me through the myriad details with thoughtfulness, patience, and care. Pam Upton shepherded the volume through the production process with great understanding of the realities of daily life.

As always, family and friends made this work possible. My children, Mariah and Micah Sieber, put up with my obsession with the study and the endless hours this project took. My daughter managed to graduate from college while I wasn't looking, and my son entered high school while telling the Tuskegee story better than I can. My colleague and companion Bill Quivers kept me focused on what is important and why it matters.

Over the years it took to put this volume together, I lost two close friends who cared deeply about ethical research and history. I am sorry that Bob Cassell did not live long enough to see this collection finished, but I am grateful for the time he took to discuss medical research and public health with me. Rachel Fruchter, a superb community public health organizer and epidemiologist, was killed tragically in a biking accident. She served as a model of a research scientist committed to ethical research and the health care of immigrants, the poor, and women.

I have tried to use all the sage advice I received in making the hard decisions over what should or should not be included in this book. I did my best to provide balance and to accept what I could or could not get permission to use. I am now an expert (alas) on the complications of the permissions process and its costs.

For those who do health-care research or are its subjects, I hope this volume serves as a warning and guidepost. For the survivors of the study and their heirs, families, and friends, I hope this book is part of the justice you deserve.

Tuskegee's Truths

α

INTRODUCTION

More Than a Metaphor:
An Overview of the Scholarship of the Study

SUSAN M. REVERBY

For more than a quarter century now, the images conjured up by the words "Tuskegee Syphilis Study" or "bad blood" have haunted our cultural landscape. Sometimes their form is highly visible to the entire country: when the study first made national news in 1972, when President Clinton offered a formal apology twenty-five years later, or when Laurence Fishburne and Alfre Woodward starred in a fictionalized television movie of the story the same year. Other times the specter becomes more faint: kept alive by memory in the African American community, in queries that circulate over the world wide web and radio talk shows, or in courses taught by historians, sociologists, or bioethicists. But whether we read James H. Jones's book, *Bad Blood*, or recoil from the fears that chill us as we vaguely recall the details, the story of the Tuskegee Syphilis Study seemingly needs to be told, and told, and told.[1]

Each telling holds onto different aspects of the story. On the surface, the "facts" of the study seem clear enough. As Jones writes:

> In late July of 1972, Jean Heller of the Associated Press broke the story: for forty years the United States Public Health Service (PHS) had been conducting a study of the effects of untreated syphilis on black men in Macon County, Alabama, in and around the county seat of Tuskegee. The Tuskegee Study, as the experiment had come to be called, involved a substantial number of men: 399 who had syphilis and an additional 201 who were free of the disease chosen to serve as controls. All the syphilitic men were in the late stage of the disease when the study began.[2]

The men, however, thought that they were patients of a joint federal and local medical and nursing program at the Tuskegee Institute and the Macon County health department for their "bad blood," a local idiom that encompassed syphilis as well as anemias.[3] They did not consider themselves subjects since they did not know the study existed. The PHS followed the men for forty years (from 1932 to

Susan M. Reverby is professor of women's studies at Wellesley College.
Printed by permission of Susan M. Reverby.

1972), actively keeping them from many forms of treatment (including penicillin when it became available in the late 1940s), never giving them a clear diagnosis, but providing them with the watchful eye of a nurse as well as exams (including a diagnostic spinal tap), placebos, tonics, aspirins, and free lunches. Burial insurance became an additional inducement for their participation. In exchange, the men or their families agreed to allow for autopsies without knowing that the researchers needed to confirm the ravages of syphilis on the men's organs and tissues. Over the years, thirteen reports of the study were published in respectable medical science journals, from the *Journal of Venereal Disease Information* to the *Archives of Internal Medicine*. The study was never hidden from the larger American medical and public-health communities.

Set up by the PHS after a Rosenwald Foundation pilot project on rural syphilis diagnosis and treatment, the ostensible purpose was to study "untreated syphilis in the male Negro." The plan was to compare it to a retrospective, not prospective, study of white men and women done in Oslo, Norway, earlier in the century when little treatment was available. Following the outrage generated by the press reports of the study in 1972, there were Senate hearings on human experimentation, federal and state investigative reports, and a $1.8 billion lawsuit filed on behalf of the survivors and their families by civil rights attorney Fred Gray that was settled for $10 million. None of the physician-researchers who ran the study were ever prosecuted. Institutional review boards (IRBs) that must examine most protocols that involve human subjects before research studies begin now exist, in part, because of the revulsion against what happened in Tuskegee. And in 1997, twenty-five years after the story of the study was exposed, President Bill Clinton finally tendered the government's apology to the remaining eight survivors, their families, and the nation's African American citizens, while promising funds for a bioethics center at Tuskegee University.[4]

There have been, of course, numerous American medical research horror stories—live hepatitis virus given to retarded children at Willowbrook, the use of servicemen to test LSD, the civilians exposed to radiation experiments at the height of the Cold War, and other misuses of groups of vulnerable subjects.[5] In this context, the Tuskegee Study could be seen as just one of many violations of basic moral codes when science goes "bad."[6] But in medical research, especially before the end of World War II, researchers often checked with the "best men" in the field before they proceeded (as the physicians in the Tuskegee Study did).[7] They were not required to do the kind of informed consent we expect now. However, as historian Martin Pernick has argued, even before a patients' rights perspective developed around informed consent there was a sense of the importance of "truth-telling and consent-seeking" in medical practice in the nineteenth and early twentieth centuries.[8] But in the context of the PHS system, where hierarchies and an officers' corps based on a military model of chain of command existed, it is not surprising that the researchers at work in Tuskegee thought what they were doing was right. Support, after all, came from the United States' surgeon general, the top "commander" for the PHS.

In a sense, the Tuskegee Study has to be seen as the doing of research, at least in the beginning, in a normal mode. And when race enters the story, and the long-standing history of the use of African Americans as research "bodies" or cadavers is understood, then the study becomes less "bad" science than what became "normative" for research in this country.[9] The problem is less what happens when science goes "bad," but what happens when it is supposed to be "good."[10] The nature of medical research, and its moral fault lines, cannot be separated from a racialized belief system. As literary critic Michael Awkward noted, with no small irony since Booker T. Washington was Tuskegee Institute's founder, "it should be clear that Washingtonian notions of a strategic separateness [between whites and blacks] are no longer tenable, if they ever were."[11]

It is not surprising that a historical experience, containing the elements of a sexually transmitted disease, African Americans, coercion and lying by government officials, violation of trust between health-care providers and patients, and fear of experimentation, wrapped into a forty-year narrative with multiple media replays, would capture our analytic focus and reach into our cultural unconscious. Playing out with all the drama of a southern gothic tale, the story of the Tuskegee Syphilis Study holds our imaginations in thrall in ways that other medical research disasters do not. It almost would have to. As scholars Geneviève Fabre and Robert O'Meally have argued, by quoting author Richard Wright's midcentury comment, " 'the Negro [sic] is America's metaphor.' "[12]

In turn, the Tuskegee Study is America's metaphor for racism in medical research. It is often paired with the Nazi doctors' experiments on Holocaust victims that were detailed at the war trials at Nuremberg. Both serve as reminders of what medicine aligned with state power can do to those defined as "other."[13] But this most powerful metaphor of racism cannot contain all the various ways the narratives about the study come to be told, as the documents in this collection demonstrate. Ultimately our attempts to create a Manichean story in literally white and black terms explains too little, leaving us without the necessary elements to attempt a more complete effort at understanding. Tuskegee's Truths is a contribution toward creating this understanding by compiling examples of the ways scholars and others have used various kinds of facts and analytic approaches about the study.

To begin, we have to examine the historically specific ways race as a social category has been both created and creates differing kinds of medical assumptions and practices. Accepted paradigms about the existence of an assumed essential "black" body, with difference embodied in muscle, sinews, and disease potential, continues to, in historian Evelynn M. Hammonds's words, "mak[e] race real . . .

[by defining] a visible economy of difference."[14] In the syphilis study case, assumptions about African Americans' supposed special sexuality and susceptibility to cardiovascular damage from syphilis underlay much of the Tuskegee research, as Jones has argued. In addition, given the 1930s debate on syphilis treatment, race was used to fill in the lacunae in medical uncertainty.[15]

Racism, medical arrogance, and state power may help us to see how the study started, but it not enough to explain how it continued. The existence of class, sexuality, and gender in a racialized medical setting needs to be explored as well.[16] Without these elements in our analytic frame, we cannot fully appreciate the dilemmas for the African American health professionals who agreed to keep the study going. An analysis of class and gender within the black community is essential to see why Tuskegee Institute officials agreed to the study and how they related to the men brought in as "subjects." The history of the politics of both accommodation *and* resistance at Tuskegee Institute is required to explain the relationships among the federal officials, local state public-health doctors, and Tuskegee's staff.

Thus the study deserves a more complex reading, a probing below the surface of an ugly and painful story of entangled violations of a moral contract between human beings. In telling these versions of the story, many of the authors whose work is represented in this volume reach for other metaphors. Some of these suggest a moral absolutism that should cover every case of medical research for all times and cultures. Others understand the historical context that would shape moral beliefs, while trying not to fall into moral relativism that excuses inexcusable behaviors. Thus for some scholars, the study is a metaphor for what happens when there is no informed consent, when medical paternalism and arrogance substitute for a consciousness about research "materials" as human beings. Other writers, focused on the black professionals, remind us that in the context of the social and race reality of Alabama, a moral high ground could not be found because of the ever-present danger of lynching and violence.[17] Some authors choose to highlight the study as a story of government power and medical bureaucracies let loose on those unable to defend themselves. Still others emphasize the stories about the difference between North and South, urban and rural, federal and state and local medical power, the compromises enforced by the necessity to gain white philanthropic support to gain black educational and political power.[18] Some even see nothing wrong with what was done.

Thus as the story of the study gets told in form after form, the multiple narratives keep changing, taking on additional or differing cultural burdens. All the documents and articles in this volume demonstrate that metaphors are more than tools of academic discourse: they shape both understanding and human survival.

For the historian, the differing ways the story of the study gets told, the various facts that get marshaled to make a particular argument, and the elements that get left out are not about false memory or necessarily bad history making. Rather, in examining what does get remembered and analyzed, we can learn about what is historically important to differing authors at specific moments in time. As oral historian Alessandro Portelli has written: "The wrong tales allow us to recognize the interests of the tellers and the dreams and desires beneath them. . . . errors, inventions and myths lead us through beyond facts to their meanings."[19] In this spirit, the many selections in this book demonstrate not only the wide variety of ways to understand the study, but also the different meanings people can make of it.

What we "read" into this study depends, too, in part not only on what the authors write but also the questions we bring to it, the knowledge and beliefs we hold. For some in the African American community, Tuskegee is about the disasters and possible conspiracies that have been lurking, and continue to lurk, behind the ostensibly benign faces of physicians. For many African American health-care researchers, Tuskegee is a sobering reminder of the dangers of co-optation and the price extracted in the name of a seemingly larger good.[20] For some nurses, the study proves one nurse's comment that "in many double-blind studies, the only one who is really blinded is the nurse."[21] Others see the dilemma as allowing for both victimization and villainy.[22] For David Feldshuh, the physician-playwright author of the fictionalized *Miss Evers' Boys*, there are the fears of what he might be doing as a physician now. As Feldshuh remarked: "Here's this reprehensible study that very caring people partook in that made me wonder what guidelines would you follow. . . . If our intentions are good, how are we to be certain that we're not engaged in something that will in the future prove to be morally reprehensible or at least morally questionable?"[23]

And for those who believe in the god of science, there is the question of what happens when its feet are sullied. The late Robert Cassell, the former medical director for the Bridgeport, Connecticut, public health department, wrote: "The goal of human experimentation must always be to advance the human condition, and to improve the lot of the subjects of the study. These are the *sine qua non* of valid medical research. . . . When I read about Tuskegee . . . I, filled with faith in the religion of good and honest investigation that we call science, was emotionally overwhelmed."[24]

Robert Cassell was right. Sometimes thinking about the study, as with work on slavery or the Holocaust or the atomic bombing of Japan, does become overwhelming. It is possible to become very angry, or to imagine that this could not have happened, or to easily just shake our heads and click our tongues over what "they" did. When President Clinton offered the federal government's apology in 1997 to the survivors, the news coverage similarly emphasized the emotionality of the event. It was almost as if only in an emotional context could the pain of racial injustice and scientific arrogance become real or discussed. The horror and perfidiousness of the study could seemingly only be communicated to a television audience in the familiar daytime format of confession and repentance. But such reliance on emotion, while critical and cathartic, will only be a temporary fix if it does not become the basis for real commitment to a rethinking of research procedures, racial injustices, ethical precepts, and the categories this introduction has suggested.[25]

Tuskegee's Truths is offered in hopes that readers will not settle for this simple emotional path, but will take the time to consider what we can learn from multiple ways of telling and understanding the story. James H. Jones's *Bad Blood* remains to date the major accounting of the study, piecing together the history from the thousands of pages of primary documents, his interviews with many of the research scientists and the survivors, and a good deal of historical acumen. Published at first in 1981, Jones's interpretation of the study provides us with a narrative that begins with a preliminary probing of racialized medical beliefs and their consequences for the study's so-called subjects. It traces out the unfolding of the study, the various turning points in its convoluted history, and the decisions and rationalizations that provided the frame for its continuation. Jones's book is a masterful touchstone used by many of the authors represented in this volume as their source for understanding and facts.

But we need not fear complicating still further our understanding of the study, or looking at it differently. The Tuskegee Study, just as with other great injustices in our history, needs to be confronted head-on, to be read in as sophisticated a way possible so that we can both understand what happened and consider what will be necessary for prevention of a contemporary repeat. In writing about modern disasters, sociologist Kai Erikson calls them "a new species of trouble" because they are, in part, made through human hands and because whole communities find it difficult to heal. When this kind of "collective trauma" happens, Erikson notes, " 'our memory repeats to us what we haven't yet come to terms with, what still haunts us.' "[26]

The story of the Tuskegee Study is a form of collective trauma because it was caused by human hands, it affected an entire community, and it continues to haunt us. Knowing about it and trying to learn its truths will never erase this trauma or lessen its impact. Knowledge, and even apology, are never enough. But in survivor Herman Shaw's words from the presidential apology ceremony in 1997: "The damage done by the Tuskegee Study is much deeper than the wounds any of us may have suffered. It speaks to our faith in government and the ability of medical science to serve us as a force for good. [But] . . . in my opinion, it is never too late to work to restore faith and trust."[27]

Tuskegee's Truths was compiled to be part of the "work to restore faith and trust." It is organized into ten sections. The opening article by Allan M. Brandt and the timetable prepared by Susan E. Bell will orient the reader to the basic "facts" of the study. In the "Contemporary Background" section, two selections from books written in the 1930s provide a sense of how a prominent black social scientist saw the culture of Macon County and how the surgeon general defined the problem of syphilis in the black community. In "Documenting the Issues," selections were made from the thousands of pages of correspondence among the research scientists, the subject men, and the local and state health officials, and Jean Heller's initial story on the study in 1972. To read a historian's account of these exchanges is one thing; it is quite another to see the actual words and the full letters. These letters and reports remain the only real evidence we have of the contemporaneous thinking of the researchers as the study unfolded. This section also includes two of the published reports on the study, interviews with the survivors after the story broke, the testimony of Peter Buxton (the venereal disease investigator at the PHS who leaked the story to journalist Jean Heller), and selections from the federal investigation's final report.

The question of what kind of "treatment" the men actually received, and what treatment was thought appropriate, is discussed in Part IV. Vanderbilt University syphilologist R. H. Kampmeier gives an explanation of why he thought journalists misunderstood the study and how he saw the researchers' obligations to their subjects. Charles J. McDonald, writing soon after in the black medical society journal, tries to find some modicum of scientific benefit to the study. Historian/physician Thomas Benedek attempts to separate the moral and methodologic aspects of the study in an effort to explore the science itself. And historian Barbara Rosenkrantz, in reviewing Jones's *Bad Blood*, provides new questions about the medical uncertainty surrounding syphilis treatment.

Part V looks at differing kinds of historical reconsiderations. Martha Solomon [Watson] focuses on the rhetoric in the actual published medical reports to explain how the study could be "public" in the medical world and yet not questioned. Susan E. Lederer examines the study in the context of other medical research, provocatively arguing that the men were identified not as subjects, nor bodies, but as "cadavers" before they died. Historian/bioethicist John C. Fletcher forces us to examine the role of the PHS more closely, even arguing that the study ought to be renamed the Public Health Service Study to intensify their blame. Physician Benjamin Roy, using some of the primary letters, focuses on the use of the sera from the subjects in the creation of venereal disease tests.

Nurse Rivers, the African American, Tuskegee-trained nurse who served as the liaison between the men and the Public Health Service for the entire length of the study, has been subjected to much speculation about her motives and dilemmas. Part VI begins with the interview she gave in 1977 with Helen Dibble, the widow of Tuskegee's medical director, and Daniel Williams, Tuskegee University's chief archivist. In the following articles, historians Evelynn M. Hammonds, Susan L. Smith, Darlene Clark Hine, and I read the extant evidence and contemporary analytic frames that shape black women's history to provide differing explanations for what Rivers did.

"The Legacy of Tuskegee" examines the ways the Tuskegee Study is remembered. The late physician Vernal G. Cave, a venereal disease specialist, public-health official, and member of the federal investigating team, begins a discussion about the impact of the study on minority communities. Health educators Stephen B. Thomas and Sandra Crouse Quinn emphasize the lasting effects of the study in the black community. Bioethicist Arthur Caplan emphasizes the moral failures of the study, while attorney Patricia A. King reminds us of the costs of difference. Historian/physician Vanessa Northington Gamble puts the study in the perspective of other realistic reasons for African American mistrust of American health care. The selections from the 1995 nomination hearings of Dr. Henry Foster for surgeon general demonstrate how much an African American physician, who was working in Tuskegee toward the end of the study, was tainted by its long reach. Journalist Carol Kaesuk Yoon reminds us of the current impact of the study on the heirs and families of the so-called subjects and controls.

In the "Key Actors Rethink the Study" section, the emphasis is on the voices of those actually involved in the study itself, or in its dismantling. The report of the 1969 meeting at the Centers for Disease Control shows the reasoning behind the researchers who decided, despite Peter Buxton's outcry, to continue the study. Civil rights activist/lawyer Fred Gray, who has been the attorney for the men in Tuskegee and their families for more than a quarter century, discusses what it was like to make law and to try to find justice for them through the courts. Harold Edgar, the Columbia University lawyer who worked with Fred Gray to create the legal framework for the lawsuit, explains how this process unfolded. John C. Cutler, another of the study's leading researchers, discusses the history of venereal disease control by health departments without ever acknowledging his own role in Tuskegee, as the letter from Yale University emeritus public-health physician George A. Silver notes in his irate retort. Journalist Tom Junod focuses on an unrepentant and unknowing Sidney Olansky, one of the final physician directors of the study from the 1950s, even after national television coverage on the study in 1993 vilified his role.

Tuskegee has also lived on in imaginations. The best-known and most controversial manifestation is physician-writer David Feldshuh's play *Miss Evers' Boys*, which has been produced worldwide in numerous major theaters and which became the basis for an Emmy award–winning movie on the HBO network in February 1997. The poem by Sadiq, focusing on the role of Nurse Rivers and using actual words from her interview with historian James H. Jones, is spoken over the wailing clarinet on the cut "Tuskegee Experiment" on Don Byron's compact disc. Essex Hemphill, a well-known contemporary poet, also focused on Nurse Rivers in his biting commentary.

In 1995, a legacy committee was formed to see if a formal apology could be obtained from the federal government along with funding for a bioethics center at Tuskegee University. The committee's request is reproduced here. The impetus for the federal apology also came from a press conference called in March 1997 by attorney Fred Gray and four of the surviving men after they saw the televised version of *Miss Evers' Boys*. The speeches from the actual apology ceremony at the White House by survivor Herman Shaw and President Clinton are next.

The last documents remind us that Tuskegee as a metaphor and as a way to describe continuing research ambiguities continues. The debate between *New England Medical Journal* editor Marcia Angell and National Institutes of Health director Harold Varmus and Surgeon General David Satcher focuses on the ethics of informed consent and the withholding of treatment from women in research studies in the Third World on AZT's use in HIV infection transmission. Historians and ethicists Amy L. Fairchild and Ronald Bayer discuss the historical specificity of Tuskegee and the problems in its use as an overall metaphor. The guide to further reading should help direct attention to still more ways to consider the study.

As I edited and selected pieces for this book, I was often torn by my desire to criticize many of the viewpoints provided, to counter arguments made, to register my repugnance or deep disagreement with positions held. It should be clear that I do not share the politics or understandings that some of these authors present. For this kind of edited collection, I decided finally to let the pieces stand without my critique and to allow readers to raise questions and draw conclusions on their own. I am in the process of writing another book that will analyze these and other documents, interviews, and stories to winnow out my own perspective on what these multiple ways of telling the study's story means.

In Tuskegee, Alabama, two different kinds of memorials to the study and the community are being created. Attorney Fred Gray, several of the survivors, and members of the community have dedicated a building that will become the Tuskegee Human and Civil Rights Multicultural Center. It will reflect the contributions made by African Americans, Native Americans, and whites to the Tuskegee community. At Tuskegee University, with assistance from the federal government as part of the formal apology, the Tuskegee University National Center for Bio-ethics in Research and Health Care has been created. The continuing debate over the study's meaning and repeatability, and the need to memorialize those who suffered under its control, seem like fitting endings to a story that should never be forgotten even as its meanings are continually reinterpreted.

NOTES

I am grateful to Evelynn M. Hammonds, Susan E. Bell, Kristel Maney, Allan M. Brandt, and James H. Jones for their ongoing conversations with me on the study that have shaped this introduction. My gratefulness to Cynthia Wilson and Daniel Williams at Tuskegee University's Washingtonian Collection knows no bounds.

1. James Jones, *Bad Blood: The Tuskegee Syphilis Experiment* (New York: Free Press, 1981; rev. ed., 1992).

2. Ibid., p. 1. I am grateful to Jim Jones for laying the extensive investigative, historical, and analytic groundwork on the study that makes it possible for me to raise other questions. There is some disagreement, however, in various papers about the exact number of men involved.

3. Some physicians, administrators, and nurses at Tuskegee Institute, at the Tuskegee Veterans Administration Hospital, and in the local medical community knew that the men were in a study for untreated syphilis (see ibid.). But this was not common knowledge in the community until 1972, see Charles G. Gomillion to Susan M. Reverby, 12 October 1994, in this volume.

4. See Susan M. Reverby, "History of an Apology: From Tuskegee to the White House," *Research Nurse* 3 (July/August 1997): 1–9.

5. See Jay Katz, *Experimentation with Human Beings* (New York: Russell Sage Foundation, 1972); David Rothman, *Strangers at the Bedside* (New York: Basic Books, 1991); and John Fletcher, "A Case Study in Historical Relativism," in this volume.

6. One of the key issues that concerned the federal Ad Hoc Committee on the Tuskegee Study was whether or not it violated understandings of informed consent and research morality in its time. For more on this concern, see selections from the report; Allan M. Brandt, "Racism and Research: The Case of the Tuskegee Syphilis Experiment"; and John Fletcher, "A Case Study," in this volume.

7. See Harry Marks, *The Progress of Experiment: Science and Therapeutic Reform in the United States, 1900–1990* (New York: Cambridge University Press, 1997); Susan E. Lederer, *Subjected to Science: Human Experimentation in America before the Second World War* (Baltimore: Johns Hopkins University Press, 1995); and Martin Pernick, "The Patient's Role in Medical Decision-Making: A Social History of Informed Consent in Medical Therapy," in *Making Health Care Decisions: The Ethical and Legal Implications of Informed Consent in the Patient-Practitioner Relationship*, vol. 3 in Appendices Studies on the Foundations of Informed Consent (Washington, D.C.: GPO, 1982), pp. 1–35.

8. Pernick, "Patient's Role in Medical Decision-Making." See also Fletcher, "Case Study."

9. See Evelynn M. Hammonds, "The Logic of Difference: A History of 'Race' in Science and Medicine in the United States, 1900–1950" (book proposal, 1997), pp. 5–6. See also Todd Savitt, "The Use of Blacks for Medical Experimentation and Demonstration in the Old South," *Journal of Southern History* 48 (August 1982): 331–48; Susan E. Lederer, "The Tuskegee Syphilis Study in the Context of American Medical Research," in this volume; and Robert L. Blakely and Judith M. Harrington, eds., *Bones in the Basement: Postmortem Racism in Nineteenth-Century Medical Training* (Washington, D.C.: Smithsonian Institution Press, 1977).

10. Beginning in the early 1970s, feminist critiques of science and medicine made clear that the problems existed not just when science was done "badly," but also when it was done "well." The differentiation between "good" and "bad" science was taught to me by Professor Diana Long, now at the University of Southern Maine.

11. Michael Awkward, *Negotiating Difference: Race, Gender and the Politics of Positionality* (Chicago: University of Chicago Press, 1995), p. 15.

12. Richard Wright, *White Man, Listen!* (New York: Doubleday, 1957), p. 109, quoted in introduction to *History and Memory in African-American Culture*, eds. Geneviève Fabre and Robert O'Meally (New York: Oxford University Press, 1994), p. 4.

13. See, for example, Ernest D. Prentice, "Nuremberg and Tuskegee: Defining Events in Research Ethics" (paper presented at "Pressure Points in Human Subject Research: University of Rochester Conference on Research Ethics," Rochester, New York, 6 August 1998).

14. Hammonds, "Logic of Difference."

15. See Barbara Rosenkrantz, "Non-Random Events," in this volume, and Susan M. Reverby, "No Treatment, No Treatment, No Treatment. The Tuskegee Syphilis Study" (paper presented at the American Public Health Association Annual Meeting, Washington, D.C., November 1994).

16. For the limitations on historical understandings of the metalanguage of race, see Evelyn Brooks Higginbotham, "African-American Women's History and the Metalanguage of Race," *Signs* 17 (Winter 1992): 251–74. As Higginbotham states: "Today, the metalanguage of race continues to bequeath its problematic legacy. While its discursive construction of reality into two opposing camps—blacks versus whites or Afrocentric versus Eurocentric standpoints—provides the basis for resistance against extrernal forces of black subordination, it tends to forestall resolution of problems of gender, class and sexual orientation internal to black communities" (p. 272).

Similarly, James H. Jones makes this much more personal when he notes, in thanking Nurse Eunice Rivers Laurie for helping him understand the study: "More than any other principal of the Tuskegee Study, she increased my tolerance for ambiguity." Jones, *Bad Blood* (1981 ed.), p. xi.

Much recent black feminist work has focused on what Kimberlé Crenshaw calls "intersectionality," or what Valerie Smith labels the "reciprocally constitutive categories of experience and analysis" that intertwine the "ideologies of race, gender . . . class and sexuality." See Crenshaw, "Demarginalizing the Intersection of Race and Sex: A Black Feminist Critique of Antidiscrimination Doctrine, Feminist Theory and Antiracist Politics," *The University of Chicago Legal Forum* (1989): 139–67, quoted in Valerie Smith, *not just race, not just gender: Black Feminist Readings* (New York: Routledge, 1998), pp. xiii–xiv.

I am grateful to Evelynn M. Hammonds for her suggestions for sources.

17. See Susan M. Reverby, "Testifying on Tuskegee: The Metalanguage of Race and the Stories of the Tuskegee Syphilis Study" (unpublished manuscript).

18. I am grateful for Susan E. Bell's suggestions on this list.

19. Alessandro Portelli, "The Death of Luigi Trastulli," in *The Death of Luigi Trastulli and Other Stories* (Albany: State University of New York Press, 1991), p. 2.

20. "Tuskegee: Could It Happen Again?" (panel discussion at the annual meeting of the Applied Research Ethics National Association [ARENA], Boston, Mass., 7 December 1997).

21. Comments made to Susan M. Reverby at Fitchberg State University Nursing School, Fitchberg, Mass., March 1993.

22. See the section in this volume on Nurse Rivers.

23. Susan M. Reverby interview with David Feldshuh, Ithaca, N.Y., 5 June 1992.

24. Robert T. Cassell, "Public Health, Then and Now. The Tuskegee Syphilis Study, 1932–1972: Implications for HIV Education and AIDS Risk Education Programs in the Black Community" (unpublished paper, 1996). I am grateful to Dr. Cassell for his discussions with me of Tuskegee's impact on a physician-researcher trained in the 1940s, and for this paper that both he and his daughter Wendy made available to me.

25. See Reverby, "History of an Apology"; and Gamble, "Under the Shadow of Tuskegee," in this volume.

26. Kai Erikson, *A New Species of Trouble: The Human Experience of Modern Disasters* (New York: W. W. Norton, 1994), p. 228; see also Kai Erikson, *Everything in Its Path* (New York: Simon and Schuster, 1976). I am grateful to Susan E. Bell for suggesting these references and this framework.

27. Herman Shaw quoted at the White House apology, reprinted in this volume.

i

Overview

RACISM AND RESEARCH

The Case of the Tuskegee Syphilis Experiment

ALLAN M. BRANDT

In 1932 the U.S. Public Health Service (USPHS) initiated an experiment in Macon County, Alabama, to determine the natural course of untreated, latent syphilis in black males. The test comprised 400 syphilitic men, as well as 200 uninfected men who served as controls. The first published report of the study appeared in 1936 with subsequent papers issued every four to six years, through the 1960s. When penicillin became widely available by the early 1950s as the preferred treatment for syphilis, the men did not receive therapy. In fact on several occasions, the USPHS actually sought to prevent treatment. Moreover, a committee at the federally operated Center for Disease Control decided in 1969 that the study should be continued. Only in 1972, when accounts of the study first appeared in the national press, did the Department of Health, Education and Welfare halt the experiment. At that time 74 of the test subjects were still alive; at least 28, but perhaps more than 100, had died directly from advanced syphilitic lesions.[1] In August 1972, HEW appointed an investigatory panel which issued a report the following year. The panel found the study to have been "ethically unjustified," and argued that penicillin should have been provided to the men.[2]

This article attempts to place the Tuskegee Study in a historical context and to assess its ethical implications. Despite the media attention which the study received, the HEW *Final Report*, and the criticism expressed by several professional organizations, the experiment has been largely misunderstood. The most basic questions of *how* the study was undertaken in the first place and *why* it continued for 40 years were never addressed by the HEW investigation. Moreover, the panel misconstrued the nature of the experiment, failing to consult important documents available at the National Archives which bear significantly on its ethical assessment. Only by examining the specific ways in which values are engaged in scientific research can the study be understood.

Allan M. Brandt is the Amalie Moses Kass Professor of the History of Medicine and Science at Harvard University and Harvard Medical School.
Originally published in The Hastings Center Report *8 (December 1978): 21–29. Reprinted by permission of the Hastings Center and Allan M. Brandt.*

Racism and Medical Opinion

A brief review of the prevailing scientific thought regarding race and heredity in the early 20th century is fundamental for an understanding of the Tuskegee Study. By the turn of the century, Darwinism had provided a new rationale for American racism.[3] Essentially primitive peoples, it was argued, could not be assimilated into a complex, white civilization. Scientists speculated that in the struggle for survival the Negro in America was doomed. Particularly prone to disease, vice, and crime, black Americans could not be helped by education or philanthropy. Social Darwinism analyzed census data to predict the virtual extinction of the Negro in the 20th century, for they believed the Negro race in America was in the throes of a degenerative evolutionary process.[4]

The medical profession supported these findings of late 19th- and early 20th-century anthropologists, ethnologists, and biologists. Physicians studying the effects of emancipation on health concluded almost universally that freedom had caused the mental, moral, and physical deterioration of the black population.[5] They substantiated this argument by citing examples in the comparative anatomy of the black and white races. As Dr. W. T. English wrote: "A careful inspection reveals the body of the negro a mass of minor defects and imperfections from the crown of the head to the soles of the feet."[6] Cranial structures, wide nasal apertures, receding chins, projecting jaws, all typed the Negro as the lowest species in the Darwinian hierarchy.[7]

Interest in racial differences centered on the sexual nature of blacks. The Negro, doctors explained, possessed an excessive sexual desire, which threatened the very foundations of white society. As one physician noted in the *Journal of the American Medical Association*, "The negro springs from a southern race, and as such his sexual appetite is strong; all of his environments stimulate this appetite, and as a general rule his emotional type of religion certainly does not decrease it."[8] Doctors reported a complete lack of morality on the part of blacks:

> Virtue in the negro race is like angels' visits—few and far between. In a practice of sixteen years I have never examined a virgin negro over fourteen years of age.[9]

A particularly ominous feature of this overzealous sexuality, doctors argued, was the black males' desire for white women. "A perversion from which most races are exempt," wrote Dr. English, "prompts the negro's inclination towards white women, whereas other races incline towards females of their own."[10] Though English estimated the "gray matter of the negro brain" to be at least 1,000 years behind that of the white races, his genital organs were overdeveloped. As Dr. William Lee Howard noted:

The attacks on defenseless white women are evidences of racial instincts that are about as amenable to ethical culture as is the inherent odor of the race. . . . When education will reduce the size of the negro's penis as well as bring about the sensitiveness of the terminal fibers which exist in the Caucasian, then will it also be able to prevent the African's birthright to sexual madness and excess.[11]

One southern medical journal proposed "Castration Instead of Lynching," as retribution for black sexual crimes. "An impressive trial by a ghost-like kuklux klan [sic] and a 'ghost' physician or surgeon to perform the operation would make it an event the 'patient' would never forget," noted the editorial.[12]

According to these physicians, lust and immorality, unstable families, and reversion to barbaric tendencies made blacks especially prone to venereal diseases. One doctor estimated that over 50 percent of all Negroes over the age of 25 were syphilitic.[13] Virtually free of disease as slaves, they were now overwhelmed by it, according to informed medical opinion. Moreover, doctors believed that treatment for venereal disease among blacks was impossible, particularly because in its latent stage the symptoms of syphilis become quiescent. As Dr. Thomas W. Murrell wrote:

They come for treatment at the beginning and at the end. When there are visible manifestations or when harried by pain, they readily come, for as a race they are not averse to physic; but tell them not, though they look well and feel well, that they are still diseased. Here ignorance rates science a fool.[14]

Even the best-educated black, according to Murrell, could not be convinced to seek treatment for syphilis.[15] Venereal disease, according to some doctors, threatened the future of the race. The medical profession attributed the low birth rate among blacks to the high prevalence of venereal disease which caused stillbirths and miscarriages. Moreover, the high rates of syphilis were thought to lead to increased insanity and crime. One doctor writing at the turn of the century estimated that the number of insane Negroes had increased 13-fold since the end of the Civil War.[16] Dr. Murrell's conclusion echoed the most informed anthropological and ethnological data:

So the scourge sweeps among them. Those that are treated are only half cured, and the effort to assimilate a complex civilization driving their diseased minds until the results are criminal records. Perhaps here, in conjunction with tuberculosis, will be the end of the negro problem. Disease will accomplish what man cannot do.[17]

This particular configuration of ideas formed the core of medical opinion concerning blacks, sex, and disease in the early 20th century. Doctors generally discounted socioeconomic explanations of the state of black health, arguing that better medical care could not alter the evolutionary scheme.[18] These assumptions provide the backdrop for examining the Tuskegee Syphilis Study.

The Origins of the Experiment

In 1929, under a grant from the Julius Rosenwald Fund, the USPHS conducted studies in the rural South to determine the prevalence of syphilis among blacks and explore the possibilities for mass treatments. The USPHS found Macon County, Alabama, in which the town of Tuskegee is located, to have the highest syphilis rate of the six counties surveyed. The Rosenwald Study concluded that mass treatment could be successfully implemented among rural blacks.[19] Although it is doubtful that the necessary funds would have been allocated even in the best economic conditions, after the economy collapsed in 1929, the findings were ignored. It is, however, ironic that the Tuskegee Study came to be based on findings of the Rosenwald Study that demonstrated the possibilities of mass treatment.

Three years later, in 1932, Dr. Taliaferro Clark, chief of the USPHS Venereal Disease Division and author of the Rosenwald Study report, decided that conditions in Macon County merited renewed attention. Clark believed the high prevalence of syphilis offered an "unusual opportunity" for observation. From its inception, the USPHS regarded the Tuskegee Study as a classic "study in nature,"* rather than an experiment.[20] As long as syphilis was so prevalent in Macon and most of the blacks went untreated throughout life, it seemed only natural to Clark that it would be valuable to observe the consequences. He described it as a "ready-made situation."[21] Surgeon General H. S. Cumming wrote to R. R. Moton, director of the Tuskegee Institute:

> The recent syphilis control demonstration carried out in Macon County, with the financial assistance of the Julius Rosenwald Fund, revealed the presence of an unusually high rate in this county and, what is more remarkable, the fact that 99 percent of this group was entirely without previous treatment. This combination, together with the expected cooperation of your hospital, offers an unparalleled opportunity for carrying on this piece of scientific research which probably cannot be duplicated anywhere else in the world.[22]

---

*In 1865, Claude Bernard, the famous French physiologist, outlined the distinction between a "study in nature" and experimentation. A study in nature required simple observation, an essentially passive act, while experimentation demanded intervention which altered the original condition. The Tuskegee Study was thus clearly not a study in nature. The very act of diagnosis altered the original conditions. "It is on this very possibility of acting or not acting on a body," wrote Bernard, "that the distinction will exclusively rest between sciences called sciences of observation and sciences called experimental."

Although no formal protocol appears to have been written, several letters of Clark and Cumming suggest what the USPHS hoped to find. Clark indicated that it would be important to see how disease affected the daily lives of the men:

> The results of these studies of case records suggest the desirability of making a further study of the effect of untreated syphilis on the human economy among people now living and engaged in their daily pursuits.[23]

It also seems that the USPHS believed the experiment might demonstrate that antisyphilitic treatment was unnecessary. As Cumming noted: "It is expected the results of this study may have a marked bearing on the treatment, or conversely the non-necessity of treatment, of cases of latent syphilis."[24]

The immediate source of Cumming's hypothesis appears to have been the famous Oslo Study of untreated syphilis. Between 1890 and 1910, Professor C. Boeck, the chief of the Oslo Venereal Clinic, withheld treatment from almost 2,000 patients infected with syphilis. He was convinced that therapies then available, primarily mercurial ointment, were of no value. When arsenic therapy became widely available by 1910, after Paul Ehrlich's historic discovery of "606," the study was abandoned. E. Bruusgaard, Boeck's successor, conducted a follow-up study of 473 of the untreated patients from 1925 to 1927. He found that 27.9 percent of these patients had undergone a "spontaneous cure," and now manifested no symptoms of the disease. Moreover, he estimated that as many as 70 percent of all syphilitics went through life without inconvenience from the disease.[25] His study, however, clearly acknowledged the dangers of untreated syphilis for the remaining 30 percent.

Thus every major textbook of syphilis at the time of the Tuskegee Study's inception strongly advocated treating syphilis even in its latent stages, which follow the initial inflammatory reaction. In discussing the Oslo Study, Dr. J. E. Moore, one of the nation's leading venereologists wrote, "This summary of Bruusgaard's study is by no means intended to suggest that syphilis be allowed to pass untreated."[26] If a complete cure could not be effected, at least the most devastating effects of the disease could be avoided. Although the standard therapies of the time, arsenical compounds and bismuth injection, involved certain dangers because of their toxicity, the alternatives were much worse. As the Oslo Study had shown, untreated syphilis could lead to cardiovascular disease, insanity, and premature death.[27] Moore wrote in his 1933 textbook:

> Though it imposes a slight though measurable risk of its own, treatment markedly diminishes the risk from syphilis. In latent syphilis, as I shall show, the probability of progression, relapse, or death is reduced from a probable 25–30 percent without treatment to about 5 percent with it; and the gravity of the relapse if it occurs, is markedly diminished.[28]

"Another compelling reason for treatment," noted Moore, "exists in the fact that every patient with latent syphilis may be, and perhaps is, infectious for others."[29] In 1932, the year in which the Tuskegee Study began, the USPHS sponsored and published a paper by Moore and six other syphilis experts that strongly argued for treating latent syphilis.[30]

The Oslo Study, therefore, could not have provided justification for the USPHS to undertake a study that did not entail treatment. Rather, the suppositions that conditions in Tuskegee existed "naturally" and that the men would not be treated anyway provided the experiment's rationale. In turn, these two assumptions rested on the prevailing medical attitudes concerning blacks, sex, and disease. For example, Clark explained the prevalence of venereal disease in Macon County by emphasizing promiscuity among blacks:

> This state of affairs is due to the paucity of doctors, rather low intelligence of the Negro population in this section, depressed economic conditions, and the very common promiscuous sex relations of this population group which not only contribute to the spread of syphilis but also contribute to the prevailing indifference with regard to treatment.[31]

In fact, Moore, who had written so persuasively in favor of treating latent syphilis, suggested that existing knowledge did not apply to Negroes. Although he had called the Oslo Study "a never-to-be-repeated human experiment,"[32] he served as an expert consultant to the Tuskegee Study:

> I think that such a study as you have contemplated would be of immense value. It will be necessary of course in the consideration of the results to evaluate the special factors introduced by a selection of the material from negro males. Syphilis in the negro is in many respects almost a different disease from syphilis in the white.[33]

Dr. O. C. Wenger, chief of the federally operated venereal disease clinic at Hot Springs, Arkansas, praised Moore's judgment, adding, "This study will emphasize those differences."[34] On another occasion he advised Clark, "We must remember we are dealing with a group of people who are illiterate, have no conception of time, and whose personal history is always indefinite."[35]

The doctors who devised and directed the Tuskegee Study accepted the mainstream assumptions regarding blacks and venereal disease. The premise that blacks, promiscuous and lustful, would not seek or continue treatment, shaped the study. A test of untreated syphilis seemed "natural" because the USPHS presumed the men would never be treated; the Tuskegee Study made that a self-fulfilling prophecy.

Selecting the Subjects

Clark sent Dr. Raymond Vonderlehr to Tuskegee in September 1932 to assemble a sample of men with latent syphilis for the experiment. The basic design of the study called for the selection of syphilitic black males between the ages of 25 and 60, a thorough physical examination including x-rays, and finally, a spinal tap to determine the incidence of neuro-syphilis.[36] They had no intention of providing any treatment for the infected men.[37] The USPHS originally scheduled the whole experiment to last six months; it seemed to be both a simple and inexpensive project.

The task of collecting the sample, however, proved to be more difficult than the USPHS had supposed. Vonderlehr canvassed the largely illiterate, poverty-stricken population of sharecroppers and tenant farmers in search of test subjects. If his circulars requested only men over 25 to attend his clinics, none would appear, suspecting he was conducting draft physicals. Therefore, he was forced to test large numbers of women and men who did not fit the experiment's specifications. This involved considerable expense, since the USPHS had promised the Macon County Board of Health that it would treat those who were infected, but not included in the study.[38] Clark wrote to Vonderlehr about the situation: "It never once occured to me that we would be called upon to treat a large part of the county as return for the privilege of making this study. . . . I am anxious to keep the expenditures for treatment down to the lowest possible point because it is the one item of expenditure in connection with the study most difficult to defend despite our knowledge of the need therefor."[39] Vonderlehr responded: "If we could find from 100 to 200 cases . . . we would not have to do another Wassermann on useless individuals."[40]

Significantly, the attempt to develop the sample contradicted the prediction the USPHS had made initially regarding the prevalence of the disease in Macon County. Overall rates of syphilis fell well below expectations; as opposed to the USPHS projection of 35 percent, 20 percent of those tested were actually diseased.[41] Moreover, those who had sought and received previous treatment far exceeded the expectations of the USPHS. Clark noted in a letter to Vonderlehr:

> I find your report of March 6th quite interesting but regret the necessity for Wassermanning [*sic*] . . . such a large number of individuals in order to uncover this relatively limited number of untreated cases.[42]

Further difficulties arose in enlisting the subjects to participate in the experiment, to be "Wassermanned," and to return for a subsequent series of examinations. Vonderlehr found that only the offer of treatment elicited the cooperation of the men. They were told they were ill and were promised free care. Offered therapy, they became willing subjects.[43] The USPHS did not tell the men that they were participants in an experiment; on the contrary, the subjects believed they were being treated for "bad blood"—the rural South's colloquialism for syphilis. They thought they were participating in a public health demonstration similar to the one that had been conducted by the Julius Rosenwald Fund in Tuskegee several years earlier. In the end, the men were so eager for medical care that the number of defaulters in the experiment proved to be insignificant.[44]

To preserve the subjects' interest, Vonderlehr gave most of the men mercurial ointment, a noneffective drug, while some of the younger men apparently received inadequate dosages of neoarsphenamine.[45] This required Vonderlehr to write frequently to Clark requesting supplies. He feared the experiment would fail if the men were not offered treatment.

> It is desirable and essential if the study is to be a success to maintain the interest of each of the cases examined by me through to the time when the spinal puncture can be completed. Expenditure of several hundred dollars for drugs for these men would be well worth while if their interest and cooperation would be maintained in so doing. . . . It is my desire to keep the main purpose of the work from the negroes in the county and continue their interest in treatment. That is what the vast majority wants and the examination seems relatively unimportant to them in comparison. It would probably cause the entire experiment to collapse if the clinics were stopped before the work is completed.[46]

On another occasion he explained:

> Dozens of patients have been sent away without treatment during the past two weeks and it would have been impossible to continue without the free distribution of drugs because of the unfavorable impression made on the negro.[47]

The readiness of the test subjects to participate, of course, contradicted the notion that blacks would not seek or continue therapy.

The final procedure of the experiment was to be a spinal tap to test for evidence of neuro-syphilis. The USPHS presented this purely diagnostic exam, which often entails considerable pain and complications, to the men as a "special treatment." Clark explained to Moore:

> We have not yet commenced the spinal punctures. This operation will be deferred to the last in order not to unduly disturb our field work by any adverse reports by the patients subjected to spinal puncture because of some disagreeable sensations following this procedure. These negroes are very ignorant and easily influenced by things that would be of minor significance in a more intelligent group.[48]

The letter to the subjects announcing the spinal tap read:

Some time ago you were given a thorough examination and since that time we hope you have gotten a great deal of treatment for bad blood. You will now be given your last chance to get a second examination. This examination is a very special one and after it is finished you will be given a special treatment if it is believed you are in a condition to stand it.

REMEMBER THIS IS YOUR LAST CHANCE FOR SPECIAL FREE TREATMENT. BE SURE TO MEET THE NURSE.[49]

The HEW investigation did not uncover this crucial fact: the men participated in the study under the guise of treatment.

Despite the fact that their assumption regarding prevalence and black attitudes toward treatment had proved wrong, the USPHS decided in the summer of 1933 to continue the study. Once again, it seemed only "natural" to pursue the research since the sample already existed, and with a depressed economy, the cost of treatment appeared prohibitive—although there is no indication it was ever considered. Vonderlehr first suggested extending the study in letters to Clark and Wenger:

At the end of this project we shall have a considerable number of cases presenting various complications of syphilis, who have received only mercury and may still be considered untreated in the modern sense of therapy. Should these cases be followed over a period of from five to ten years many interesting facts could be learned regarding the course and complications of untreated syphilis.[50]

"As I see it," responded Wegner, "we have no further interest in these patients *until they die*."[51] Apparently, the physicians engaged in the experiment believed that only autopsies could scientifically confirm the findings of the study. Surgeon General Cumming explained this in a letter to R. R. Moton, requesting the continued cooperation of the Tuskegee Institute Hospital:

This study which was predominantly clinical in character points to the frequent occurrence of severe complications involving the various vital organs of the body and indicates that syphilis as a disease does a great deal of damage. Since clinical observations are not considered final in the medical world, it is our desire to continue observation on the cases selected for the recent study and if possible to bring a percentage of these cases to autopsy so that pathological confirmation may be made of the disease processes.[52]

Bringing the men to autopsy required the USPHS to devise a further series of deceptions and inducements. Wenger warned Vonderlehr that the men must not realize that they would be autopsied:

There is one danger in the latter plan and that is if the colored population become aware that accepting free hospital care means a post-mortem, every darkey will leave Macon County and it will hurt [Dr. Eugene] Dibble's hospital.[53]

"Naturally," responded Vonderlehr, "It is not my intention to let it be generally known that the main object of the present activities is the bringing of the men to necropsy."[54] The subjects' trust in the USPHS made the plan viable. The USPHS gave Dr. Dibble, the director of the Tuskegee Institute Hospital, an interim appointment to the Public Health Service. As Wenger noted:

> One thing is certain. The only way we are going to get post-mortems is to have the demise take place in Dibble's hospital and when these colored folks are told that Doctor Dibble is now a Government doctor too they will have more confidence.[55]*

After the USPHS approved the continuation of the experiment in 1933, Vonderlehr decided that it would be necessary to select a group of healthy, uninfected men to serve as controls. Vonderlehr, who had succeeded Clark as chief of the Venereal Disease Division, sent Dr. J. R. Heller to Tuskegee to gather the control group. Heller distributed drugs (noneffective) to these men, which suggests that they also believed they were undergoing treatment.[56] Control subjects who became syphilitic were simply transferred to the test group—a strikingly inept violation of standard research procedure.[57]

The USPHS offered several inducements to maintain contact and to procure the continued cooperation of the men. Eunice Rivers, a black nurse, was hired to follow their health and to secure approval for autopsies. She gave the men noneffective medicines—"spring tonic" and aspirin—as well as transportation and hot meals on the days of their examinations.[58] More important, Nurse Rivers provided continuity to the project over the entire 40-year period. By supplying "medicinals," the USPHS was able to continue to deceive the participants, who believed that they were receiving therapy from the government doctors. Deceit was integral to the study. When the test subjects complained about spinal taps one doctor wrote:

---

*The degree of black cooperation in conducting the study remains unclear and would be impossible to properly assess in an article of this length. It seems certain that some members of the Tuskegee Institute staff such as R. R. Moton and Eugene Dibble understood the nature of the experiment and gave their support to it. There is, however, evidence that some blacks who assisted the USPHS physicians were not aware of the deceptive nature of the experiment. Dr. Joshua Williams, an intern at the John A. Andrew Memorial Hospital (Tuskegee Institute) in 1932, assisted Vonderlehr in taking blood samples of the test subjects. In 1973 he told the HEW panel: "I know we thought it was merely a service group organized to help the people in the area. We didn't know it was a research project at all at the time." (See "Transcript of proceedings," Tuskegee Syphilis Study Ad Hoc Advisory Panel, Feb. 23, 1973, unpublished typescript, National Library of Medicine, Bethesda, Maryland.) It is also apparent that Eunice Rivers, the black nurse who had primary responsibility for maintaining contact with the men over the 40 years, did not fully understand the dangers of the experiment. In any event, black involvement in the study in no way mitigates the racial assumptions of the experiment, but rather, demonstrates their power.

They simply do not like spinal punctures. A few of those who were tapped are enthusiastic over the results but to most, the suggestion causes violent shaking of the head; others claim they were robbed of their procreative powers (regardless of the fact that I claim it stimulates them).[59]

Letters to the subjects announcing an impending USPHS visit to Tuskegee explained: "[The doctor] wants to make a special examination to find out how you have been feeling and whether the treatment has improved your health."[60] In fact, after the first six months of the study, the USPHS had furnished no treatment whatsoever.

Finally, because it proved difficult to persuade the men to come to the hospital when they became severely ill, the USPHS promised to cover their burial expenses. The Milbank Memorial Fund provided approximately $50 per man for this purpose beginning in 1935. This was a particularly strong inducement as funeral rites constituted an important component of the cultural life of rural blacks.[61] One report of the study concluded: "Without this suasion it would, we believe, have been impossible to secure the cooperation of the group and their families."[62]

Reports of the study's findings, which appeared regularly in the medical press beginning in 1936, consistently cited the ravages of untreated syphilis. The first paper, read at the 1936 American Medical Association annual meeting, found "that syphilis in this period [latency] tends to greatly increase the frequency of manifestations of cardiovascular disease."[63] Only 16 percent of the subjects gave no sign of morbidity as opposed to 61 percent of the controls. Ten years later, a report noted coldly, "The fact that nearly twice as large a proportion of the syphilitic individuals as of the control group has died is a very striking one." Life expectancy, concluded the doctors, is reduced by about 20 percent.[64]

A 1955 article found that slightly more than 30 percent of the test group autopsied had died *directly* from advanced syphilitic lesions of either the cardiovascular or the central nervous system.[65] Another published account stated, "Review of those still living reveals that an appreciable number have late complications of syphilis which probably will result, for some at least, in contributing materially to the ultimate cause of death."[66] In 1950, Dr. Wenger had concluded, "We now know, where we could only surmise before, that we have contributed to their ailments and shortened their lives."[67] As black physician Vernal Cave, a member of the HEW panel, later wrote, "They proved a point, then proved a point, then proved a point."[68]

During the 40 years of the experiment the USPHS had sought on several occasions to ensure that the subjects did not receive treatment from other sources. To this end, Vonderlehr met with groups of local black doctors in 1934, to ask their cooperation in not treating the men. Lists of subjects were distributed to Macon

County physicians along with letters requesting them to refer these men back to the USPHS if they sought care.[69] The USPHS warned the Alabama Health Department not to treat the test subjects when they took a mobile VD unit into Tuskegee in the early 1940s.[70] In 1941, the army drafted several subjects and told them to begin antisyphilitic treatment immediately. The USPHS supplied the draft board with a list of 256 names they desired to have excluded from treatment, and the board complied.[71]

In spite of these efforts, by the early 1950s many of the men had secured some treatment on their own. By 1952, almost 30 percent of the test subjects had received some penicillin, although only 7.5 percent had received what could be considered adequate doses.[72] Vonderlehr wrote to one of the participating physicians, "I hope that the availability of antibiotics has not interfered too much with this project."[73] A report published in 1955 considered whether the treatment that some of the men had obtained had "defeated" the study. The article attempted to explain the relatively low exposure to penicillin in an age of antibiotics, suggesting as a reason: "the stoicism of these men as a group; they still regard hospitals and medicines with suspicion and prefer an occasional dose of time-honored herbs or tonics to modern drugs."[74] The authors failed to note that the men believed they already were under the care of the government doctors and thus saw no need to seek treatment elsewhere. Any treatment which the men might have received, concluded the report, had been insufficient to compromise the experiment.

When the USPHS evaluated the status of the study in the 1960s they continued to rationalize the racial aspects of the experiment. For example, the minutes of a 1965 meeting at the Center for Disease Control recorded:

Racial issue was mentioned briefly. Will not affect the study. Any questions can be handled by saying these people were at the point that therapy would no longer help them. They are getting better medical care than they would under any other circumstances.[75]

A group of physicians met again at the CDC in 1969 to decide whether or not to terminate the study. Although one doctor argued that the study should be stopped and the men treated, the consensus was to continue. Dr. J. Lawson Smith remarked, "You will never have another study like this; take advantage of it."[76] A memo prepared by Dr. James B. Lucas, assistant chief of the Venereal Disease Branch stated: "Nothing learned will prevent, find, or cure a single case of infectious syphilis or bring us closer to our basic mission of controlling venereal disease in the United States."[77] He concluded, however, that the study should be continued "along its present lines." When the first accounts of the experiment appeared in the national press in July 1972, data were still being collected and autopsies performed.[78]

The HEW Final Report

HEW finally formed the Tuskegee Syphilis Study Ad Hoc Advisory Panel on August 28, 1972, in response to criticism that the press descriptions of the experiment had triggered. The panel, composed of nine members, five of them black, concentrated on two issues. First, was the study justified in 1932 and had the men given their informed consent? Second, should penicillin have been provided when it became available in the early 1950s? The panel was also charged with determining if the study should be terminated and assessing current policies regarding experimentation with human subjects.[79] The group issued their report in June 1973.

By focusing on the issues of penicillin therapy and informed consent, the *Final Report* and the investigation betrayed a basic misunderstanding of the experiment's purposes and design. The HEW report implied that the failure to provide penicillin constituted the study's major ethical misjudgment; implicit was the assumption that no adequate therapy existed prior to penicillin. Nonetheless medical authorities firmly believed in the efficacy of arsenotherapy for treating syphilis at the time of the experiment's inception in 1932. The panel further failed to recognize that the entire study had been predicated on nontreatment. Provision of effective medication would have violated the rationale of the experiment—to study the natural course of the disease until death. On several occasions, in fact, the USPHS had prevented the men from receiving proper treatment. Indeed, there is no evidence that the USPHS ever considered providing penicillin.

The other focus of the *Final Report*—informed consent—also served to obscure the historical facts of the experiment. In light of the deceptions and exploitations which the experiment perpetrated, it is an understatement to declare, as the *Report* did, that the experiment was "ethically unjustified," because it failed to obtain informed consent from the subjects. The *Final Report*'s statement, "Submitting voluntarily is not informed consent," indicated that the panel believed that the men had volunteered *for the experiment*.[80] The records in the National Archives make clear that the men did not submit voluntarily to an experiment; they were told and they believed that they were getting free treatment from expert government doctors for a serious disease. The failure of the HEW *Final Report* to expose this critical fact—that the USPHS lied to the subjects—calls into question the thoroughness and credibility of their investigation.

Failure to place the study in a historical context also made it impossible for the investigation to deal with the essentially racist nature of the experiment. The panel treated the study as an aberration, well intentioned but misguided.[81] Moreover, concern that the *Final Report* might be viewed as a critique of human experimentation in general seems to have severely limited the scope of the inquiry. The *Final Report* is quick to remind the reader on two occasions: "The position of the Panel must not be construed to be a general repudiation of scientific research with human subjects."[82] The *Report* assures us that a better designed experiment could have been justified:

> It is possible that a scientific study in 1932 of untreated syphilis, properly conceived with a clear protocol and conducted with suitable subjects who fully understood the implications of their involvement, might have been justified in the pre-penicillin era. This is especially true when one considers the uncertain nature of the results of treatment of late latent syphilis and the highly toxic nature of therapeutic agents then available.[83]

This statement is questionable in view of the proven dangers of untreated syphilis known in 1932.

Since the publication of the HEW *Final Report*, a defense of the Tuskegee Study has emerged. These arguments, most clearly articulated by Dr. R. H. Kampmeier in the *Southern Medical Journal*, center on the limited knowledge of effective therapy for latent syphilis when the experiment began. Kampmeier argues that by 1950, penicillin would have been of no value for these men.[84] Others have suggested that the men were fortunate to have been spared the highly toxic treatments of the earlier period.[85] Moreover, even these contemporary defenses assume that the men never would have been treated anyway. As. Dr. Charles Barnett of Stanford University wrote in 1974, "The lack of treatment was not contrived by the USPHS but was an established fact of which they proposed to take advantage."[86] Several doctors who participated in the study continued to justify the experiment. Dr. J. R. Heller, who on one occasion had referred to the test subjects as the "Ethiopian population," told reporters in 1972:

> I don't see why they should be shocked or horrified. There was no racial side to this. It just happened to be in a black community. I feel this was a perfectly straightforward study, perfectly ethical, with controls. Part of our mission as physicians is to find out what happens to individuals with disease and without disease.[87]

These apologies, as well as the HEW *Final Report*, ignore many of the essential ethical issues which the study poses. The Tuskegee Study reveals the persistence of beliefs within the medical profession about the nature of blacks, sex, disease—beliefs that had tragic repercussions long after their alleged "scientific" bases were known to be incorrect. Most strikingly, the entire health of a community was jeopardized by leaving a communicable disease untreated.[88] There can be little doubt that the Tuskegee researchers regarded their subjects as less than human.[89] As a result, the ethical canons of experimenting on human subjects were completely disregarded.

The study also raises significant questions about professional self-regulation and scientific bureaucracy. Once the USPHS decided to extend the experiment in the summer of 1933, it was unlikely that the test would be halted short of the men's deaths. The experiment was widely reported for 40 years without evoking any significant protest within the medical community. Nor did any bureaucratic mechanism exist within the government for the periodic reassessment of the Tuskegee experiment's ethics and scientific value. The USPHS sent physicians to Tuskegee every several years to check on the study's progress, but never subjected the morality or usefulness of the experiment to serious scrutiny. Only the press accounts of 1972 finally punctured the continued rationalizations of the USPHS and brought the study to an end. Even the HEW investigation was compromised by fear that it would be considered a threat to future human experimentation.

In retrospect the Tuskegee Study revealed more about the pathology of racism than it did about the pathology of syphilis; more about the nature of scientific inquiry than the nature of the disease process. The injustice committed by the experiment went well beyond the facts outlined in the press and the HEW *Final Report*. The degree of deception and damages have been seriously underestimated. As this history of the study suggests, the notion that science is a value-free discipline must be rejected. The need for greater vigilance in assessing the specific ways in which social values and attitudes affect professional behavior is clearly indicated.[90]

NOTES

1. The best general accounts of the study are "The 40-year death watch," *Medical World News*, Aug. 18, 1972; 15–17; and Dolores Katz, "Why 430 blacks with syphilis went uncured for 40 years," Detroit *Free Press*, Nov. 5, 1972. The mortality figure is based on a published report of the study which appeared in 1955. See Jesse J. Peters, James H. Peers, Sidney Olansky, John C. Cutler, and Geraldine Gleeson, "Untreated syphilis in the male Negro: pathologic findings in syphilitic and nonsyphilitic patients," *J. Chron. Dis.*, Feb. 1955, 1:127–148. The article estimated that 30.4 percent of the untreated men would die from syphilitic lesions.

2. *Final Report* of the Tuskegee Syphilis Study Ad Hoc Advisory Panel, Department of Health, Education, and Welfare (Washington, D.C.: Government Printing Office, 1973). (Hereafter, HEW *Final Report*).

3. See George M. Frederickson, *The Black Image in the White Mind* (New York: Harper and Row, 1971), pp. 228–255. Also, John H. Haller, *Outcasts From Evolution* (Urbana: Univ. of Illinois Press, 1971), pp. 40–68.

4. Frederickson, *The Black Image*, pp. 247–249.

5. "Deterioration of the American Negro," *Atlanta J.-Rec. Med.*, July 1903, 5:287–288. See also J. A. Rodgers, "The effect of freedom upon the psychological development of the Negro." *Proc. Am. Medico-Psychological Assn.*, 1900, 7:88–99. "From the most healthy race in the country forty years ago," concluded Dr. Henry McHatton, "he is today the most diseased." "The sexual status of the Negro—past and present," *Am. J. Dermatology & Genito-Urinary Dis.*, Jan. 1906, 10:7–9.

6. W. T. English, "The Negro problem from the physician's point of view," *Atlanta J.-Rec. Med.*, Oct. 1903, 5:461. See also "Racial anatomical peculiarities," *N.Y. Med. J.*, Apr. 1896, 63:300–501.

7. "Racial anatomical peculiarities," p. 501. Also, Charles S. Bacon, "The race problem," *Medicine* (Detroit), May 1903, 9:338–343.

8. H. H. Hazen, "Syphilis in the American Negro," *J.A.M.A.*, Aug. 8, 1914, 63:463. For deeper background into the historical relationship of racism and sexuality, see Winthrop D. Jordan, *White Over Black* (Chapel Hill: Univ. of North Carolina Press, 1968; Pelican Books, 1969), pp. 32–40.

9. Daniel David Quillian, "Racial peculiarities: a cause of the prevalence of syphilis in Negroes," *Am. J. Dermatology & Genito-Urinary Dis.*, July 1906, 10:277.

10. English, "The Negro problem . . . ," p. 463.

11. William Lee Howard, "The Negro as a distinct ethnic factor in civilization," *Medicine* (Detroit), June 1903, 9:424. See also, Thomas W. Murrell, "Syphilis in the American Negro," *J.A.M.A.*, Mar. 12, 1910, 54:848.

12. "Castration instead of lynching," *Atlanta J.-Rec. Med.*, Oct. 1906, 8:457. The editorial added: "The badge of disgrace and emasculation might be branded upon the face or forehead, as a warning, in the form of an 'R,' emblematic of the crime for which this punishment was and will be inflicted."

13. Searle Harris, "The future of the Negro from the standpoint of the southern physician," *Alabama Med. J.*, Jan. 1902, 14:62. Other articles on the prevalence of venereal disease among blacks are: H. L. McNeil, "Syphilis in the southern Negro," *J.A.M.A.*, Sept. 30, 1916, 67:1001–1004; Ernest Philip Boas, "The relative prevalence of syphilis among Negroes and whites," *Social Hygiene*, Sept. 1915, 1:610–616. Doctors went to considerable trouble to distinguish the morbidity and mortality of various diseases among blacks and whites. See, for example, Marion M. Torchia, "Tuberculosis among American Negroes: medical research on a racial disease, 1830–1950," *J. Hist. Med.*, July 1977, 32:252–279.

14. Thomas W. Murrell, "Syphilis in the Negro: its bearing on the race problem," *Am. J. Dermatology & Genito-Urinary Dis.*, Aug. 1906, 10:307.

15. "Even among the educated, only a very few will carry out the most elementary instructions as to personal hygiene. One thing you cannot do, and that is to convince the negro that he has a disease that he cannot see or feel. This is due to lack of concentration rather than lack of faith; even if he does believe, he does not care; a child of fancy, the sensations of the passing hour are his only guides to the future." Murrell, "Syphilis in the American Negro," p. 847.

16. "Deterioration of the American Negro," *Atlanta J.-Rec. Med.*, July 1903, 5:288.

17. Murrell, "Syphilis in the Negro; its bearing on the race problem," p. 307.

18. "The anatomical and physiological conditions of the African must be understood, his place in the anthropological scale realized, and his biological basis accepted as being unchangeable by man, before we shall be able to govern his natural uncontrollable sexual passions." See "As ye sow that shall ye also reap," *Atlanta J.-Rec. Med.*, June 1899, 1:266.

19. Taliaferro Clark, *The Control of Syphilis in Southern Rural Areas* (Chicago: Julius Rosenwald Fund, 1932), pp. 53–58. Approximately 35 percent of the inhabitants of Macon County who were examined were found to be syphilitic.

20. See Claude Bernard, *An Introduction to the Study of Experimental Medicine* (New York: Dover, 1865, 1957), pp. 5–26.

21. Taliaferro Clark to M. M. Davis, Oct. 29, 1932. Records of the USPHS Venereal Disease Division, Record Group 90, Box 239, National Archives, Washington National Record Center, Suitland, Maryland. (Hereafter, NA-WNRC). Materials in this collection which relate to the early history of the study were apparently never consulted by the HEW investigation. Included are letters, reports, and memoranda written by the physicians engaged in the study.

22. H. S. Cumming to R. R. Moton, Sept. 20, 1932, NA-WNRC.

23. Clark to Davis, Oct. 29, 1932, NA-WNRC.

24. Cumming to Moton, Sept. 20, 1932, NA-WNRC.

25. Bruusgaard was able to locate 309 living patients, as well as records from 164 who were deceased. His findings were published as "Ueber das Schicksal der nicht specifizch behandelten

Luetiken," *Arch. Dermatology & Syphilis*, 1929, 157:309–332. The best discussion of the Boeck-Bruusgaard data is E. Gurney Clark and Niels Danbolt, "The Oslo Study of the natural history of untreated syphilis," *J. Chron. Dis.*, Sept. 1955, 2:311–344.

26. Joseph Earle Moore, *The Modern Treatment of Syphilis* (Baltimore: Charles C. Thomas, 1933), p. 24.

27. *Ibid.*, pp. 231–247; see also John H. Stokes, *Modern Clinical Syphilology* (Philadelphia: W. B. Saunders, 1928), pp. 231–239.

28. Moore, *Modern Treatment of Syphilis*, p. 237.

29. *Ibid.*, p. 236.

30. J. E. Moore, H. N. Cole, P. A. O'Leary, J. H. Stokes, U. J. Wile, T. Clark, T. Parran, J. H. Usilton, "Cooperative clinical studies in the treatment of syphilis: latent syphilis," *Venereal Disease Information* (Sept. 20, 1932), 13:351. The authors also concluded that the latently syphilitic were potential carriers of the disease, thus meriting treatment.

31. Clark to Paul A. O'Leary, Sept. 27, 1932, NA-WNRC. O'Leary, of the Mayo Clinic, misunderstood the design of the study, replying: "The investigation which you are planning in Alabama is indeed an intriguing one, particularly because of the opportunity it affords of observing treatment in a previously untreated group. I assure you such a study is of interest to me, and I shall look forward to its report in the future." O'Leary to Clark, Oct. 3, 1932, NA-WNRC.

32. Joseph Earle Moore, "Latent syphilis," unpublished typescript, n.d., p. 7. American Social Hygiene Association Papers, Social Welfare History Archives Center, University of Minnesota, Minneapolis.

33. Moore to Clark, Sept. 28, 1932, NA-WNRC. Moore had written in his textbook, "In late syphilis the negro is particularly prone to the development of bone or cardiovascular lesions." See Moore, *The Modern Treatment of Syphilis*, p. 35.

34. O. C. Wenger to Clark, Oct. 3, 1932, NA-WNRC.

35. *Ibid.*, Sept. 29, 1932.

36. Clark memorandum, Sept. 26, 1932, NA-WNRC. See also Clark to Davis, Oct. 29, 1932, NA-WNRC.

37. As Clark wrote: "You will observe that our plan has nothing to do with treatment. It is purely a diagnostic procedure carried out to determine what has happened to the syphilitic Negro who has had no treatment." Clark to Paul A. O'Leary, Sept. 27, 1932, NA-WNRC.

38. D. G. Gill to O. C. Wenger, Oct. 10, 1932, NA-WNRC.

39. Clark to Vonderlehr, Jan. 25, 1933, NA-WNRC.

40. Vonderlehr to Clark, Feb. 28, 1933, NA-WNRC.

41. *Ibid.*, Nov. 2, 1932. Also, *ibid.*, Feb. 6, 1933.

42. Clark to Vonderlehr, Mar. 9, 1933, NA-WNRC.

43. Vonderlehr later explained: "The reason treatment was given to many of these men was twofold: First, when the study was started in the fall of 1932, no plans had been made for its continuation and a few of the patients were treated before we fully realized the need for continuing the project on a permanent basis. Second it was difficult to hold the interest of the group of Negroes in Macon County unless some treatment was given." Vonderlehr to Austin V. Diebert, Dec. 5, 1938, Tuskegee Syphilis Study Ad Hoc Advisory Panel Papers, Box 1, National Library of Medicine, Bethesda, Maryland. (Hereafter, TSS-NLM.) This collection contains the materials assembled by the HEW investigation in 1972.

44. Vonderlehr to Clark, Feb. 6, 1933, NA-WNRC.

45. H. S. Cumming to J. N. Baker, Aug. 5, 1933, NA-WNRC.

46. Vonderlehr to Clark, Jan. 22, 1933; Jan. 12, 1933, NA-WNRC.

47. Vonderlehr to Clark, Jan. 28, 1933, NA-WNRC.

48. Clark to Moore, Mar. 25, 1933, NA-WNRC.

49. Macon County Health Department, "Letter to subjects," n.d., NA-WNRC.

50. Vonderlehr to Clark, Apr. 8, 1933, NA-WNRC. See also Vonderlehr to Wenger, July 18, 1933, NA-WNRC.

51. Wenger to Vonderlehr, July 21, 1933, NA-WNRC. The italics are Wenger's.

52. Cumming to Moton, July 27, 1933, NA-WNRC.

53. Wenger to Vonderlehr, July 21, 1933, NA-WNRC.

54. Vonderlehr to Murray Smith, July 27, 1933, NA-WNRC.

55. Wenger to Vonderlehr, Aug. 5, 1933, NA-WNRC.

56. Vonderlehr to Wenger, Oct. 24, 1933, NA-WNRC. Controls were given salicylates.

57. Austin V. Diebert and Martha C. Bruyere, "Untreated syphilis in the male Negro, III," *Venereal Disease Information*, Dec. 1946, 27:301–314.

58. Eunice Rivers, Stanley Schuman, Lloyd Simpson, Sidney Olansky, "Twenty-years of fol-lowup experience in a long-range medical study," *Public Hlth. Rep.*, Apr. 1953, 68:391–395. In this article Nurse Rivers explains her role in the experiment. She wrote: "Because of the low educa-tional status of the majority of the patients, it was impossible to appeal to them from a purely scientific approach. Therefore, various methods were used to maintain their interest. Free medi-cines, burial assistance or insurance (the project being referred to as 'Miss Rivers' Lodge'), free hot meals on the days of examination, transportation to and from the hospital, and an oppor-tunity to stop in town on the return trip to shop or visit with their friends on the streets all helped. In spite of these attractions, there were some who refused their examinations because they were not sick and did not see that they were being benefitted" (p. 393).

59. Austin V. Diebert to Raymond Vonderlehr, Mar. 29, 1939, TSS-NLM, Box 1.

60. Murray Smith to subjects, 1938, TSS-NLM, Box 1. See also Sidney Olansky to John C. Cutler, Nov. 6, 1951, TSS-NLM, Box 2.

61. The USPHS originally requested that the Julius Rosenwald Fund meet this expense. See Cumming to Davis, Oct. 4, 1934, NA-WNRC. This money was usually divided between the undertaker, pathologist, and hospital. Lloyd Isaacs to Raymond Vonderlehr, Apr. 23, 1940, TSS-NLM, Box 1.

62. Stanley H. Schuman, Sidney Olansky, Eunice Rivers, C. A. Smith, Dorothy S. Rambo, "Untreated syphilis in the male Negro: background and current status of patients in the Tuskegee study," *J. Chron. Dis.*, Nov. 1955, 2:555.

63. R. A. Vonderlehr and Taliaferro Clark, "Untreated syphilis in the male Negro," *Venereal Disease Information*, Sept. 1936, 17:262.

64. J. R. Heller and P. T. Bruyere, "Untreated syphilis in the male Negro: II. Mortality during 12 years of observation," *Venereal Disease Information*, Feb. 1946, 27:34–38.

65. Jesse J. Peters, James H. Peers, Sidney Olansky, John C. Cutler, and Geraldine Gleeson, "Untreated syphilis in the male Negro: pathologic findings in syphilitic and non-syphilitic pa-tients," *J. Chron. Dis.*, Feb. 1955, 1:127–148.

66. Sidney Olansky, Stanley H. Schuman, Jesse J. Peters, C. A. Smith, and Dorothy S. Rambo, "Untreated syphilis in the male Negro, X. Twenty years of clinical observation of untreated syphilitic and presumably nonsyphilitic groups," *J. Chron. Dis.*, Aug. 1956, 4:184.

67. O. C. Wenger, "Untreated syphilis in male Negro," unpublished typescript, 1950, p. 3. Tuskegee Files, Center for Disease Control, Atlanta, Georgia. (Hereafter TF-CDC).

68. Vernal G. Cave, "Proper uses and abuses of the health care delivery system for minorities with special reference to the Tuskegee syphilis study," *J. Nat. Med. Assn.*, Jan. 1975, 67:83.

69. See for example, Vonderlehr to B. W. Booth, Apr. 18, 1934; and Vonderlehr to E. R. Lett, Nov. 20, 1933, NA-WNRC.

70. "Transcript of proceedings—Tuskegee Syphilis Ad Hoc Advisory Panel," Feb. 23, 1973, unpublished typescript, TSS-NLM, Box 1.

71. Raymond Vonderlehr to Murray Smith, Apr. 30, 1942; and Smith to Vonderlehr, June 8, 1942, TSS-NLM, Box 1.

72. Stanley H. Schuman, Sidney Olansky, Eunice Rivers, C. A. Smith, and Dorothy S. Rambo, "Untreated syphilis in the male Negro: background and current status of patients in the Tuskegee study," *J. Chron. Dis.*, Nov. 1955, 2:550–553.

73. Raymond Vonderlehr to Stanley H. Schuman, Feb. 5, 1952, TSS-NLM, Box 2.

74. Schuman and others, "Untreated syphilis . . .," p. 550.

75. "Minutes, April 5, 1965," unpublished typescript, TSS-NLM, Box 1.

76. "Tuskegee Ad Hoc Committee meeting—minutes, February 6, 1969," TF-CDC.

77. James B. Lucas to William J. Brown, Sept. 10, 1970, TF-CDC.

78. Elizabeth M. Kennebrew to Arnold C. Schroeter, Feb. 24, 1971, TSS-NLM, Box 1.

79. See *Medical Tribune*, Sept. 13, 1972: 1, 20; and Report on HEW's Tuskegee Report, *Medical World News*, Sept. 14, 1973: 57–58.

80. HEW *Final Report*, p. 7.

81. The notable exception is Jay Katz's eloquent "Reservations about the panel report on Charge 1," HEW *Final Report*, pp. 14–15.

82. HEW *Final Report*, pp. 8, 12.

83. *Ibid.*

84. See R. H. Kampmeier, "The Tuskegee Study of untreated syphilis." *Southern Med. J.*, Oct. 1972, 65:1247–1251; and "Final report on the 'Tuskegee Syphilis Study,'" *Southern Med. J.*, Nov. 1974, 67:1349–1353.

85. Leonard J. Goldwater, "The Tuskegee Study in historical perspective," unpublished typescript, TSS-NLM; see also "Treponemes and Tuskegee," *Lancet*, June 23, 1973: 1438; and Louis Lasagna, *The VD Epidemic* (Philadelphia: Temple Univ. Press, 1975), pp. 64–66.

86. Quoted in "Debate revives on the PHS study," *Medical World News*, Apr. 19, 1974: 37.

87. Heller to Vonderlehr, Nov. 28, 1933, NA-WNRC; quoted in *Medical Tribune*, Aug. 23, 1972: 14.

88. Although it is now known that syphilis is rarely infectious after its early phase, at the time of the study's inception latent syphilis was thought to be communicable. The fact that members of the control group were placed in the test group when they became syphilitic proves that at least some infectious men were denied treatment.

89. When the subjects are drawn from minority groups, especially those with which the researcher cannot identify, basic human rights may be compromised. Hans Jonas has clearly explicated the problem in his "Philosophical reflections on experimenting with human subjects," *Daedalus*, Spring 1969, 98:234–237. As Jonas writes: "If the properties we adduced as the particular qualifications of the members of the scientific fraternity itself are taken as general criteria of selection, then one should look for additional subjects where a maximum of identification, understanding, and spontaneity can be expected—that is, among the most highly motivated, the most highly educated, and the least 'captive' members of the community."

90. Since the original publication of this article, a full-length study of the Tuskegee Experiment has appeared. See James H. Jones, *Bad Blood: The Tuskegee Syphilis Experiment* (New York: Free Press, 1981).

EVENTS IN THE TUSKEGEE SYPHILIS STUDY

A Timeline

SUSAN E. BELL

November 1929

The Rosenwald Fund votes to spend up to $50,000 from January through December 1930 for syphilis-control demonstration programs. The Public Health Service (PHS) recommends six locations for the program: Macon County, Alabama; Scott County, Mississippi; Tipton County, Tennessee; Glynn County, Georgia; Pitt County, North Carolina; Albemarle County, Virginia.

January 1930

The program begins in Macon County, Alabama, and the five other recommended sites in the South.

May 1930

Dr. H. L. Harris Jr. makes a site visit for the Rosenwald Fund to Macon County, Ala.

Fall 1930

Harris visits the Macon County site again, and he recommends that the project be discontinued (it is) and a comprehensive health plan be implemented (it is not).

September 1932

The PHS proposes to study untreated syphilis in Macon County, since the prevalence of syphilis is 35 percent, the highest of all demonstration programs. Tuskegee Institute officials and the local health department agree to the study. Nurse Eunice Rivers is appointed to the study as a liaison to the men.

October 1932

The PHS study of untreated syphilis begins in and around Macon County. The projected length of the study is 6–8 months and includes black men at least 25 years old who have had positive Wassermans (confirmed by a second test), who have had syphilis for at least five years (determined by onset of chancres), and who have not been treated. Subjects are then administered less than the recommended amount of therapy.

Susan E. Bell is professor of sociology at Bowdoin College.
Printed by permission of Susan E. Bell.

May 1933

The study's participants are subjected to spinal taps to diagnose neural syphilis.

June 1933

Dr. Taliaferro Clark retires from the PHS; Dr. Raymond A. Vonderlehr succeeds him and continues the study. Vonderlehr hospitalizes terminally ill subjects at Tuskegee Institute Hospital and adds autopsies to the study's protocol. The only further treatment the men receive from the PHS is aspirin, protiodide, iron, and placebos. Over the next four decades the head of the Division of Venereal Disease (VD) is usually recruited from a man who has worked on the Tuskegee Syphilis Study.

November 1933–March 1934

Vonderlehr begins selecting a group of men as subjects and controls for the study.

May 1935

The Milbank Memorial Fund gives the first annual award of $500 to the PHS to use for the burial stipends for families of subjects consenting to autopsies ($50/subject).

1936

The first report of the study is published: R. A. Vonderlehr et al., "Untreated Syphilis in the Male Negro: A Comparative Study of Treated and Untreated Cases," *Venereal Disease Information* 17 (1936): 260–65.

1943

The PHS begins administering penicillin to people with syphilis in several U.S. treatment centers.

1946

The second and third reports of the study are published: John R. Heller et al., "Untreated Syphilis in the Male Negro: Mortality during Twelve Years of Observation," *Venereal Disease Information* 27 (1946): 34–38; A. V. Deibert et al., "Untreated Syphilis in the Male Negro: III. Evidence of Cardiovascular Abnormalities and Other Forms of Morbidity," *Journal of Venereal Disease Information* 27 (1946): 301–14.

1950

The fourth report on the study is published: Pasquale J. Pesare et al., "Untreated Syphilis in the Male Negro: Observation of Abnormalities over Sixteen Years," *American Journal of Syphilis, Gonorrhea, and Venereal Diseases* 34 (1950): 201–13.

1951

The PHS reviews the Tuskegee Study procedures and recommends changes.

1952

The study's files are reorganized, autopsy reports are transferred to punch cards, and a single set of diagnostic standards for syphilis and syphilitic heart disease are adopted.

A study of aging is added to the original syphilis study.

1953

The fifth report on the study is published: Eunice Rivers et al., "Twenty Years of Followup Experience in a Long-Range Medical Study," *Public Health Reports* 68 (1953): 391–95.

1954

The sixth and seventh reports on the study are published: J. K. Shafer et al., "Untreated Syphilis in the Male Negro: A Prospective Study of the Effect on Life Expectancy," *Public Health Reports* 69 (1954): 691–97; Sidney Olansky et al., "Environmental Factors in the Tuskegee Study of Untreated Syphilis," *Public Health Reports* 69 (1954): 691–98.

1955

The eighth and ninth reports on the study are published: Jesse J. Peters et al., "Untreated Syphilis in the Male Negro: Pathologic Findings in Syphilitic and Nonsyphilitic Patients," *Journal of Chronic Diseases* 1 (1955): 127–48; Stanley H. Schuman et al., "Untreated Syphilis in the Male Negro: Background and Current Status of Patients in the Tuskegee Study," *Journal of Chronic Diseases* 2 (1955): 543–58.

1956

The tenth and eleventh reports on the study are published: Sidney Olansky et al., "Untreated Syphilis in the Male Negro: X. Twenty Years of Clinical Observation of Untreated Syphilitic and Presumably Nonsyphilitic Groups," *Journal of Chronic Diseases* 4 (1956): 177–85, and "Untreated Syphilis in the Male Negro: Twenty-two Years of Serological Observation in a Selected Syphilis Study Group," *A.M.A. Archives of Dermatology* 73 (1956): 519–22.

1958

The PHS distributes certificates of appreciation and cash payments of $25 to the subjects.

Nurse Rivers (Laurie) wins the Third Annual Oveta Culp Hobby Award, the highest commendation the United States Department of Health, Education, and Welfare (HEW) can bestow on an employee.

Early 1960s

The PHS begins a regular distribution of small cash payments of $1–2 per subject to induce cooperation.

1961

The twelfth report on the study is published: Donald H. Rockwell et al., "The Tuskegee Study of Untreated Syphilis: The Thirtieth Year of Observation," *Archives of Internal Medicine* 114 (1961): 792–98.

1962

Pure Food and Drug Act Amendments order doctors to inform patients when they are being given drugs experimentally.

1964

World Health Organization issues the Declaration of Helsinki, which contains stringent provisions regarding informed consent.

1965

For the first time, a member of the medical profession objects to the study in a letter to the PHS.

1966

The surgeon general issues Policy and Procedure Order No. 129 establishing guidelines for, among other things, peer review for publicly funded research (revised in 1969 and 1971).

1966, 1968

Peter Buxton, a PHS venereal disease interviewer and investigator, expresses grave moral concerns about the study to the Centers for Disease Control (CDC).

1969

The Alabama State Board of Health and the Macon County Medical Society support continuation of the study. The Tuskegee Institute again becomes actively involved with the study, and a new nurse is appointed in addition to Nurse Rivers (Laurie).

February 1969

The CDC convenes a panel of physicians and scientists to investigate the study. The panel recommends continuation. One panelist objects to the decision.

1970

The assistant chief of the VD Branch of the PHS says the study is incongruous with the goals of PHS and is bad science, but he opposes ending it.

July 1972

Buxton tells an Associated Press reporter about the study.

25 July 1972

The Associated Press sends the story about the study to major newspapers.

August 1972

After a public outcry, the HEW appoints an ad hoc panel to review the study.

1973

The thirteenth and last report on the study is published: Joseph G. Caldwell, "Aortic Regurgitation in the Tuskegee Study of Untreated Syphilis," *Journal of Chronic Diseases* 26 (1973): 187–94.

February / March 1973

Senator Edward Kennedy holds hearings on human experimentation before the Subcommittee on Health of the Committee of Labor and Public Welfare, U.S. Senate.

New HEW guidelines including treatment and compensation are established regarding research projects involving human subjects.

March 1973

The HEW halts the study by authorizing treatment.

April 1973

The CDC offers to find subjects, treat them, and pay for their medical care, but does not offer the study's participants compensation.

23 July 1973

A $1.8 billion class-action lawsuit is filed against the United States, HEW, PHS, CDC, the State of Alabama, the State Board of Health of Alabama, the Milbank Fund, and some individuals connected with the study.

December 1974

A settlement is reached and the government agrees to pay approximately $10 million. Each living syphilis subject receives $37,500, the heirs of each deceased subject with syphilis are awarded $15,000, each living control is granted $16,000, and each deceased control is awarded $5,000.

1975

The U.S. government extends treatment to the subjects' wives and children who have contracted syphilis.

1996

The last payments are made to survivors, controls, and their heirs. Medical care continues.

1997

President Bill Clinton and Vice President Al Gore offer a formal apology in a White House ceremony.

Contemporary Background

THE SHADOW OF THE PLANTATION
Survival

CHARLES S. JOHNSON

Macon County ranked third in Negro mortality in a list of 67 rural Alabama counties, according to the 1929 mortality census. There were 406 deaths and these gave a rate of 18.4. This rate was exactly the same as that for the white population in this county. There is, however, something unexplained about the figures. Just one year before the Negro mortality was 22.1 and in 1925 it was 22.2 and second highest in the state. The ratio between white and Negro deaths has remained approximately the same, and the mortality of the white population of this county has exceeded that of Negroes in the majority of counties of the state. This may indeed be a reflection of the hard life of the northern section of the county where most of the white residents live (in the shadow of their own past).

One of the unexplained circumstances in the number of Negro deaths for 1929 may possibly be connected with the discrepancy between the numbers of Negroes dying as reported by the federal census, on the one hand, and the county health officer, on the other. The records of the latter show 60 white and 154 Negro death certificates while the census shows 87 whites and 406 Negroes, residents and nonresidents. This would presumably include deaths at the Negro Veterans Hospital located in the county near Tuskegee. During the same year 119 white and 574 Negro babies were added to the population. The white population, thus, it seems, had 98 per cent more birth survivals than deaths and the Negroes about 3.6 per cent more. The extent to which the lower Negro rates of survival are related to inadequate birth registration is not evident in the figures alone, nor does the county health officer know what proportion of the total was registered. There is some evidence that the number of Negro births registered is less than the actual number of births. In our 612 families, which might be taken as an average, there were 69 children under one year of age. These were 2.7 of the total population. If this rate may be assumed for the entire population, it would be expected that 600 of the children born during a given twelve months' period would be alive. Such an

Charles Johnson was president of Fisk University and a well-known sociologist. This study was funded by the Rosenwald Fund to provide a sociological analysis of the African American community in Macon County.
Originally published in Shadow of the Plantation *(Chicago: University of Chicago Press, 1934), 186–207. Reprinted by permission of the University of Chicago Press.*

41

estimate, however, would not take into account those who were born and died during the first few months of the year. If these were included it would point to a somewhat greater discrepancy. Since the fecundity rate is known to be high, a situation exists which emphasizes the high infant mortality rate as well as the rate for stillbirths and nonviable abortions.

In order of numerical importance the chief causes of death, as listed by the county health officer, were violence, heart disease, stillbirths, tuberculosis, influenza, nephritis, cancer, pellagra, and malaria. The distribution is unusual. Little confidence can be placed in the figures available on this mortality. In the first place, diseases are not adequately diagnosed because of the uncertain relation of doctors to sick persons, the rather general ignorance of disease, the reliance upon folk diagnosis and cures, and the exceedingly high rate of venereal infection in the population. The relative inaccessibility of many of the families leaves them very largely to the informal agencies of the community for handling both sickness and death. When violence is responsible for death it becomes a matter of both health and crime registration, and the state steps in with considerably more determination and insists on greater accuracy in the record.

The only index to sickness among the families studied was the non-technical one of persons being treated for malaria, pellagra, and syphilis, the latter under a special demonstration instituted as an experiment by the Rosenwald Fund. The county health service provided some mass treatment for persons with malaria. In 100 of the 612 families, or 16.3 per cent, all members of the family had been treated for malaria; in 194, or 31.6 per cent of the families, one or both of the parents had been treated; and in 50 more families, or about 5 per cent of them, some of the children and one or both parents had been treated. Twenty-eight of the families, or 4 per cent, reported that some of the children had been treated. In 212 families, or 43.6 per cent, there was no record of treatment for malaria. This does not measure the extent of malarial infection. Pellagra is similarly a common malady as indicated by the scaly, cracking skins, but there was no medical appraisal of the extent, since this would have required professional examination. Forty-one families were receiving, or had received, some treatment for pellagra. With respect to syphilis, however, the opportunity for determining the extent was unparalleled for studies of this type.

The Julius Rosenwald Fund, in co-operation with the United States Public Health Service, had undertaken a study of the prevalence of syphilis among Negroes in selected areas of the South. The health officers of six southern states were brought in co-operation with the Fund, through the Public Health Service and demonstrations were set up in six areas. The purpose of the demonstration was to provide a basis for determining the practicability and effectiveness of measures for the mass control of syphilis. Macon County was selected as one of these areas because of the proximity of Tuskegee Institute, the John A. Andrews Hospital, and the United States War Veterans Hospital, and because the administrative controls of the county and state, particularly in the health and welfare divisions, were co-operative. A thorough campaign was made to include as large a number of families as possible within a limited section of the country, in examinations which included Wassermann tests. All ages of both sexes were examined, and as many treated as would accept. The results of the medical examinations provide perhaps one of the most complete samples of a total population anywhere available. In this county 3,684 Wassermanns were taken, of which 1,474, or 35 per cent, were positive. This rate, incidentally, was the highest of the six demonstrations. A county in Georgia stood next with 26 per cent, on the basis of 5,775 tests; a county in Mississippi was next in order with 20 per cent on 9,753 tests; a county in North Carolina ranked fourth with only 12 per cent positives on a basis of 10,196 examinations. The average for the 30,000 serological examinations was 20 per cent positives.

In Macon County the large number of positive Wassermanns for children pointed to heridito-syphilis. The large number of positive reactions in men and women of advanced ages presented a problem for the medical men, since it is usually expected that the disease would have manifested itself in the advanced ages in other and more violent results.

The highest positive rates for men were found in the age group twenty-five to twenty-nine, with 32 per cent of their cases, and the women in the age group twenty to twenty-four, with 34 per cent of the cases.

Most of these families were not burdened by defectives so far as it was possible to ascertain. In 588 families, or 96 per cent of the total, there were no defectives. There was a blind child in 2 of the families. Two families had what appeared to be an imbecile, and 5 families had a person subject to "spells." A crippled person was found in 13 families, while 1 family had a ten-year-old child that had been crippled and an imbecile because of infantile paralysis since he was two or three years old.

The number of stillbirths and miscarriages in these families also served as an index to the health of the people in these communities. In the 612 families there were 490 known stillbirths. Less than half of the wives were responsible for the 490 stillbirths and miscarriages. There were 368 families in which none was reported.

To understand the somewhat unusual incidence of certain diseases and causes of death it is necessary to go back again to the life of the families.

Violent Deaths

There is a tradition of violence which seems to mark personal relations to a high degree. Although strictly speaking not a matter of health, reference to the setting in which these violent deaths take place is important as a phase of the social life as well as the mortality. They include accidents of various sorts as well as homicides. The violence of life was an inescapable fact in a large number of families of the county. In another connection reference has been made to the violence attending jealousy in sex relations, but violence is not confined to love affairs. The large amount resulting in death in this group of 612 families may be considered simply another index to its cultural status. A woman who was asked about sleeping with her windows open replied that "people do's so much killin' round here, I'se scared to leave 'em open." Another, referring to their recreation, explained why they stopped attending the dances: "Dere's so much cutting and killing going on." One notes either casualness or fatalism in recounting deaths in the family by violence.

My little grandchild what dead got a grain of corn down her throat, I think. She was shelling corn when she started coughing and she look jest like she had whooping cough, and never did get well. My other boy got kilt. He was jest stabbed to death. Oh, they sent the boy what done it to the reformatory.

Playing with Weapons

My brother wuz killed accidentally by his wife. He had gone to see 'bout my oldest sister who had gone crazy. He took my brother-in-law's automatic pistol back to Birmingham with him 'cause he was 'fraid my sister would get holt to it and hurt somebody. He had promised to teach his wife to shoot it, so one mornin' he was learnin' her. He took all the cartridges out and give it to her to shoot but he had left one in. He didn't know one wuz in the barrel. She took the pistol and 'cose she wuz scared to shoot it, and she throw her head on the side and her hand out and shot it and it hit my brother right in the head.

Juvenile Murders

My brother got killed out there by the creek. He was coming home from a ball game one evening and two boys grabbed him. I spose they got to fussing and the boys got mad and kilt him. We found him dead over there. They caught the boys. . . . One was a little boy 'bout twelve. They sent him to the 'formatory. The other one they sent to the mines for seven years.

Absent Sons

My boy got killed in Birmingham. They say he got shot—I don' know.

A White Gentleman Shot Him

My boy dead now. A white gentleman shot him. He went to his house to see his sister working there, and the gentleman told him to stay 'way. 'Twas his fault, I reckon. The man said, "Stay 'way."

A Baseball Bat

Our preacher's brother just got killed. He was at a ball game and a boy was batting and instead of hitting the ball he turned the bat loose and it went and struck him. The boy batting musta had something in him [corn whiskey].

All of this suggests the rough-handed closeness of a frontier community before adequate control of personal relations have been developed. There is the significant difference that social control in this community is related only vaguely to law. The courts are outside of the scheme of life; adjustment of relations in the past has been very largely the province of the white planter. Such unanimity of sentiment on law as exists is a common disposition to remain as far as possible out of contact with the courts whether as plaintiff or accused. Where these traditional forms of control over all phases of Negro social life by the white proprietor are weakening, as is apparent in the younger generation, or where there are no protectors available, the adjustment of disputes becomes a matter of the individuals involved. Instead of providing security as the arbitrator of personal differences, the courts are an institution to be feared, a medium through which justice is to be secured only by recourse to some individual white protector. Thus, differences tend to be settled on a personal and face-to-face basis. This sentiment helps further to account for the prevalence of weapons of defense.

One of the most frequently asserted evidences of respectability is that "we ain't been in no trouble yet." It is sufficiently difficult to avoid, in the community setting, to make avoidance a virtue.

Woofter reports an interesting situation among St. Helena Negroes, who live relatively isolated but very largely under their own social controls. There is similar attitude toward the "law," which they refer to as "the unjust law," in contradistinction to their own extra-legal machinery centered largely in the church. The local magistrates, recognizing this, encourage settlements through their own agencies. Cases of violence are thus very often avoided. A consequence is that there is very little crime and extremely few civil suits. Out of a population of about five thousand there were only about thirty-five cases annually brought before the local magistrate and most of these were cases of nonresidents.

Folk Knowledge of Disease

Except on the basis of a general health examination it would be impossible to estimate the extent of sickness from various diseases. Complaints are generalized into merely "feelin' kinda poorly" or "I ain't no good," and generalized complaints call for the generalized measures of patent medicines, or home herb remedies. "Black Draught," "666," salts, and castor oil make up a large part of the treatment of disease. Other standard remedies are "White Wonder Salve," calomel, and quinine.

Unless there is some folk pattern of treatment, death may result from sickness which in all probability could be avoided or intelligently treated. As one illiterate mother stated: "I had one child to die when it was just three days old, but I ain't never knowed what the trouble was. It just cried an' cried for three days and nights and then died."

Children die in great numbers and mothers accept their death with a dull and uninquiring fatalism. Some of the expressions back of the infant mortality rates are thus most casual and uninformed: The mother of eleven children sighed when she recalled "I don' had lots of chillun to die. I don't know what ailed them." Another, referring to her stillbirths, said, "I birthed eleven chillun. I got two living, six was born dead, and three lived a little while. That boy that died when he was three days old bled to death at the navel."

All that another mother knew about her infant's death was that "he just keep on spitting up blood and then died." "The granny" explained that "strainers" [meaning constipation] killed one infant, and eating too much dirt while carrying twins killed both of them for another of her patients. Then came this accident, which left a heavy memory for the mother:

> I was washing and my little baby asked for some water. I said, "Wait, honey; mammy busy," and I plumb forgot him till he scream. He done drunk my lye. He die so pitiful and hard I wisht I'da stop and give him a drink.

By some good fortune there are those who survive serious attacks without the aid of physicians. A man and his wife, aged fifty-three and forty-six respectively, live alone and pay $65 for rent of their farm. One daughter of the husband died of tuberculosis. The husband said:

> Don't ask me if we've been sick; that's all we bees. Last year I paid nigh over one hundred dollars for my sickness alone, and then my old lady there she's all time sick. Got so once we thought we was losing her for fair. All one side was paralyzed. She didn't speak for twenty-four hours. All the church folks come. Some give money, some give food, and she just lay there and hold 'em. Didn't know who gie'd 'em. She don't know yet. Well, I got busy. God and myself worked, rubbed, and twisted her till she finally come 'round. I tell you I believe in the Lord. He just didn't mean for me to lose her. . . . I has all kinds of trouble with my stomach. That's why I'm sick.

The following is an account of one woman's "miseries" as she described them. She had been sick for three years.

> I was in the field plowing one day and I felt something jerkin' my head around. Then I tried to spit and I couldn't. I said to my sister, "Can yo spit?" And she did, but I couldn't. I been sick and not able to work for three years. I has miseries in my stomach.

Indigestion ("indijestus") is a frequent complaint among the families, and this is a description of it:

My boy's out there is sick. He got indijestus. It jest takes him that way every time he gets a little cold in him. He'll start coughing and it hurts him all in there [lungs and chest], and you kin hear him trying to git his breath and he just has that indijestus with it every time.

My girl is sick too. The boy ain't sick as the girl. He only gits that way when he takes cold, but she dat way all the time.

This mother had thirteen children, and most of them had had trouble with "indijestus." The family gave evidence of being wracked with tuberculosis without the least suspicion of the lethal character of the ailment. Each successive death was an accidentally ill effect of "indijestus." Other descriptions of ailments suggest serious maladies, but in the absence of both diagnosing physicians or adequate treatment of these disorders they usually take this fatal issue, and perhaps affect others through contagion.

My husband he got sores all over him and I ain't got but one sore.

This child takes fits after his daddy. He ain' long stopped having them.

All my chillen is fond of having fevers.

They tell me its "two bumps" [tuberculosis]; anyhow he keep a terrible misery in his throat so he can't swallow water.

Two of my chillen die with "yellow thrash." I gived them thread salve made from yellow berries but they die right on.

I been sick a year going on two months. I ain't nobody, honey. See all these here sores on my legs [pointing to open sores as large as one's hand], water runs out of my legs there like that all the time. I can't lay down. I have to set up all the time. I can't lay down. If I lay down this here water you see running out will overflow my heart. I ain't nobody to be depended on. Liable to be dead tomorrow. I jest set here all day and fan flies. All this begin when I was four years old; now I'm at changing life. Sometimes I'm so hot look like I'm gonna run out of my skin, but in the evenings I get jest as cold as ice.

My wife here she out of her mind; jest come and go you know. She been sick so long.

My boy there [aged eleven] he had tumors—you know, a risin' come out on his head. In three weeks them doctors got sixty dollars but they saved him. For myself you see I ain't got no teeth. I tooks a dose of calomoy and 'fore I know it my teeth all start dropping out. I has the ear run, too, but that ain't so bad. Now my wife she died 'cause she had some tumors in her stomach. Them folks at the hospital [in Montgomery] just killed her. How I knows 'cause one of them nurses is my friend and she tole me herself they jest feeled around and couldn't find the tumor so they jest out and out and cut the wrong vescicule.

I been sick about four years. I have shortness of breath and fulness of the chest.

I got plenty chillen dead. One eleven months old died with fever; one the thrase run over him and one girl sixteen died in 1915. She got wet the wrong time. Doctor claim she had pellagacy. She said she could hear something inside her head, and she break out with great big old red bumps. Then they went in an' where they left was just as black. She didn't live no time. She was sick four weeks to the day she died.

I been so sick with my back and running bladder.

My daughter died with the fever. I don't know 'zackly what kind of fever it was. Dr. —— say it was swamp fever, but Dr. —— say it was malaria. My son die with heart trouble. That what Dr. —— say, but Dr. —— say it was bad blood. Dr. ——'s father was my husband's father's master. That's wha' he gets the same name.

That child there has spells since she was a little baby. Jest one right after another from eight to four o'clock every day for two years. I dosed her with calomel and I sent to Montgomery and got some worm powder and got nineteen worms from her in one day. But she can't learn nothing in school now. She jest sets with her mouth open and her tongue doubled back most of the time.

The heavy fall of death prompts to reliance upon both herbs and something akin to magic, in the attempt to bring about cures. The little granddaughter of one of the older women became ill.

I done all I could. Then one of them nurses in Tuskegee says to me I weren't doing the right thing by the child. Honey, I sho' was hurted so much 'cause I done everything for the little motherless thing. So I got me a bottle of castoria and fed it to her but hit didn't help her none. By and by I was told to wash her in dish water, so I done that every night for a long time. Then when I fear'd it warn't no use, my dead friend she come to me in a dream. She and me was dear friends together. She stood right there at the bed like real and she washed up a big sheet till hit was pure white. She ain't never spoke till she got done. Then she hung it up and spoke for the first time. She said, "Dat child ain't gonna die; she gwine live and grow up from there restrenkened." I got some more castoria and worked on the baby and here she am—well and healthy. It sho' was a miraculous sent from God.

Whooping cough is treated by tying a leather string around the child's neck. A necklace of cork and moles' feet is used to make teething easy. "White Wonder Salve" softens up old injuries; "Thread Salve" cures "yellow thrash." A woman said:

"Papa died with pneumonia. He wouldn't use nothing but rubbing medicine, and wouldn't never call no doctor." Another woman, with enormous sores of long standing on her arm and breast, was trying to nurse her baby. "Dese boils hurt so bad," she complained. "Dey's sore from de kernel. I been so sick I could hardly stand up." She put sulphur and vaseline on these sores. There was, however, a sense of the possibility of contagion. She talked of weaning the baby "so de boils won't turn on it." Still another woman kept a string around the children's necks to keep off disease. Pomegranate hull tea and broom-straw root tea are used for "back weakness." Peach-tree leaves and elephant tongue are good for fever. The woman who gave this formula said "doctor ain't no good when it comes to fevers." Boiled fireweed and lard make an excellent salve for burns. Sheep-nanny tea, kerosene, and sugar may be used for whooping cough, or red onions alone. If swollen feet are sweated first in pine top and mullen, then in cedar water, they will give no more trouble. Pepper and salt will cure spasms.

Use of Physicians

Rural calls are expensive and time consuming to make, whether the physicians take into account the ability of patients to pay or not. During the past year 258 of the 612 Negro families used the professional services of physicians, 322 did not use them, and in 32 cases the information could not be secured.

The expenditures for health as nearly as they could be estimated were as shown in Table 1.

The fee for an office consultation is $2.50 and $3.00. Fees for rural calls appear to vary according to distance and accessibility, sometimes amounting to $12. A curious practice of using proxies in the diagnosis of disease is noted in the following case:

> I fell mighty low sick. I don't know exactly what the trouble. Think the doctor says it was an abscess on my bladder and it busted. The doctor didn't come to see me 'cause he was busy wid a label case, but he sent Mr. —— over to see me and he took down my complaint and written up my case. No, Mr. —— ain't no doctor but he writes up my case and takes it back to Dr. —— and he sent me some medicine.

All of the physicians serving the Negroes of this part of the country are white, save one who lives in the town of Greenwood. Some of the physicians are also landowners. One doctor, in particular, seems to be greatly liked and admired by the Negroes. He extends them credit, does not exact exorbitant fees, and is sympathetic with their complaints. A few of the plantation-owners will send doctors to their good workers when they are ill, or guarantee the payment of their bills. This

TABLE 1. *Health Expenditures*

None	248
Amount unknown	115
Under $5	112
$5–$9	45
$10–14	33
$15–19	17
$20–24	13
$25–29	5
$30–34	1
$35–39	0
$40–44	5
$45–49	1
$50 and over	17
Total	612

is sufficient security since the doctor's bill can be taken out of the crop. For the most part, however, the doctors insist upon some security for the debt before calling. Ownership of a cow, or mule, or other property will suffice, and these are taken in if the bills are not paid within a reasonable time. Some of the objection to doctors was based upon their insistence upon prompt payment in cash.

> They just gets all our money when we is sick. A poor nigger has a hard time. You phones them and they say, "Is you got the money?" If you ain't, you need not 'spect them. You gotta have that money right on the table or you just lies here and dies.

Adjustments are made around the necessity for doctors. One woman, in speaking of her husband, said:

> When I get sick, he don't take me to no doctor. He'll buy medicine and bring it to me. He'll go to the doctor hisself, but he won't take me. Last time I was sick I had stomach trouble and he kept getting me medicine and I got worse, so he got a midwife and she said my womb had fallen. She fixed it up and I got all right. He had been giving me "666" and castor oil.

As serious as any other factor, however, in the attitude toward and frequently fatal result of disease is the air of resignation toward sickness when it comes. It explains to some extent the frequent lack of faith in doctors and the diffidence about certain public health measures.

> Old man B— took dropsy. His legs bust open and his feet bust open. He had money enough to buy fifty-cent socks, but he ruint so many they had to put ten-

cent socks on him. They take him to springs but it didn't do no good. When God get hold of you, you can go to any kind of springs but it won't help you none.

An old man and his wife, both devoutly religious, sat waiting for death. Said the husband:

The Marster [God] give me notice about six months ago for me to wind up my portion of this world's goods and to go in secret prayer. I was in the room and he come in too and just look like I could shake hands with him. I don't feel sick but I'm painful.

Said the wife:

The Lord come to me about three or four weeks ago. I was in bed and I look up and saw him just like I'm seeing you, and he was in a book. I got up and put on my burial clothes and he was waiting for me. I called my son to come in there and look at him but couldn't nobody see him but me. I kept waiting all day dressed for I thought he done come to take me. I'm prepared to die when he do come to get me. I ain't dead yet and I thought good God done come after me long time ago.

Midwives

The rôle of the midwife and her method can be best understood in the account of one of the best-known "grannies" of the county:

How Training Was Acquired

These old people 'round here learned me how to deliver babies. Long before I ever thought 'bout it we was at Mr. ——'s sister's house and she got confined and they sent for the granny and she didn't come. I didn't know and mammy didn't know what to do. So I measured the baby's navel and cut it off and I cut it off too much and that baby died, but the doctor didn't do nothing about it but he said that old granny ought to be stopped for not coming to see about her and I couldn't help it 'cause I was doing the best I could. Then after that, when I was living down on the hill a girl got confined and her brothers got on the horses and started for the granny and 'fore she could get there the baby begin to come on and I told her I wan't gonna let it drap, to let it come on that I wan't gonna let it hit the floor. I put the girl to bed good as I could, and I didn't put a cloth to her but I seed after the baby.

Treatment of the Mother

You know you don't put a cloth to a woman till after three days; it is best to let it drain for that long. It will kill her if you bound her up before that time. I don't like to have a crowd around when I am bringing a baby; somebody might go out and say one thing and some will go out and say another. Some of them will go out and talk about how the woman carried on and I just don't like to have them around. You turn the baby on the right side so as to give the blood chance to go all through his body. Then you turn the mother on her right side and let her lay on her right side for 'bout a hour.

A Knife To Cut the Pain

I usually put a sharp knife under the pillow; they say that cuts the pain, but I don't know whether it do or not. Some people say they can tell how many children you gonna have by the number of rings on the cord, but I don't believe that's so 'cause the old granny told me I was gonna have 'bout ten chillen and I ain't never had but one. After that I said I was done with that saying.

Mighty few of the chillen glad to see you come, for they 'fraid they will have to give you a little bread. Now when I lived in Birmingham all the little chillen used to see me coming and holler, "Yon come my mammy," and they all say, "Don't you stay down there and suffer for nothing to eat."

Cutting the Cord with Scissors

I always cut the cord with scissors and when I get through I just slip them under the pillow. They tells us you ought to get hold of what you charge before you hit a lick of work. These folks don't want to pay you for nothing. I heard that Mrs. F—— was telling all the women to use G——. G—— is a right nice seamstress and I reckon she do sewing for Mrs. F—— and Mrs. F—— tell the women to use her, but I reckon the Lord will straighten things out. I loses more than I make trying to get my money.

Causes of Deformity

Plenty women's chillen is deformed 'cause its the way they do in carrying them and they always trying to lay it on the fever, 'cause fever don't cause you to be deformed 'cause I try to hold the jints together so close so that they won't be deformed. I had a brother who was deformed; he was marked by a turtle. My mamma was plowing one day and plowed up a turtle and she stuck a plow in the back of his head. He sets his feet out like a turtle and walks and slides them back like one. I got one of his shoes in here now and it don't look like it was ever straight. I was a plow hand when my first child was born and I plowed up to the time and it didn't hurt it none; its just all right if you don't let the plow kick you. That woman over yonder plows all the time and it don't hurt her, and that other woman said she went over to her mama's and picked a bag of peas and carried them home and that's what caused her to have him deformed.

Dirt-Dauber Tea for Labor Pains

Some folks say if you pick the dirt out of dirt-dauber holes and make tea out of it, it will cut the pains, but I don't know whether that will do any good or not.

I sometimes give them a little weak camphor to force the pains and that is mighty weak too. Sometimes when folks eat dirt and when the baby comes its a whole lot of dirt on his back where they have been eating too much. I don't believe in using so many of these old things 'cause I believe some of them is pizen.

White-Flannel Weed for "Whites"

There is a weed grows out there called "white flannel" that is mighty good for whites [leucorrhea]. A woman asked me once, "Ain't you a doctor woman?" And I told her yes, and she told me her daughter don't never have no health and said she can't hardly get over the floor, and I told her to go get her some white flannel and make her a tea off it; and she wanted to know if a yard would be enough to get and I told her it wasn't no cloth but a weed. So I went up on the hill and found her some and give it to her. That woman got all right. Her husband had to stop work every week one day and stay home with her and help her scrub, but after she started taking the white-flannel tea she got all right. That white flannel sho' is good.

How To Reduce Water

Another thing, some women when they has babies they drink so much water that their stomach's get large and poke way out and get pot-gutted; well, if you fix up some corn bread with a heap of salt in it and put it on the fire and let it burn right black and then split it open and put it in a bucket and let her drink off that, her stomach will come down jest as nice.

Hot Ginger Tea for Retarded Menstruation

Heap of them come to me for female trouble but I tell them to go on to the doctor 'cause I'm 'fraid to fool with so many things. When the flowers is clogged I give them hot ginger tea.

Bad Blood and Corn Bread

When I went to the clinic they said my blood was good, but I told the doctor my blood might be good but there was something the matter with my body 'cause I can't eat corn bread no more. I used to eat corn bread all the time and I believe I eat too much 'cause one day something come and said to me just like somebody talking, "That corn bread is killing you." It done that twice and I quit eating it 'cause I didn't want it to kill me, and I told the doctor about it and told him to give me some medicine for it.

The county has been attempting to give some instruction to the Negro midwives, recognizing that most of the deliveries are made by them. The health officer has corralled sixty-seven of these midwives and has been talking to them about cleanliness and essential though elementary hygiene for mother and child, and about the necessity of records, although most of the midwives are illiterate. From the record of the health officer's work it appears that each midwife had been talked to once in individual conference.

Attitude toward Syphilis

In the entire 612 families interviewed there was not a single expression which seemed to connect syphilis with the sexual act. The fact of "bad blood" carried little social stigma and was spoken of in about the same manner as one speaks of having a "bad heart" or "bad teeth." The violent expressions of jealousy, manifested toward women suspected of transferring affections to other men, reflected no relation to transmitted infection. In one instance only was "bad blood" associated with heredity. "I knowed I had bad blood 'cause my mamma had scrofula when I was born." In but few instances was "bad blood" associated with syphilis as a venereal disease. Where there were obvious physical manifestations of the disease the persons were referred to as being afflicted, but this was generalized. Often no distinction was made between complaints and the symptoms of "bad blood." Accordingly, treatments for bad blood were expected to cure headaches, indigestion, pellagra, sterility, sores of various sorts, and general run-down condition.

Attitude toward the Health Demonstration

The Rosenwald Fund experiment in mass control of syphilis was probably more successful in bringing a large number of persons to have blood tests made than any similar venture. The reasons for this lie in the character and habits of the population. There was a lack of social embarrassment in being examined and treated for syphilis. The directors of the experiment succeeding in giving a medical rather than a social stress to the connotation of "bad blood."

> My blood was drawed twice but they never sent me no invitation about it. I bet my blood ain't good 'cause I hear everybody say they blood is bad. I think mine ought to be bad too. I just went down there one day and said I wanted shots and they shot me.

The tradition of dependence and obedience to the orders of authority, whether these were mandatory or not, helps to explain the questionless response to the invitation to examination and treatment. In the conduct of the demonstration, however, the greatest kindliness was shown the patients, and the invitations were in no sense supported by force, either direct or implied.

The extent of sickness among the Negro families and the hope of relief without cost were means of drawing and holding them. "Me and my wife went over to the schoolhouse and they drawed our blood and say it was good, but I can't understand why we are always so painful." The familiarity of some of the Negro families with the method of giving "shots" by physicians for which comparatively large sums were paid had given them a "set" for the demonstration. Free "shots" were taken as a boon. The fitting of "salves" and red medicine of the old clinic into old habits of getting relief gave confidence. Some of the persons attempted to get the salves for general complaints, even though their blood was reported "good." "They said my blood was good. You don't get no treatment if your blood is good, but sometimes I wish it was bad 'cause they gives away a salve up there and I wanted some of it so bad." The "shots" were indeed expected to cure all complaints.

They drawed my blood twice last year but I never did get no hearing from it. Look like mine ought to be bad 'cause I was bothered with pellagacy sometime ago.

I goes down to the clinic last Wednesday for the doctor to give me a shot but he didn't give me none. I had a roaring in my head for four or five years.

Good effects observed prompted many to continue treatment and others to seek examination and treatment.

I never knowed women to have babies like they do this year. Them shots is making them have babies. I knowed women who been married a long time and this year they are all poking out. There is K—— W——; she about thirty-odd years old and been all about different places too and she been taking them shots and now she is 'way out yonder. You reckon them shots make you have babies? I sho' don't want no more and if they do I rather have bad blood.

Just think of Sister S—— up there. Her husband was as raw as a piece of meat the first of this year, but he done got better since he been taking these shots.

The medicine I took helped me 50 per cent. I had a terrible misery in my throat. I was sorry for the time to come to drink water, it hurt me so bad. I have taken twenty shots and it certainly has helped me.

The cost of doctors has helped attendance at the clinics:

I tell you dem doctors done de people a whole lot of good 'cause heap of people wan't able to pay a doctor. They have done this country good 'cause heaps of dem was in a bad fix. The doctors done git tight on de people since dese clinics been through here. They won't come to see you less you got the money or will pay something. See these folks is knocking them. They charge seven, eight, nine, and ten dollars 'cording how far they have to come.

Finally there was the attitude of appreciation for the gesture of helpfulness which the demonstration represented, and a response on that basis. Many of the families are enthusiastic in their praise of the work being done by the clinic. The wife in a family consisting of mother and father and ten children said:

Them shots really hoped me. 'Til last May I ain't layed down a night the whole night and slept without getting up and staying wake in twenty years. I can lay down and go to sleep with the chickens and never wake up. When I got so I could rest, I got scared. I used to get up and no feel like working, but now I can get up and feel good. . . . This baby [a little girl five years old] has taken twenty and she don't cry none hardly. That little boy [aged seven] was born sick, and he has taken all his shots and he is so much better. He used to get off and hide and never did run and play like the rest of the children. We would have to hunt for him all the time. I was jest expecting to find him dead any time 'cause he would go 'way off somewhere and hide all the time. Now he runs round jest like the rest of them. [The mother and father and eight of the ten children gave positive Wassermanns.]

The figures for mortality, morbidity, illegitimacy, illiteracy, poverty, insufficiency of food and clothing, are barren records for an understanding of the human struggle behind them. They all come to a focus in the story of Mary Hardy, a very sad and very bewildered woman, whose career follows the pattern of life around her, because she could not understand how or why her children continued to die from some strange, persistent malady. She was not married but had wanted the security of a husband and a family.

The first man I liked real well give me a baby. My grandmother made me lave home, and I went and lived with another woman till the baby came, then grandma let me come back home, but he stole me again one night. I had to wait till my grandmother was sleep, so it was about nine o'clock and I slipped out of the window and he was down in the woods waiting for me. I went with him to his people and I stayed with his sister. I never did stay with him, but my grandmother would not let me come back home after I'd done run away and he kept putting me off. He promised to marry me the next morning. I never would a run off with him if he hadn't promised to marry me, but kept putting me off and I wanted to go back to grandma, but she told me not to come back there less she tell me so, so I just had to stay. I stayed there with his sister three years and got these other two chillen. His mother kept the oldest boy and raised him.

When my third baby was coming, his father jumped up and married another girl. She was in a family way and I wondered why he married her 'cause she was in a family way and he didn't marry me when I was in a family way too.

This girl was a school teacher and he married her one month before she got down. Then when he started coming back 'round, I told him, "I ain't going to fool with you no more; you done fooled me enough. I got real mad. I got mad about him, so I told him to stay away 'cause I felt bad about it . . . and I was 'specting to marry him.

He left here and went to Montgomery. Then he sent me money to come to him but I was so hungry that I took the money and bought us something t'eat. I guess I'd a went if we hadn't been so hungry. After he married, he would give me rice and things for the chillen every time he saw me in town. He just seemed to be in love with the chillen. They say now that he is living with another woman. His wife died when she was getting down the second time. He had left and went to Montgomery to work but they wasn't separated. It was after she died that he sent for me to come to him.

Now my youngest boy is sickly and got bumps breaking out on his face—you know, fever blisters, but big ones, and when they burst they leave a sore. The sore leaves a black place when it dries up. I took him to the doctor once and he said he charge $2.50. I didn't have but $2.00, so he said he would charge me that. Then we had to send for him once and I ain't never paid him for that. He usually charge $12.50 to come out here.

Just when I thought I got my chillen well, my oldest boy die. He just rotted to death. This is how he got sick. He started with a headache. He said his head nearly bust open and Br'er [brother] got some salts and give him and he didn't complain no more for about two weeks; then he went to school one morning and the next morning they didn't have no school and he got up and it started with a hurting right here [just inside the elbow bend]. He said it was itching first, then hurting, and he just started running 'round having fits. He just went crazy. We rubbed and greased his arms and we rubbed him good, but he just went crazy and tore up the things in the house. The doctor give him some medicine when we took him to him and he said it was pellagacy but I ain't seed where it done him a bit of good. He told one man down here that it was the curriest pellagacy he ever seed in his life, and he told somebody up there that he didn't know what it was; but he told me it was pellagacy. Well, that boy would run away and I'd hear him calling way up on the hill. He just come unjointed. It all just rotted off—all his hands and arms. He bit one of his fingers off and he never was in his right mind after he first went crazy. He would take the bed down and when you ask him what he was doing it for, he's say he wanted to put it up on a hill. He swold up and just come in two. He died in two weeks.

When I got sick I went to Dr. —— and he told me I needed shots but that he couldn't give them to me 'cause I wasn't able to pay. He asked me if I had any property and I told him no. He said he just couldn't give 'em to me then. He said, "If you just had a cow to put up against it!"

The experimental health demonstration set up by the Rosenwald Fund in a portion of the county in 1930 has made certain social discoveries vital to other than the venereal problem. The adequate treatment of specific luetic conditions demanded preliminary general physical examinations and these laid bare an extravagant incidence of other disabilities. Some 7,500 blood examinations and 3,200 urine analyses were made on those under treatment, and a total of 2,042 prescriptions dispensed during the first year. Apart from this, however, 3,500 typhoid inoculations were given, and 600 children immunized against diphtheria, and 200 vaccinated against smallpox. This altogether, with the Red Cross distribution of seeds for gardens and yeast to be used in combating pellagra, constituted one of the most intense concentrations upon a reconstructive health campaign of any rural section in the South.

It was evident, however, that that dependent relationship of the Negro tenants to white landowners called for education of the landowner as well as the tenant. And although this has not yet become common in either direction, there are indications that some of the white planters are recognizing time off for health as profitable in the end. One of them commented thus to an official of the demonstration: "The year before this demonstration was put on I paid out over fifteen hundred dollars to doctors for medical service. This year I have had a doctor on the place only twice and those were for new babies. The men work better."

The startling inbreeding of disease among the Negroes, the violent eruption of nutritional disorders, and the rapid contagion of infectious diseases are intricately bound up with their isolation, their low literacy, and their cultural backwardness. They have little or no knowledge of the diseases responsible for their excessive deaths, and little access to physicians when the seriousness of ailments exceeds their simple folk remedies. With these, however, goes a life-organization which permits neither the full responsibility of the planter for their troubles nor the free development among and for themselves of controls over their most common disabilities. The situation has fostered a striking disorganization.

As in other respects, the most far-reaching changes in habits are proceeding at most rapid pace in the work done with and through the children. This suggests that along with the programs of adult education, social work, and compulsory health regulations, the elementary schools demand foremost attention if these changes are to be given permanence and significance.

SHADOW ON THE LAND

Syphilis, the White Man's Burden

THOMAS PARRAN

Syphilis is the white man's disease. He may, as medical historians tell us, have contracted it from the American Indian following Columbus' discovery. But the brown, the yellow, and the black races seem to have been infected with it only after the visits of the white explorers to their native lands, and it has continued to decimate the white populations of the earth.

It has been said that the negro slave brought to America malaria and hookworm disease. If he did, the white man paid him back with usury by giving him tuberculosis and syphilis. The fact that he is at the bottom of the economic ladder contributes to his abnormally high death rate. For among the third of our population which is ill fed, ill clothed, and ill housed, as a race, north and south, and especially in the rural south, his house is the most miserable, his clothing the scantiest, and his food ration the most poorly balanced.

Scattered evidence accumulated over a period of years had indicated a high prevalence of venereal disease, and especially syphilis, among the Negroes. Wenger[1] had shown this in several Mississippi counties. He had shown also that the Negroes welcomed these blood tests. "Holding high Wassermann in the market place," Keyes[2] called it after seeing Wenger at work on Saturday afternoon in a crossroads store. Until 1929, however, when the Rosenwald Fund of Chicago began a study of syphilis and a demonstration of treatment among the Negroes of six counties in five southern states, exact knowledge on the subject justified only generalizations concerning it.

For many years the late Julius Rosenwald was interested in giving the Negro a better chance for an education. Having been interested in the problem by their director of medical service, Dr. Michael M. Davis, the philanthropic corporation bearing Rosenwald's name expanded its activities in 1928 to include the improvement of health status for the race. Joining with the U.S. Public Health Service and the state and local departments of health, the studies supported by the Fund attempted to find the answer to eight questions:

Dr. Thomas Parran was the director of the Public Health Service's Division of Venereal Disease when the study began and the U.S. surgeon general when his book on syphilis was published. Originally published in Shadow on the Land: Syphilis, the White Man's Burden *(New York: Waverly Press, 1937): 160–81.*

1. What is the incidence of syphilis as shown by the Wassermann tests among the rural negro population of all ages?
2. Can rural Negroes be induced to accept Wassermann tests and those with syphilis induced to take an amount of treatment sufficient to render them noninfectious?
3. Can satisfactory treatment of syphilis be given under field conditions?
4. Can these special activities for syphilis control be integrated with the general health program of the community?
5. At what cost can the case-finding and treatment methods be carried out?
6. To what extent can funds be secured from state and local tax sources to bear the cost of this project?
7. What are the direct and indirect effects of syphilis upon these negro populations in terms of sickness and death? And finally, the most important question,
8. Can syphilis be controlled by these intensive medical methods; and if so, how soon and at what rate can its prevalence be reduced?

At the time these studies were begun, I was an assistant surgeon general of the U.S. Public Health Service in charge of the Division of Venereal Diseases. During the discussion of practical methods to be used in conducting the studies, we were guided largely by Wenger's successful study of prevalence. Also, I recalled reports of intensive syphilis control a few years earlier in areas of Eastern Europe overrun by armies during the World War and where, in many of the villages, syphilis was almost pandemic—practically everybody had it. The method followed here was to make routine Wassermann tests on whole population groups in one community after another. A similar Wassermann dragnet was determined upon as a starting point among the southern Negroes.

But the practical problem was how to do it. We realized that many of these people had never in their lives been treated by a doctor. Few of them had even seen a hypodermic needle. How, then, without the exercise of brute force could we get blood specimens for diagnosis? For the group with latent syphilis, who felt well, who had no "misery" to bring them to the doctor, how persuade them to take the long-continued, somewhat uncomfortable treatments which would protect them against late, serious symptoms? How start the job among folk who did not even know the word syphilis?

From the beginning it was decided to use as many Negroes as possible in the professional personnel. Although methods in each of the counties differed some-what in detail, the general plan was to provide a syphilis control unit consist-ing of a physician, a nurse, and a clerk in each area, working with the local health departments under state supervision, the Public Health Service acting as a co-ordinator.

In selecting the counties in which studies were to be made, two factors were taken into consideration: First, their unlikeness; for little would be learned concerning syphilis among Negroes unless as many different types as possible were brought into the demonstration and from communities varying as widely as possible as to industry, literacy, and economic status. The second and very important factor, however, was one of similarity; for, unless both the state and local health departments were interested in carrying out the study and concerned about the basic problem of syphilis control, failure was inevitable.

On these bases, the following locations for the studies were agreed upon:

1. Scott, Mississippi, on the plantation of the Delta & Pine Land Company.
2. Albemarle County, Virginia, a community above the average in literacy and where good medical care has been available.
3. Macon County, Alabama, the most primitive of the communities studied and the most poverty ridden.
4. Brunswick, Georgia, and the turpentine forests back of it in Glynn County.
5. Tipton County, Tennessee, a cotton-growing section normally above the average in economic status.
6. Pitt County, North Carolina, a tobacco-growing section in the eastern part of the state.

Not only was it necessary in beginning this work to get the co-operation of state and local health officers, but it was vitally necessary to sell the idea of testing and treatment to the Negro concerned.

In the first place, it is true in the South, by and large, that the Negro instinctively trusts the white man, except where he has suffered from sharp dealing and has good reason to be suspicious. He trusts the doctor—thanks to the fine character of many of our rural southern physicians. He trusts the Government, because in spite of clumsy dealing and mistakes since the post–civil war period, he has believed that the Government is a friend of his and tries to help him. The "government health doctor" therefore has an entreé. If he deals fairly and is considerate, it is not too difficult to get co-operation.

The Negro trusts the elders of his own race. Their older generation has an influence with the young that is far greater than among us. He trusts the educated man and woman of his race; except, again, when he has suffered from some attempt of theirs to take advantage of his lack of education. The negro preacher, the school-teacher, the occasional doctor are the acknowledged leaders of their race. Arrangements were made through them for talks in the schools and churches.

Though most of the audience did not know the word syphilis, many of them were familiar with what they called "bad-blood" disease and the miseries it brought. After the talk came the call for testing. Sometimes it was done on the spot, blood specimens taken from everybody in the place, and a date set for a second clinic to which each person present was asked to bring all members of his own family and his friends. Usually it was not difficult to get blood specimens from the whole crowd, once a leader among them had been persuaded to submit to the first test. When testing was done at a school session, a lollypop apiece helped to motivate the timid small fry.

We had some good arguments to use in conferences with the plantation owners and white leaders of the community. Public health in the South has done some impressive things in the reduction of typhoid fever, malaria, and pellagra. Some of the old-timers could remember the terror of yellow fever and how it had vanished. In asking help for syphilis control, I am not ashamed of the fact that we made a great point of the improved labor efficiency that would result from healthy Negroes, though I am glad to say that every doctor and nurse who worked on the project was thinking in the more human terms of relief from suffering, prevention of needless deaths, and the addition to human happiness.

After all, however, whether it is public health or sewing machines you have to sell, you must talk to your customer in his own language. I knew that the majority of these plantation owners, fine fellows that they were, would give us their sympathetic good wishes in whatever we ourselves chose to do to improve the welfare and promote the happiness of the Negroes on their plantations. But if we expected them to do anything about it, I knew we had to use the argument that it would be more profitable to work a healthy field hand than a sick one.

Usually we got a prompt response. "Tell those niggers the health doctor will be at the Possom Hollow school tonight. He's got some government medicine to cure the blood disease. A lot of these niggers have got blood trouble, sickly, no 'count, lazy; but maybe it's not their fault. This doctor will find out." Or again, "Yes, Doc, go ahead, I've got about forty of them here pickin' cotton. Can you test them here? How long does it take?"

Man, woman, or child, as one after another reached the end of the cotton row, there was the doctor to take the blood test and a brief history. Some would hold back, only to be joshed by the more courageous fellows who had found the test not to be much of an ordeal.

We debated at length one question: Should we disregard the cases of late syphilis, concentrating on the early infectious case? Public health theory said, "Yes. The old syphilitic can't hurt anyone but himself. Concentrate on the infectious cases and try to slow up the spread." The practical psychology of Wenger said, "No. Treat the old syphilitic with 'rheumatism,' give him the painless mercury rubs. He will feel better and will bring in the whole family for the treatment they need. Don't forget, they listen to their granddaddies."

It was decided not to give intravenous (arsphenamine) treatment to those over 50, or whose history of syphilis antedated 20 years. It was early decided, too, that intramuscular injections of bismuth or mercury in the buttocks could not be used.

Except with very careful management, they may cause painful lumps which, it had been observed in clinics, the Negro particularly dislikes. How, then, could the heavy metals be given effectively?

Mercury ointment is effective if rubbed in properly. The rural Negroes wear no shoes, so ointment in the sock was out of the question. On ships in the early days it was traditional for the syphilitic sailors to sit on stools in a circle, backs bare, and rub each other with mercury ointment.

Could the same plan be used here? Get them together in the church, sitting in a circle, have the pastor lead them in a spiritual, keeping time to the up-and-down and round-and-round rubbing of mercury ointment into the backs. This was tried, but with indifferent success; partly, someone said, because the pastor thought he didn't get rubbed hard enough.

The best method proved to be the use of a mercury ointment on a rubber and canvas belt—endowed by the doctor, it is true, with all the white magic of health and strength-giving qualities his tongue could contrive.

"Take this package of salve, cut it into six pieces. Every morning, smear one piece on the belt; like this. Tie the belt tightly around your waist; on the seventh day, wash yourself thoroughly and meet me here. Don't forget, one week from today, and you'll feel strong as a mule."

At first, we cast about for a place where we could get such belts, cheaply, because the budget was small. There were no W.P.A. sewing rooms then. But then, as now, there was the Red Cross. In half a dozen county seats, the local chapters made the canvas and rubber belts in their sewing rooms by the hundreds, at a cost of only a few cents for the materials.

How much syphilis was found in these rural negro groups? In Albemarle County, Virginia (Charlottesville), the ratio was less than among many white groups—8.9 per cent. Here for a hundred years, the University of Virginia Hospital has furnished good medical care to the Negroes. Through rendering domestic and other services, they have been in close contact with the whites. They have better than the average schools; their general economic conditions were much better than in the deep South. The result was little syphilis.

At the other extreme was Macon County, Alabama, where in spite of the wholesome influence of Tuskegee Institute, very primitive conditions exist. Even in prosperous times, the poverty exceeded anything most of us have seen. The houses were tumble-down shacks, many without floors, with no furniture, and only a few rags for bedding; there were no screens, a privy only when underbrush was not conveniently close.

One reaction to their dreary surroundings was their constant wandering about in search of something better, with respect both to housing and labor terms.

They ate a pellagrous diet—salt pork, hominy grits, and molasses. They had no green vegetables, no fruit, no milk, no red meat. What they had was usually insufficient in amount. The only well-fed Negroes I saw in Macon County were the students in Tuskegee Institute and the patients in the nearby Veterans Hospital, many paretics among these last.

Southern counties in those days had little idea of public relief for the destitute. When I was there in 1932 a devoted social worker who combined the positions of county truant officer, welfare commissioner, and children's aid official in this county of 30,000 said: "I think they have done very well in this county in taking care of the poor. The county appropriated $300 for me to use this year. Then, too, I can get some clothes and things from the church groups, which helps out."

Destitution, ignorance, lack of medical care—the Wassermann dragnet showed a different record from that in Albemarle County, Virginia, where the Negroes' environment more nearly approached the white man's. In all age groups 39.8 per cent were positive. That represents almost the saturation point when one considers that in older age groups, the blood of some syphilis patients spontaneously became negative, even though symptoms of late syphilis may persist; that the congenital syphilitics presumably are immune to acquired infection, and some of them show negative tests in early adult life; and that in the age group under puberty, infection usually has not yet been acquired.

With so many of the population infected, only a limited section of Macon County could be included in the demonstration. Even in this limited area, the prevalence of syphilis was not uniform. There was one plantation where most of the tests were negative. The medical officer thought something had gone wrong in the laboratory with this batch of specimens, but a re-check confirmed the results. There were about 30 families here, nearly all of whose ancestors had been slaves on the same place. Very few had moved away. The owner and his father both had been doctors. The sick Negroes had been treated by the best of the existing medical knowledge. Lack of migration and good treatment were the only observable factors differentiating this group from the rest of Macon County. Is it not likely that here as in Charlottesville if the white man gives the Negro a chance the result is less syphilis?

In general, it was found that work was being done with syphilis in its native state, without the modifications that arise from treatment in any quantity, no matter how inadequate.

Of the 1,400 cases admitted to treatment in Macon County, only 33 had ever taken any previous treatment and these had had an average of 4.3 doses of neoarsphenamine.

The Wassermann dragnet method of case finding showed that from a total of 33,234 persons who were tested in the six counties, 6,800 or 20.5 per cent were found to be positive. Of the total patients for whom the time of infection was ascertained, 14.4 per cent were congenital. This means that today, syphilis is a more important factor in the southern states than malaria, pellagra, or hookworm. The

Public Health Service census shows only 7.2 per 1,000 of cases under treatment. In other words, there are 25 times as many Negroes with positive Wassermann tests for syphilis as there are syphilitic Negroes receiving care.

A treatment goal of 20 arsphenamines and 192 mercury rubs was set, requiring 34 weeks of treatment. Forty per cent of this goal was reached; or an average of 8.4 arsphenamines and 72.6 mercury rubs. Two-thirds of the patients received seven or more doses of arsphenamines. This is as good a record as one sees in the average public health clinic or hospital dispensary. It is not good enough, but even so, many infectious cases were eliminated and many person-to-person epidemics stopped.

What about results? In one community, the plantation owner and the doctor had records to show that the total amount of sickness among the negro workers had been cut in half following the syphilis control work. Here the plantation owner—an exception to the rule—for several years had provided medical treatment for all his negro workers, and the number of the doctor's calls could be compared from year to year.

In Bolivar County, Mississippi, however, we had the best example of labor efficiency resulting from the syphilis-control work. Here is one of the largest cotton plantations in the world, 60 square miles and almost 40,000 acres, owned by the Delta & Pine Land Company, on which live 3,500 to 4,000 negro sharecroppers. There is a resident doctor and hospital; also a veterinarian to take care of the mules. The plantation is conducted like a large-scale industrial enterprise.

The year after the demonstration, the resident manager said to me:

This is a matter of dollars and cents for our company. We have found that it doesn't pay to keep sick livestock. But the sickly nigger is another problem. We have screened their cabins to keep our malaria mosquitoes, and when they kicked out the screens to let the dog through, we gave them quinine, instead. We have vaccinated them against typhoid fever, and built sanitary privies to avoid hookworm. We require that each family make a garden, and we sell canned salmon in the commissary to prevent pellagra. But never before have we been able to do anything about the syphilis.

You remember that one in four had a positive blood test. I called the croppers together and told 'em I had the healthiest mules in Mississippi and I didn't want 'em driven by men dying of syphilis. I said, "You ought to want to be as good as a mule. You go down and get the blood test and take all the treatment the doctors tell you to."

As a result, I never had so little sickness as last year, nor so many live babies born. The death rate used to be higher than the birth rate but we've reversed it. This is the best thing we have ever done. See that old man over there? Last year he could hardly drag himself around, sores all over his legs, crippled up with rheumatism; now he does as good a day's work as any man on the place.

The average cost in all six demonstrations of case finding, plus treatment of positives, was $8.60 per case on an annual basis, or $2.30 per capita of the population tested.

Studies show that syphilis cuts in half the ability to do a full day's work, doubles the load of the unemployables. Yet the cost of finding and treating a case of syphilis among rural Negroes is less than one week's relief wages. If the Government were to take one fifty-second of the annual average wage, one week's pay, and spend it in finding and treating syphilis, the results would more than pay for the cost in better labor efficiency. The delayed deaths and lessened disability would be a net gain.

Started under good auspices, using methods soundly conceived and well executed, these demonstrations gave promise of excellent and lasting results. But when the depression came the Rosenwald Fund was unable to carry on. At the same time the communities themselves were faced with the acute depression problem of six-cent cotton and could not possibly take up the added load.

The spirochetes, however, were only temporarily depressed. They have continued to thrive since the demonstrations closed. Syphilitic Negroes continue to drag their diseased bodies across the cotton fields. The relief rolls are swelled by the disabling effects of late syphilis.

The Negro is not to blame because his syphilis rate is six times that of the white. He was free of it when our ancestors brought him from Africa. It is not his fault that the disease is biologically different in him than in the white; that his blood vessels are particularly susceptible so that late syphilis brings with it crippling circulatory diseases, cuts his working usefulness in half, and makes him an unemployable burden upon the community in the last years of his shortened life. It is through no fault of hers that the colored woman remains infectious two and one-half times as long as the white woman. In the white man, diseases of the central nervous system are more likely to occur; but though there are some racial differences in the type of disablement suffered by white and black in late syphilis, both pay the extreme penalty.

It has been argued that greater sexual promiscuity accounts for the increased prevalence of syphilis among the Negro. Even if this were true, and it is certainly not the whole truth, whose fault is it? Promiscuity occurs among the black race as it does among the white in groups and communities of the underprivileged. It is the smug citizen, satisfied with the *status quo*, who is to blame for the children, black or white, without moral standards, brought up in the slums, without decent education, wholesome play, or useful work, without ambition because without hope.

We are apt to think of slums as belonging to the congested districts of the great cities. The rural slums where many Negroes live in this country are far more miserable. They are tucked away where complacent white folks are not reminded of them. They are teeming with disease. There are no school doctors to find sick children; no clinics where the sick and the handicapped receive help; no visiting nurses to look after the sick in their homes. There is no control over polluted milk or water and there is very little milk. There is no money to buy medical service, and only a little offered through charity.

In many sections of the deep South, until some very recent efforts to improve his economic status without doing much to improve the Negro to take advantage of it, the only wholesome influence the Negro has enjoyed has been the influence of his religion. And simple-minded folk, no matter what their color, would be apt to find religion more convincing if they saw more of it practiced by the white people they know who seem to have enough to eat. As it stands, the restrictions of a good life are preached to the Negro, while the rewards of a good life invariably seem to go to someone else. Even the exhortation is likely to be sporadic, for most of the great churches apparently take more real interest in saving the souls of the brown or yellow heathen in far countries than in services to the souls within our immediate boundaries.

Wherever education and living conditions among the negro race approximate that of the white race, the syphilis rate approximates that of the white. The most recent evidence comes from physicians at the Meharry Medical College in Nashville, who find that among the professional students, there was a blood-positive rate of 5.9. They found that in one college, the negro girls showed a rate of less than 2 per cent.

Promiscuity, with its admitted impetus to the spread of syphilis, occurs among both white and black where we permit children to grow up ignorant among depraved surroundings. I cannot see how the white man may divest himself of his burden of responsibility for syphilis among the Negro by being sanctimonious about it.

Ignoring the psychological advantage of facing our problems squarely, however, there may be those who are comforted by feeling superior to the poor, ignorant, unmoral creatures, who fall sick and die so readily from the disease we gave them. Such superior beings need to be frightened within an inch of their lives, however, about their own lack of safety from infection if this is allowed to continue. For it is my firm belief that no man or woman, no family, can be so highly placed, so surrounded by privilege, as to be safe from syphilis if we permit it to saturate the deep strata of the less privileged, white and black, in our civilization.

That is a hypothetical situation, however. From the end of the fifteenth century when syphilis was called the "court disease" in Spain, the rich and the powerful have suffered from it. It is true that they have suffered less, for the best medical service of the day always has been ready to their call.

There are those who are afraid to employ Negroes because of the syphilis from which so many of them suffer. In the first place, without examination, one cannot be sure that the white employee is not suffering from the same condition; and further, a syphilitic under treatment is completely safe to have about one's business or household in any ordinary capacity. The risks are much less than in employing an unexamined person in any walk of life. The thing for an employer to do is to set a good example by taking a blood test himself and require it of every person employed, making clear—and sticking to it—that the results will be without prejudice if proper medical treatment is taken.

The first national organization formally to vote cooperation with the syphilis control campaign of the Public Health Service was the National Medical Association, composed of the negro physicians. This Association at its meeting last summer appointed a Commission on the Eradication of Syphilis, which came to Washington in September to present a tentative program and to ask how their cooperation could be made most effective.

They offered "unremitting efforts to enlist the services of all colored physicians, dentists, pharmacists, nurses, social workers, and affiliated women's organizations, aggregating over 15,000."

Dr. D. W. Byrd, of Norfolk, Virginia, chairman of the Commission, brought with him letters from his senators and congressmen who spoke of him as a leading citizen of his city and a physician devoted wholeheartedly to solution of the health problems of his race.

Ways and means of reaching the negro population were discussed. One handicap is the shortage of institutions for the training of negro physicians in syphilis control. Negro leaders are keenly aware of the importance of the syphilis problem to their race and are anxious to do something about it. At our National Conference on Venereal Disease Control held in Washington last winter, Dr. Byrd told the story of his own volunteer work in Norfolk, and lifted the audience to real enthusiasm:

> I was drawn into this fight more than 20 years ago when someone I loved fell an innocent victim to the silent, insidious, relentless, devastating spirochete of syphilis. When I realized it—too late—death was written in the heart muscles and claimed the young man, trained in one of our best colleges and well fitted for the fight of life. So for 20 years a blood test has been made of every patient entering my office or attended. . . . In these years what a fearful picture has been mine to see; no age, no sex, no condition of life is exempt. The innocence of babyhood, the strength of learned manhood and womanhood have paid, are paying a horrible toll. Crime, economic waste, sickness and insanity are stalking the land, throwing out a challenge to this conference, to every citizen of America, "Why don't we stamp out syphilis?"
>
> With a determination born, not only of knowledge, but of personal injury, I answer the challenge; this conference, all America must answer the challenge.

Dr. Byrd then described how his clinic was started, with the encouragement of the Norfolk City Health Department and the Public Health Service, and continued:

In the last three years our little clinic has taken bloods and physically examined over 15,000 patients and has found about one-third positive. These have been classified and are receiving treatment. The clinic has not received a penny from city or other sources, except services of W.P.A. social workers, through whom follow-up has been done.

Physicians and others most generously have given their services. The small charge of 25 cents, with no one lacking funds turned away,[3] has helped in the purchase of arsenicals, heavy metals and other drugs. Dark-field equipment has been placed; especial attention also is given to expectant mothers.

The Negro is a firm believer in God. We believe that God is in this work, that he will permit attainment of our object—a nation free from the ravages of this disease.

The white man, let me reiterate it, gave syphilis to the Negro. He controls the purse strings and dominates the medical services which can eradicate it as a public health menace to white and colored alike. Aside from the elemental justice involved, it will be cheaper, easier, safer for the individual and the nation, white citizen and colored citizen together, to institute practical measures for the control of the disease, than for us all to muddle along, as we have in the past, with the dead weight of it upon public tax rolls and constituting an unnecessary stumbling block to our movements for social betterment.

The whole nation owes the negro doctors a debt of gratitude for the enthusiasm and courage with which they take up their share of the load. I hope that the rest of us may measure up as well to our share of the responsibility.

NOTES

1. Surgeon O. C. Wenger of the U.S. Public Health Service, long-time chief of the Federal Venereal Disease Clinic at Hot Springs, Ark.

2. Dr. E. L. Keyes of New York; former President, American Social Hygiene Association.

3. Others have told me how Dr. Byrd at each clinic session moves about from one to another of those applying for treatment; his pockets full of quarters, giving one to each patient who really did not have the money, in order that all may be treated.

SOURCES

Taliaferro Clark, M.D., "The Control of Syphilis in Southern Rural Areas," Julius Rosenwald Fund, Chicago, 1932; Prof. Charles S. Johnson, Shadow of the Plantation, University of Chicago Press, Chicago, 1934; K. F. Maxey, M.D., & W. A. Brumfield, M.D., "A Serological Survey for Syphilis in a Negro Population," So. Medical Journal, 1934; P. S. Carley & O. C. Wenger, "The Prevalence of Syphilis in Apparently Healthy Negroes in Miss.," Journal of the A.M.A., 1930; D. G. Gill, "Syphilis in the Rural Negro," Southern Med. Journal, 1932; O. C. Wenger, The Pitt Co., N.C., Demonstration—Venereal Disease Information, 1932; J. A. Crabtree & E. L. Bishop, "Syphilis in a Rural Negro Population in Tenn.," Am. Jour. of Public Health, 1932; G. D. Holloway, W. H. Grant & M. J. Bent, "The Incidence of Syphilis in the Negro as Indicated by Serologic Tests," American Jour. of Syphilis, Gonorrhea & Venereal Disease, 1937.

Documenting the Issues

SELECTED LETTERS BETWEEN THE UNITED STATES PUBLIC HEALTH SERVICE, THE MACON COUNTY HEALTH DEPARTMENT, AND THE TUSKEGEE INSTITUTE, 1932–1972

It is almost impossible to capture what it is like to sit in an archive, whether in Tuskegee, Washington, or Atlanta, and sift through all the extant letters and reports of the Tuskegee Syphilis Study. Even for a seasoned historian, the experience can be overwhelming as the assumptions, beliefs, and convoluted reasoning of those involved in the creation and perpetuation of the study are visible.

Since the contemporary reader begins by knowing what happened in the end in this quintessential American tragedy, the inexorable progress of the study, in its seeming banality and scientific neutrality, is painful to read. For the scientist, researcher, historian, or citizen, these documents are humbling reminders of how much medical research and treatment decisions are inextricably intertwined with assumptions about medical uncertainty, scientific progress, racial and gender stereotypes, and class power.

The thousands of pages of primary documents cannot be reprinted here (but they can be found in the collections cited in the Guide to Further Reading). The selections were made with an eye toward capturing a sense of the range of discussion over the course of the study's history. The sifting was a difficult task and is meant to capture some of the study's unfolding and complexity.

Taliaferro Clark, Assistant Surgeon General, Public Health Service, to Dr. J. N. Baker, State Health Officer, Montgomery, Alabama, August 29, 1932

August 29, 1932
Doctor J. N. Baker
State Health Officer
Montgomery, Alabama

Dear Doctor Baker:
I have for some time wished to talk over with you a piece of research work that might be carried out on syphilitic Negroes in Macon County, the expense of which

is to be borne by the Public Health Service. If you are likely to be in Montgomery about the middle of September I should like to arrange to leave Washington on the afternoon of September 12th en route for Montgomery to talk this matter over with you in person and then proceed to Tuskegee with a view of securing the cooperation of the Andrews Memorial Hospital of Tuskegee Institute.

In working up the data for the final report to the Julius Rosenwald Fund I was particularly impressed with the fact that a negligible number, something less than 35, of the Negroes under treatment in Macon County during the period of the demonstration had ever had any previous treatment. It seems to me that this situation in a very heavily infected population group affords an unparalleled opportunity of studying the effect of untreated syphilis on the human economy. If you think you will be interested in this subject, but nevertheless cannot arrange to be in Montgomery on the date or dates specified above, I shall arrange to visit you on any date that may be mutually satisfactory.

Very sincerely yours,

Taliaferro Clark

Assistant Surgeon General

Division of Venereal Diseases

TC:AMM

United States Public Health Service Division of Venereal Diseases, Record Group 90 (1918–1936), Box 239, Folder 1, Macon County, National Archives.

J. N. Baker to Assistant Surgeon General Taliaferro Clark, September 23, 1932

September 23, 1932

Assistant Surgeon General, Taliaferro Clark

United States Public Health Service

Washington, D.C.

Dear Dr. Clark:

In accordance with our previously discussed plans, Dr. Gill met with the Macon County Board of Health this morning. At this meeting he presented the proposed study in Macon County and asked for their approval. The Board was quite enthusiastic about the previous project, and was quite willing for this new undertaking to proceed along the suggested lines. Accordingly, they passed a motion approving the project, but with the distinct understanding that treatment be provided for these people. The Board approved the idea of internes from Tuskegee Institute giving this treatment under the general supervision of Dr. Smith, County Health Officer.

The County Board of Health speaks for the organized medical profession in

Macon County, so with their endorsement it is now possible to proceed with your further plans.

Kindest personal regards, I am

Very sincerely yours,

J. N. Baker, M.D.

State Health Officer

United States Public Health Service Division of Venereal Diseases, Record Group 90 (1918–1936), Box 239, Folder 1, Macon County, National Archives.

Eugene H. Dibble, Jr., Medical Director, Tuskegee Institute, to Dr. R. R. Moton, Principal, Tuskegee Institute, September 17, 1932

September 17, 1932

Dr. R. R. Moton, Principal

Tuskegee Inst., Alabama

My dear Dr. Moton:

Dr. Taliaferro Clark, Assistant Surgeon General, Division of Venereal Diseases, U.S. Public Health Service came to Tuskegee last Tuesday evening and remained over until Wednesday night. He tried to wait until you returned to the Institute, but he had to catch a train out of Montgomery, so I took him to Montgomery about seven o'clock Wednesday evening.

He was very sorry that he was not able to have a conference with you, and asked me to express to you his very best regards and in the meantime to take up with you his mission to Tuskegee.

The U.S. Public Health Service in connection with the Julius Rosenwald Fund and the Alabama State Board of Health conducted in Macon county a survey of the syphilis problem together with its treatment.

This experiment was very successful but was discontinued due to the lack of funds. The U.S. Public Health Service however, is very anxious to extend its research further into this problem, so that they can find out just what effect syphilis is having on people who have been untreated over a period of years. As you know, there are hundreds of people in this section who probably have certain forms of syphilis and have never had any treatment whatever. This would occur of course, in people from 25 to 70 years of age.

The cost of the treatment of this disease is very high, so that it would be of world wide significance to have this study made. The study, of course would have a special attention paid to the effects of this disease on the cardiovascular system and the nervous system.

It is the desire of Surgeon General Cummings and Dr. Clark that this study should be made at our Hospital. There would be no cost, as I understand it from

Dr. Clark, to the Institute. This would necessitate of-course, the use of the facilities of the hospital including the use of a section of the clinical building, the use of the minor operating room for the taking of blood wassermans and spinal fluids.

They would furnish the necessary dressings, cotton, X-Ray films and the Neo-Salvarsan for any treatment given. In a conference with Dr. Ward at the U.S. Veterans Hospital, he has consented with the approval of the Veterans Bureau, for the use of the electro-cardiograph for the taking of heart tracings.

The personnel would be supplied from the Public Health Service, and paid from that service also. This would include one of the Specialists in the Venereal Disease Control Work who would be detailed to Tuskegee for the purpose of directing this course. In addition, Dr. Clark has authorized me, if the thing goes thru' to appoint one of our own nurses to assist in carrying on this work. The salary of the nurse would be approximately $1200.00 per year, plus $50.00 per month for the maintainence of her car.

In thinking over this and especially in connection with the Alabama State Board of Health, we feel that we could give Miss Eunice Rivers leave from her work at the hospital for the purpose of this service. She, as you know has been connected with the State Department for the past ten years, and has personally done more effective Public Health work with that department than any of our group.

Of course, our Internes and Nurses would be greatly benefited by this training. In addition, Dr. Clark has asked that one of our Internes be allowed two after-noons a week to accompany the Nurse during this course, into the country for the further treatment of these cases.

While this would not bring any additional compensation to our hospital, it would certainly not cost us any more and would offer very valuable training for our students as well as for the Internes. As Dr. Clark said, our own hospital and Tuskegee Institute would get credit for this piece of research work. He also predicts that the results of this study will be sought after the world over. Personally, I think we ought to do it and I would be very glad to talk with you personally or to confer with any committee you desire me to meet.

I am quite sure that you will be hearing from Dr. Clark immediately upon his return to Washington further about this. I am taking the liberty to inclose to you a copy of a letter from Dr. Clark to me.

Yours very truly,
Eugene H. Dibble, Jr.
Medical Director
EHD/J
Incl.

R. R. Moton Papers, General Correspondence, Box 180, Folder 1516, Public Health Service, Tuskegee University Archives. Permission granted by Tuskegee University.

H. S. Cumming, Surgeon General, to Dr. R. R. Moton, September 20, 1932

September 20, 1932
Doctor R. R. Moton
Tuskegee Institute
Alabama

Dear Doctor Moton:

I regret your unavoidable absence from Tuskegee that prevented your meeting Assistant Surgeon General Taliaferro Clark at the time of his recent visit to Tuskegee because I wanted him to explain to you at firsthand the proposed study of the effects of untreated syphilis on the human economy with the cooperation of your hospital. It is expected the results of this study may have a marked bearing on the treatment, or conversely the non-necessity for treatment, of cases of latent syphilis. For this reason I shall be grateful if you shall be able to extend the splendid cooperation offered by Doctor Dibble contingent on your approval.

The recent syphilis control demonstration carried out in Macon County, with the financial assistance of the Julius Rosenwald Fund, revealed the presence of an unusually high prevalence rate in this county and, what is still more remarkable, the fact that approximately 99 per cent of this population group was entirely without previous treatment. This combination, together with the expected cooperation of your hospital, offers an unparalleled opportunity for carrying on this piece of scientific research which probably cannot be duplicated anywhere else in the world.

No doubt Doctor Dibble has explained our plan of procedure to you that contemplates, among other things, an intensive physical and serological examination of untreated cases having positive Wassermann, which may not be carried out in the necessary scientific detail except in a hospital. You can readily see, therefore, that the success of this important study really hinges on your cooperation.

Sincerely,
H. S. Cumming
Surgeon General
TC:AMM

R. R. Moton Papers, General Correspondence, Box 180, Folder 1516 Public Health Service, Tuskegee University Archives. Permission granted by Tuskegee University.

**Joseph Earle Moore, M.D., Johns Hopkins University Medical School,
to Dr. Taliaferro Clark, Assistant Surgeon General, September 28, 1932**

Sept. 28, 1932
Doctor Taliaferro Clark, Assistant Surgeon General
United States Public Health Service
Washington, D.C.

Dear Doctor Clark:

I have given considerable thought to the problem which you raise of the investigation of the course of untreated syphilitic infection in the negroes of Macon County, Alabama. You state that there are in this county about 8000 negroes in a rural area far removed from medical care, and that Wassermann surveys have shown about half the adult population to be infected with syphilis. In order to study the effects of treated syphilitic infection with any accuracy, it would be necessary, it seems to me, to survey the entire adult male population of the county without reference to whether or not their blood Wassermanns were positive or negative. This inclusion of all males is essential, because of the fact that the spontaneous evolution of untreated syphilis may lead to the spontaneous production of a negative Wassermann reaction in a considerable proportion, perhaps twenty-five per cent, of cases. If you rely on a Wassermann survey only, you will miss this group entirely when, as a matter of fact, they may prove to be the most important group of the lot.

Second, the study should be limited to males since only males as compared with females can usually give a definite history of infection.

Third, it should be limited to males who can give a definite history of infection so that the duration of syphilitic infection can be dated with at least approximate accuracy.

Fourth, it should be limited to males over the age of 30 so as to obtain the clinical material composed of patients who have had syphilis for 10 years or longer.

I visualize the selection of this material somewhat as follows: It may be necessary to do a Wassermann survey on the entire population of the county, men, women and children. At the time this Wassermann survey is made, males over the age of 30 should be carefully questioned for a history of syphilitic infection. A history should be accepted as positive only if it includes a story of the lesions of secondary syphilis following at an appropriate interval after a genital sore. A mere history of a penile sore only would not be adequate, inasmuch as the average negro has had as many penile sores as rabbits have offspring. Furthermore, the patient should be able to date, at least with approximate accuracy, the onset of his syphilitic infection. And finally, there must be a definite history of the absence of antisyphilitic treatment. Patients who have been previously treated should be excluded from the detailed survey. I should imagine that in going over the entire 8000 population you might find perhaps two or three hundred males in whom such an adequate history could be obtained. These patients should be selected for special study and the remainder completely disregarded.

In the patients selected for special study, a complete medical history should be taken and a complete physical examination carried out. The history should lay particular stress on the possible occurrence of bone or cardiovascular symptoms, since involvement of these two systems is especially common in the negro. Under the head of the symptoms of cardiovascular syphilis, each patient should be specifically questioned for the presence of dyspnea on exertion, paroxysmal dyspnea, nocturnal or otherwise, and substernal pain.

From the physical standpoint, particular emphasis should be laid by the examiner on the following features of the examination:

- The pupils
- The fundus of the eye
- Simple hearing tests for air and bone conduction (Watch and tuning fork).
- The reflexes
- Deep pain sense in Achilles' tendons and testes
- Generalized enlargement of the lymph nodes
- Inspection and palpation of all accessible long bones and the skull
- Complete examination of the skin and mucous membranes of the stripped body for lesions or scars (note particularly the palms and soles)
- The presence or absence of retrosternal dulness
- The presence or absence of an accentuated tympanitic, bell-like aortic second sound, especially in patients without hypertension or peripheral arteriosclerosis.
- The presence or absence of visible or palpable pulsation in the episternal notch.
- The presence or absence of cardiac murmurs, particularly in a systolic murmur in the aortic area or a diastolic murmur down the left sternal border.
- The blood pressure
- Palpation and percussion of the abdomen with particular reference to the size of the liver
- Inspection of the genitalia for scar and palpation of the scrotal contents.

In addition to these physical investigations, which should be specifically noted, both in positive and negative form, the following laboratory tests should be carried out:

- Urine
- blood Wassermann

- spinal fluid
- teleroentgenographic and fluoroscopic examination of the chest.

It is understood that this very detailed study will be applicable only to a very small group of the inhabitants and that the remainder may be dismissed with a Wassermann survey and subsequent anti-syphilitic treatment when the Wassermann is found to be positive. It is also understood that where such outspoken lesions as tabes, paresis, aortic insufficiency, aortic aneurysm, etc., exist, it will not be necessary to provide the details of all of the physical findings suggested above. Positive or negative statements as to such a minute examination are intended to pick up particularly those patients with minor abnormalities in the central nervous system and those with syphilitic aortitis uncomplicated by aortic regurgitation or aneurysm.

I think that such a study as you have contemplated would be of immense value. It will be necessary of course in a consideration of results to evaluate the special factors introduced by a selection of the material from negro males. Syphilis in the negro is in many respects almost a different disease from syphilis in the white.

If I or any of the members of my staff can be of any further service to you with reference to this proposed investigation, I should be only too glad to have you call upon me, either for advice or for more concrete assistance.

Respectfully yours,

JEM:G

United States Public Health Service Division of Venereal Diseases, Record Group 90 (1918–1936), Box 239, Folder 1, Macon County, National Archives.

R. A. Vonderlehr, Passed Assistant Surgeon, Public Health Service, to Assistant Surgeon General Taliaferro Clark, January 22, 1933

Tuskegee, Jan. 22, 1933

Dear Dr. Clark:

For some time I have been planning to take up with you the matter of supply of anti-syphilitic drugs and the present scarcity of mercury forces the problem rather acutely upon us. We have received none of the oleate of mercury as yet but I believe that this shipment will be somewhat inadequate except for immediate demands. A recent inventory of our neoarsphenamine shows that this supply also is rapidly becoming exhausted.

The need for the strictest economy in this project is and has been fully appreciated from its inception, but, as you know, unusual and unexpected conditions have complicated the problem and made it much more expensive than originally anticipated. The positive Wassermann prevalence is perhaps the most outstanding example but the number of individuals receiving previous treatment is higher than we believed it to be.

At the present time it is probably that the number of patients under antisyphilitic treatment approximates 500. I have completed about 1175 physical examinations on negro men in the desired group, and experience has taught us that these men constitute about 33.3% of the syphilitic individuals uncovered. I do not believe that the number of negroes under treatment will go much above the present peak but if we are to continue the study the number will remain at about that figure. The completion of the course of arsenic will automatically eliminate large numbers of patients each month, equalizing the new numbers acquired. It is desirable and essential if the study is to be a success to maintain the interest of each of the cases examined by me through to the time when the spinal puncture can be completed. Expenditure of several hundred dollars for drugs for these men would be well worth the while if their interest and cooperation could be maintained in so doing. Our serious mistake made in the beginning was that patients receiving neo-arsphenamine were given heavy metal treatment concomitantly instead of following the course of arsenic with mercury treatment and prolonging the therapeutic period without any additional cost. I only learned of this concomitant treatment a few days ago from Dr. Smith and have given him strict instructions to give treatment with both drugs simultaneously in the early communicable cases of syphilis only. This will lengthen the treatment period in late syphilis 50% without extra cost and decrease the probability of injury to vital organs already discussed. We are also cutting the dose of neoarsphenamine in all late cases of syphilis from 0.6 grams to 0.4 grams, any action which I feel will not be detrimental to the welfare of those under treatment. It would be a great economic aid if the number of women applying for treatment could be decreased and Smith and myself have under consideration various methods to accomplish this end without injury to the project. We are at present endeavoring to bring in the husbands of the infected women, and already show special consideration to such female patients. Any drastic attempt to separate the sexes would be productive of more harm than good as I informed you in my December report.

I should like to give you some idea of the amount of antisyphilitic drugs which we will need if 400 cases are to be examined. I previously estimated that it would take until March 15th to complete 300 examinations, and, if the tilling of the soil does not offer too many difficulties, we should finish the 400 by May 1st. The spinal punctures should be carried out in one month and treatment could be stopped about June 1st. This gives us a period of four months—about 18 weeks—during which we must treat an average of 500 patients once a week. We shall, therefore, need for the 300 patients on mercury about 75,000 doses (300 patients X 18 weeks X 14 doses per week for mercury administered per [unclear]=75,600 doses). If mercury inunctions are given in the oleate, a ¼ lb. jar lasts a pt. with a belt one month, and one would need approximately 300 lbs. of oleate of mercury in ¼ lb. (300 patients X 4 months=1200 one fourth pound jars). Two hundred of the weekly patients receive neoarsphenamine, and without committing myself as to the amount of treatment we would administer I have the promise of Dr. Gill, after a visit to Montgomery yesterday, for a supply of neoarsphenamine sufficient to treat 100 cases weekly. We have at present 300 grams of the first arsenic sent or enough with Dr. Gills supply to last six weeks to carry on treatment until June first—12 additional weeks—we shall need 50 grams per week or 600 more grams. Recapitulating then we shall need the following drugs to carry the study to completion on approximately June 1st:

600 grams neoarsphenamine

150—3.0 gram ampules

150—0.6   "   "

75000 pill of protiodide of mercury *or* 300 lbs. oleate of mercury in ¼ lb. jars.

I realize that this request is very much greater than we originally thought it would be, but am certain that our experiment cannot be carried out without treatment. If we are to retain the services of Dr. Smith after Jan. 31st the question of the administration of these drugs is settled, and without Smith or someone of his ability we could not carry on. In making the request for these drugs I believe that the added expense is justifiable for the great amount of good, which they will do per se to the negroes of the county, irrespective of the effect their administration will have on the study of untreated syphilis.

Sincerely yours,

R. A. Vonderlehr

P.A. Surgeon

United States Public Health Service Division of Venereal Diseases, Record Group 90 (1918–1936), Box 239, Folder 2, Macon County, National Archives.

R. A. Vonderlehr to Dr. Clark, April 8, 1933

Tuskegee, Ala, April 8, 1933

Dear Doctor Clark:

For some I have been thinking of an aspect of the study of untreated syphilis being conducted here, which may not have occurred to you. I do not submit this idea with the desire that it even be considered a suggestion but rather that you keep it [in] mind until I return to my work in Washington.

At the end of this project we shall have a considerable number of cases presenting various complications of syphilis who have received only mercury and may still be considered untreated in the modern sense of therapy. Should these cases be followed over a period of from five to ten years many interesting facts could be learned regarding the course of complications [of] untreated syphilis. The longevity of these syphilitics could be ascertained, and if properly administered I believe that many necropsies could be arranged through the hospital at the Institute with the cooperation of the National Institute of Health. A part time social worker should be able to see the cases as often as necessary and the whole scheme could be supervised by one of our officers occasionally. Undoubtedly other interesting points for study could be worked out should this follow-up work be considered seriously. I realize, of course, the difficulties in the way of the projection of such a plan in view of the unsettled conditions and the urgent need for economy. However, it seems a pity to me to lose such an unusual opportunity.

Sincerely yours,

R. A. Vonderlehr

P.A. Surgeon

United States Public Health Service Division of Venereal Diseases, Record Group 90 (1918–1936), Box 239, Folder 2, Macon County, National Archives.

R. A. Vonderlehr to Surgeon O. C. Wenger, July 18, 1933

July 18, 1933

PERSONAL AND CONFIDENTIAL

Dear Doc:

During the past 6 weeks I have been busily engaged in reviewing the literature in connection with our recent study of untreated syphilis in Alabama. I have also discussed the matter with a number of the officers here in Washington and everyone is agreed that the proper procedure is the continuance of the observation of the Negro men used in the study with the idea of eventually bringing them to autopsy. I realize that this may be impracticable in connection with some of the younger cases, but those more advanced in age with serious complications of the vital organs should have to be followed for only a period of a few years.

Some time ago I submitted a memorandum to the Surgeon General outlining the activities in which I believed the Division should take part and one of these activities was the continued observation of our untreated syphilis cases. I have reason to believe that this program will be approved by the Surgeon General. I am taking this matter up with you primarily to ascertain whether or not you have any member of your staff whose services could be dispensed with without serious harm to the work at Hot Springs. Here in Washington the Division has lost (including Doctor Clark) 3 of the 15 former members of the personnel and there is also a possibility that 2 of our statistical workers, whose salaries are at present being paid by a philanthropic organization, may be discontinued on January first. While it might be possible to drop one of the clerks in the statistical section, this work would be greatly handicapped if we lost the support of the philanthropic organization.

Briefly my plan in Tuskegee is to obtain the cooperation of the state and local health departments and, most important of all, the Tuskegee Institute Hospital. Doctor Dibble would probably accept the appointment of Acting Assistant Surgeon and act in an advisory capacity as far as the nurse was concerned. As you know, the nurse I plan to use was the previous one employed during the untreated syphilis project last winter, and I feel that we could employ her on a two-thirds time basis, having her furnish transportation, for $1,000 a year. I believe that $200 per month additional would furnish incidental needs, such as small amounts of medicines, et cetera.

I would like for you to give this matter your careful attention and let me hear from you in the next few days.

Doctor Pierce has promised to detail an Assistant Surgeon in the regular corps to Hot Springs for a period of 8 months in order to familiarize him with work in the venereal diseases. It is my aim, if possible, to keep a young Service officer at all times stationed with you.

With best wishes from all in Washington,

Sincerely yours,

(Sgd) R. A. Vonderlehr

R. A. Vonderlehr

Passed Assistant Surgeon

RAV:AMM

Surgeon O. C. Wenger
U.S. Public Health Service
Hot Springs, Arkansas

United States Public Health Service Division of Venereal Diseases, Record Group 90 (1918–1936), Box 239, Folder 2, Macon County, National Archives.

O. C. Wenger to R. A. Vonderlehr, July 21, 1933

July 21, 1933
Personal and Confidential

Dear Von:

In reply to your personal letter of the 18th., let me explain the duties of our staff so you will understand how understaffed we are.

My own time is taken up as the executive officer and filling in where ever needed [Letter continues to list the staff and their duties at the Public Health Service Venereal Disease Clinic in Hot Springs, Arkansas]

You can readily see that we are understaffed. Further more, none of the staff, with the exception of myself, has had any experience in the field. We certainly could not spare any of the doctors for the work in Macon County and no other member of the staff, even if available could handle this field work.

I remember we discussed this matter when together in Tuskegee and I agreed with you it would be a good plan. I believed at that time and still do that you can carry out your program without the aid of the nurse at $1,000 per annum. I don't see that she can do anything else than use up gasoline making weekly calls on these patients, which does not seem to me to be necessary.

As I see it, we have no further interest in these patients *until they die* [underlining in the original]. To secure the post-mortems two plans present themselves. When these patients die, some one of the dozen or more physicians in Macon County must sign a death certificate, which goes to the County Health Officer, Doctor Murray Smith. Doctor Smith could then notify Doctor Dibble who could make arrangements for the post-mortem. Or, thru the cooperation of Doctor Dibble, we could arrange with the doctors in Macon County to turn over to Doctor Dibble any of our demonstration cases applying to them for treatment. This would enable Doctor Dibble to keep more complete notes on these cases and in the event of a death he would have more time to persuade the family to have a post-mortem performed. I know the doctors of Macon County well enough to believe they will cooperate.

There is one danger in the latter plan and that is if the colored population becomes aware that accepting free hospital care means a post-mortem, every darkey will leave Macon county and it will hurt Dibble's hospital. This can be prevented, however, if the doctors of Macon County are brought into our confidence and requested to be very careful not to let the objective of the plan be known.

It may be several months or longer before any of these cases need medical attention and I cannot see how the nurse would be profitably employed all of the time. In fact it seems to me that nurse might do more harm than good by making weekly visits to these families in the hope of finding them in extremis and ready for a postmortem. If the nurse continues to call and give these patients medicines, some of the local doctors might object and embarrass the State Board of Health and local health unit.

I am sure that Doctor Dibble will cooperate and that he will accept a position as Acting Assistant Surgeon at $1.00 per annum as you suggest.

Now there is something else. Who will do the post-mortems? Certainly not Dibble or any of his internes because their findings would be of no more scientific value than if you or I did the post-mortem. So why not bring into the picture the pathologist at the U.S. Veterans Bureau Hospital? Then we will have a post-mortem record that is worth while.

summarize:

We have no personnel available at this clinic.

A nurse does not seem necessary to this program.

Doctor Dibble and the Macon County doctors will cooperate.

Patients decease may either be reported thru the County Health Officer when death certificate is filed, or the local physicians may refer patients to Doctor Dibble when they report to him for treatment.

Now let me have your reaction to this. Perhaps you can run to Montgomery and Tuskegee yourself and see Baker, Gill, Dibble and the local men. If you can't go yourself and want me to go down there for a few days I can arrange to do so. I do wish, however, you would go yourself and then come on to Hot Springs for a few days visit.

The best news I have heard is that Doctor Pierce and you are planning on sending a young regular officer here for training.

Best regards to everybody, including Lady Vonderlehr.

Sincerely,

O. D. Wenger, Surgeon

Acting Medical Officer in Charge

ow/cr

Centers for Disease Control Papers, Tuskegee Syphilis Study Administrative Records, 1930–80, Box 5, Folder Correspondence, National Archives–Southeast Region, East Point, Georgia.

R. A. Vonderlehr to Dr. H. T. Jones, Tallassee, Alabama, November 20, 1933

November 20, 1933
Doctor H. T. Jones
Tallassee, Alabama

Dear Doctor Jones:

A week or two ago I paid a visit to Tallassee for the purpose of contacting you in connection with the study of untreated syphilis in the Negro, which the Public Health Service is conducting in Macon County with the cooperation of the Alabama State Health Department, the Macon County Health Unit, and the Tuskegee Institute. About 400 cases of syphilis in Negro males 25 years of age and over have been found and subjected to thorough clinical and roentgenological examinations. Preliminary analysis of the records of this group shows that cardiovascular disease is extremely frequent although it is impossible to say just how much syphilis is responsible for the cardiovascular disease. Hypertension and arteriosclerosis were frequent complications and a control group of 200 Negroes is now being examined with the idea of noting the prevalence of arteriosclerosis and hypertension in this nonsyphilitic group.

This study should give valuable information to the scientific world in indicating the efficacy of present-day antisyphilitic treatment. The Public Health Service already has on hand records of a fairly large number of Negroes who have been both adequately and inadequately treated for syphilis and it is our desire to use the untreated group now being examined in Macon County as a comparison to indicate the value of treatment.

In order that the observation of this untreated group may be completed, it has been decided to attempt to follow the clinical course in the 600 syphilitic and nonsyphilitic Negroes and in case of death attempt to obtain a necropsy. Arrangements for the necropsy have been made with the Tuskegee Institute but if the attempt is to be most successful it is believed that it will be necessary to hospitalize those cases in the event of a terminal illness. The Tuskegee Institute has agreed to furnish free hospitalization to each one of these patients should he become seriously ill, and your cooperation is sought in reporting the serious illness of any one of these Negroes who may consult you. This can probably be best worked out if you will ask Negroes past the age of 25, in the neighborhood of Realtown on the Macon-Tallapoosa County border who consult you for a serious illness, whether they were examined for bad blood by the "Government doctor" at Tuskegee Institute. Your alertness in detecting these cases and immediately notifying Doctor Eugene H. Dibble, Jr., Tuskegee Institute, Alabama, will do much to make this study a success. It is doubtful whether a great deal can be accomplished without your cooperation.

By direction of the Surgeon General:

Respectfully,

(Sgd) R. A. Vonderlehr

R. A. Vonderlehr

Passed Assistant Surgeon for Division of Venereal Diseases

RAV:AMM

United States Public Health Service Division of Venereal Diseases, Record Group 90 (1918–1936), Box 239, Folder 3, Macon County, National Archives.

Patient X, Auburn, Alabama, to The Public Health Service, June 4, 1934

Auburn, Ala
June 4, 1934
The Public Health Service

Dear Sirs your answer to my letter of May 12 Stating that you would try to arrange to have Doctor Dibble of the John A hospital to give my wife some treatment it was suggested that I take her to Doctor Dibble in the near future that he would tell me whether he would be able to treat her or not so I have been to see him and he said that he could and would Just as soon as you sent the Medicines and was to let me know as soon as he got it but have fail to here from him so if you have not sent it please send it because my wife is haves a lot of trouble with blood. [I told] Doctor Dibble said they come [here] that bad blood Please let me hear from you but at once and if you all send the medicines tell Doctor Dibble to notify me my wife is [blanked out in original]

Your

[subject name blanked out in original]

United States Public Health Service Division of Venereal Diseases, Record Group 90 (1918–1936), Box 239, Folder 3, Macon County, National Archives.

R. A. Vonderlehr to Patient X, June 7, 1934

June 7, 1934
R.F.D. 2, Box 76
Auburn, Alabama

Dear Rubin:

Your letter of June 4, making further request that treatment be given your wife, has been received. The medicine which Doctor Dibble required for the treatment of your wife's bad blood has been furnished him and if you will take her to John A. Andrew Hospital I am sure treatment will be started immediately. On the day that you take her go in the morning and tell her not to eat any breakfast before she leaves home.

It has been possible for the Public Health Service to give your wife this treatment because we are cooperating with the Tuskegee Institute and the Macon County Board of Health.

Very truly yours,

(Sgd) R. A. Vonderlehr

R. A. Vonderlehr

Passed Assistant Surgeon

Division of Venereal Diseases

RAV:KNV

United States Public Health Service Division of Venereal Diseases, Record Group 90 (1918–1936), Box 239, Folder 3, Macon County, National Archives.

Austin V. Deibert, Passed Assistant Surgeon, to Dr. R. A. Vonderlehr, November 26, 1938

Nov. 28, 1938
Doctor R. A. Vonderlehr
Assistant Surgeon General
Division Venereal Disease
United States Public Health Service
Washington, D.C.

Dear Doctor Vonderlehr:

In the two months which have passed since I began the resurvey of our un-treated syphilis study, I noticed the increasing incidence of cases who received some arsenical therapy on their admission to the study. Recently I analyzed statistically from the files that I have here, and according to age groups, the amount of treatment they received. I was quite amazed to discover that fully 40% of the group had received some treatment, even though inadequate. The grouping is as follows:

AGE	NUMBER OF INJECTIONS	
	1–5	6–9
25–29	28	51
30–34	16	19
35–39	9	15
40 plus	6	19
	59	104
		59
		163 TOTAL

I understand that our study is, in spirit, an introspective one in contradistinction to the retrospective study of Bruusgaard. I firmly believe that we cannot obtain a true reflection of the course of untreated syphilis in view of 40% of the cases having had some treatment.

I have made no attempt to divide the 163 cases into early and late syphilis as inadequate treatment reacts in various ways. Apparently in early syphilis a few injections of an arsenical suffices to greatly lower, if not prevent, late syphilitic cardiovascular disease. Again, inadequate treatment in early syphilis greatly increases the incidence of neurorecurrence and other forms of relapse. The effect of inadequate treatment on late syphilis is problematical. In view of the foregoing statements I acutely fear that adverse criticism of the study would be justifiable, viewing it as an "untreated group."

With your approval, and if reasonably statistically sound, I would like very much to supplement the present study with the following plan, believing that it would not cause an appreciable increase in expenditure of time or money: 1) Maintain the syphilitic cases who have received some treatment as a study group of inadequately treated cases and on whom subsequent periodic observations can be made. 2) Replace these cases with strictly new untreated men of comparable ages and infection dates.

I am assured here that little trouble would be encountered in finding suitable cases as numbers have stated they would like very much to get on the "government list," and Dr. Smith advises that I could, with comparative ease, locate many cases in his files with positive blood tests who have never received any therapy.

Hoping that such a plan as this will meet with your approval, I am,

Sincerely yours,

Austin V. Deibert

Passed Assistant Surgeon

Tuskegee, Ala.

Centers for Disease Control Papers, Tuskegee Syphilis Study Administrative Records, 1930–80, Box 7, Folder 1938, National Archives–Southeast Region, East Point, Georgia.

R. A. Vonderlehr to Austin V. Deibert, December 5, 1938

December 5, 1938

P.A. Surgeon Austin V. Deibert

U.S. Public Health Service

c/o County Health Department

Tuskegee, Alabama

Dear Doctor Deibert:

Your letter of November 28th has been received and I am sorry that you were surprised to learn that a considerable group of the individuals included in the untreated syphilis study in Macon County had actually received treatment. I had the impression that we had discussed this matter with you before you went to Alabama. The reason treatment was given to many of these individuals was two-fold: First, when the study was started in the fall of 1932, no plans had been made for its continuation and a few patients were treated before we fully realized the need for continuing the project on a permanent basis. Second, it was difficult to hold the interest of the group of Negroes in Macon County unless some treatment was given. This was particularly true in the patients with early syphilis. In consequence, we treated practically all of the patients with early manifestations and many of the patients with latent syphilis.

I have discussed with Miss Usilton your plans for examining additional Negro males in the proper age groups to replace those who were previously treated. If you can find the Negro males in these age groups who have been untreated without a great deal of additional work, I see no reason why they should not be carefully examined. It is desirable to increase the number of individuals included in this study because the number is already small for the purpose of statistical analysis.

If it is not possible to add to the number of untreated syphilitic Negro males included in the study, it will, of course, be necessary to exclude all of those who were treated some years ago in the future. I doubt the wisdom of bothering to examine the treated individuals carefully because we already have in the clinics of the Cooperative Clinical Group a considerable number of Negro males in the proper age groups who have received inadequate treatment and who are under observation.

Sincerely yours,

(Sgd) R. A. Vonderlehr

R. A. Vonderlehr

Assistant Surgeon General

Division of Venereal Diseases

RAV:MCK

Centers for Disease Control Papers, Tuskegee Syphilis Study Administrative Records, 1930–80, Box 7, Folder 1938, National Archives–Southeast Region, East Point, Georgia.

Austin V. Deibert to R. A. Vonderlehr, March 20, 1939

March 20, 1939

Asst. Surgeon General R. A. Vonderlehr

Division of Venereal Disease

U.S. Public Health Service

Washington, D.C.

Dear Doctor Vonderlehr:

I was very much disappointed that your trip South was cancelled but realize how necessary was your presence in Washington at that time.

My chief reason for wanting to talk to you was regarding spinal punctures on the group. I know now that if I had not deferred obtaining spinal taps, we wouldn't have examined half the cases we have to date. They simply do not like spinal punctures. A few of those who were tapped are enthusiastic over the results but to most, the suggestion of another causes violent shaking of the head; others claim they were robbed of their procreative powers (regardless of the fact that I claim it stimulates them); some experienced memorable headaches. All in all and with no attempt at humor, it is a headache to me.

As a consequence of those primary taps, Nurse Rivers has had some difficulty getting patients in when breaking into a new community. After the word passes along sufficiently that we are not giving "back shots" they come out of the cane-brakes. I hope I know something of the psychology of the negro but at any rate I try my best to send them forth happily shouting the praises of the clinic to their friends at home.

If we repuncture, or try to, I gravely fear that they will not be persuaded to come in a third time and the study would collapse. Those cases who have not had punctures and those whose fluids were positive, I think should be punctured.

I don't believe that any information relative to neurosyphilis on this group would be of much value as it would be open to criticism in that malaria is so wide-spread here. Doctor Smith tells me a survey here last year of 1,600 people revealed the presence of parasites in 20%. No one can say how many have had or will be in-fected with malaria before the study is over. Malaria probably is the best treatment for neurosyphilis and nearly every patient I have seen so far gives a good history of having had it. So far in the study I have found only a few neurosyphilitics and they were vascular affairs and optic atrophies with not a case of tabes or paresis.

With the exception of new patients, those old ones who have not been punc-tured and in cases who had positive fluids, I personally feel that repuncture is inadvisable. The danger of jeopardizing the future of the study by lack of coopera-tion of the patients far outweighs the importance of obtaining information about the spinal fluid, which information at best would be open to adverse criticism. I would like very much to have your reaction to this.

Sincerely yours,
Austin V. Deibert
P.A. Surgeon
Tuskegee, Ala.

Centers for Disease Control Papers, Tuskegee Syphilis Study Administrative Records, 1930–80, Box 7, Folder 1939, National Archives–Southeast Region, East Point, Georgia.

R. A. Vonderlehr to Special Consultant C. A. Walwyn, John Andrew Memorial Hospital, June 13, 1939

June 13, 1939
Special Consultant C. A. Walwyn
U.S. Public Health Service
c/o John Andrew Memorial Hospital
Tuskegee, Alabama

Dear Doctor Walwyn:
Within the next month or two the Public Health Service proposes to make available on loan to the Macon County Health Department a mobile treatment unit for the control of syphilis in this area. If the usefulness of the mobile unit is

demonstrated, it may be extended to include one or two counties adjacent to Macon County.

Some time ago Doctor J. N. Baker requested that Nurse Eunice Rivers be assigned to duty on this unit, and because I feel that it will facilitate the follow-up of patients included in our study of untreated syphilis, I have recommended to the Surgeon General that this assignment be made. Consequently, official orders have been requested assigning Nurse Rivers to duty with the Macon County Health Department. I trust that this action meets with your approval.

Sincerely yours,

(Sgd) R. A. Vonderlehr

R. A. Vonderlehr

Assistant Surgeon General

Division of Venereal Diseases

RAV:MCK

cc: Dr. Deibert

Centers for Disease Control Papers, Tuskegee Syphilis Study Administrative Records, 1930–80, Box 12, Folder Personnel 1938–39, National Archives–Southeast Region, East Point, Georgia.

Murray Smith, M.D., to R. A. Vonderlehr, November 27, 1941

Tuskegee, Alabama

November 27, 1941

Dr. R. A. Vonderlehr

U.S. Public Health Service

Washington, D.C.

Dear Doctor Vonderlehr:

When it comes time for you to renew the Milbank appropriation for taking care of autopsies in the untreated syphilis study, I wish that you would give some consideration to placing the Fund with the Macon County Health Department instead of the Tuskegee Institute. The officials at Tuskegee Institute are not the same ones that you and I had such fine cooperation with a few years ago. They know nothing about the study, they do nothing for the patients, and for two years autopsies have been done in undertaker parlors. This proved to be more convenient for undertakers, and for us. The Institute will pay no bills that Dr. J. A. Kenny does not approve. Dr. Kenney knows nothing of what is going on, is always hard to find and is out of town a good deal of the time.

If you will allow us to disburse the fees, it will give us a closer tie-in with the families and undertakers, whereas at present, they feel that Tuskegee Institute is giving them this help. They have lost sight of the fact that the Health Department is still doing its part in keeping the study going along according to plans.

Please advise me of your reaction to this proposition. Its sole aim is to place the Health Department more in the "spot light" than Tuskegee Institute.

Sincerely yours,

Murray Smith, M.D.

Special Expert, V.D.

Tuskegee Syphilis Study, HEW Report Documents, Bound Book II, Tuskegee University Archives.

D. G. Gill, Bureau of Preventable Diseases, Department of Public Health, State of Alabama, to R. A. Vonderlehr, July 3, 1942

July 3, 1942

Dr. R. A. Vonderlehr

Assistant Surgeon General

U.S. Public Health Service

Washington, D.C.

Dear Doctor Vonderlehr:

Dr. Murray Smith has called my attention to the fact that in our program of getting all selectees who are rejected for syphilis under treatment we are encroaching on some of your study material. Apparently a few of the untreated cases of syphilis have been called for army duty and rejected on account of a positive blood. In conjunction with the draft boards we are insisting on all these men taking treatment. I am wondering if we should make an exception of these few individuals. There should not be many of them involved since most of your group are beyond draft age by this time. I would appreciate your advice on this matter.

Very sincerely yours,

D. G. Gill, M.D., Director

Bureau of Preventable Diseases

DGG/h

Tuskegee Syphilis Study, HEW Report Documents, Bound Book II, Tuskegee University Archives.

Vonderlehr to Gill, July 10, 1942

Bethesda Station

July 10, 1942

Dr. D. G. Gill

Director

Bureau of Preventable Diseases

Department of Public Health

Montgomery, Alabama

Dear Doctor Gill:

Receipt is acknowledged of your letter of July 3rd regarding the treatment of some of the men included in the study of untreated syphilis in Macon County under the provisions which have been set up for the treatment of selectees in connection with the current mobilization program.

Some time ago Doctor Murray Smith wrote to me about this matter. I suggested to him that he confer with the chairman of the local Selective Service Board, Mr. J. F. Segrest, and explain to him that this study of untreated syphilis is of great importance from a scientific standpoint. It represents one of the last opportunities which the science of medicine will have to conduct an investigation of this kind.

Doctor Smith replied that he had furnished the local board a list containing 256 names of men under 45 years of age and asked that these men be excluded from the list of draftees needing treatment. During his conference with the board they agreed to this arrangement in order to make it possible to continue this study on an effective basis.

Sincerely yours,

(Sgd.) R. A. Vonderlehr

R. A. Vonderlehr

Assistant Surgeon General

Division of Venereal Diseases

RAV:LR

Tuskegee Syphilis Study, HEW Report Documents, Bound Book II, Tuskegee University Archives.

Murray Smith to R. A. Vonderlehr, August 6, 1942

Tuskegee, Alabama

August 6, 1942

Dr. R. A. Vonderlehr

U.S. Public Health Service

Washington, D.C.

Dear Doctor Vonderlehr:

A new situation has arisen with reference to the untreated syphilis study patients. Some of the Control cases who have developed syphilis, are getting notices from the draft boards to take treatment. So far, we are keeping the known positive patients from getting treatment. Is a control case of any value to the study, if he has contracted syphilis? Shall we withhold treatment from a control case who has developed syphilis? Please let me have your wishes with reference to handling this type patient and I shall carry them out as best I can.

Sincerely yours,

Murray Smith, M.D.

Special Expert, V.D.

MS/S

Tuskegee Syphilis Study, HEW Report Documents, Bound Book II, Tuskegee University Archives.

R. A. Vonderlehr to Dr. Murray Smith, August 11, 1942

Bethesda Station

August 11, 1942

Dr. Murray Smith

Macon County Health Dept.

Tuskegee, Alabama

Dear Doctor Smith:

Replying to your letter of August 6th, it seems to me that the non-syphilitic control cases in the study of untreated syphilis in the Negro who have acquired syphilis since the time the study began have lost their value to the study.

There is no reason why these patients should not be given appropriate treatment unless you hear from Doctor Austin V. Deibert who is in direct charge of this study and who may foresee some objection with which I am not familiar.

Sincerely yours,

(Sgd) R. A. Vonderlehr

R. A. Vonderlehr

Assistant Surgeon General

Division of Venereal Diseases

RAV:LR

CC: Dr. Deibert

Centers for Disease Control Papers, Tuskegee Syphilis Study Administrative Records, 1930–80, Box 17, Folder Vonderlehr, National Archives–Southeast Region, East Point, Georgia.

Dr. Wenger, "Untreated Syphilis in Negro Male," September 18, 1950

Dr. Wenger

Hot Springs Seminar

In this series of meetings there has been much discussion about finding people with syphilis, how to treat them and how to evaluate the results of that treatment.

This is good and it is proper. But in the few minutes I have, I wish to focus your attention on another aspect of the broad study of syphilis, that of its effect on those you don't find, don't treat and don't follow.

This subject of untreated syphilis is not something new. The study of it was started some twenty years ago and has been plodding quietly along ever since, with parts of the findings coming to print sporadically. I would like briefly to review the matter.

Among the many interests of the late Julius Rosenwald was the health and welfare of the American Negro. From the Fund that now carries his name came money which was used in cooperation with Federal, State and local health departments for a survey of the prevalence of syphilis among negroes. One county in each of six southern states was chosen for study. The highest rate was found in Macon County, Alabama. Not only was the prevalence higher, but it was found that only one out of 25 had received treatment. With this as a start, Drs. Vonderlehr, Heller, Taliaferro Clark, Austen Diebert and myself, along with others, got together to organize a study of the syphilitic process when uninfluenced by treatment and to compare those findings with results after treatment had been given.

We decided to limit the study to negro males 25 years old or more. In the winter months of 1931–32 and 32–33 a group of 399 negro males with untreated syphilis was selected together with a group of 201 negro males who were presumably non-syphilitic to be used as a control. The age distributions in the two groups were comparable.

I won't bother you with minor details of how the study was to operate except to say that all were to have regular blood tests, and physical examinations. In addition it was planned to secure autopsies at death whenever possible. The Milbank Memorial Fund agreed to contribute money for necropsy. Part of the money goes to the physician doing the work and part of it goes to the family to aid in burial expenses.

The first physical examinations were made in 1932–33 with the findings published in September 1936. In 1938–39, a second physical examination was made at which time it was found that a considerable proportion of the younger men had received some but inadequate treatment.

From the second examination came two papers in 1946—one covering mortality, in February and one on cardiovascular abnormalities and other forms of morbidity, in December.

A third physical examination was made in the fall of 1948. In May of this year, 1950, the findings were published, covering abnormalities observed under 16 years.

Now, what have these findings been, in terms of generalities? First, that untreated syphilis apparently shortens the life expectancy by 20 percent. Second, that there is a greater involvement of the cardiovascular system and third, that syphilitics without treatment appear to be subject to a higher rate of other types of morbidity. Thus there are more potentially disabling defects among them and they die earlier. This is probably what most people might expect from general knowledge or assumption, but it is important to have the facts documented.

I heartily support the work that has been done, but it does not go far enough. When the third examinations were done in 1948–49, 26 percent of the syphilitics had been lost from observation and 35 percent of the controls. This is not counting known deaths. One of the reasons for selecting Macon county as a study area, aside from its high prevalence rate, was that it seemed remarkably suitable for the study purposes. It had the broad extremes of development of the Negro race, from those connected with Tuskegee Institute to those with the lowest of living standards. Health facilities ranged from a Veterans hospital to nothing, transportation from 3 railway centers and a main highway to inaccessible winter roads. But most of all, the county's principal industry is agriculture of a type which tends to provide a stable population for a long term study such as this. What became of this third or so that dropped from observation? Were they in the county but just didn't respond to a written notice? Would they have responded if they could read? Did they stay away because they were no longer interested or were they too ill to come in? Perhaps they had moved out of the county. Some have, I am sure. But if they've moved—are they living and well? If they are dead, what was the cause?

These questions are important to the value of the study. There is a nurse in the county whose salary is paid to keep track of these patients but I think more is necessary. Remember, these patients wherever they are, received no treatment on our recommendation. We know now, where we could only surmise before, that we have contributed to their ailments and shortened their lives. I think the least we can say is that we have a high moral obligation to those that have died to make this the best study possible.

This is the last chance in our country to make an investigation of this sort. You may say, if that's so isn't the point rather academic. I don't think so. It may be academic so far as the patient who is treated, but you know even better than I, that you are not yet finding and treating all of the cases. Your casefinding publicity makes a point for the public to "Know for Sure" whether the disease has been contracted. I say it behooves the medical profession to "Know for Sure" what happens if the disease is not treated.

I urge in the strongest possible way that the Public Health Service place a full time male investigator in Macon county whose sole job is to locate those persons who were first selected and examined. Sure, they may have moved, perhaps moved and died, but arrangements can be made for them to be examined wherever they may be, if living. If they've died, let's trace them through vital statistics to see when, where and why. And if humanly possible, arrange for autopsy of those who die in the future.

This matter of autopsies is of tremendous importance. There are, as you know, only two other studies that even remotely resemble this—the one started by Bruusgaard in Norway and the study of Rosahn at Yale. So far, of the 1/3 deaths recorded for the Alabama group 67 percent have come to autopsy. The correlation of postmortem findings with periodic clinical findings can be done only in the Alabama group. What other way will we ever be able to learn the meaning of our clinical findings?

Once again let me emphasize the importance of this quiet undertaking and urge that steps be taken so that it doesn't slip through our fingers.

9-18-50
KHJ/mrb

Tuskegee Syphilis Study, HEW Report Documents, Bound Book II, Tuskegee University Archives.

Sidney Olansky, Sr. Surgeon, Public Health Service, Venereal Disease Research Laboratory, Chamblee, Georgia, to Dr. John C. Cutler, Washington, D.C., November 6, 1951

November 6, 1951
Chief, Division of Venereal Disease
U.S. Public Health Service
Federal Security Building (South)
Washington 25, D.C.

Attn: Dr. John C. Cutler

Dear John:

I received your letter of October 22, 1951. Stanley and I have both studied and discussed your outline. We agree wholeheartedly with your premises for the validity of the study, your arguments for the importance of this follow-up, and your recommendations for the clinical examination.

Enclosed is our outline of the Tuskegee project which you have requested, in as much detail as possible at this time. Much of this will merely be repetition of what Dr. Bauer has already received in our progress reports. (Reference is made to letters dated September 24, 1951 and October 18, 1951, especially.)

Please pardon the length of the outline. Some of the details may be more useful than superfluous to any future investigators on this project.

Yours sincerely,
SIDNEY OLANSKY
Sr. Surgeon, USPHS
Director
Encl.—1
CC: Dr. Bauer

Outline of Problems to Be Considered in Tuskegee Study

A. Even though there is real and reasonable doubt as to the original diagnosis of many of the patients, it seems to me that it may be necessary to consider the diagnosis as probably correct and to work on. While malaria may have played a role in false positivity and while other factors may have been operative, the same factor was working in all groups of patients considered—untreated, treated, and controls. Furthermore, the lower level of sensitivity of tests of those days gives good reason to assume that the level of false reactivity was lower than would be expected today.

The very large differences in morbidity of syphilitic and control groups suggests a real difference in the two "universes" with possible economic and social differences which, however, cannot be resolved now.

So regardless of our present feeling, I feel that we must utilize the material available with knowledge that the diagnoses were made by very competent syphilologists, utilizing the best information available at the time.

B. Assuming the diagnostic validity of the material, it is felt advisable to get all the information possible from the material. We have an investment of almost 20 years of Division interest, funds, and personnel; a responsibility to the survivors both for their care and really to prove that their willingness to serve, even at risk of shortening of life, as experimental subjects. And finally, a responsibility to add what further we can to the natural history of syphilis.

Out of what we have, the following avenues of exploration remain:

1. It is assumed that complete studies will be done, i.e., physical and history, with attention to intercurrent illness, administration of penicillin, etc. In other words, a medical school type work-up.

2. When the follow-up worker is assigned, one of the first bits of information obtained may be further study of the progression in the observed and non-observed groups. Compare with Iskrant hypothesis that both are same.

Knowing the type of cardiovascular studies done earlier, it is felt that the same techniques of measurements, etc. should be repeated to observe changes. For the cardiovascular work-up, it is felt that the services of a cardiologist should be secured and that full advantage should be taken of the technical diagnostic measures.

Careful studies of spinal fluid and neuromuscular system are advised. For this the type of work-up to fill the new CNS evaluation forms are recommended so as to get material comparable with that from the research participants.

From this type of work-up it is anticipated that data comparable with the Bruusgaard material may be obtained.

3. Serologic studies relative to spontaneous cure, correlation between STS

and clinical, and pathological findings may be productive of much valuable information.

4. The pathologic studies made to date must be gathered together and worked up. Shall Rosahn's protocol for tabulation be followed.

5. There is much valuable material here for aid in evaluation of the TPI procedure.

Centers for Disease Control Papers, Tuskegee Syphilis Study Administrative Records, 1930–80, Box 7, Folder 1951, National Archives–Southeast Region, East Point, Georgia.

Eleanor N. Walker to Dr. John C. Cutler, December 4, 1952

TO: Dr. John C. Cutler

DATE: December 4, 1952

FROM: Eleanor N. Walker

SUBJECT: Study of Untreated Syphilis in the Male Negro, Macon County, Alabama

It seems to me that after 20 years we have too much of a stake in this study to let it slide now for the sake of a few more dollars. I have never felt that Nurse Rivers was an adequate "policeman" for these people. I know the colored people in the South and one shouldn't expect 100% effort from any of them unless they are under constant supervision. In a community of this type where everyone knows everybody's business I can't see how we could have lost from contact so many of the group if Nurse Rivers had been even moderately interested in perpetuating this study.

I would like to spend several weeks with her and prepare from the records and from whatever other source available, an informative list of the "lost" study individuals and try to locate some of them through a series of letters to the various local health departments. In the case of those residing in Alabama it should be simple to have them located and examined.

The assignment of a young investigator to the County Health Department to absorb some of Nurse Rivers duties doesn't appear to be the answer, because he is here today and gone tomorrow. Would it be possible to think about tying in more closely with the Institute staff in some way. Certainly something should be done right now to put this study on a firmer foundation if it is determined it should be continued.

Centers for Disease Control Papers, Tuskegee Syphilis Study Administrative Records, 1930–80, Box 7, Folder 1952, National Archives–Southeast Region, East Point, Georgia.

Public Health Service to Dear Sir, October 18, 1955

Tuskegee, Alabama
October 18, 1955

Dear Sir:

The Government doctor will be here next week. Be sure to meet him at the time and place listed below that is nearest your home.

Tuesday, November 1, 1955

Cooper's Chapel	8:30 A.M.
Creek Stand	9:30 A.M.
Cross Roads	10:45 A.M.
Swanson	11:30 A.M.
Hannon	12:00 Noon
Robe	12:30 P.M.
Armstrong	12:45 P.M.
Ft. Davis	1:15 P.M.
Cotton Valley	2:00 P.M.
Mt. Nebo	2:30 P.M.

Wednesday, November 2, 1955

Nebraska	8:45 A.M.
Chesson	9:45 A.M.
Prairie Farm Clinic	10:15 A.M.
Pinkston's Store	10:45 A.M.
Milstead	11:30 A.M.
Bethal Grove	12:45 P.M.
Walker's Chapel	1:00 P.M.

Thursday, November 3, 1955

Simmons' Chapel	8:30 A.M.
Mt. Zion	9:00 A.M.
Shiloh	9:30 A.M.
McCray's Chapel	10:00 A.M.
Brown Hill	10:30 A.M.
Oak Grove	11:00 A.M.
Brownville #2	11:45 A.M.
Brownville #1	12:30 P.M.
Pine Grove	1:15 P.M.
Mt. Pleasant	1:45 P.M.

Friday, November 4, 1955

Macon County Health Office	8:30–12:00

Centers for Disease Control Papers, Tuskegee Syphilis Study Administrative Records, 1930–80, Box 16, Folder Alabama Miscellaneous, National Archives–Southeast Region, East Point, Georgia.

Eunice Rivers Laurie to Dear Sir, July 16, 1963

July 16, 1963

Dear Sir:

The Public Health Service doctor who was here last fall plans to return to Tuskegee about the 23rd of July for a visit of several weeks. During that time he would like to see you at the Veterans Administration Hospital, if you are able, if not, he will visit you at your home.

I will notify you 2 or 3 days in advance of the exact day on which the doctor will expect you and I will let you know at that time when and where I will meet you to take you to the hospital. Since the examination will take a little time, lunch will be provided at the hospital before you are returned home.

In appreciation of your cooperation during the last 30 years and for your valuable contribution to medical research, you will be presented a cash award. I sincerely hope, therefore, that you will make every effort to see the doctor when you are notified.

Sincerely yours,

Eunice Rivers Laurie, R.N.

Public Health Service

Centers for Disease Control Papers, Tuskegee Syphilis Study Administrative Records, 1930–80, Box 16, Folder Alabama-Miscellaneous, National Archives–Southeast Region, East Point, Georgia.

Irwin J. Schatz, M.D., Henry Ford Hospital, Detroit, Michigan, to Donald H. Rockwell, Venereal Disease Research Laboratory, Public Health Service, Atlanta, Georgia, June 11, 1965

June 11, 1965

Donald H. Rockwell, M.D.

Venereal Disease Research Laboratory

Communicable Disease Center

United States Public Health Service

Atlanta, Georgia 30333

Dear Dr. Rockwell:

I have recently read your paper on the Tuskegee Study of Untreated Syphillis appearing in the Archives of Internal Medicine in December, 1964.

I am utterly astounded by the fact that physicians allow patients with potentially fatal disease to remain untreated when effective therapy is available. I assume you feel that the information which is extracted from observation of this untreated group is worth their sacrifice. If this is the case, then I suggest that the United States Public Health Service and those physicians associated with it in this study need to re-evaluate their moral judgements in this regard.

Yours sincerely,

IRWIN J. SCHATZ, M.D.

Head, Section of Peripheral Vascular Disease

IJS:cao

Centers for Disease Control Papers, Tuskegee Syphilis Study Administrative Records, 1930–80, Box 8, Folder 1965, National Archives–Southeast Region, East Point, Georgia.

Anne R. Yobs, M.D., to Dr. E. J. Gillespie, June 15, 1965

NOTE—DO NOT USE THIS ROUTE SLIP TO SHOW FORMAL CLEARANCES OR APPROVALS

DATE: 6/15/65

TO: AGENCY   BLDG.   ROOM

Dr. E. J. Gillespie   Buckhead   500

APPROVAL   REVIEW   PER CONVERSATION

SIGNATURE   NOTE AND SEE ME   AS REQUESTED

COMMENT   NOTE AND RETURN   NECESSARY ACTION

FOR YOUR INFORMATION

PREPARE REPLY FOR SIGNATURE OF

REMARKS: This is the first letter of this type we have received. I do not plan to answer this letter.

(Fold here for return)

To

From Anne R. Yobs, M.D.

PHONE   BUILDING   ROOM

Centers for Disease Control Papers, Tuskegee Syphilis Study Administrative Records, 1930–80, Box 8, Folder 1965, National Archives–Southeast Region, East Point, Georgia.

Peter J. Buxtun to Dr. William J. Brown, Chief, Venereal Disease Branch, Communicable Disease Center, November 24, 1968

11/24/68

Dr. William J. Brown

Chief, Venereal Disease Branch

Communicable Disease Center

Atlanta, Georgia

Dear Dr. Brown:

I again am writing you with regard to the study of untreated Syphilis in the male negro. It has been well over a year since I last communicated with you in this regard. In that period of time, I have left the USPHS, and so am no longer informed as to CDC projects.

When we discussed the matter in Atlanta, I told you that I had grave moral doubts as to the propriety of this study. While I could see the justification and propriety of the study at its inception, and even up to the time of the widespread use of penicillin, I could not condone the continuation of this study up to the present day. While I must grant the danger of treating aged syphilitics, and while I am sure medical science has benefitted by the study, I still must advocate the following points:

1.) The group is 100% negro. This in itself is political dynamite and subject to wild journalistic misinterpretation. It also follows the thinking of negro militants that negros have long been used for "medical experiments" and "teaching cases" in the emergency wards of county hospitals.

2.) The group is not composed of "volunteers with social motives." They are largely uneducated, unsophisticated, and quite ignorant of the effects of untreated syphilis.

3.) Today it would be morally unethical to begin such a study with such a group. Probably not even the suasion of belonging to the "Nurse Rivers Burial Society" would be sufficient inducement.

I earnestly hope that you will inform me that the study group has been, or soon will be, treated.

Very truly yours,

Peter J. Buxtun

1730 Kearny St.

San Francisco

CC:DI

Centers for Disease Control Papers, Tuskegee Syphilis Study Administrative Records, 1930–80, Box 6, Folder Buxtun, National Archives–Southeast Region, East Point, Georgia.

Ira L. Myers, M.D., State Health Officer, State of Alabama, to William J. Brown, M.D., Chief Venereal Disease Branch, Public Health Service, March 13, 1969

March 13, 1969
William J. Brown, M.D.
Chief, Venereal Disease Branch
Department of Health, Education and Welfare
Public Health Service
National Communicable Disease Center
Atlanta, Georgia 30333

Dear Dr. Brown:

I have discussed the Macon County Untreated Syphilis Project with Dr. Ruth R. Berrey, the County Health Officer, and she knows of no opposition to the project at this time. She feels that it is not generally known or publicized. She doubts if the Medical Society is aware of its existence but hopes they will be sympathetic with the desires of the Public Health Service.

This matter has been discussed with the State Board of Health and as we discussed at the Advisory Meeting, the Alabama State Board of Health refers this matter to the Macon County Medical Society for its decision regarding continuity. The present officers of the Society are as follows:

Luther Curtis McRae, Jr., M.D., President
Henry Wendell Foster, M.D., Vice-President
Sheridan Howard Settler, Jr., M.D., Secretary Treasurer

I shall attempt to discuss this matter and this action with Dr. McRae later today. You may proceed to make your contacts directly with local officers. Please keep us informed and if a visit is made we will provide someone to go along or meet you there, if possible.

Dr. W. H. Y. Smith is improving and out of intensive care. We are encouraged by his progress.

With kindest personal regards, I am
Sincerely yours,
Ira L. Myers, M.D.
State Health Officer
ILM:fs

[handwritten addendum]
4/16 - Dr. Sencer was advised that Dr. Myers had talked to Dr. McRae and that Dr. McRae was receptive to the idea of bringing the Med. Society "on board" and suggested Mon May 19th for appearance before the Society. WJB

Centers for Disease Control Papers, Tuskegee Syphilis Study Administrative Records, 1930–80, Box 1, Folder Ad Hoc, National Archives–Southeast Region, East Point, Georgia.

James B. Lucas, M.D., Assistant Chief, Venereal Disease Branch, Public Health Service, to William J. Brown, M.D., Chief, Venereal Disease Branch, September 10, 1970

Date: September 10, 1970

Subject: An analysis of the current status of the Tuskegee Study

To: William J. Brown, M.D.

Chief, Venereal Disease Branch

1. In recent years the Tuskegee Study has become an increasingly emotionally charged subject. This aura has in large measure prevented a rational appraisal of the situation. It is hoped that these remarks will aid in restoring our prospectives and lead to a reasonable course of future action.

2. *Priority*—Resources must follow priorities. While some medical knowledge has been gained from this study its volume and quality has been less than gleaned from the preceding Boeck-Bruusgaard study. This is largely because effective and undocumented treatment has been given to the vast majority of patients in the syphilitic group. Most received this therapy in the "happenstance" manner while under treatment for other conditions. The impact of this inadvertent treatment will be almost impossible to assess, but without question the course of untreated syphilis (which the study was supposed to have delineated) has been radically altered. This is not to suggest that some contributions to medical knowledge do not yet lurk in the information gathered to date. However, it must be fully realized that the remaining contribution from this study will be largely of *historical* interest. Nothing learned will prevent, find, or cure a single case of infectious syphilis or bring us closer to our basic mission of controlling venereal disease in the United States.

3. Probably the greatest contribution that the Tuskegee Study has made and can continue to provide has been documented sera for study in our laboratory. Without those sera the problem of evaluating new serologic tests becomes much more difficult and the results less certain. In a great measure the development and our endorsement, of the FTA-ABS test rested on Tuskegee sera. The collection of future specimens hardly requires a special unit for that purpose.

4. To point up how obtunded the medical findings are currently one must only look to the special study carried out in 1967 by Dr. J. Lawton Smith. We permitted him to study these patients, but insisted on a "blind" study so he would not know who were syphilitic and who were controls. All available patients were rather elaborately studied for neurologic and ophthalmologic defects. When Dr. Smith presented his clinical findings we broke the code. Absolutely no correlation was discovered between the pathology uncovered in his study and the status of the patients.

5. All of this simply serves to point out that neither major medical revelations nor program benefits are likely to be forthcoming irregardless of who supervises

the study, and thus the overall priority of the Tuskegee Study from these viewpoints is relatively low.

6. *Moral Obligation*—Any question of termination hinges upon an obligation to the remaining syphilitic patients. This is both an implied and expressed obligation. The long continued assignment of Mrs. Laurie and now Mrs. Kennebrew to Tuskegee demonstrates our good faith and sincerity. The annual examination of survivors and referral of those with significant physical findings also clearly demonstrates our position and good will. Several recent pieces of correspondence indicate that termination is now desirable since many of the patients are now dead or that the deaths of those remaining will bring the study to a natural termination within the next few years. Certainly we are obligated to maintain our present level of observation as long as a significant number of patients remain alive.

7. A point may be reached where the number of survivors no longer justifies continued surveillance, but this might expose the program to justifiable criticism on grounds of the moral issue. What number of survivors would justify such a decision?

8. A more definite answer can be made concerning natural termination. One merely needs to know the current number of survivors, their average age, and have access to a life table for non-white males to definitely determine the number who will be living for any future year. Currently 149 syphilitics are alive and their average age is 71. In five years, 101 can be expected to still be alive. In 1980, sixty-eight of the syphilitics will still be living. In the years that follow the annual mortality will probably be no greater than 9–10 percent so that approximately 25 individuals may reasonably be expected to survive yet another decade (1990). This exercise simply points out that natural termination in the forseeable future is an unlikely event.

9. It is also suggested that a lack of continuity on the part of VD personnel is a valid excuse for termination. I would like to point out that this study has not had a fulltime person (other than Nurse Laurie) handling this study for a great many years. Periodically medical officers have become interested or were assigned for short periods to the project, but there has been very little medical continuity since the inception of the study. It is true that Mrs. Price has handled the record keeping for many years, but this was only a small part of her duties. She is still readily available as a consultant should questions concerning the records arise. In essence then, there has long been a lack of medical continuity and the need for this now is debatable at best.

10. Due to our present financial duress it hardly seems feasible to commit $150,000 over a three or four-year period or even hire a GS-14 pathologist to oversee the study. It has also been suggested that a summary monograph obstensively authored by appropriate experts be prepared. This raises several questions. Why outside experts, who have not been involved in the study? Such experts may very well prefer not to be associated with this study because of its sensitive nature. In any event there remains very little expertise on late syphilis.

11. More importantly, what would be the value of an elaborate and expensive monograph? The "green book" certainly adequately covers the pertinent aspects of late syphilis. Distribution of such a monograph might well cause more harm than good to the program.

12. A much more realistic approach would involve the preparation of a series of "in-house reports." Any findings of special interest or importance might then be published in appropriate journals as has been done in the past.

13. In summary, three distinct courses of action appear to be open:

(1) The study may be terminated. This is clearly not justified from the foregoing discussion. In fact the assignment of a new nurse already indicates our dedication to this study and its subjects.

(2) The study may be continued along its present lines with periodic clinical observation and serologic surveillance. On occasion the publication of any new significant finding may be considered. This can be handled by the present staff in clinical research with occasional supplementation by VDRL or VD Branch medical officers.

(3) A special unit with a fulltime director may be created. The costs, value and long term nature of this option have been discussed.

14. In my opinion, when all factors are considered, the second option appears to be the wisest course of action.

James B. Lucas, M.D.
Assistant Chief
Venereal Disease Branch
State and Community Services Division

U.S. Department of Health, Education and Welfare, Tuskegee Syphilis Study Ad Hoc Advisory Panel, Box 2, Ad Hoc Committee Folder, MSC 264, National Library of Medicine, History of Medicine Division, Bethesda, Maryland.

Don W. Printz, M.D., Chief, Clinical Research Activity, Venereal Disease Branch, Center for Disease Control, to Mrs. Elizabeth M. Kennebrew, Macon County Health Department

April 27, 1972
Mrs. Elizabeth M. Kennebrew
Macon County Health Department
Tuskegee, Alabama 36083

Dear Mrs. Kennebrew:
From time to time it is customary to review the duties and responsibilities of our field assignees who serve principally with state and local health departments. I

notice I have not corresponded with you about this since I assumed the position of Chief, Clinical Research Activity.

My predecessor, Dr. Arnold L. Schroeter, was especially pleased with your new system of record keeping for patients being followed in Tuskegee. I too feel it is imperative with the average age of the patients involved well in excess of 70 years that we maintain as close contact with them as possible. Therefore, I suggest you make personal contact with every patient being followed in the Tuskegee area at least once every 2 months. The excellent rapport which Mrs. Laurie had with these patients cannot be achieved overnight, but I believe a regular system of visitation will aid you in doing this. In addition, patients who are hospitalized for any reason should be followed daily with visits. Because of the great age of the patients now in the study, the regular physical examination, with good patient participation, will loom even more important in the future.

I envision at least 80 percent of your working time, that is 4 out of 5 working days, should be spent working exclusively with the Tuskegee patients. It may be that from time to time during illness of other nurses or during exceptional circumstances, such as epidemics, you may have some duties assigned to you by the Macon County Health Department. However, these should be the exception rather than the rule. I feel to justify the Federal Government paying 100 percent of your salary we should expect you to devote 80 percent of your time exclusively to work with the Tuskegee patients on our Venereal Disease Branch sponsored program. The remaining 20 percent of your time should be devoted to venereal disease control programs in the Macon County area in cooperation with and with direction from VD control officials of the State of Alabama.

Sincerely yours,
Don W. Printz, M.D.
Chief, Clinical Research Activity
Venereal Disease Branch
State and Community Services Division

JOB DESCRIPTION OF "PROGRAM REPRESENTATIVE" WITH TUSKEGEE STUDY

The "Tuskegee Study" is a research study of Negro males, all of whom resided in the Macon County, Alabama area when the study began in 1933. Participants of the project fall in one of two categories: (1) untreated, acquired syphilitics; (2) non-syphilitic controls. Average age of participants is approximately 74. This project is being conducted by the Venereal Disease Program, Division of Special Health Services, United States Public Health Service.

The public health nurse, or "program representative," is to provide specialized nursing services to a group of study patients, most of whom reside in Macon County and surrounding Bullock, Lee, Russell and Tallapoosa Counties.

Long-range nursing care planning will include following the patients for life;

establishing and maintaining good rapport with patients and their families; promoting optimal health; maintaining present caseload and continuing caseholding efforts of "lost" patients; making preparations and assisting (Communicable Disease Control) public health physicians with routine physical examinations; and obtaining permission for autopsy from family when death occurs.

Regular home visits should be made at least every three months on each patient; more often, if necessary.

Advice and assistance should be provided in Venereal Disease other health problems and problems not related to health, if possible and guidance patient's condition should be kept for information of Communicable Disease Control physicians.

Families are requested to inform nurse when serious illness or death occurs; follow-up care, as deemed necessary is initiated.

When necessary, patients are to be taken by automobile to private physicians for medication and/or examination.

Inquiries should be made of friends, relatives and older citizens of the communities as to lead where abouts of inactive participants as caseholding efforts.

When not needed on the v-d project the nurse will assist with the general Public Health Nursing program of Macon County.

Centers for Disease Control Papers, Tuskegee Syphilis Study Administrative Records, 1930–80, Box 12, Folder Personnel Arrangements, National Archives–Southeast Region, East Point, Georgia.

SDS Leaflet

SYPHILIS STUDY "DEFENSIBLE"?

DAVID SENCER, DIRECTOR OF CDC (Center for Disease Control) SAYS "YES!!"

SDS (Students for a Democratic Society) SAYS "NO!!"

A 40-year-old syphilis research program, otherwise known as the "Tuskegee Study," has taken the lives of 150 black men in Alabama. These men could have been spared their sufferings from the dreaded disease, syphilis: however, they were among over 400 men who were denied treatment by the government "in the interest of science." These men were told only that they had "bad blood"—but the real nature of the disease was not explained.

Such acts of racist genocide must be stopped *NOW!*"

DEMONSTRATE: Saturday, August 12, 1:00 PM, outside the Public Health Service Building at 60 Eighth St. NE.

PICKET the CENTER FOR DISEASE CONTROL: Thursday, August 17 at 3:00 PM. If you need a ride, or for more information, call 373-0713 or 875-5350.

WE INVITE ALL GROUPS AND INDIVIDUALS TO JOIN US IN DEMANDING (1) $600,000 REPARATIONS FOR FAMILIES OF VICTIMS, AND (2) SENCER RETRACT HIS STATEMENT THAT THE STUDY WAS "DEFENSIBLE."

Join us—TO PROTEST this RACIST STUDY—and BUILD a LASTING MOVEMENT against RACISM

(See other side for the Anti-Racism Bill, sponsored by SDS, which we want to bring to Miami to present to the Republicans).

Centers for Disease Control Papers, Tuskegee Syphilis Study Administrative Records, 1930–80, Box 8, Folder 1972, National Archives–Southeast Region, East Point, Georgia.

Robert H. Huffaker, Biohazards Control Officer, Memorandum for the Record, August 24, 1972

TO: Memorandum for the Record
DATE: August 24, 1972
FROM: Biohazards Control Officer
SUBJECT: Implementation of Emergency Plans; Picketing by SDS

Late on Thursday, August 10, 1972, the CDC Executive Office received copies of a handbill (exhibit 1) printed by the Students for a Democratic Society (SDS) which announced plans to "Demonstrate August 12, 1972, in front of the PHS building at 60 Eighth Street N.E." (this houses FDA) and to "Picket CDC on Thursday, August 17, at 3:00 p.m."

What followed provided a test of CDC disaster preparedness emergency plans. (The formal plans were never referred to during the "exercise"; probably because it was felt that decisions and actions had to be applicable to the specific situation and "cook-book" guides would not be valuable. Probably the greatest value of the formal plan was in preparing the people who compiled them to make decisions during an actual emergency situation).

Friday, August 11, 1972—The following were notified of the planned picketing:

FBI Atlanta Office   Mr. Stan Maurio
DeKalb County Police   Sgt. Roderick
HEW—Washington   Mr. Don Dick
U.S. Attorney's Atlanta Office Mr. Gene Madori
U.S. Magistrate's Atlanta Office Mr. Al Chancey
FDA—Atlanta Office   Mr. Dawson (to warn them that they were
                                scheduled to have a "demonstration.")

All chiefs of programs, offices, etc. of CDC. Each was contacted by telephone and told:

1. That SDS was planning to picket, and the date and time.
2. That the information was provided to counteract rumors and enable them to answer questions.
3. That the information was not an invitation from management for employees to participate and that it was expected there would be business as usual.

Later on, the question of employee participation in the demonstration was raised, and it was decided that each inquirer should be sent to personnel (Dr. George Glover) where they would be shown the applicable rules and regulations. The decision to participate would have to be made by each individual. This information should have been given in the initial contact with the supervisors but was not. No written statement was made by CDC to our personnel regarding the picketing. NMAV should have been contacted but was not.

Monday, August 14 - Reports from FDA were that seven people had come to demonstrate on Saturday; these went into the hippy area and got four recruits and returned. The eleven presented demands to a closed building and hung Dr. Sencer in effigy. (The body was cut down for reuse.)

Plans were made to secure the Clifton Road facility. Buckhead and Lawrenceville were informed but were to take no special action. Atlanta City Police were asked to "look in" on Buckhead. Because of the proximity of the Chamblee facility to IRS (known to be demonstration prone), it was decided to close and lock gates in the perimeter fence on Thursday afternoon. One of these gates is card controlled, and an Engineering Branch man was to operate the gate for non-cardholders.

Tuesday, August 15 - Atlanta Police Intelligence said that an appeal to help picket had been placed in the "Great Speckled Bird." According to the Atlanta Police, the FBI felt there might be a large gathering at CDC on Thursday, August 17.

Wednesday, August 16

Messrs. Gunn and Paine stated that CDC has "proprietorial interest" in the facility and that DeKalb Police have jurisdiction *on* and *in* the grounds and buildings. (This point had been researched earlier for another reason.)

Sgt. Brooks (DeKalb County Police) came to Clifton Road and went over the buildings and security plans.

Thursday, August 17

All gates to the parking area were locked just after 1:00 p.m. A guard remained at the upper gate with the key and to admit cars with CDC stickers and also to let traffic out. All building doors were locked at this time with the exception of the doors on the basement level of B (Clinic entrance) and the main front entrance of Building 1. These doors were attended by guards. All other doors "above" the fence that could be opened from the inside were attended by personnel from Engineering Services. Signs were made asking people to use the front door, and these were posted on locked doors.

Captain James Stanley, in charge of the DeKalb County Police, made his headquarters in the front lobby.

Dr. Rafe Henderson invited SDS representatives to come to CDC and discuss the Tuskegee Study. Four people came and talked with him for 2½ hours, and when they left they appeared to be satisfied with the information. This discussion was probably very important in aborting the picketing.

CDC people behaved very well; there was extra traffic to the cafeteria during the time scheduled for picketing but little loitering and no interference with guards, etc. NO PICKETS CAME.

A complaint was received that the basement door of Building 4 could not be opened from the inside when locked. This will be changed by installing a crash bar.

Increased security will be continued at night; two of the three outside doors which have often been blocked open will be secured as it is impossible to control access to the facility while these doors are unlocked. The third back door of CDC is open until midnight. Further evaluation of building security must be made and deficiencies corrected as soon as possible.

Friday, August 18

The Information Office had reports of picketing of the Regional Office in Chicago by SDS. In addition, the syphilis study in Chicago is getting very bad press. None of this has appeared on the wire service as yet.

Robert H. Huffaker, D.V.M.

Centers for Disease Control Papers, Tuskegee Syphilis Study Administrative Records, 1930–80, Box 8, Folder 1972, National Archives–Southeast Region, East Point, Georgia.

Charles G. Gomillion to Susan M. Reverby, October 12, 1994

September 20 1994

Dear Dr. Reverby:

I was in Tuskegee during the period of the "Tuskegee Syphilis Experiment," and I was aware that Miss Eunice Rivers was a nurse employed in the program, but, like many other citizen in Macon County, I thought that the persons being treated by the physicians and nurses were being treated in order to cure them of their ailment. We did not know that the program was a scientific/medical experiment until we read about it in the newspapers. So, we made no inquiries about it. We were glad that those affected with syphilis were being treated.

Miss Rivers might have been a dues-paying member of the Tuskegee Civic Association, but I do not remember her as having been an active participant on any program, or a member of any committee.

I regret that I was very ignorant of what was actually being done to the syphilitic persons in the program. After the suit was filed by Mr. Fred D. Gray, I was informed that a Mr. Pollard, who was an officer in the Macon County Democratic Club, of which I was president, was one of the syphilitic participants. For several years, he and I had worked together in a program of civic and political education. He was the precinct leader for Notasulga [just outside Tuskegee]. At the time, I did not know Mr. Pollard was a participant in the "health" program. He never mentioned it to me. I have not talked with him about it.

Sincerely,

Charles G. Gomillion

October 12, 1994

Dear Ms. Reverby:

Before the newspapers reported that the Federal health project on which Miss Eunice Rivers worked was a research project, I had heard that those who were being "treated" for "bad blood" had syphilis. I think that few persons in the TCA [Tuskegee Civic Association] who talked with me about the project thought as I did, namely, that the project was one to improve the health of the participants, and reduce the mortality rate.

In the '30s, '40s, and 50s, the TCA was almost as active in doing what it could to improve the public health and educational opportunities and services as it was in increasing voter registration and voting. If any of the officials in the TCA had known that the syphilitic persons did not know that the project was a research project, and that some (half) of those were *not* being treated to improve their health, we (the TCA) would have engaged in some kind of action. There might have been some persons in the community, in addition to Miss Rivers, who knew that the project was a research project, but they did not talk with me about it.

I do not know how Miss Rivers was treated in the community by those who knew that the project was a research one, after the newspapers reported the nature of the project, and after Mr. Fred D. Gray became involved, I heard that some blamed Miss Rivers for having participated in the project, if she knew that some of the syphilitic patients did not know that they were not being given health-improving drugs.

Sincerely,

Charles G. Gomillion

Charles Gomillion was a sociology professor at Tuskegee University and the longtime head of the Tuskegee Civic Association which led the struggle for voting and other civil rights in Tuskegee. Permission granted by Lawrence A. Sims, grandson and executor of the Estate of Charles G. Gomillion.

SYPHILIS VICTIMS IN U.S. STUDY
WENT UNTREATED FOR 40 YEARS

JEAN HELLER

WASHINGTON, July 25—For 40 years the United States Public Health Service has conducted a study in which human beings with syphilis, who were induced to serve as guinea pigs, have gone without medical treatment for the disease and a few have died of its late effects, even though an effective therapy was eventually discovered.

The study was conducted to determine from autopsies what the disease does to the human body.

Officials of the health service who initiated the experiment have long since retired. Current officials, who say they have serious doubts about the morality of the study, also say that it is too late to treat the syphilis in any surviving participants.

Doctors in the service say they are now rendering whatever other medical services they can give to the survivors while the study of the disease's effects continues.

Dr. Merlin K. DuVal, Assistant Secretary of Health, Education and Welfare for Health and Scientific Affairs, expressed shock on learning of the study. He said that he was making an immediate investigation.

The experiment, called the Tuskegee Study, began in 1932 with about 600 black men, mostly poor and uneducated, from Tuskegee, Ala., an area that had the highest syphilis rate in the nation at the time.

Four hundred of the group had syphilis and never received deliberate treatment for the venereal infection. A control group of 200 had no syphilis and did not receive any specific therapy.

Some subjects were added to the study in its early years to replace men who had dropped out of the program, but the number added is not known. At the beginning of this year, 74 of those who received no treatment were still alive.

As [i]ncentives to enter the program, the men were promised free transportation to and from hospitals, free hot lunches, free medicine for any disease other than syphilis and free burial after autopsies were performed.

Jean Heller was the reporter who broke the story of the study on the Associated Press wireservice, as printed in the New York Times *on July 26, 1972. Reprinted by permission of the Associated Press.*

The Tuskegee Study began 10 years before penicillin was found to be a cure for syphilis and 15 years before the drug became common, and while its use probably could have helped or saved a number of the experiment subjects, the drug was denied them, Dr. J. D. Millar says.

Dr. Millar is chief of the venereal disease branch of the service's Center for Disease Control in Atlanta and is now in charge of what remains of the Tuskegee Study. He said in an interview that he has serious doubts about the program.

Dr. Millar said that "a serious moral problem" arose when penicillin therapy, which can cure syphilis in its early stages, became available in the late nineteen-forties and was withheld from patients in the syphilis study. Penicillin therapy became, Dr. Millar said, "so much more effective and so much less dangerous" than pre-existing therapies.

"The study began when attitudes were much different on treatment and experimentation." Dr. Millar said, "At this point in time, with our current knowledge of treatment and the disease and the revolutionary change in approach to human experimentation, I don't believe the program would be undertaken."

Members of Congress reacted with shock to the disclosure today that the syphilis experimentation on human guinea pigs had taken place.

"A Moral Nightmare"

Senator William Proxmire, Democrat of Wisconsin, a member of the Senate Appropriations subcommittee that oversees Public Health Service budgets, called the study "a moral and ethical nightmare."

Syphilis is a highly contagious infection spread by sexual contact. If untreated, it can cause bone and dental deformations, deafness, blindness, heart disease, and deterioration of the central nervous system.

No figures were available as to when the last death in the program occurred. One official said that no conscious effort was apparently made to halt the program after it got under way.

A 1969 study of 276 untreated syphilitics who participated in the Tuskegee Study showed that seven had died as a direct result of syphilis. The 1969 study was made by the Atlanta center, whose officials said they could not determine at this late date how many additional deaths had been caused by syphilis.

However, of the 400 men in the original syphilitic group, 154 died of heart disease that officials in Atlanta said was not specifically related to syphilis. Dr. Millar said that this rate was identical with the rate of cardio-vascular deaths in the control, or non-syphilis group.

Dr. Millar said that the study was initiated in 1932 by Dr. J. R. Heller, assistant Surgeon general in the service's venereal disease section, who subsequently became division chief.

Of the decision not to give penicillin to the untreated syphilitics once it became widely available, Dr. Millar said, "I doubt that it was a one-man decision. These things seldom are. Whoever was director of the VD section at that time, in 1946 or 1947, would be the most logical candidate if you had to pin it down."

"Never Clandestine"

The syphilis study "was never clandestine" and 15 scientific reports were published in the medical literature, Dr. Millar said in a telephone interview yesterday from Atlanta.

Officials who [initiated] the study in 1932 had informed the syphilis victims that [they] could get treatment for the infection at any time, Dr. Millar said.

"Patients were not denied drugs," Dr. Millar stressed. Rather they were not offered drugs.

When the study began, doctors could offer only what now is regarded as poor therapy—injections of metals like bismuth, arsenic and mercury. Such treatments were known to be toxic.

Many doctors, Dr. [Millar] said, then thought "it better not to treat syphilis cases because of the mortality from" the metal therapies.

The critical period in ethics was in the late nineteen forties and early nineteen-fifties when antibiotics could have been but were not prescribed for the syphilis patients.

UNTREATED SYPHILIS IN THE MALE NEGRO
Mortality During 12 Years of Observation

J. R. HELLER & P. T. BRUYERE

This paper is the second of a series of studies of untreated acquired syphilis in the male Negro. It deals particularly with the effect of the disease on the life span of the human host. Subsequently in more detailed analyses of the material attempts will be made to describe and evaluate specific changes brought about by the disease in the infected individual, with particular reference to the cardiovascular system.

The material upon which the study is based consists of records of 410 Negro men with untreated syphilis and a comparable group of 201 uninfected Negro men. In a previous report (1) the population under study was described, considerable attention being given to the methods of diagnosis and to the physical and roentgenologic findings in the two groups, syphilitic and control. The individuals were carefully chosen, the decision as to the presence or absence of syphilis being based on history, physical examination, and serologic tests of the blood and spinal fluid. X-ray examinations of the heart were made on all the individuals selected for study, and additional roentgenologic studies were made when indicated. The syphilitic group was chosen first, and the control group was selected in such a way as to have a nearly identical age distribution. All members of both groups were inhabitants of a rural area in Alabama.

The examinations were made and the study population selected during the winter seasons of 1931–32 and 1932–33, the time of year being chosen in order not to interfere with the usual agricultural occupations of the individuals involved. Since that time there has been an annual visit to the region by a physician for the purpose of obtaining specimens of blood for serologic examination, and a second complete examination was made of the majority of the group in 1938–39. In addition, a nurse in the local health department has kept in constant touch with the members of the group. Some of these have left the area from time to time, but most of them return eventually and the whereabouts of practically every one is

Dr. John Heller was medical director chief of the Venereal Disease Division of the Public Health Service when this was published. Dr. P. T. Bruyere was a statistician also with the division. Originally published in Journal of Venereal Disease Information *27 (1946): 34–38. Reprinted by permission of* Public Health Reports.

known through relatives and friends still living in the region. It is felt that as yet not one individual still living has been completely lost from observation.

An important part of the study has been the performance of autopsies on those who have died. Through the end of 1944, 129 were known to have died. Of these, 93 were examined post mortem. The majority not so examined lived in far outlying areas so that news of their death was not received promptly. In a few cases death occurred while the patient was living outside the area; however, news of the event was obtained from relatives. Since, as has already been pointed out, all of the individuals not reported as dead are either still residing in the area or are heard of, at least occasionally, through relatives and friends, it is reasonably sure that there have been no other deaths than the 129 recorded.

From the foregoing remarks it can be seen that very little error can result from basing mortality rates on the assumption that the entire study group, syphilitic and control, has been under continuous observation from Jan. 1, 1933, to the present time. Because there is occasionally a time lag, however, between the occurrence of death and its report, and also because this analysis was commenced before the end of 1945, the study was limited to the events between Jan. 1, 1933, and Dec. 31, 1944, a period of 12 years. The original study group consisted of 410 syphilitics, of whom 101 died during the period mentioned, and 201 controls, of whom 28 died. It will be seen at once that there was a much greater mortality among the syphilitics than among the controls, 24.6 percent as compared with 13.9 percent.

As has already been stated, the control group was selected so as to conform to the syphilitic group with regard to sex and age, so that these factors cannot account for any part of the difference. It is known that some of the control group have acquired syphilis, although the exact number cannot be accurately determined at present, and that about one-fourth of the syphilitic individuals received some treatment for their infection. Most of these, however, received no more than 1 or 2 arsenical injections; only 12 received as many as 10. The exact effect of these circumstances on the relative mortality of the 2 groups is not known. It is evident that infection with syphilis of members of the control group would tend, if anything, to make the mortality of this group more nearly like that of the syphilitic group. The effect of treatment on the mortality of the syphilitic group is open to question. However, the amount of treatment was small and certainly could not have accounted for any appreciable increase in mortality. Therefore, the fact that nearly twice as large a proportion of the syphilitic individuals as of the control group has died is a very striking one.

The foregoing observations led us, as a preliminary step in the analysis of the material, to attempt to measure more exactly the relative mortality of the 2 groups. The most efficient statistical procedure for that purpose, the construction of life tables, was adopted. The results are presented in the table and charts.

Since the period of the study was 12 years, from the beginning of 1933 to the end

TABLE 1. *Abridged Life Tables for Negro Males Aged 25–74 with Untreated Syphilis and Not Infected with Syphilis, Macon County, Ala., 1933–44*

	Syphilitics					Controls				
	Observed population		Theoretical life table population			Observed population		Theoretical life table population		
Age period	Person-years of observation	Number of deaths	Number surviving to beginning of age period out of 1,000 alive at age 25	Number dying in central year of age period per 1,000 alive at beginning of that year	Average number of years of life through age 74 remaining to an individual alive at beginning of age period	Person-years of observation	Number of deaths	Number surviving to beginning of age period out of 1,000 alive at age 25	Number dying in central year of age period per 1,000 alive at beginning of that year	Average number of years of life through age 74 remaining to an individual alive at beginning of period
			l_x	$1000q_x$	$°e_x$			l_x	$1000q_x$	$°e_x$
25–29	308.25	3	100,000	10.81	34.09			100,000	5.87	42.37
30–34	564.00	9	94,706	16.36	30.83	748.50	3	97,081	4.13	38.58
35–39	616.50	4	87,489	6.06	28.18			95,072	3.33	34.34
40–44	455.00	4	84,455	8.21	24.12			93,483	3.45	29.88
						502.50	2			
45–49	499.75	12	80,600	24.20	20.13			91,863	4.26	25.37
50–54	588.75	15	71,765	25.35	17.28			89,905	5.91	20.86
						612.50	5			
55–59	521.25	11	63,285	20.38	14.28			87,228	10.44	16.42
60–64	324.50	11	56,777	33.35	10.63			82,689	19.75	12.17
						281.50	8			
65–69	192.50	13	47,530	67.14	7.17			74,737	36.83	8.18
70–74	79.75	7	33,694	83.82	4.06			61,856	62.35	4.33

of 1944, each individual who survived into 1945 contributed 12 person-years of observation, at ages depending on his age on Jan. 1, 1933. Likewise those who died contributed varying numbers of person-years of observation at various ages, depending on their ages in 1933 and the date of their deaths. The number of deaths at each age related to the number of person-years of observation at that age yielded a set of age-specific mortality rates which could be determined separately for the syphilitic and the control groups. Because of the relatively small number of individuals, rates could not be computed for single years of age and groupings had to be made. Estimated rates for the individual ages were obtained by a process of interpolation, using third degree polynomials. These were then adjusted, where necessary, so that they would apply to persons exactly at a given birthday rather than halfway between two birthdays, as is the case with the usual age-specific mortality rates computed by relating the number of persons at a given age, say 25 years old (that is between their 25th and 26th birthdays), to the number of living

CHART 1. *Mortality Rates among Negro Men with Untreated Acquired Syphilis and among Nonsyphilitic Control Population*

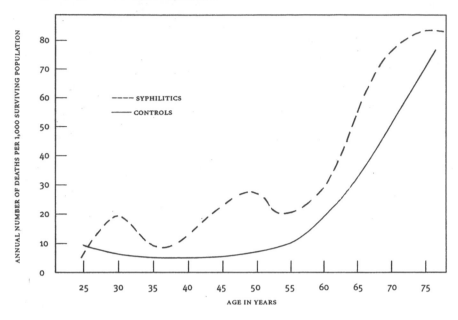

persons of that age. The rates finally resulting from this process are indicated by the curves in chart 1 and those for every fifth year between 25 and 75 are listed in the column q_x in the table. In the charts, the large dots indicate the basic points between which interpolation was made. The table and charts start with age 25 because at the time of the original selection all the men in the study group were 25 or older. Data for ages 75 and up are not shown because the number of person-years of life and the number of deaths occurring beyond that age were so small that the rates were not reliable.

There are several points of interest about the mortality rates obtained. The curve for the control group lies entirely below that for the syphilitic group. The control group curve is smooth, without peaks or irregularities, which is what one expects in a normal population. The curve for the syphilitic group has 2 marked peaks. The first occurs at about age 30. There is no obvious explanation for this, but it may be associated with the fact that the control group curve is also slightly higher at its beginning than later on. Possibly there is some factor operating on Negro men living in the region which accounts for both curves, or possibly both are merely the result of chance. The second peak in the curve for the syphilitic group reaches its highest point at about age 50. A similar peak, or at least accelerated upward trend, has been found by Usilton and Miner (2) who ascribed it to the fact that deaths from cardiovascular syphilis are most frequently observed at about this age.

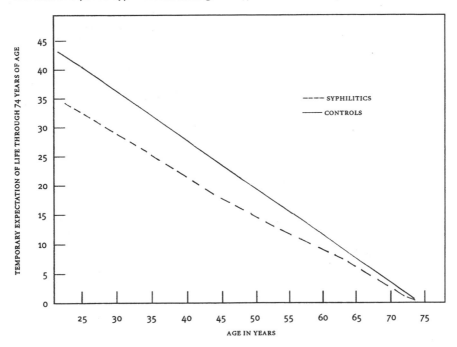

The mortality rates for single years of life estimated from the observed data were applied successively to a hypothetical group of 100,000 persons aged 25. By this means was calculated the number of persons who would still be alive at each age from 25 to 74 if they had been subjected to these particular mortality rates. The results for every fifth year are shown in the columns headed l_x in the table. And finally the so-called "temporary expectation of life" through age 74 was calculated. This value, shown in the columns headed $°e_x$ in the tables and plotted in chart 2, is the average number of years of life under age 75 remaining to individuals reaching a given age.

From chart 2 and the corresponding data in the table it can be seen that the syphilitic individuals had a much shorter life expectancy than did the normal controls. At age 25 the normal individual averaged 8 more years of life than did the syphilitic of the same age. In other words, syphilis shortened the lives of its hosts by almost 20 percent. A similar percentage reduction in life expectancy is found at ages up to about 45, after which the difference between the 2 groups decreases with increasing age.

The experience upon which the life tables are based is quite limited in comparison with the material used for the construction of most complete life tables for human populations. However, the differences between the syphilitic and control groups are so large that there can be no doubt of their significance. Furthermore, comparison with the recent standard life tables for the United States (3) reveals that the results are at least reasonable, in that the mortality rates for our control group are quite similar to those for all Negro men in the United States. The discrepancies which do exist are readily accounted for by regional differences and chance fluctuation in a group as small as ours, where a single death, more or less, causes a large difference in the results.

For these reasons we feel that our results are valid, and that the general levels of the mortality rates of the 2 groups, as reflected in the average expectation of life, are reliable. The location and size of the "humps" observed in the mortality curves are, of course, approximations since they are based on a somewhat small experience.

In conclusion, it can be said that the life expectancy of a Negro man between the ages of 25 and 50 who is infected with syphilis and receives no treatment for his infection is on the average reduced by about 20 percent.

REFERENCES

1. Vonderlehr, R. A.; Clark, T.; Wenger, O. C.; Heller, J. R., Jr.: Untreated syphilis in the male Negro. Ven. Dis. Inform., 17: 260–265, 1936.

2. Usilton, L. J.; Miner, J. R.: A tentative death curve for acquired syphilis in white and colored males in the United States. Ven. Dis. Inform., 18:231–239, 1937.

3. Bureau of the Census: United States life tables, 1939–1941. Vital Statistics—Special Reports, 19: 31–45, 1944.

TWENTY YEARS OF FOLLOWUP EXPERIENCE IN A LONG-RANGE MEDICAL STUDY

EUNICE V. RIVERS, STANLEY H. SCHUMAN,

LLOYD SIMPSON, & SIDNEY OLANSKY

One of the longest continued medical surveys ever conducted is the study of untreated syphilis in the male Negro. This study was begun by the Public Health Service in the fall of 1932 in Macon County, Ala., a rural area in the eastern part of the State, and is now entering its twenty-second year (1–4). This paper is the first report dealing with the nonmedical aspects of the study. The experiences recounted may be of value to those who are planning continuing studies in other fields.

In beginning the study, schedules of the blood-drawing clinics throughout the county were announced through every available source, including churches, schools, and community stores. The people responded willingly, and 600 patients were selected for the study—400 who had syphilis and, for controls, 200 who did not. The patients who had syphilis were all in the latent stage; any acute cases requiring treatment were carefully screened out for standard therapy.

At Tuskegee, each of the 600 patients initially was given a complete physical examination, including chest X-rays and electrocardiograms. Careful histories were taken and blood tests were repeated. Thereafter, each of the patients was followed up with an annual blood test and, whenever the Public Health Service physicians came to Tuskegee, physical examinations were repeated.

There have been four surveys: in 1932, 1938, 1948, and 1952. Between surveys contact with the patients was maintained through the local county health department and an especially assigned public health nurse, whose chief duties were those of followup workers on this project. The nurse also participated in a generalized public health nursing program, which gave her broad contact with the families of the patients and demonstrated that she was interested in other aspects of their welfare as well as in the project. The nurse was a native of the county, who had lived near her patients all her life, and was thoroughly familiar with their local ideas and customs.

Eunice Rivers was the "scientific assistant" and public-health nurse associated with the study for its entire forty years.
Originally published in Public Health Reports 68 (1953): 391–95. Reprinted by permission of Public Health Reports.

A most important phase of the study was to follow as many patients as possible to postmortem examination, in order to determine the prevalence and severity of the syphilitic disease process. Cooperation of patients with this plan was sought by offering burial assistance (through a private philanthropy, the Milbank Memorial Fund) on condition that permission be granted for autopsy. For the majority of these poor farmers such financial aid was a real boon, and often it was the only "insurance" they could hope for. The Federal Government offered physical examinations and incidental medication, such as tonics and analgesics, but was unable to provide financial assistance on a continuing basis. The Milbank Memorial Fund burial assistance made it possible to obtain a higher percentage of permissions for postmortem examination than otherwise would have been granted.

Transportation to the hospital for X-rays and physical examination was furnished by the nurse. Her car was too small to bring in more than two patients at one trip; therefore, two men were scheduled for examination in the morning and two for the afternoon. During the early years of the study, when the county was strictly a rural one, the roads were very poor, some being impassable during the rainy season. Very often, the patients spent hours helping to get the car out of a mudhole. Now, with modern conveniences (telephones, electricity, cars, and good roads) the nurse's problems are fewer than in the early days.

Having a complete physical examination by a doctor in a hospital was a new experience for most of the men. Some were skeptical; others were frightened and left without an examination. Those who were brave enough to remain were very pleased. Only one objection occurred frequently: the "back shot," never again! There are those who, today, unjustifiably attribute current complaints (backaches, headaches, nervousness) to those spinal punctures.

Followup

The patients have been followed through the years by the same nurse but by different doctors. Some doctors were liked by all the patients: others were liked by only a few. The chief factor in this was the length of time doctor and patients had to get to know each other. If the doctor's visit to the area was brief, he might not have time to learn and to understand the habits of the patients. Likewise, the patients did not have an opportunity to understand the doctor. Because of their confidence in the nurse, the patients often expressed their opinion about the doctor privately to her. She tried always to assure them that the doctor was a busy person interested in many things, but that they really were first on his program.

It is very important for the followup worker to understand both patient and doctor, because she must bridge the gap between the two. The doctors were concerned primarily with obtaining the most efficient and thorough medical examination possible for the group of 600 men. While they tried to give each patient the personal interest he desired, this was not always possible due to the pressure of time. Occasionally, the patient was annoyed because the doctor did not pay attention to his particular complaint. He may have believed that his favorite home remedy was more potent than the doctor's prescription, and decided to let the whole thing go. It then became the task of the nurse to convince him that the examinations were beneficial. If she failed, she might find that in the future he not only neglected to answer her letters but managed to be away from home whenever she called. Sometimes the doctor grumbled because of the seemingly poor cooperation and slowness of some of the patients; often the nurse helped in these situations simply by bridging the language barrier and by explaining to the men what the doctor wanted.

Sometimes the nurse assisted the physician by warning him beforehand about the eccentricities of the patients he was scheduled to see during the day. For example, there was the lethargic patient with early cancer of the lip who needed strong language and grim predictions to persuade him to seek medical attention. On the other hand, there was the hypochondriac who overheard the doctor mention the 45° angle of rotation of his body during the X-ray examination; the next day, the entire county was buzzing with gossip about their remarkable friend who was "still alive, walking around with his heart tilted at a 45° angle."

Following a group of patients in a specialized field over a period of years becomes monotonous to patient and nurse, and both could lose interest easily. For the patients, the yearly visits by the "Government doctor," with free medicines, revived their interest. The annual blood tests and the surveys were always scheduled at "slack" times, between fall harvest and spring planting. The patients congregated in groups at churches and at crossroads to meet the nurse's car in the morning. As the newness of the project wore off and fears of being hurt were relieved, the gatherings became more social. The examination became an opportunity for men from different and often isolated parts of the county to meet and exchange news. Later, the nurse's small car was replaced with a large, new Government station wagon. The ride to and from the hospital in this vehicle with the Government emblem on the front door, chauffeured by the nurse, was a mark of distinction for many of the men who enjoyed waving to their neighbors as they drove by. They knew that they could get their pills and "spring tonic" from the nurse whenever they needed them between surveys, but they looked forward happily to having the Government doctor take their blood pressure and listen to their hearts. Those men who were advised about their diets were especially delighted even though they would not adhere to the restrictions.

Because of the low educational status of the majority of the patients, it was impossible to appeal to them from a purely scientific approach. Therefore, various methods were used to maintain and stimulate their interest. Free medicines, burial

Miss Rivers knows her patients well. She was born in Georgia and has lived in that vicinity her entire life. After graduation from the Tuskegee Institute School of Nursing in 1922, she joined the Alabama State Department of Health. There she was assigned to the bureau of maternal and child welfare where she helped farmers and their wives in the rural areas of Alabama with problems of home nursing and home hygiene. In a later assignment with the Alabama bureau of vital statistics, she assisted midwives in problems of rural nursing and in their vital statistics reports. After 8 years of work for the State, she returned to Tuskegee to be night supervisor of the John A. Andrew Memorial Hospital.

In 1932, Miss Rivers was offered a position as night supervisor in a New York general hospital. She chose, instead, to stay in Alabama as a scientific assistant with the Division of Venereal Disease of the Public Health Service. Miss Rivers still holds this position, in which she cooperates with the physicians and contact investigators on the Tuskegee untreated syphilis study. She also is the contact worker with the venereal disease control program in addition to assisting in the general nursing service of the Macon County Health Department.

Among her deepest convictions is the belief that rural areas desperately need good and sympathetic nurses to participate in and carry out effectively public health programs, as well as private medical care. She feels very strongly, on the basis of her own experience, that the girl who is trained in nursing in a rural area is much more likely to live and practice nursing in that area. Miss Rivers feels that, had she taken the offer to go to New York City many years ago, she probably would never have returned to the people with whom she is so familiar and for whom she feels she now can do her small part to contribute to better health and advances in public health.

assistance or insurance (the project being referred to as "Miss Rivers' Lodge"), free hot meals on the days of examination, transportation to and from the hospital, and an opportunity to stop in town on the return trip to shop or visit with their friends on the streets all helped. In spite of these attractions, there were some who refused their examinations because they were not sick and did not see that they were being benefited. Nothing provoked some of the patients more than for a doctor to tell them that they were not as healthy as they felt. This attitude sometimes appeared to the examining physician as rank ingratitude for a thorough medical workup which would cost anyone else a large amount of money if sought at personal expense. At these times the nurse reminded the doctor of the gap between his education and health attitudes and those of the patients.

When a patient asks the nurse for help because he is a "Government patient" and she explains there are no funds for this, he may point out that he needs assistance while he is living, not after he is dead. Whenever the nurse heard this complaint, she knew that there was danger of a lost patient. She appealed to him from an unselfish standpoint: What the burial assistance would mean to his family, to pay funeral expenses or to purchase clothes for his orphaned children. Even though a large number wished they might derive more benefits from being "Government patients," most of them answered the call to meet the doctor, some willingly, others after much persuasion.

The study group was composed of farmers who owned their homes, renters who were considered permanent residents, and day laborers on farms and in sawmills. The laborers were the hardest to follow. Some of the resident farmers traveled to other sections seeking work after their own crops had been harvested, but they came back when it was time to start planting. An effort was made continually through relatives to keep informed of the patients' most recent addresses, and this information regularly has been placed in their records. During the 20 years of the study, 520 of the original 600 men have been followed consistently if living, or to autopsy. It is possible that some of the 80 now considered lost will at some time return to the county or write the nurse from distant places for medical advice.

Autopsies

The excellent care given these patients was important in creating in the family a favorable attitude which eventually would lead to permission to perform an autopsy. Even in a friendly atmosphere, however, it was difficult for the nurse to approach the family, especially in the early years of the project, because she herself was uneasy about autopsies. She was pleasantly surprised to receive fine response from the families of the patients—only one refusal in 20 years and 145 autopsies obtained. Finally, the nurse realized that she and not the relatives had been hesitant and squeamish.

Sometimes the family asked questions concerning the autopsy, but offered no objections when they were assured that the body would not be harmed. If the patient had been ill for a long time and had not been able to secure any relief from his symptoms, they were anxious to know the reason. If he had died suddenly, they were anxious for some explanation. They also feared that some member of the family might have the same malady, and that information learned from the autopsy might aid them. Now, after many years, all of the patients are aware of the autopsies. When a member of "Miss Rivers' Lodge" passes, his surviving colleagues often will remind the family that the doctor wants "to look at his heart." Autopsies today are a routine; neither nurse nor family objects.

One cannot work with a group of people over a long period of time without becoming attached to them. This has been the experience of the nurse. She has had an opportunity to know them personally. She has come to understand some of their problems and how these account for some of their peculiar reactions. The ties are stronger than simply those of patient and nurse. There is a feeling of complete confidence in what the nurse advises. Some of them bring problems beyond her province, concerning building, insurance, and other things about which she can give no specific advice. She directs them always to the best available sources of guidance. Realizing that they do depend upon her and give her their trust, she has to keep an open mind and must be careful always not to criticize, but to help in the most ethical way to see that they get the best care.

Conclusions

Experience with this project has made several points clear which may benefit anyone now engaged in planning or executing a long-range medical research study:

1. Incentives for maximum cooperation of the patients must be kept in mind. What appears to be a real incentive to an outsider's way of thinking may have little appeal for the patient. In our case, free hot meals meant more to the men than $50 worth of free medical examination.
2. The value of rapport and sympathy between patient and physician, and between patient and nurse or followup worker never can be overestimated. Material incentives can merely supplement and support a basic feeling of good will. A kind word is often worth a carton full of free medicines. A single home visit is worth more than a dozen letters on impressive stationery.
3. Change in key personnel over the years in a long-range project can seriously weaken the project by upsetting continuity and familiar routine. It is not amiss to start a long-range study with young personnel who should then be around for the conclusion of the project. On the other hand, some new personnel may bring fresh ideas and energies to a lagging effort.
4. Teamwork between all members of the research staff is essential: doctor, nurse, investigator, technicians, and clerks all must work together for a common goal. They must appreciate the importance of each other's efforts to the success of the whole.
5. As difficult as it may be to maintain patient interest and personnel efficiency in a long-term study, there is still the advantage of momentum which gathers slowly but increasingly, until patient cooperation becomes so routine as to be habitual. Difficulties often can be anticipated due to previous experience, and thereby avoided.

6. The gains to medical knowledge derived from the horizontal, long-term study of illness and health are only just beginning to be realized. As public health workers accumulate experience and skill in this type of study, not only should the number of such studies increase, but a maximum of information will be gained from the efforts expended.

REFERENCES

1. Vonderlehr, R. A., Clark, T., Wenger, O. C., Heller, J. R., Jr.: Untreated syphilis in the male Negro. A comparative study of treated and untreated cases. Ven. Dis. Inform. 17: 260–265 (1936).

2. Heller, J. R., Jr., and Bruyere, P. T.: Untreated syphilis in the male Negro. II. Mortality during 12 years of observation. J. Ven. Dis. Inform. 27: 34–38 (1946).

3. Deibert, A. V., Bruyere, M. C.: Untreated syphilis in the male Negro. III. Evidence of cardiovascular abnormalities and other forms of morbidity. J. Ven. Dis. Inform. 27: 301–314 (1946).

4. Pesare, P. J., Bauer, T. J., and Gleeson, G. A.: Untreated syphilis in the male Negro. Observation of abnormalities over 16 years. Am. J. Syph., Gonor. & Ven. Dis., 34: 201–213 (1950).

INTERVIEW WITH FOUR SURVIVORS, DEPARTMENT OF HEALTH, EDUCATION AND WELFARE STUDY, 1973

Four subjects were interviewed in sequence.

Interview #1

Subject was asked what the study meant to the people involved, how it started, etc.

Subject—Started with a blood test. Clinic met at Shiloh Church. They gave us shots. Nurse (Rivers) came out and took us in (to John Andrews Hospital). One time I had a spinal puncture—had to stay in bed for 10 days afterward. Had headaches from that. Several others did too (and stayed in bed awhile). I wore a rubber belt for a long time afterward. Had ointment to run in under the belt.

Doctors came every year or so. After 25 years they gave everyone in the study $25.00 and a certificate. They told him he was in pretty good health.

At the beginning he thought he had "bad blood." They said that was syphilis. (He) just thought it was an "incurable disease." He was booked for Birmingham for "606" shots but "nurse stopped it." Some other doctor took blood that time and he was signed up to go to Birmingham. Nurse Rivers said he wasn't due to take the shots . . . he went to get on the bus to Birmingham and they turned him down. This was some time between 1942–1947.

He did not know he was sick before 1932. They gave them a bunch of shots—about once a month. Then they did a spinal. Nurse would notify them about the blood tests and bring them down.

He had not talked to any of the other participants lately.

He had the shots in his arm. In 1961 he had a growth removed from his bladder. (He is 66). Health insurance paid for it. He paid his bill and his insurance paid back all but $20.

These interviews were done as part of the work of the U.S. Department of Health, Education and Welfare Tuskegee Syphilis Study Ad Hoc Advisory Panel in 1973.
U.S. Department of Health, Education and Welfare, Tuskegee Syphilis Study MSC 264, Advisory Panel, Box 2, Ad Hoc Committee Folder, National Library of Medicine, History of Medicine Division, Bethesda, Maryland.

Question—could all the people in the group afford hospitalization? What would others have done?

Subject—I don't know. I asked the (government) doctors about it (the growth) and they sent me to my family doctor. The government people didn't know I had insurance.

He didn't know of any others in the study who had been in the hospital although one man had become blind after awhile. He hadn't thought much about whether his disease had been cured. The doctor was seeing him every year, and he was feeling pretty good. He was not told what the disease might do to him. He stayed in the program because they asked him to. Nurse came and got him. He thought they all had the same disease. The blind man had been blind nearly 20 years—had worn glasses awhile, then had become blind.

Question—Did anyone do anything about the blind man's eyes?

Subject—I think he told nurse. They talked one time about sending him somewhere. Wasn't treated that he knew of. He (the blind man) never went anywhere and he (subject) didn't know the details. The blind man is about 75 now.

He knew maybe 15–20 people in the study. The only time they got together as a group was when the government doctors came in.

Interview #2

(This subject was a control)

Subject had come into the program when "they were recruiting up people." Nurse got him in. He was never told what was wrong with him. He had rheumatism. He has (and had at the time) swollen fingers. He has heart disease—his heart "skips." When he says "they" he is referring to "that government affair."

He didn't always come up to the clinics. Sometimes he was away. He thought maybe Nurse Rivers came and got him because someone told her where he lived.

When asked if he had been sick, the subject said no—he had never been sick. Just slight rheumatism all his life. He really thought they were interested in his fingers. Then he thought they were interested in his heart.

Before Nurse Rivers came to see him no one had tested him. Then he was examined and his blood tested. Nothing was said about his blood although his peculiar heart was later commented on.

He had "never been in the hospital." But I was for my hernia. Had a pain in my side once. Doctor gave me pills. I'm a pretty unusual person. Two or three years ago I had a headache that lasted about three weeks. Slowed down all my work.

He had known several others in the program. All now dead. He is now 66.

Interview #3

Subject is 81 years old. Had farmed all his life (up to three years ago) and had gone through the third grade. When he got into the program he had been sick. Nurse Rivers said he could get treatments. He was told he had "some funny name thing." Main thing though was his cataracts. He had them out in 1953 at John Andrews Hospital.

Nurse Rivers had told him to be at the school and they would check them up. Every couple of years (they came.) Nurse Rivers came to the plantation to get them. He first saw her at the hospital clinic (after she suggested that he go to the clinic.)

Subject's wife interjected that the nurse had said government doctors were coming from the north and had suggested that he join the program. Later he got notices.

The doctors told him different things. They never said he had any diseases. Once they gave him shots in his back. He just got up and left.

They took blood every time. Said they sent it off. Never told him anything. Said the first test was good. Later said it was not so good. The doctors gave them pills and medicines and shots—hip and arm mostly. He didn't know why they were giving him shots. The doctor told him he had a bad heart, bad circulation, arthritis. He also had falling spells.

Lots of people went to the clinic with him. He didn't know them all. They all got the same medicine. Nobody ever said anything about his blood. They never told them what was wrong with them. They got a lot of pills. He took some of the pills, not all. He had never been hospitalized before his operation for cataracts. He took a lot of home remedies. Nurse would tell him to come in and get checked over. He saw different doctors over the years. Sometimes private doctors. When he went to private doctors, he had to pay. He didn't know if they knew he was in the program.

The doctor (he was seeing) now said his blood was good. He had had different shots over the years. Some hip shots. He didn't know if he had ever heard of penicillin or if he had ever had any. He said he had never heard of syphilis. He had heard of "bad blood" but didn't know what it meant.

Interview #4

Subject had gotten into the program when people were going around giving treatment. He didn't know what kind of treatment or what the treatment was for. They drew blood. Had them come up at different times. They never told him anything. Never said they tested the blood. Never said anything was wrong. Did not say why they were testing (the subjects).

The first contact he had with the study was in church. "Lady came down talking about what they would do." It was on a Sunday. Said go to city hall for blood tests. He went. Then he got a letter saying they wanted to see him. He got a letter each year.

Each year they took blood. Sat down and talked. Gave them some medicine. He went every time. No one said anything to him about his health. Nurse Rivers asked him how he was.

Asked about his health, subject said he'd been getting along o.k. He had had shots (sometime) in his arm. He had seen no private doctors. Nothing was said about his blood. He had no good friends in the program. Had known some—all dead and gone. He didn't know the causes of death (of his friends).

He didn't know why they wanted him to be in the program. He didn't think it was helping him. He just went along.

The subject is in his 70's. He had gone through the second grade.

TESTIMONY BY FOUR SURVIVORS FROM THE UNITED STATES SENATE HEARINGS ON HUMAN EXPERIMENTATION, 1973

SENATOR KENNEDY: Maybe we could talk a little bit with Mr. Scott and Mr. Pollard.

Maybe both of you gentlemen would be kind enough to tell us a little bit how you were first enrolled in the study, how you heard about it, if you can remember back to those days, how you became enrolled.

Let's start with you, Mr. Pollard. Would you tell us a little bit about how you heard about this study, how you became involved?

MR. POLLARD: Back in 1932, I was going to school back then and they came around and said they wanted to have a clinic blood testing up there.

SENATOR KENNEDY: How old were you then?

MR. POLLARD: How old was I? Well, I was born in 1906. I had been married— no, I hadn't been married. Anyhow, they came around give us the blood tests. After they give us the blood tests, all up there in the community, they said we had bad blood. After then they started giving us the shots and give us the shots for a good long time. I don't remember how long it was. But after they got through giving us those shots, they give me a spinal tap. That was along in 1933. They taken me over to John Henry Hospital.

SENATOR KENNEDY: That is rather unpleasant, isn't it, a spinal tap!

MR. POLLARD: It was pretty bad with me.

SENATOR KENNEDY: I have had a spinal tap myself. They stick that big, long needle into your spine.

MR. POLLARD: That is right, at John Andrew Hospital. After that, we went over early that morning, a couple of loads of us, and they taken us upstairs after giving us the spinal shot. They sit me down in the chair and the nurse and the doctor got behind and give me the shot. Then they take us upstairs in the elevators, our heels up and head down. They kept us there until five o'clock that evening, and then the nurse brought us back home.

These hearings were convened by Senator Edward Kennedy in 1973 over widespread concern with abuse in human experimentation, including the Tuskegee Study.
Originally published in Quality of Health Care: Human Experimentation, 1973, *Hearings before the Subcommittee on Health of the Committee on Labor and Public Welfare, 93rd Cong. (Washington, D.C., 1973), 3:1036–43, 1210–14.*

After then, I stayed in the bed. I had taken down a day or two after I got through with the spinal tap. I stayed in bed 10 days or two weeks and the nurse came out there and give me some pills. I don't think she give me any of the medicine at that time, but just gave me some of the pills. Anyhow, she made several trips out there and I finally got in pretty good shape afterwards. It looked like my head was going back.

So after then they went to seen us once a year. They sent out notices for us to meet at Shiloh School. Sometimes they would just take the blood sample and give us some medicine right there at the school, under the oak tree where we met at Shiloh.

SENATOR KENNEDY: This is a small community?

MR. POLLARD: It is a small community.

SENATOR KENNEDY: How many people are in the community?

MR. POLLARD: Well, Tuskegee is about 12,000, but this other little place up there I imagine is a couple thousand people there. I am about three and a half miles out.

SENATOR KENNEDY: What would you do, come into town?

MR. POLLARD: That is right, go into town.

SENATOR KENNEDY: Did they have a little clinic there or a little hospital?

MR. POLLARD: They didn't have any of that.

SENATOR KENNEDY: What did you do, just meet under the tree?

MR. POLLARD: Yes, at Shiloh School. It was about two and a half miles out. It is 10 miles between there and Tuskegee.

SENATOR KENNEDY: What did they do, ask you to come back once in a while or every couple of weeks?

MR. POLLARD: That is it. They would give us the date to come back and take those shots.

SENATOR KENNEDY: What were the shots for, to cure the bad blood?

MR. POLLARD: Bad blood, as far as I know of.

SENATOR KENNEDY: Did you think they were curing bad blood?

MR. POLLARD: I didn't know. I just attended the clinic.

SENATOR KENNEDY: They told you to keep coming back and you did?

MR. POLLARD: When they got through giving the shots, yes. Then they give us that spinal puncture.

SENATOR KENNEDY: Did they tell you why they were giving a spinal puncture?

MR. POLLARD: No.

SENATOR KENNEDY: Did you think it was because they were trying to help you?

MR. POLLARD: To help me, yes.

SENATOR KENNEDY: You wanted some help?

MR. POLLARD: That is right. They said I had bad blood and they was working on it.

SENATOR KENNEDY: How long did they keep working on it?

MR. POLLARD: After that shot, that spinal shot—

SENATOR KENNEDY: When was that?

MR. POLLARD: That was in 1933.

SENATOR KENNEDY: 1933?

MR. POLLARD: That is right. I don't remember what month it was in, but I know it was in 1933.

SENATOR KENNEDY: Did they treat you after that? Did they treat you after 1933?

MR. POLLARD: Yes. They treat me every year. They would come down and see us every year. Of course, during that time, after I taken that spinal puncture, I wore a rubber belt around my stomach. It had a long strand around it and I would run it around, come back in front and tie it in a bow knot. They used a little ointment or salve that I rubbed on my stomach. I reckon I wore it a year or six months, something like that. After then they would see us once a year up to 25 years.

SENATOR KENNEDY: During this time, did they indicate to you what kind of treatment they were giving you, or that you were involved in any kind of test or experiment?

MR. POLLARD: No, they never did say what it was.

SENATOR KENNEDY: What did you think they were doing, just trying to cure the bad blood?

MR. POLLARD: That is all I knew of.

SENATOR KENNEDY: Did they ever take any more blood and examine it and tell you the blood was getting better?

MR. POLLARD: They would take out blood, though.

SENATOR KENNEDY: What did they tell you after they would take the blood?

MR. POLLARD: They would just give us the pills and sometimes they would give us a little tablet to put under our tongue for sore throats. Then they would give us the green medicine for a tonic to take after meals.

SENATOR KENNEDY: You thought they were treating the bad blood?

MR. POLLARD: That is right.

SENATOR KENNEDY: During this time did they ever give you any compensation or any money?

MR. POLLARD: After that 25 years they gave me $25, a $20 and a $5 bill.

SENATOR KENNEDY: After 25 years?

MR. POLLARD: That is it. They give me a certificate.

SENATOR KENNEDY: They gave you a what?

MR. POLLARD: They gave me a certificate and a picture with six of us on there.

SENATOR KENNEDY: What did the certificate say, do you remember?

MR. POLLARD: This is one of them here in my hand.

SENATOR KENNEDY: It is a certificate of merit, is it?

"U.S. Public Health Service. This certificate is awarded in grateful recognition of 25 years of participation in the Tuskegee Medical Research Study."

MR. POLLARD: I have one of these and then I have one with a picture of five more on it.

SENATOR KENNEDY: Were you glad to get it? Were you glad to get that certificate?

MR. POLLARD: Yes.

SENATOR KENNEDY: You were glad to get the $25.

MR. POLLARD: That is right. I used the $25.

SENATOR KENNEDY: Did they ever offer you anything else? Did they ever offer you any kind of free meals or free rides, anything like that?

MR. POLLARD: No. We would have a lunch when we would go over to the Veterans Hospital. We would go to the canteen and have lunch. A lot of times I went in my own car and I would help the nurse carry the boys down there sometimes, a lot of times. I would always go in my car a lot of times.

SENATOR KENNEDY: Sometime last fall did you hear or read about the experiment that was taking place, the study that was taking place on you and some of the others that were supposed to have bad blood?

MR. POLLARD: Back last year?

SENATOR KENNEDY: Yes.

MR. POLLARD: Yes.

SENATOR KENNEDY: Would you tell us a little bit about that, how you first heard about it, and what your reaction was to it?

MR. POLLARD: The people that contacted me at the stockyard—

SENATOR KENNEDY: Is that where you worked?

MR. POLLARD: That is where I worked when they contacted me. A heavy built lady contacted me.

SENATOR KENNEDY: How long have you worked at the stockyard.

MR. POLLARD: I wasn't working out there. I was taking some cows down there last summer, my grandboy and myself.

SENATOR KENNEDY: How old is he?

MR. POLLARD: The grandboy?

SENATOR KENNEDY: Yes.

MR. POLLARD: He is 17.

SENATOR KENNEDY: So you were taking some cows down to the stockyard?

MR. POLLARD: That is it. I was taking the cows down there. A lady came up to me and asked about Charles Pollard. I looked at my grandboy and said, "I didn't know Charles Pollard. I knew Charles Wesley Pollard," and she said, "Yes, you are the one." She said she had been all over and asked about me but nobody had seen me. But I had been on the payroll bringing cows down there.

Afterwards, she told me to go ahead and get my cows unloaded and to come back out there, that she wanted to talk with me. So that is what I did.

SENATOR KENNEDY: So you went out and talked to her?

MR. POLLARD: That is right.

SENATOR KENNEDY: What did she tell you?

MR. POLLARD: She asked me wasn't I in a study or a clinic back 40 years ago. I looked at my grandboy then and he looked back. I had done forgot about it. I said, "Yes, I was in a clinic back in that time but I have done forgot about it." So she wanted to know the story of it.

You see, after them 25 years, the doctors started them two years and after that went for about three years. I haven't seen them in the last three or four years.

SENATOR KENNEDY: You haven't seen them in the last three or four years?

MR. POLLARD: No. I told her the best I could about it, what I could remember.

SENATOR KENNEDY: Were you surprised when you heard about it?

MR. POLLARD: That is right. I was surprised.

SENATOR KENNEDY: Were you a little mad that you were sort of being used in a test that you didn't know about?

MR. POLLARD: Well, at that time, you see, I didn't know nothing about it until well after I got back home. I had taken the Birmingham News. I have been taking it for 25 or 30 years. It was there. What I told her was in the Birmingham News that evening. So we read it, got to reading it, and talking about black men in Macon County. Of course, the week before then they had told in the news there about 400 or 600 men, whatever it was, the black men in Macon County, but I didn't give it even a thought, until after she told me that. That was on a Tuesday when she saw me.

SENATOR KENNEDY: Have you seen any doctors since then? Have any doctors come down to see you and help you at all recently?

MR. POLLARD: Not lately.

SENATOR KENNEDY: In the last few months?

MR. POLLARD: No. The Government doctors, no. I had been visiting a doctor, some individual doctors. Of course, I had a bad case of arthritis last year, in the last week in January. I went to Montgomery to a doctor for a month. He give an X-ray on me and sent me back to the bone specialist in Tuskegee. He doctored on me for about a month and I got on crutches and stayed on them. He finally told me to go back home. If it never did get no worse, don't come back. So I am still taking medicine, capsules that he give me. That was after he give me that shot in the hip.

SENATOR KENNEDY: Did you get any bill from the doctor for seeing him about your arthritis?

MR. POLLARD: Did I get a bill from him?

SENATOR KENNEDY: Yes.

MR. POLLARD: No, because I paid him each time.

SENATOR KENNEDY: You paid him?

MR. POLLARD: Yes, each time. That was my doctor.

SENATOR KENNEDY: How much do you pay for a visit down there?

MR. POLLARD: The X-ray cost me $25 and the medicine one time cost me $15.

SENATOR KENNEDY: That one X-ray was equivalent to the $25 you got from the Government.

MR. POLLARD: That is right. And after then I went back and got some medicine. I think I had to pay him $10 that trip. He didn't make the X-ray until to wind it up. Then he sent me back to Dr. Hume, in Tuskegee.

SENATOR KENNEDY: Did you pay him, too?

MR. POLLARD: Dr. Hume? That is right.

SENATOR KENNEDY: Do you remember how much that was?

MR. POLLARD: I paid him $15, I think, the first time. On the next trip I think I paid him $10. But I have been buying the medicine. I bought the medicine and I paid for the medicine at the desk.

SENATOR KENNEDY: It runs into a lot of money, doesn't it?

MR. POLLARD: Yes, when you go to these hospitals. Of course, back in 1961 I had an operation. I had a gland operation.

SENATOR KENNEDY: Mr. Scott, would you tell us a little bit about how you heard about this?

MR. SCOTT: Yes. In 1932, we were all on the farm and going to school and Miss Rivers came out and Dr. Smith. He said he wanted to see all of us people around there, to meet at the school. So we went out and he said the purpose was to take the test of blood. So he drew blood and we went back home.

He said to be out here next Wednesday. We went back and he said, "You have bad blood and we will have to give you shots." So we would go up every week or sometimes every other week, and take shots. That is how I got involved in that. I had taken the shots for a good long while and then left the county to go to another community, but we would meet with him.

SENATOR KENNEDY: How long did you take the shots?

MR. SCOTT: We were taking those shots for about a year, almost a year.

SENATOR KENNEDY: Did you receive any compensation for this?

MR. SCOTT: I was away up in Ohio. At the time they wrote a letter to my sister and they sent $25. They said it was for the study, with Miss Rivers.

SENATOR KENNEDY: Is that the first time that you knew you were involved in a study?

MR. SCOTT: I was involved in it before I left. This time, this study now, I got involved through Miss Rivers, I believe it was.

SENATOR KENNEDY: What did you think they were giving the shots for?

MR. SCOTT: Bad blood.

SENATOR KENNEDY: They just told you it was for bad blood?

MR. SCOTT: Yes.

SENATOR KENNEDY: Did you think the shots were making you better?

MR. SCOTT: I thought they would at that time.

SENATOR KENNEDY: Is that what the doctor told you who gave you the shots?

MR. SCOTT: Yes. He told me it was for bad blood.

SENATOR KENNEDY: And sometime later you got the $25?

MR. SCOTT: Yes. It was six or seven years after I left.

SENATOR KENNEDY: Did you get a certificate of appreciation, too?

MR. SCOTT: No, I did not.

SENATOR KENNEDY: But you heard that some of the others got it.

How did you feel after you read in the newspapers that you had been involved in this kind of study or experiment? Did that bother you at all?

MR. SCOTT: Well, not too much at that time because I was thinking of my health, figuring they were doing me good. So I didn't think too much of it. I thought it would be all right.

And then when this study came along. I don't think much of it because I think they were just using me for something else, as an experiment.

SENATOR KENNEDY: Do you think that is right?

MR. SCOTT: No, I don't think that is right.

SENATOR KENNEDY: Do you think they should have told you about it?

MR. SCOTT: I think they should have told. If they had told, I would have resorted to a family doctor or some other doctor.

SENATOR KENNEDY: You would have gone to your family doctor and got treated?

MR. SCOTT: Yes.

SENATOR KENNEDY: You thought you were being treated?

MR. SCOTT: I thought I was being treated then.

SENATOR KENNEDY: And you were not?

MR. SCOTT: I was not.

SENATOR KENNEDY: That is not right, is it?

MR. SCOTT: No, it is not right.

SENATOR KENNEDY: What do you think the Government ought to do now?

MR. SCOTT: I think the Government ought to do something as they were using us. They ought to give us compensation or something like that, where we can see other doctors and continue our health. That is what I think.

SENATOR KENNEDY: You want to make sure that the next time you see a Government doctor that he is treating you to get you better.

MR. SCOTT: That is right.

SENATOR KENNEDY: That is what you want.

MR. SCOTT: And I can be sure I go to the right doctor.

SENATOR KENNEDY: What about you, Mr. Pollard? What would you like?

MR. POLLARD: This I read in the paper I don't want no parts of it.

I was fixing to say I was booked to go to Birmingham when this penicillin come out, but the nurse told me I wasn't able to go up there. So they turned me down. I don't want no more part of it.

SENATOR KENNEDY: Mr. Scott and Mr. Pollard, when you were talking to these doctors that were giving you these shots, did they ever suggest to you or recommend to you that you not have a family?

MR. SCOTT: No, they did not.

MR. POLLARD: Not what?

SENATOR KENNEDY: Not have a family. Did they ever recommend to you that you not have a family?

MR. POLLARD: No, they never said anything about that.

SENATOR KENNEDY: They never mentioned that?

MR. POLLARD: No.

SENATOR KENNEDY: Mr. Gray, have you any further comments?

MR. GRAY: I would simply like to say, Senator Kennedy, on behalf of these participants we certainly want to express our genuine appreciation for being able to come. At least now this committee knows the views of the participants, and we certainly hope that this subcommittee and the Congress will take appropriate action to see that these people are adequately compensated.

Thank you.

SENATOR KENNEDY: I want to thank you very much for coming. As you know several months ago, some four months ago, the Department of HEW indicated that they were going to move on this to try and remedy or rectify the situation.

The commission met on March 1 and indicated that still there had been no care forthcoming. We had another commitment pledge by the Secretary that there would be action. I want to indicate to you that we are going to make sure, as far as the power of this Senate Subcommittee, that there will be help and assistance and care for all of those individuals.

It is absolutely an outrageous and intolerable situation which this Government never should have been involved in. That is bad enough, but we are going to do everything in our power to work with Mr. Pollard and Mr. Scott, and all of the others who still need the help, and the heirs of the others as well.

I want to give those assurances to you, Mr. Pollard and Mr. Scott. We will look forward to working with you.

MR. GRAY: We have waited really, Senator, about nine months on the Government to take some action before we would take any legal action. The Government simply moves very slowly and time is beginning to run out on us.

Thank you.

SENATOR KENNEDY: We are going to stay after it and we will work with you.

I want to thank both of you gentlemen for your appearance here, for your willingness to share with us your experience. It has been very, very helpful.

SENATOR KENNEDY: Could we hear from either Mr. Shaw or Mr. Howard.

Mr. Shaw, did you sometimes leave Tuskegee County and travel to another place, and did the Public Health Service offices in the new county attempt to treat the syphilis?

MR. SHAW: No sir.

MR. GRAY: He lives right on the county line, just out of Macon County in an adjoining county. That is how he ended up being sent to Birmingham.

SENATOR KENNEDY: Maybe he could just tell us a little bit about his experience.

MR. SHAW: Mr. Chairman, would you like to know how I became involved in the study?

SENATOR KENNEDY: Yes, in your own words.

MR. SHAW: For those who are living and remember, and for those who just read about it, in 1932 we began to emerge from what was known as the Hoover panic. We did not have adequate money, in other words, to care for our families. This offer was made in 1932 as free medication known as a blood test. I entered it in 1932 and was affiliated with it ever since.

Every 4 years they would take our blood. They would transport us to the Tuskegee VA hospital and give us a thorough examination.

In the late 1940's—I do not remember the exact date—they sent me to Birmingham. We left about 2 o'clock and we got to Birmingham before dark. They gave us our supper and put us to bed. The next morning they gave us breakfast. I saw a nurse roaming through the crowd. She said she had been worried all night. She said that she had been looking for a man that was not supposed to be here and his name is Herman Shaw. Naturally I stood up. She said come here.

She said what are you doing up here? I said I do not know, they sent me here. They got me a bus and sent me back home. When I notified the nurse of what happened in Macon County, I did not get any response.

SENATOR KENNEDY: Did you feel during this period that you were being cured, that they were looking after your medical needs?

MR. SHAW: I have never had any treatment whatever.

SENATOR KENNEDY: What did they tell you when they looked at your blood? Did they tell you it looked good or looked bad?

MR. SHAW: I just got a slap on the back and they said you are good for 100 years. That is all I ever had.

SENATOR KENNEDY: How many years have they been slapping you on your back?

MR. SHAW: Forty years.

SENATOR KENNEDY: You were in this study for 40 years?

MR. SHAW: Yes, sir.

SENATOR KENNEDY: Did they give you any kind of compensation while they were doing this study?

MR. SHAW: No sir, with the exception of a 25-year certificate.

SENATOR KENNEDY: Twenty-five year what?

MR. SHAW: Twenty-five year health certificate. They gave us a dollar a year, $25.

SENATOR KENNEDY: A dollar a year?

MR. SHAW: Yes sir. Up to that time, from 1932, up until the time the 25-year limit ran out.

SENATOR KENNEDY: So the only compensation you have received has been the $25?

MR. SHAW: That is right.

SENATOR KENNEDY: And the certificate of merit?

MR. SHAW: Yes, sir.

SENATOR KENNEDY: What was the certificate of merit for?

MR. SHAW: I do not know, sir. It was for regular attendance, that is all I can figure.

SENATOR KENNEDY: Do you think it is because you kept going back to the nurse or the doctor and letting them take your blood as they told you to do?

MR. SHAW: Yes, sir.

SENATOR KENNEDY: When you were told to go back, did you think this was a check up and that since they didn't prescribe medication, that therefore you were healthy? What did you assume?

MR. SHAW: Every year they would give us a white tablet for pain and a little vial—I guess it was some type of tonic. Every year for 40 years up to now, we had two different doctors. We would never get the same doctor back each time.

SENATOR KENNEDY: Different doctors?

MR. SHAW: Different doctor every year.

SENATOR KENNEDY: When was the last time you were at a clinic?

MR. SHAW: Last year.

SENATOR KENNEDY: What did they tell you last year?

MR. SHAW: Slap on the back and said I was good for 100 years. I guess it was routine.

SENATOR KENNEDY: They gave you tablets in case you had any pain?

MR. SHAW: Yes.

SENATOR KENNEDY: Did you ever have to take those tablets?

MR. SHAW: Sometimes. Sometimes they would stay in the bottle until they were brown as that wall.

SENATOR KENNEDY: What did you think when you read about the news of the story, when the story broke about this experiment that you were a part of? What was your reaction to it?

MR. SHAW: Being personally acquainted with Attorney Gray, I went to his office for advice and carried him the information I had received.

SENATOR KENNEDY: Were you surprised to read that this experiment was taking place and that you had been a part of it?

MR. SHAW: Yes, sir; I certainly was surprised.

SENATOR KENNEDY: Were you happy or were you sad?

MR. SHAW: I was sad in a way, and I was happy with the consolation that Mr. Gray gave me.

SENATOR KENNEDY: Have your lives changed very much down there, Mr. Shaw, after the publicity in the community?

MR. SHAW: Beg pardon?

SENATOR KENNEDY: Have the people in the town or community treated you any differently after the news came out?

MR. SHAW: No, sir. In a way they seemed to be very hopeful, those in the study that I have talked with.

SENATOR KENNEDY: What do you think that the Federal Government ought to do now?

MR. SHAW: Having made the sacrifices, I think we should be paid.

SENATOR KENNEDY: Fair compensation for this?

MR. SHAW: Yes, sir.

SENATOR KENNEDY: They have had this experiment with you, you have been a part of it 40-odd years?

MR. SHAW: Yes, sir.

SENATOR KENNEDY: I suppose you realize that when the Federal Government participates in these other studies they compensate people. All you are trying to get is the same kind of compensation?

MR. SHAW: That is right.

SENATOR KENNEDY: At this time you want to make sure you get some decent health care, too, I imagine.

MR. SHAW: I am glad you mentioned that. The man that came offered me medicare, medication, and what have you.

SENATOR KENNEDY: Which man is this?

MR. SHAW: I do not know who he was. He came and left a letter at my house and left a card. I work from 2 until 10.

SENATOR KENNEDY: Where do you work?

MR. GRAY: Tallassee Mill.

SENATOR KENNEDY: How long have you worked there?

MR. SHAW: Forty-four years and working there now. I am 70.

SENATOR KENNEDY: You are 70?

MR. SHAW: Yes, sir.

SENATOR KENNEDY: I think you are going to live to be 100 years.

MR. SHAW: I told the man that I have Medicare. I have medication and hospital insurance. I can walk. I do not see any need for anybody holding my arm. I can stand on my own feet and walk. I had everything they offered me and so compensation is what I need now.

SENATOR KENNEDY: Mr. Howard, we want to welcome you here. Maybe you could tell us a little about your experience.

MR. HOWARD: About who has been at my place?

SENATOR KENNEDY: Tell us a little bit about how you got involved.

MR. HOWARD: I hardly know how I got involved in it. I was involved in it in 1932. They were having school in the church, and I think the teacher put out a notice for everybody in the community to meet out there on a certain date. Dr. Smith and I were the first two, I remember. At the end of a 2 hour meeting, they started taking blood, checking temperatures, heartbeat, blood system, and all of that. I got the same thing for about 40 years, I guess. I did get $25, and I do not know if it was for appreciation or they just decided they would give me something because I was so good about meeting them every time.

SENATOR KENNEDY: You met with them every time you were supposed to?

MR. HOWARD: Yes, sir.

SENATOR KENNEDY: They gave you $25 too?

MR. HOWARD: They gave me $25 and a 25-year certificate for being with them that long. I think I got that in 1958.

SENATOR KENNEDY: When was the last time you saw the doctor?

MR. HOWARD: I saw him last year in June.

SENATOR KENNEDY: June of this past year?

MR. HOWARD: Yes, sir, last year in June.

SENATOR KENNEDY: What did the doctor tell you?

MR. HOWARD: He just gave me some pills and some medicine out of a bottle and said she would see me soon. That was last year in June, and I have not seen her since.

SENATOR KENNEDY: What did you think was happening when you saw these doctors over the period of these years? Did you think they were giving you a clean bill of health?

MR. HOWARD: I hardly know. I had bad blood and they said they were working on it.

SENATOR KENNEDY: Did they indicate to you your blood was getting better?

MR. HOWARD: No, sir, they didn't say—or getting worse—

SENATOR KENNEDY: When you heard about the study what did you do? Were you very much concerned about it?

MR. HOWARD: Yes. When I first heard about it, I did not give it too much attention. I first read it in the paper. The next time I heard it broadcast on the TV. Every time they would come by, I would read something, but I could not understand what it meant.

SENATOR KENNEDY: What did you do about it? Did you try to find Mr. Gray?

MR. HOWARD: I went to hunt Mr. Gray several different times, but it was a long time before I could catch him.

SENATOR KENNEDY: He is a busy man working in the legislature, and I am sure tries to help the people.

Then you had either a letter or visit from somebody recently, as I understand, telling you that your medical bills were going to be looked out after. Do you remember that?

MR. HOWARD: Yes. A man came to my house—

SENATOR KENNEDY: How long ago was that?

MR. HOWARD: About 3 weeks ago. He left me a letter to read. Everything he promised me I already had, medicaid and medicare, and private insurance.

He said he would be back Thursday about 12 o'clock. But he came back Thursday about 9 o'clock that morning, and I told him I did not need that because I already had it. He did not say anything.

SENATOR KENNEDY: So you already had what the Public Health Service was offering you, is that right?

MR. HOWARD: Yes, I already had that.

SENATOR KENNEDY: What do you think you need? What do you want them to do for you?

MR. HOWARD: I need some money, that is what I need.

SENATOR KENNEDY: You think you ought to be compensated like others in the country are compensated when they are made a part of tests like that? You are asking that you be treated the same as other people are treated in this respect, is that right?

MR. HOWARD: Yes.

SENATOR KENNEDY: I want to thank both of you gentlemen, Mr. Howard and Mr. Shaw, for coming up here. As we indicated, we are going to pursue this issue and work with you to make sure that justice is done in this case.

We want to let you know personally that I and the committee are committed to making sure that you get the things which you need now and in the future. We are very glad that you are here.

MR. GRAY: Thank you very much.

SENATOR KENNEDY: We want to thank you, Representative Gray, for being with us. You have effectively pushed this issue, and I know the people involved value highly your counsel and guidance. We want to tell you how much we have appreciated working with you on this matter.

MR. GRAY: Thank you very much.

TESTIMONY BY PETER BUXTON FROM THE UNITED STATES SENATE HEARINGS ON HUMAN EXPERIMENTATION, 1973

Statement of Peter Buxton, Law Student, San Francisco, Calif.

MR. BUXTON: Thank you, Mr. Chairman. In hearing the statements that the gentlemen who just left made, I have a copy of that 25-year certificate of appreciation if you would care to see it. I do not know if you have seen one previously. Perhaps later I could show it to you.

I could read it to you if you would like to have it in your record.

SENATOR KENNEDY: All right.

MR. BUXTON: It is a form copy of what I have here, a Xerox, large type at the top. It says the U.S. Public Health Service, and then there is a circle about the size of a half dollar with the number 25 in it. It says: "This certificate is awarded to"—and then a participant's name is typed in—"in grateful recognition of 25 years of active participation in the Tuskegee medical research study."

At the bottom it says "Awarded 1958."

There is a seal of the U.S. Public Health Service and a signature of the Surgeon General.

Now as to my involvement, being that I was a resident in San Francisco, physically removed from Tuskegee, I suppose the best way that I would have giving this would be to read the statement that I prepared, which is a brief synopsis.

In December of 1965 I was hired as an interviewer/investigator by the U.S. Public Health Service and was assigned to the Venereal Disease Clinic then operated by the city of San Francisco at 33 Hunt Street. I was given a training course in the medical effects, diagnosis, and treatment of VD and was given further on-the-job training at the clinic. While my work dealt primarily with patients in the early—infectious—stages of syphilis, I saw numbers of patients undergoing diagnosis and treatment for late syphilis.

Peter Buxton, now an attorney in San Francisco, was a venereal disease investigator with the Public Health Service in San Francisco in the 1960s. His persistent questioning of the study and the information he provided to the Associated Press led to the study's public exposure in 1972.
Originally published in Quality of Health Care: Human Experimentation, 1973, *Hearings before the Subcommittee on Health of the Committee on Labor and Public Welfare, 93rd Cong. (Washington, D.C., 1973), 3:1223–28.*

In the fall of 1966 I overheard an older fellow worker discussing the Tuskegee study. As I recall, most of us had heard something of this and the earlier—1891–1910 Oslo, Norway, study of untreated human syphilis. The effects of untreated syphilis figured prominently in both my prejob training and the information we helped disseminate to doctors and the public.

On this occasion, however, I was startled by being told of a Tuskegee participant who had gone insane and had been diagnosed syphilitic and then treated by a private physician. My friend said that CDC—the Communicable Disease Center, USPHS, Atlanta—had been annoyed by this as it jogged their statistics. He said that private physicians and public clinics in the Tuskegee area had been notified not to treat men participating in the study that this insane individual had been brought to a doctor out of the geographic area of this notification.

Part of my job was to write a bimonthly research narrative on some subject related to our work. I wrote to CDC in Atlanta requesting information on the Tuskegee study and was surprised to receive what seemed to be the entire, nearly complete file of published reports. I did not request nor did I receive any individual medical data.

Upon reading the reports, I was shocked by the statements such as: "An important phase of the study has been the performance of autopsies." "Mortality and morbidity are consistently higher among the untreated syphilitics," and other passages which indicated the participants did not realize what was happening to them. There were some comments which talked about one of the participants being asked about pains in his chest. Perhaps you know one of the effects, one of the deadly effects of those who are killed by syphilis is chest pain, perhaps caused by enlargement of the aorta. One of the public health documents that we used to hand out to physicians had a fantastic picture of an individual with a lump on his chest the size of his fist. This was his aorta having eaten itself way out of the front of his chest.

These participants were asked about these chest pains and in the report which I was at that time reading, it said, well this man when asked if he had any chest pains, any difficulty walking upstairs, heavy labor, he made a comment that with his old mule he could plow all day, but with his new or younger mule he could not do that.

That was the level that the people seemed to understand, their physical involvement, that they seemed not to comprehend or even care much about syphilis, that they were more concerned with the weather and how it effected their crops. That is sort of path raising what was in there.

Upon reflection, I excerpted sections from these reports and from other sources, including the Proceedings of the International Military Tribunal, Nuremburg, into an attack upon the moral justification for the study. I pointed out that the Tuskegee study could be compared to the German medical experiments at Dachau and that public disclosure of such a scandal could jeopardize congressional funding for other beneficial PHS projects.

My superiors were shocked at what I had done, afraid of losing my job—my boss thought he was going to be fired along with me—but after warning me that I would probably be fired, they agreed to forward my report to CDC.

SENATOR KENNEDY: Why did they feel you were going to be fired, and why did your boss fear for the loss of security?

MR. BUXTON: I was possibly the lowest cog on the wheel of the organization at that time.

SENATOR KENNEDY: Would they not want to find out about this kind of situation? Would they not welcome this kind of suggestion?

MR. BUXTON: That is a difficult question for me to answer, sir. Nobody in the position in a bureaucracy likes to rock the boat. This was very definitely boat rocking of the type that was not ever expected, was not encouraged, was not discouraged, just was not thought to be a thing to have happened.

Also my boss did not think that anyone in CDC would appreciate the comparison of their work to the work of Dachau. It was a pretty drastic thing that I did.

I did not however feel that the report would attract enough attention, so on November 9, 1966, I wrote a personal letter to Dr. William J. Brown, Chief of the Venereal Disease Branch of CDC. This letter preceded my report by about 1 week and was written as a private citizen. In it, I questioned the volunteer status of the participants and, among other things, asked whether untreated syphilitics were still being followed for autopsy. I have a copy of this letter with me.

The initial reaction seemed to be shocked silence. Recently when I testified before the DHEW ad hoc investigation I was given a draft copy of a reply to my letter which I never received. Instead, I was informally interviewed by a high-level administrator from CDC who was spending Christmas with relatives in San Francisco. I elaborated to him what I felt was wrong and he said he would convey my stand to Dr. Brown. Nothing happened for a couple of months.

About 3 months later I was flown to CDC Atlanta where I met with Dr. William J. Brown, three other administrators, and one of the doctors who had set up the Tuskegee study. I have a copy of Dr. Brown's memo on this meeting. I recall being ushered into a large conference room and getting a rather stern lecture from the doctor who had been instrumental in setting up the study. After he outlined the details and supposed benefits, he asked if I had any questions.

I then read excerpts from the Tuskegee reports and I vividly recall his reaction to hearing one part. He jumped up saying: "Let me see that, I didn't write that, it must have been written by one of my colleagues."

The excerpt mentioned that without the "suasion"—that is the word used in the report—without the suasion of free transportation, free hot lunches, burial benefits, and treatment for other disease, it would have been impossible to secure the cooperation of the participants and their families.

At that point the conversation changed more from a lecture—they were sort of placating me; they could not understand why I brought all of this up. Apparently none of them was aware of it, including the doctor who had originally participated in setting up the study. We then had maybe a 10-minute discussion of what should be done. I said I thought the people should be treated. I was then told that people who are elderly and have syphilis, that there is a certain risk. I do not know if you are familiar with the reaction that often or sometimes follows treatment for active syphilis. I have seen a number of patients go through this reaction, headache, chills, and fever, and some people become quite frightened that they are dying.

I was told this is often enough to preclude treatment of elderly persons, who otherwise do not have any visible symptoms of long-term syphilis.

About a year later I left the Public Health Service and went to law school. I continued a correspondence with Dr. Brown and suggested continually these people either be treated or something be done about the study. I have copies of this correspondence. In this correspondence I have a letter from Dr. Brown which I believe misstates a few facts. If you would like, I could either read this letter for you or submit it to be put into your record.

SENATOR KENNEDY: We will put it in the record.

[The letter referred to follows:]

February 27, 1969
Mr. Peter J. Buxtun
1730 Kearny Street
San Francisco, California 94133
Dear Mr. Buxtun:

I have delayed answering your letter of late November 1968 until a planned review of the Tuskegee Study was completed.

Following the review we assembled a committee of professionals from outside the National Communicable Disease Center to consider all aspects of this long-term study, including the point you have made in your letter; namely: treating the remaining persons in the study group.

After an examination of the data and a very lengthy discussion regarding treatment, our committee of highly competent professionals did not agree nor recommend that the study group be treated. The youngest living member of the study group is 69 years old. The question of treating persons of this age and older, unless it is demonstrated that active disease is present, is a matter of medical judgment since the benefits of such therapy must be offset against the risks to the individual.

We will be working with the State Health Department, the Macon County Health Department and the local Medical Society of Tuskegee to assure that all possible individual attention be given to people who participated in the study. To this end we will continue to augment the staff available in Macon County.

You can be assured that competent professionals have studied the point you made and that each person still in the study will be evaluated fully.
Sincerely yours,
William J. Brown, M.D.
Chief, Venereal Disease Branch

MR. BUXTON: Beyond that, there is not much that I have to say. While I was in law school, I contacted several professors and told them this story. I told the story a number of times to many people. Dean Prosser, who was until his death one of the country's authorities on torts, discouraged me and said it would merely be stirring up litigation to do anything about this study. I finally in desperation mentioned the story to a friend of mine in the Associated Press and she in cooperation with Ms. Heller broke the story to the public and we now have the current situation.

When the story was broken, I did travel to Tuskegee. Ms. Heller and I interviewed some people there, and I was quite bothered by the fact that these people, participants, probably now are absolutely noncontagious, probably were noncontagious at the time the study was begun, but nobody seems to care to publicize this. I tried to get some publicity for it in the local Tuskegee paper. I think this was done. I asked Mr. Gray about it earlier. He said, yes, there had been a small amount of publicity on this fact. I did not want the population of Tuskegee to shun these participants because they had had or at that time still had syphilis, and of course there were the controls.

SENATOR KENNEDY: What bothered you most about the study?

MR. BUXTON: The fact that the participants really did not seem to be consulted. They were being used. It was difficult for me to tell really what was going on from the geographical distance, from only the technical medical reports that I had to work on. It seemed apparent to me that these people had been told that they had a disease and that they could receive some benefits as they did some things, and in some sort of hazy way their cooperation was induced.

I do not use the word "consent." I felt that what was being done was very close to murder and was, if you will, an institutionalized form of murder and something the Public Health Service should have no part at. At that time I was an employee of the Public Health Service, and I felt that good work was being done and I could only see this damaging work of the Public Health Service.

SENATOR KENNEDY: Why do you think there was such reluctance, even going back to 1966, for others in the Department to move on this issue? This is not 1932 or 1934.

MR. BUXTON: Sir, I feel that it had become an accepted thing within the Public Health Service. Oh, yes, so and so over in that office is working on Tuskegee, and here is some data that we got, and nobody had paid any attention to it for years. It was just an ongoing thing, not subject to any review.

I think the review of 1969 was due to this confrontation that I just described to you. I think that was the first time it had occurred, to see what circumstances differed after the advent of penicillin, and before 1932, and they were shooting arsenic into people's veins, and anywhere from 1 out of every 2,000, 1 out of every 7,000 injections would cause death or other different things, I am sure you have had testimony on that. Nobody seemed to think of it.

There was one other factor, which if I might mention in conversations at the time the story was broken, I called various people at CDC, and I was told that there had been a great lack of leadership at that time in that particular area and that certain individuals had actually been demoted as a result of basic incompetence having nothing to do with Tuskegee. I cannot speak of any personal knowledge of this, but this was said to me in a telephone conversation.

SENATOR KENNEDY: Why did you come to feel that you had to take the route that you took in order to get some action?

MR. BUXTON: Sir, I got the idea that this is accepted, that it was published regularly, the Public Health Service wished to call some attention to the usefulness of the data that were being gained. The publications were not terribly interesting. They were generally in an obscure medical journal. I, on reflection, today, think what I did was a bit rash, but eventually it did lead to these results. I thought something needed to be done immediately, and I felt people were dying at that time. I did not feel that 1 or 2 years was an acceptable length of time to wait.

I, at the time, was eager to get something done then.

SENATOR KENNEDY: Did you find any other studies that were as troublesome as this to you?

MR. BUXTON: No, sir. The other thing that did bother me, quite far afield from here, I, at the time, was also bothered that I felt the Public Health Service statistics were being misused.

SENATOR KENNEDY: In what respect?

MR. BUXTON: I felt that there was an active program to sell the public on venereal disease epidemic and the extent to which this epidemic involved teen-agers. I found that there had been an extensive public relations job done with our statistics. Part of my job was to gather statistics. Part of my job was to go around and make sure the doctors reported every case that came through their office.

Then later I would notice that, say, a certain city perhaps in California, perhaps elsewhere would suddenly publicize—we have had a 45 percent increase in re-ported venereal disease. I would know that maybe three Federal investigators had been assigned to that city, and making them report. The doctors merely previously would treat someone, would not report, and would sort of neglect California statutes that would say these cases had to be reported, particularly with gonorrhea, not so much with syphilis—a large part of syphilis was reported. I felt a rather concerted program to harp on the fact that there was a lot of VD. I think the word

VD should be thrown out. I think it is basically misleading to the nature of the problem.

Most of the infection is gonorrhea, and nobody really dies of gonorrhea, and a small amount of syphilis. The information is packaged and says VD kills. Yes, syphilis kills, but most of it was gonorrhea. This was a report of estimated cases.

Then I noticed things like the National Hospital Association coming out with a big anti-VD program. I have contacted them. I found that they gathered most of their statistics from official Public Health Service reports.

They then tried to enlist volunteers to organize chapters or whatever and to pressure Congress to increase appropriations for Public Health treatment of venereal disease. It strikes me that somehow public money is being used to pump up and alter statistics into sort of handholding organizations that then pressure Congress. In other words, tax money is being used to lobby Congress. It is a long way around the circle, but I think somebody should look into it.

I have not had sufficient contact with it. I think what we have here is multimillion-dollar industry keeping charitable organizations and secretaries office space, and high priced personnel.

Again I am sorry if this had wandered off the field of Tuskegee, but you asked me what other problems I saw.

SENATOR KENNEDY: Thank you very much. We appreciate your appearance here and thank you for sharing your experience with us.

MR. BUXTON: Thank you, sir.

SELECTIONS FROM THE FINAL REPORT OF THE AD HOC TUSKEGEE SYPHILIS STUDY PANEL, DEPARTMENT OF HEALTH, EDUCATION AND WELFARE, 1973

April 28, 1973
Dr. Charles C. Edwards
Assistant Secretary for Health
U.S. Department of Health, Education, and Welfare
Washington, D.C. 20202

Dear Doctor Edwards:

The final report of the Tuskegee Syphilis Study Ad Hoc Advisory Panel is transmitted herewith. The Chairman specifically abstains from concurrence in this final report but recognizes his responsibility to submit it.

Sincerely yours,

Broadus N. Butler, Ph.D.
President
Dillard University

Charter

Tuskegee Syphilis Study Ad Hoc Advisory Panel to the Assistant Secretary for Health and Scientific Affairs

Purpose
To fulfill the public pledge of the Assistant Secretary for Health and Scientific Affairs to investigate the circumstances surrounding the Tuskegee, Alabama, study

The Ad Hoc Advisory Panel was convened by the U.S. Secretary for Health, Education and Welfare (now the Department of Health and Human Services) to investigate the circumstances surrounding the study.
Originally published as Final Report of the Tuskegee Syphilis Study Ad Hoc Advisory Panel *(Washington, D.C.: U.S. Department of Health, Education and Welfare, Public Health Service, 1973), 1–3, 6–15, 23–24, 47.*

of untreated syphilis in the male Negro initiated by the United States Public Health Service in 1932.

Authority

The committee is established under the provisions of Section 222 of the Public Health Service Act, as amended, 42 US Code 217a, and in accordance with the provisions of Executive Order 11671, which sets forth standards for the formation and use of advisory committees.

Function

The committee will advise the Assistant Secretary for Health and Scientific Affairs on the following specific aspects of the Tuskegee Syphilis Study:

Determine whether the study was justified in 1932 and whether it should have been continued when penicillin became generally available.

Recommend whether the study should be continued at this point in time, and if not, how it should be terminated in a way consistent with the rights and health needs of its remaining participants.

Determine whether existing policies to protect the rights of patients participating in health research conducted or supported by the Department of Health, Education, and Welfare are adequate and effective and to recommend improvements in these policies, if needed.

Structure

The committee will consist of nine members, including the Chairman, not otherwise in the full-time employ of the Federal Government. Members will be selected by the Assistant Secretary for Health and Scientific Affairs from citizens representing medicine, law, religion, labor, education, health administration, and public affairs.

The Panel members will be invited to serve for a period not to extend beyond December 31, 1972, unless an extension beyond that time is approved by the Assistant Secretary for Health and Scientific Affairs. The Assistant Secretary for Health and Scientific affairs will designate the Chairman.

Management and staff services will be provided by the Office of the Assistant Secretary for Health and Scientific Affairs.

Meetings

Meetings will be held at the call of the Chairman, with the advance approval of a Government official who shall also approve the agenda. A Government official will be present at all meetings.

Meetings shall be conducted, and records of the proceedings kept as required by Executive Order 11671 and applicable Departmental regulations.

Compensation

Members who are not full-time Federal employees will be paid at the rate of $100 per day for time spent at meetings, plus per diem and travel expenses in accordance with Standard Government Travel Regulations.

Annual Cost Estimate

Estimated annual cost for operating the committee, including compensation and travel expenses of members but excluding staff support, is $74,000. Estimate of annual man years of staff support required is one year at an estimated annual cost of $16,000.

Report

A final report based on the committee's investigation will be made to the Assistant Secretary for Health and Scientific Affairs. A copy of this report shall be provided to the Department Committee Management Officer.

The Tuskegee Syphilis Study Ad Hoc Advisory Panel to the Assistant Secretary for Health and Scientific Affairs will terminate on December 31, 1972, unless extension beyond that date is requested an approved.

FORMAL DETERMINATION

By authority delegated to me by the Secretary on September 29, 1969, I hereby determine that the formation of the *Tuskegee Syphilis Study Ad Hoc Advisory Panel to the Assistant Secretary for Health and Scientific Affairs* is in the public interest in connection with the performance of duties imposed on the Department by law, and that such duties can best be performed through the advice and counsel of such a group.

8/28/72(sgd.) Merlin K. DuVal, M.D.

Date Assistant Secretary for Health and Scientific Affairs

Charter

Tuskegee Syphilis Study Ad Hoc Advisory Panel to the Assistant Secretary for Health

Purpose

To fulfill the public pledge of the Assistant Secretary for Health to investigate the circumstances surrounding the Tuskegee, Alabama, study of untreated syphilis in the male Negro initiated by the United States Public Health Service in 1932.

Authority

The committee is established under the provisions of Section 222 of the Public Health Service Act, as amended, 42 US Code 217a; the Panel is governed by provisions of Executive Order 11671, which sets forth standards for the formation and use of advisory committees.

Function

The committee will advise the Assistant Secretary for Health on the following specific aspects of the Tuskegee Syphilis Study:

Determine whether the study was justified in 1932 and whether it should have been continued when penicillin became generally available.

Recommend whether the study should be continued at this point in time, and if not, how it should be terminated in a way consistent with the rights and health needs of its remaining participants.

Determine whether existing policies to protect the rights of patients participating in health research conducted or supported by the Department of Health, Education, and Welfare are adequate and effective and to recommend improvements in these policies, if needed.

Structure

The Tuskegee Syphilis Study Ad Hoc Advisory Panel to the Assistant Secretary for Health consists of nine members, including the Chairman, not otherwise in the full-time employ of the Federal Government. Members are selected by the Assistant Secretary for Health from citizens representing medicine, law, religion, labor, education, health administration, and public affairs. The Chairman is designated by the Assistant Secretary for Health.

The Panel members are invited to serve for a period not to extend beyond March 31, 1973, unless an extension beyond that time is approved by the Assistant Secretary for Health.

Management and staff services will be provided by the Office of the Assistant Secretary for Health which supplies the Executive Secretary.

Meetings

Meetings will be held at the call of the Chairman, with the advance approval of a Government official who shall also approve the agenda. A Government official will be present at all meetings.

Meetings are open to the public except as determined otherwise by the Secretary; notice of all meetings is given to the public.

Meetings shall be conducted, and records of the proceedings kept, as required by applicable laws and Departmental regulations.

Compensation

Members who are not full-time Federal employees will be paid at the rate of $100 per day for time spent at meetings, plus per diem and travel expenses in accordance with Standard Government Travel Regulations.

Annual Cost Estimate

Estimated annual cost for operating the Panel, including compensation and travel expenses of members but excluding staff support, is $74,000. Estimate of annual man years of staff support required is one year, at an estimated annual cost of $16,000.

Report

A final report based on the Panel's investigation will be made to the Assistant Secretary for Health, not later than April 30, 1973, which contains as a minimum a list of members and their business addresses, the dates and places of meetings, and a summary of the Panel's activities and recommendations. A copy of this report shall be provided to the Department Committee Management Officer.

Termination Date

Unless renewed by appropriate action prior to its expiration, the Tuskegee Syphilis Study Ad Hoc Advisory Panel to the Assistant Secretary for Health will terminate on March 31, 1973.

APPROVED:

1/4/73 (sgd.) Richard L. Seggel
Date Acting Assistant Secretary for Health

Panel Members

Chairman:
Broadus N. Butler, Ph.D.
    President, Dillard University
    2601 Gentilly Boulevard
    New Orleans, Louisiana 70122

Members:
Mr. Ronald H. Brown
    General Counsel
    National Urban League
    55 East 52nd Street
    New York, New York 10022

Vernal Cave, M.D.
    Director, Bureau of Venereal Disease Control
    New York City Health Department
    93 Worth Street
    New York, New York 10013
Jean L. Harris, M.D., F.R.S.H.
    Executive Director
    National Medical Association Foundation, Inc.
    1150 17th Street, N.W.
    Washington, D.C. 20036
Seward Hiltner, Ph.D., D.D.
    Professor of Theology
    Princeton Theological Seminary
    Princeton, New Jersey 08540
Jay Katz, M.D.
    Professor (Adjunct) of Law and Psychiatry
    Yale Law School
    127 Wall Street
    New Haven, Connecticut 06520
Jeanne C. Sinkford, D.D.S.
    Associate Dean for Graduate and Postgraduate Affairs
    College of Dentistry
    Howard University
    600 W Street, N.W.
    Washington, D.C. 20001
Mr. Fred Speaker
    Attorney at Law
    2 North Market Square
    Harrisburg, Pennsylvania 17108
Mr. Barney H. Weeks
    President, Alabama Labor Council
    AFL-CIO
    1018 South 18th Street
    Birmingham, Alabama 35205

Final Report

Tuskegee Syphilis Study Ad Hoc Advisory Panel
Report on Charge 1-A
Statement of Charge 1-A: Determine whether the study was justified in 1932

Background Data

The Tuskegee Study was one of several investigations that were taking place in the 1930's with the ultimate objective of venereal disease control in the United States. Beginning in 1926, the United States Public Health Service, with the cooperation of other organizations, actively engaged in venereal disease control work.[1] In 1929, the United States Public Health Service entered into a cooperative demonstration study with the Julius Rosenwald Fund and state and local departments of health in the control of venereal disease in six southern states:[2] Mississippi (Bolivar County); Tennessee (Tipton County): Georgia (Glynn County); Alabama (Macon County); North Carolina (Pitt County); Virginia (Albermarle County). These syphilis control demonstrations took place from 1930–1932 and disclosed a high prevalence of syphilis (35%) in the Macon County survey. Macon County was 82.4% Negro. The cultural status of this Negro population was low and the illiteracy rate was high.

During the years 1928–1942 the Cooperative Clinical Studies in the Treatment of Syphilis[3] were taking place in the syphilis clinics of Western Reserve University, Johns Hopkins University, Mayo Clinic, University of Pennsylvania, and the University of Michigan. The Division of Venereal Disease, USPHS provided statistical support, and financial support was provided by the USPHS and a grant from the Milbank Memorial Fund. These studies included a focus on effects of treatment in latent syphilis which had not been clinically documented before 1932. A report issued in 1932 indicated a satisfactory clinical outcome in 35% of untreated latent syphilitics.

The findings of Bruusgaard of Oslo on the results of untreated syphilis became available in 1929.[4] The Oslo study was a classic retrospective study involving the analysis of 473 patients at three to forty years after infection. For the first time, as a result of the Oslo study, clinical data were available to suggest the probability of spontaneous cure, continued latency, or serious or fatal outcome. Of the 473 patients included in the Oslo study, 309 were living and examined and 164 were deceased. Among the 473 patients, 27.7 percent were clinically free from symptoms and Wassermann negative; 14.8 percent had no clinical symptoms with Wassermann positive; 14.1 percent had heart and vessel disease; 2.76 percent had general paresis and 1.27 percent had tabes dorsalis. Thus in 1932, as the Public Health Service put forth a major effort toward control and treatment much was still unknown regarding the latent stages of the disease especially pertaining to its natural course and the epidemiology of late and latent syphilis.

Facts and Documentation Pertaining to Charge 1-A

1. There is no protocol which documents the original intent of the study. None of the literature searches or interviews with participants in the study gave any evidence that a written protocol ever existed for this study. The theories

postulated from time to time include the following purposes either by direct statement or implication:[5–7]

a. Study of the natural history of the disease.
b. Study of the course of treated and untreated syphilis (Annual Report of the Surgeon General of the Public Health Service of the United States 1935–36).
c. Study of the differences in histological and clinical course of the disease in black versus white subjects.
d. Study with an "acceptance" of the postulate that there was a benign course of the disease in later stages vis-a-vis the dangers of available therapy.
e. Short term study (6 months or longer) of the incidence and clinical course of late latent syphilis in the Negro male (From letter of correspondence from T. Clark, Assistant Surgeon General, to M. M. Davis of the Rosenwald Fund, October 29, 1932)—Original plan of procedure is stated herein.
f. A study which would provide valuable data for a syphilis control program for a rural impoverished community.

In the absence of an original protocol, it can only be assumed that between 1932 and 1936 (when the first report[5] of the study was made) the decision was made to continue the study as a long-term study. The Annual Report of the Surgeon General for 1935–36 included the statement: "Plans for the continuation of this study are underway. During the last 12 months, success has been obtained in gaining permission for the performance of autopsies on 11/15 individuals who died."

2. There is no evidence that informed consent was gained from the human participants in this study. Such consent would and should have included knowledge of the risk of human life for the involved parties and information re possible infections of innocent, non-participating parties such as friends and relatives. Reports such as "Only individuals giving a history of infection who submitted voluntarily to examination were included in the 399 cases" are the only ones that are documentable.[5] Submitting voluntarily is not informed consent.

3. In 1932, there was a known risk to human life and transmission of the disease in latent and late syphilis* was believed to be possible. Moore[3] 1932 reported satisfactory clinical outcome in 85% of patients with latent syphilis that were treated in contrast to 35% if no treatment is given.

4. The study as announced and continually described as involving "untreated" male Negro subjects was not a study of "untreated" subjects. Caldwell[8] in

*Vonderlehr to T. Clark—Memorandum—June 10, 1932.

1971 reported that: All but one of the originally untreated syphilitics seen in 1968–1970 have received therapy, although heavy metals and/or antibiotics were given for a variety of reasons by many non-study physicians and not necessarily in doses considered curative for syphilis. Heller[6] in 1946 reported "about one-fourth of the syphilitic individuals received treatment for their infection. Most of these, however, received no more than 1 or 2 arsenical injections; only 12 received as many as 10." The "untreated" group in this study is therefore a group of treated *and* untreated male subjects.

5. There is evidence that control subjects who became syphilitic were transferred to the "untreated" group. This data is present in the patient files at the Center for Disease Control in Atlanta. Caldwell[8] reports 12 original controls either acquired syphilis or were found to have reactive treponemal tests (unavailable prior to 1953). Heller,[6] also, reported that "It is known that some of the control group have acquired syphilis although the exact number cannot be accurately determined at present." Since this transfer of patients from the control group to the syphilitic group did occur, the study is not one of late latent syphilis. Also, it is not certain that this group of patients did in fact receive adequate therapy.

6. In the absence of a definitive protocol, there is no evidence or assurance that standardization of evaluative procedures, which are essential to the validity and reliability of a scientific study, existed at any time. This fact leaves open to question the true scientific merits of a longitudinal study of this nature. Standardization of evaluative procedures and clinical judgment of the investigators are considered essential to the valid interpretation of clinical data.[9] It should be noted that, in 1932, orderly and well planned research related to latent syphilis was justifiable since a. Morbidity and mortality had not been documented for this population and the significance of the survey procedure had just been reported in findings of the prevalence studies for 6 southern counties;[1] b. Epidemiologic knowledge of syphilis at the time had not produced facts so that it could be scientifically documented "just how and at what stage the disease is spread."* c. There was a paucity of knowledge re clinical aspects and spontaneous cure in latent syphilis[3] and the Oslo study[4] had just reported spontaneous remission of the disease in 27.7% of the patients studied. If perhaps a higher "cure" rate could have been documented for the latent syphilitics, then the treatment priorities and recommendations may have been altered for this community where funds and medical services were already inadequate.

*Letter from L. Usilton, VD Program 1930–32 and memorandum from Vonderlehr to T. Clark (Assistant Surgeon General) June 10, 1932.

The retrospective summary of the "Scientific Contributions of the Tuskegee Study" from the Chief, Venereal Disease Branch, USPHS (dated November 21, 1972) includes the following merits of the study:

Knowledge already gained or potentially able to be gained from this study may be categorized as contributing to improvements in the following areas:
1. Care of the surviving participants,
2. Care of all persons with latent syphilis,
3. The operation of a national syphilis control program,
4. Understanding of the disease of syphilis,
5. Understanding of basic disease producing mechanisms.

Panel Judgments on Charge 1-A
1. In retrospect, the Public Health Service Study of Untreated Syphilis in the Male Negro in Macon County, Alabama, was ethically unjustified in 1932. This judgment made in 1973 about the conduct of the study in 1932 is made with the advantage of hindsight acutely sharpened over some forty years, concerning an activity in a different age with different social standards. Nevertheless one fundamental ethical rule is that a person should not be subjected to avoidable risk of death or physical harm unless he freely and intelligently consents. There is no evidence that such consent was obtained from the participants in this study.
2. Because of the paucity of information available today on the manner in which the study was conceived, designed and sustained, a scientific justification for a short term demonstration study cannot be ruled out. However, the conduct of the longitudinal study as initially reported in 1936 and through the years is judged to be scientifically unsound and its results are disproportionately meager compared with known risks to human subjects involved. Outstanding weaknesses of this study, supported by the lack of written protocol, include lack of validity and reliability assurances; lack of calibration of investigator responses; uncertain quality of clinical judgments between various investigators; questionable data base validity and questionable value of the experimental design for a long term study of this nature.

   The position of the Panel must not be construed to be a general repudiation of scientific research with human subjects. It is possible that a scientific study in 1932 of untreated syphilis, properly conceived with a clear protocol and conducted with suitable subjects who fully understood the implications of their involvement, might have been justified in the pre-penicillin era. This is especially true when one considers the uncertain nature of the results of treatment of late latent syphilis and the highly toxic nature of therapeutic agents then available.

Report on Charge 1-B

Statement of Charge 1-B: Determine whether the study should have been continued when penicillin became generally available

Background Data

In 1932, treatment of syphilis in all stages was being provided through the use of a variety of chemotherapeutic agents including mercury, bismuth, arsphenamine, neoarsphenamine, iodides and various combinations thereof. Treatment procedures being used in the early 1930's extended over long periods of time (up to two years) and were not without hazard to the patient.[10] As of 1932, also, treatment was widely recommended and treatment schedules specifically for late latent syphilis were published and in use.[3-10] The rationale for treatment at that time was based on the clinical judgment "that the latent syphilitic patient must be regarded as a potential carrier of the disease and should be treated for the sake of the Community's health."[3] The aims of treatment in the treatment of latent syphilis were stated to be: 1) to increase the probability of "cure" or arrest, 2) to decrease the probability of progression or relapse over the probable result if no treatment were given and 3) the control of potential infectiousness from contact of the patient with adults of either sex, or in the case of women with latent syphilis, for unborn children.

According to Pfeiffer (1935),[11] treatment of late syphilis is quite individualistic and requires the physician's best judgment based upon sound fundamental knowledge of internal medicine and experience, and should not be undertaken as a routine procedure. Thus, treatment was being recommended in the United States for all stages of syphilis as of 1932 despite the "spontaneous" cure concept that was being justified by interpretations of the Oslo study, the potential hazards of treatment due to drug toxicity and to possible Jarisch-Herxheimer reactions in acute late syphilis.[12]

Documented reports of the effects of penicillin in the 1940's and early 1950's vary from outright support and endorsement of the use of penicillin in late and latent syphilis,[13-15] to statements of possible little or no value,[16-17] to expressions of doubts and uncertainty[18-19] related to its value, the potency of penicillin, absence of control of the rate of absorption, and potential hazard related to severe Herxheimer effects.

Although the mechanism of action of penicillin is not clear from available scientific reports of late latent syphilis, the therapeutic benefits were clinically documented by the early 1950's and have been widely reported from the mid 1950's to the present. In fact, the Center for Disease Control of the USPHS has reported treatment of syphilitic mothers in all stages of infection with penicillin as of 1953[20] and has demonstrated that penicillin is the most effective treatment yet known for neurosyphilis (1960).[21]

Facts and Documentation re Charge 1-B

1. Treatment schedules recommending the use of arsenicals and bismuth in the treatment of late latent syphilis were available in 1932.[3] Penicillin therapy was recommended for treatment of late latent syphilis in the late 1940's[14-15] which was *before* it became readily available for public use (estimated to have been 1952–53).

2. It was "known as early as 1932 that 85% of patients treated in late latent syphilis would enjoy prolonged maintenance of good health and freedom from disease as opposed to 35 percent if left untreated."[3] Scientists in this study,[5] reported in 1936, that morbidity in male Negroes with untreated syphilis far exceeds that in a comparable nonsyphilitic group and that cardiovascular and central nervous system involvements were two or three times as common. Moreover, Wenger,[22] in 1950, reported: "We know now, where we could only surmise before, that we have contributed to their ailments and shortened their lives. I think the least we can say is that we have a high moral obligation to those that have died to make this the best study possible." The effect of syphilis in shortening life was published from observations made by Usilton et al. in 1937.[23] The study by Rosahn[24] at Yale in 1947 reported strong clinical evidence that syphilis ran a more fatal course in Negroes than in Caucasians.

3. Reports regarding the withholding of treatment from patients in this study are varied and are still subject to controversy. Statements received from personal interviews conducted by Panel members with participants in this study cannot be considered as conclusive since there are varied opinions concerning what actually happened. In written letters and in open interviews, the panel received reports that treatment was deliberately withheld on the one hand and on the other, we were told that individuals seeking treatment were not denied treatment (in transcript and correspondence documents).

What is clearly documentable (in a series of letters between Vonderlehr and Health officials in Tuskegee taking place between February 1941 and August 1942) is that known seropositive, untreated males under 45 years of age from the Tuskegee Study had been called for army duty and rejected on account of a positive blood. The local board was furnished with a list of 256 names of men under 45 years of age and asked that these men be excluded from the list of draftees needing treatment! According to the letters, the board agreed with this arrangement in order to make it possible to continue this study on an effective basis. It should be noted that some of these patients had already received notices from the Local Selective Service Board "to begin their antisyphilitic treatment immediately."

According to Wenger,[22] the patients in the study "received no treatment on our recommendation." At the present time, we know that most of the participants in this study received some form of treatment with heavy metals and/or antibiotics.[8] Although the adequacy of treatment received is not known, it is clear that the treatment received was provided by physicians who were not a part of the study and who were individually sought by the individual patients related to their own medical symptoms and pursuit of treatment.

4. The five survey periods in this study occurred in 1932, 1938–39, 1948, 1952–53 and 1968–70.[8–25] This study lacks continuity except through the public health nurse and at these isolated survey periods. In 1969 an Ad Hoc Committee reviewed the Tuskegee Study with the purpose: to examine data from the Tuskegee Study and offer advice on continuance of this study.

Participants of the February 6, 1969 meeting included:

Committee Members:

Dr. Gene Stollerman
    Chairman, Dept. of Medicine
    University of Tennessee, Memphis

Dr. Johannes Ipsen, Jr.
    Professor
    Dept. of Community Medicine
    University of Pennsylvania, Philadelphia

Dr. Ira Myers
    State Health Officer
    Montgomery

Dr. J. Lawton Smith
    Associate Professor of Ophthalmology
    University of Miami

Dr. Clyde Kaiser
    Senior Member Technical Staff
    Milbank Memorial Fund
    New York City

Resource Persons:

Dr. Bobby C. Brown, VDRL, NCDC
Mrs. Eleanor V. Price, VD Branch, NCDC
Dr. Joseph Caldwell, VD Branch, NCDC
Dr. Paul Cohen, VDRL, NCDC
Dr. Sidney Olansky
    Professor of Medicine
    Dept. of Internal Medicine
    Emory University Clinic, Atlanta

Recorders:

Dr. Leslie Norins
    Chief, VDRL, NCDC
Mrs. Doris J. Smith
    Secretary to Dr. Norins, VDRL, NCDC

Attending:

Dr. David J. Sencer
  Director, NCDC
Dr. William J. Brown
  Chief, VD Branch, NCDC
Dr. U. S. G. Kuhn, III, VDRL, NCDC
Miss Genevieve W. Stout, VDRL, NCDC
Dr. H. Bruce Dull
  Assistant Director, NCDC

The meeting was convened at 1:00 p.m. and adjourned at 4:10 p.m.

A summary report of the meeting includes the following:

The purpose of the meeting was to determine if the Tuskegee Study should be terminated or continued.

Considerations were:

1. How the study was setup in 1932
2. Are the participants all available
3. How are the survivors faring

At the time of this study there were only seven patients whose primary cause of death was ascribed to syphilis.

It was determined that benefits to be achieved from the study at this time were:

1. Relationship of serology to morbidity from syphilis
2. Relationship of known pathology to syphilis
3. Various epidemiological considerations

Full treatment of the survivors was also considered and the following liabilities listed.

Danger of late Herxheimer's reaction which would worsen or possibly kill those syphilitic patients suffering from cardiovascular or neurological conditions.

At this time it was mentioned that both Macon County Health Department and Tuskegee Institute were cognizant of the study.

The meeting was terminated with several salient points.

1. This type of study would never be repeated.
2. There were certain medical facts to be learned by continuing the present study.
3. Treatment for these patients was not indicated unless they had signs of active syphilitic disease.
4. More contact should be established between PHS and Macon County Health Department and Medical Society so they would cooperate in the continuance of the study.

It should be noted that the Committee was eminently represented from the medical community. However, legal representatives and others from the non-medical community of scholars were not adequately represented for so sensitive a study. This is especially true since the Tuskegee Study was being continued at a time when Department of Health, Education, and Welfare guidelines for the Protection of Human Subjects were being widely disseminated for compliance by all institutions receiving grant support. The three hours and ten minutes were not adequate for in-depth study of the broad issues, implications and ramifications of this study.

In 1970, Drs. Anne Yobs and Arnold L. Schroeter in separate memoranda (to the Director, Center for Disease Control and to the Chief, Venereal Disease Branch) recommended procedures for orderly termination of this study. Dr. James Lucas, Assistant Chief of the Venereal Disease Branch, in a memorandum to the Chief of the Venereal Disease Branch dated September 10, 1970 states: It must be fully realized that the remaining contribution from this study will be largely of *historical* interest. Nothing learned will prevent, find, or cure a single case of infectious syphilis or bring us closer to our basic mission of controlling venereal disease in the United States.

5. There is a crucial absence of evidence that patients were given a "choice" of continuing in the study once penicillin became readily available. This fact serves to amplify the magnitude of encroachment on the human lives and well-being of the participants in this study. This is especially significant when there is uncertainty as to the whole issue of "consent" of the participants.

Panel Judgments on Charge 1-B

The ethical, legal and scientific implications which are evoked from the facts presented in the previous section led the Panel to the following judgment:

That penicillin therapy should have been made available to the participants in this study especially as of 1953 when penicillin became generally available.

Withholding of penicillin, after it became generally available, amplified the injustice to which this group of human beings had already been subjected. The scientific merits of the Tuskegee Study are vastly overshadowed by the violation of basic ethical principles pertaining to human dignity and human life imposed on the experimental subjects.

Report on Charge 1

Summary

This section of the Advisory Panel's report deals specifically with Charge Codes 1-A and 1-B.

Statement of Charge Codes

Charge 1-A. Determine whether the study was justified in 1932, and

Charge 1-B. Determine whether it should have been continued when penicillin became generally available.

Introduction

The Background Paper on the Tuskegee Study, prepared by the Venereal Disease Branch of the Center for Disease Control, July 27, 1972, included the following statements:

"Because of the lack of knowledge of the pathogenesis of syphilis, a long-term study of untreated syphilis was considered desirable in establishing a more knowledgeable syphilis control program."

"A prospective study was begun late in 1932 in Macon County, Alabama, a rural area with a static population and a high rate of untreated syphilis. An untreated population such as this offered an unusual opportunity to follow and study the disease over a long period of time. In 1932, a total of 26 percent of the male population tested, who were 25 years of age or older, were serologically reactive for syphilis by at least two tests, usually on two occasions. The original study group was composed of 399 of these men who had received no therapy and who gave historical and laboratory evidence of syphilis which had progressed beyond the infectious stages. A total of 201 men comparable in age and environments and judged by serology, history, and physical examination to be free of syphilis were selected to be the control group."

Panel Conclusions re Charge 1-A and 1-B of the Tuskegee Study

After extensive review of the available documents, interviews with associated parties and pursuit of various other avenues of documentation, the Panel concludes that:

1. In retrospect, the Public Health Service Study of Untreated Syphilis in the Male Negro in Macon county, Alabama was ethically unjustified in 1932.
2. Because of the paucity of information available today on the manner in which the study was conceived, designed and sustained, scientific justification for a short-term demonstration study in 1932 cannot be ruled out. However, the conduct of the longitudinal study as initially reported in 1936 and through the years is judged to be scientifically unsound and its results are disproportionately meager compared with known risks to the human subjects involved.
3. Penicillin therapy should have been made available to the participants in this study not later than 1953.

The Panel qualifies its conclusions with several position statements summarized as follows.

a. The judgments in 1973 about the conduct of the Tuskegee Study in 1932 are made with the advantage of hindsight, acutely sharpened over some forty years concerning an activity in a different age with different social standards. Nevertheless one fundamental ethical rule is that a person should not be subjected to avoidable risk of death or physical harm unless he freely and intelligently consents. There was no evidence that such consent was obtained from the participants in this study.

b. History has shown that certain people under psychological, social or economic duress are particularly acquiescent. These are the young, the mentally impaired, the institutionalized, the poor and persons of racial minority and other disadvantaged groups. These are the people who may be selected for human experimentation and who, because of their station in life, may not have an equal chance to withhold consent.

c. The Tuskegee Syphilis Study, placed in the perspective of its early years, is not an isolated event in terms of the generally accepted conditions and practices that prevailed in the 1930's.

d. The position of the Panel must not be construed to be a general repudiation of scientific research with human subjects. It is possible that a scientific study in 1932 of untreated syphilis, properly conceived with a clear protocol and conducted with suitable subjects who fully understood the implications of their involvement, might have been justified in the pre-penicillin era because of the uncertain nature of results of treatment of late latent syphilis with the highly toxic therapeutic agents then available.

REFERENCES

1. Clark, T. *The Control of Syphilis in Southern Rural Areas.* Julius Rosenwald Fund, Chicago, 1932, p. 27.

2. Ibid., pp. 6–36.

3. Moore, Joseph Earle. Latent Syphilis Cooperative Clinical Studies in the Treatment of Syphilis. Reprint No. 45 from *Venereal Disease Information*, Vol. XIII, Nos. 8–12, 1932 and Vol. XIV, No. 1, 1933, pp. 1–56.

4. Bruusgaard, E. The Fate of Syphilitics Who are not Given Specific Treatment. *Archiv tur Dermatologie und Syphilis* 1929, 157, p. 309.

5. Vonderlehr, R. A., et al. Untreated Syphilis in the Male Negro. *Venereal Disease Information* 17:260–265, 1936.

6. Heller, J. R. and Bruyere, P.T.: Untreated Syphilis in Male Negro: II. Mortality During 12 Years of Observation. *Venereal Disease Information* 27: 34–38, 1946.

7. Shafer, J. K., Usilton, L. J., and Gleason, G. A. Untreated Syphilis in Male Negro: Prospective Study of Effect on Life Expectancy. *Public Health Reports* 69:684–690, 1954; *Milbank Memorial Fund Quarterly*, 32:262–274, July 1954.

8. Caldwell, J. G., Price, E. V., Shroeter, A. L., and Fletcher, G. F. Aortic Regurgitation in a

Study of Aged Males with Previous Syphilis. Presented in part at American Venereal Disease Association Annual Meeting, 22 June 1971.

9. Feinstein, A. R. *Clinical Judgment*. Baltimore, William and Wilkins Co., 1967, pp. 45–48.

10. Gaupin, C. E. The Treatment of Latent Syphilis. *Kentucky Medical Journal* 30: 74–77, February 1932.

11. Pfeiffer, A. Medical Aspects in the Prevention and Management of Late and Latent Syphilis. *Psychiatric Quarterly* 9: 185–193, April 1935.

12. Greenbaum, S. C. The "Bismuth Approach" in the Treatment of Acute (Late) Syphilis. *Journal of Chemotherapy* 13: 5–8, April 1936.

13. Stokes, J. H., et al. The Action of Penicillin in Late Syphilis. *J.A.M.A.* 126: 73–79, September 1944.

14. Dexter, D. C. and Tucker, H. A. Penicillin Treatment of Benign Late Gummatous Syphilis, Report of Twenty-one Cases. *American Journal of Syphilis, Gonorrhea, and Venereal Disease* 30: 211–226, May 1946.

15. Committee on Medical Research: The Changing Character of Commercial Penicillin with Suggestions as to the Use of Penicillin in Syphilis. U.S. Health Service and Food and Drug Administration. *J.A.M.A.* 131: 271–275, May 1946.

16. Barnett, C. W. The Public Health Aspects of Late Latent Syphilis. *Stanford Medical Bulletin* 10: 152–156, August 1952.

17. Reynolds, F. W. Treatment Failures Following the Use of Penicillin in Late Syphilis. *American Journal of Syphilis, Gonorrhea, and Venereal Disease* 32: 233–242, May 1948.

18. McElligott, G. L. M. The Management of Late and Latent Syphilis. *British Medical Journal* 1: 829–830, April 1953.

19. Barnett, C. W., Epstein, N. J., Brewer, A. F. et al. Effect of Treatment in Late Latent Syphilis. *Arch Dermat Syph* 69: 91–99, January 1954.

20. *VD Fact Sheet*, No. 10. U.S. Public Health Service Publication, December 1953, p. 20

21. *VD Fact Sheet*, No. 17. U.S. Public Health Service Publication, December 1960, p. 19.

22. Wenger, O. C. Untreated Syphilis in Negro Male. Hot Springs Seminar, 9-18-50 (From CDC Files).

23. Usilton, L. et al. A Tentative Death Curve for Acquired Syphilis in White and Colored Males in the United States. *Venereal Disease Information* 18: pp. 231–234, 1937.

24. Rosahn, P. D. Autopsy Studies in Syphilis. *Journal of Venereal Disease Information* 28: Supplement No. 21, pp. 32–39, 1949.

25. Rivers, E., Schuman, S., Simpson, L., and Olansky, S. Twenty Years of Follow-up Experience in a Long-Range Medical Study. *Public Health Reports* 68: (4), 391–395, April 1953.

Respectfully Submitted,

Ronald H. Brown

Jean L. Harris, M.D.

Seward Hiltner, Ph.D., D.D.

Jeanne C. Sinkford, D.D.S., Ph.D.

Fred Speaker

Barney H. Weeks

Approval with Reservations:
(See addendum for reservation statement)
    Jay Katz, M.D.
    Vernal Cave, M.D.

Abstention:
Broadus N. Butler, Ph.D.

Yale Law School, New Haven, Connecticut 06520

TO: THE ASSISTANT SECRETARY FOR HEALTH AND SCIENTIFIC AFFAIRS

FROM: JAY KATZ, M.D.

TOPIC: RESERVATIONS ABOUT THE PANEL REPORT ON CHARGE 1

I should like to add the following findings and observations to the majority opinion:

(1) There is ample evidence in the records available to us that the consent to participation was not obtained from the Tuskegee Syphilis Study subjects, but that instead they were exploited, manipulated, and deceived. They were treated not as human subjects but as objects of research. The most fundamental reason for condemning the Tuskegee Study at its inception and throughout its continuation is not that all the subjects should have been treated, for some might not have wished to be treated, but rather that they were never fairly consulted about the research project, its consequences for them, and the alternatives available to them. Those who for reasons of intellectual incapacity could not have been so consulted should not have been invited to participate in the study in the first place.

(2) It was already known before the Tuskegee Syphilis Study was begun, and reconfirmed by the study itself, that persons with untreated syphilis have a higher death rate than those who have been treated. The life expectancy of at least forty subjects in the study was markedly decreased for lack of treatment.

(3) In addition, the untreated and the "inadvertently" (using the word frequently employed by the investigators) but inadequately treated subjects suffered many complications which could have been ameliorated with treatment. This fact was noted on occasion in the published reports of the Tuskegee Syphilis Study and as late as 1971. However the subjects were not apprised of this possibility.

(4) One of the senior investigators wrote in 1936 that since "a considerable portion of the infected Negro population remained untreated during the entire course of syphilis . . . an unusual opportunity (arose) to study the untreated syphilitic patient from the beginning of the disease to the death of the infected person." Throughout, the investigators seem to have confused the study with an "experiment in nature." But syphilis was not a condition for which no beneficial treatment was available, calling for experimentation to learn more about the condition in the hope of finding a remedy. The persistence of the syphilitic disease from which the victims of the Tuskegee Study suffered resulted from the unwillingness or incapacity of society to mobilize the necessary resources for treatment. The investigators, the USPHS, and the private foundations who gave support

to this study should not have exploited this situation in the fashion they did. Unless they could have guaranteed knowledgeable participation by the subjects, they all should have disappeared from the research scene or else utilized their limited research resources for therapeutic ends. Instead, the investigators believed that the persons involved in the Tuskegee Study would *never* seek out treatment; a completely unwarranted assumption which ultimately led the investigators deliberately to obstruct the opportunity for treatment of a number of the participants.

(5) In theory if not in practice, it has long been "a principle of medical and surgical morality (never to perform) on man an experiment which might be harmful to him to any extent, even though the result might be highly advantageous to science" (Claude Bernard 1865), at least without the knowledgeable consent of the subject. This was one basis on which the German physicians who had conducted medical experiments in concentration camps were tried by the Nuremberg Military Tribunal for crimes against humanity. Testimony at their trial by official representatives of the American Medical Association clearly suggested that research like the Tuskegee Syphilis Study would have been intolerable in this country or anywhere in the civilized world. Yet the Tuskegee study was continued after the Nuremberg findings and the Nuremberg Code had been widely disseminated to the medical community. Moreover, the study was not reviewed in 1966 after the Surgeon General of the USPHS promulgated his guidelines for the ethical conduct of research, even though this study was carried on within the purview of his department.

(6) The Tuskegee Syphilis Study finally was reviewed in 1969. A lengthier transcript of the proceedings, not quoted by the majority, reveals that one of the five members of the reviewing committee repeatedly emphasized that a moral obligation existed to provide treatment for the "patients." His plea remained unheeded. Instead the Committee, which was in part concerned with the possibility of adverse criticism, seemed to be reassured by the observation that "if we established good liaison with the local medical society, there would be no need to answer criticism."

(7) The controversy over the effectiveness and the dangers of arsenic and heavy metal treatment in 1932 and of penicillin treatment when it was introduced as a method of therapy is beside the point. For the real issue is that the participants in this study were never informed of the availability of treatment because the investigators were never in favor of such treatment. Throughout the study the responsibility rested heavily on the shoulders of the investigators to make every effort to apprise the subjects of what could be done for them if they so wished. In 1937 the then Surgeon General of the USPHS wrote: "(f) or late syphilis no blanket prescription can be written. Each patient is a law unto himself. For every syphilis patient, late and early, a careful physical examination is necessary before starting treatment and should be repeated frequently during its course." Even prior to that, in 1932,

ranking USPHS physicians stated in a series of articles that adequate treatment "will afford a practical, if not complete guaranty of freedom from the development of any late lesions."

In conclusion, I note sadly that the medical profession, through its national association, its many individual societies, and its journals, has on the whole not reacted to this study except by ignoring it. One lengthy editorial appeared in the October 1972 issue of the Southern Medical Journal which exonerated the study and chastised the "irresponsible press" for bringing it to public attention. When will we take seriously our responsibilities, particularly to the disadvantaged in our midst who so consistently throughout history have been the first to be selected for human research?

Respectfully submitted,

(sgd.) Jay Katz, M.D.

II. Summary of Conclusions and Recommendations

A. Evaluation of Current DHEW Policies for the
Protection of Human Research Subjects

1. No uniform Departmental policy for the protection of research subjects exists. Instead one policy governs "extramural" research—research supported by DHEW grants or contracts to institutions outside the Federal Government and conducted by private researchers—and another policy governs "intramural" research—research conducted by personnel of the Public Health Service. Furthermore, Food and Drug Administration (FDA) regulations promulgated to protect subjects in drug research, whether or not supported by DHEW or conducted by the PHS, incorporate variations of their own. The lack of uniformity in DHEW policies creates confusion, and denies some subjects the protection they deserve.

Moving to the next higher level, no uniform Federal policies exist for the protection of subjects in Government-sponsored research. Other agencies wholly separate from DHEW—most notably, the Department of Defense—support or conduct human research. DHEW policies do not govern such research. Here too, the Federal Government's failure to develop a uniform policy has been detrimental to the welfare of research subjects.

2. Under current DHEW policies for the protection of research subjects, regulation of research practices is largely left to the biomedical professions. Since the conduct of human experimentation raises important issues of social policy, greater participation in decision-making by representatives of other professions and of the general public is required.

3. The present reliance by DHEW on the institutional review committee as the primary mechanism for the protection of research subjects was an important advance in the continuing effort to guarantee ethical experimentation. Prior peer review of research protocols is a requirement which should be retained.

4. The existing review committee system suffers from basic defects which seriously undermine the accomplishment of the task assigned to the committees:

   a. The governing standards promulgated by DHEW which are intended to guide review committee decisions in specific cases are vague and overly general.
   b. No provisions are made for the dissemination or publication of review committee decisions. Their low level of visibility hampers efforts to evaluate and learn from committee attempts to resolve the complex problems of human research.
   c. Although the informed consent of the research subject is one of the most important requirements of research ethics, DHEW policies for obtaining consent are poorly drafted and contain critical loopholes. As a result, one crucial task of institutional review committees—the implementation of the informed consent requirement—is commonly performed inadequately. In particular, consent is far too often obtained in form alone and not in substance.
   d. DHEW policies do not give sufficient attention to the protection of such special research subjects as children, prisoners and the mentally incompetent. The use of these subjects in human experimentation presents grave dangers of abuse.
   e. The obligation of institutional review committees to conduct continuing review of research projects after their initial approval is undefined and as a consequence often neglected.
   f. Inefficient utilization of institutional review committees contributes to their ineffectiveness. Committees are overburdened with a variety of separate functions, and could operate best if their tasks were narrowly defined to encompass mainly the implementation of research policies adequately formulated by others.
   g. Effective procedures for enforcing DHEW policies, when those policies are disregarded, have not been devised.

5. No policy for the compensation of research subjects harmed as a consequence of their participation in research has been formulated, despite the fact that no matter how careful investigators may be, unavoidable injury to a few is the price society must pay for the privilege of engaging in research which ultimately benefits the

many. Remitting injured subjects to the uncertainties of the law court is not a solution.

B. Policy Recommendations

1. Congress should establish a permanent body with the authority to regulate *at least* all Federally supported research involving human subjects, whether it is conducted in intramural or extramural settings, or sponsored by DHEW or other government agencies, such as the Department of Defense. Ideally, the authority of this body should extend to all research activities, even those not Federally supported. But such a proposal may raise major jurisdictional problems. This body could be called the National Human Investigation Board. The Board should be independent of DHEW, for we do not believe that the agency which both conducts a great deal of research itself and supports much of the research that is carried on elsewhere is a position to carry out dispassionately the functions we have in mind. The members of the Board should be appointed from diverse professional and scientific disciplines, and should include representatives from the public at large.

2. The primary responsibility of the National Human Investigation Board should be to formulate research policies, in much greater detail and with much more clarity than is presently the case. The Board must promulgate detailed procedures to govern the implementation of its policies by institutional review committees. It must also promulgate procedures for the review of research decisions and their consequences. In particular, this Board should establish procedures for the publication of important institutional committee and Board decisions. Publication of such decisions would permit their intensive study both inside and outside the medical profession and would be a first step toward the case-by-case development of policies governing human experimentation. We regard such a development, analogous to the experience of the common law, as the best hope for ultimately providing workable standards for the regulation of the human experimentation process.

3. The National Human Investigation Board should develop appeals procedures for the adjudication of disagreements between investigators and the institutional review committees.

4. The National Human Investigation Board should also develop a "no fault" clinical research insurance plan to assure compensation for subjects harmed as a result of their participation in research. Institutions which sponsor Federally supported research activities should be required to participate in such a plan.

5. With the establishment of adequate policy formulation and review mechanisms, the structure and functions of the institutional review committee should be altered

to enhance the effectiveness of prior review. In place of the amorphous institutional review committee as it now exists, we propose the creation of an Institutional Human Investigation Committee (IHIC) with two distinct subcommittees. The IHIC should be the direct link between the institution and the National Human Investigation Board, and should establish local regulations consistent with national policies. The IHIC should also assume an educational role in its institutions, informing participants in the research enterprise of their rights and obligations. The implementation of research polices should be left to the two subcommittees of the IHIC:

a. A Protocol Review Group (PRG) should be responsible for the prior review of research protocols. The PRG should be composed mainly of competent biomedical professionals.

b. A Subject Advisory Group (SAG) should be responsible for aiding subjects in their decision-making whenever they request its services. Subject must be made aware of the existence of the SAG. The primary concern of the SAG should be with procedures for obtaining consent, and with the quality of consents obtained. The SAG should be composed of both professionals and laymen.

Conclusion

Human experimentation reflects the recurrent societal dilemma of reconciling respect for human rights and individual dignity with the felt needs of society to overrule individual autonomy for the common good. Throughout this report we have expressed our concern for the lack of attention which has been given to the protection of the rights and welfare of human subjects in research. Society can no longer afford to leave the balancing of individual rights against scientific progress to the scientific community alone. The revelations of the Tuskegee Syphilis Study once again dramatically confirmed this conclusion.

We offer our far-reaching proposals in the hope that the decision-making process for human research will become more open and more effectively regulated. We have amply documented the need for implementing this most basic recommendation. Precise rules and efficient procedures, however, are not by themselves proof against a repetition of Tuskegee. For, however well designed the system of regulation, the danger of token adherence to ethical standards and evasion in the guise of flexibility will persist. Ultimately, the spirit in which an aware society undertakes to use human beings for research ends will determine the protection which those human beings will receive. Therefore, we have urged throughout a greater participation by society in the decisions which affect so many human lives.

Respectfully submitted,

Ronald H. Brown
Vernal Cave, M.D.
Jean L. Harris, M.D.
Seward Hiltner, Ph.D., D.D.
Jay Katz, M.D.
Jeanne C. Sinkford, D.D.S., Ph.D.
Fred Speaker
Barney H. Weeks

Abstention:

Broadus N. Butler, Ph.D.

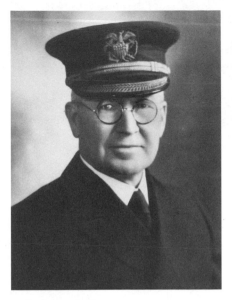

Taliaferro Clark.
(Images from History of Medicine,
National Library of Medicine)

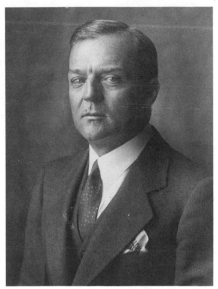

Oliver C. Wenger.
(Images from History of Medicine,
National Library of Medicine)

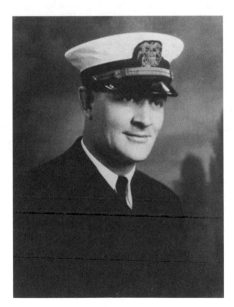

Austin V. Diebert.
(Images from History of Medicine,
National Library of Medicine)

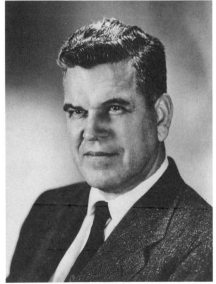

John R. Heller.
(Images from History of Medicine,
National Library of Medicine)

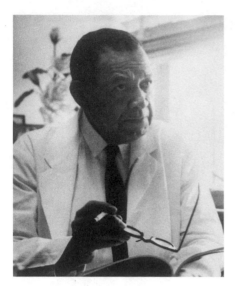

*Eugene H. Dibble.
Dr. Dibble was medical
director of the John A. Andrew
Hospital at Tuskegee Institute
when the study began in 1932.*

(Eugene H. Dibble Papers,
Tuskegee University Archives,
Tuskegee University; reprinted
by permission of Tuskegee
University)

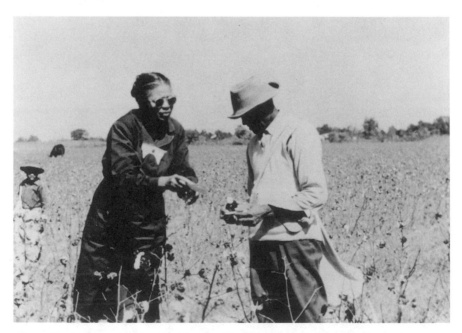

Nurse Eunice Rivers and an unidentified "subject" in the cotton fields, no date.
(Centers for Disease Control Papers, Tuskegee Syphilis Study Administrative Records, 1930–80,
Box 33, negative no. 18939, National Archives–Southeast Region, East Point, Ga.)

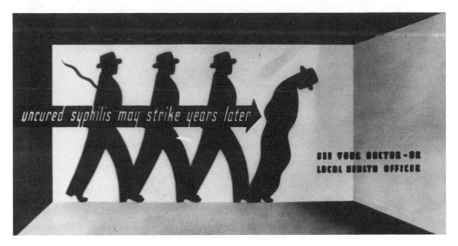

Poster, ca. 1930s.
(Images from History of Medicine, National Library of Medicine)

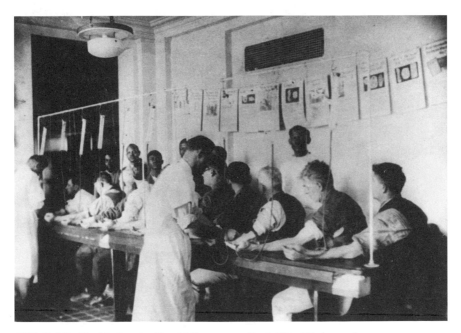

U.S. Public Health Service Rapid Treatment Penicillin Clinic, ca. late 1940s.
(Images from History of Medicine, National Library of Medicine)

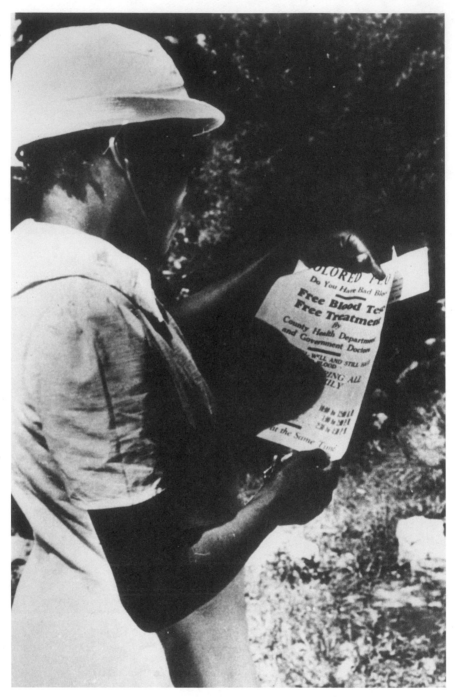

"Colored People, Bad Blood, Free Blood Test, Free Treatment,"
campaign flyer, ca. 1930s.
(Images from History of Medicine, National Library of Medicine)

Macon County Health Department

ALABAMA STATE BOARD OF HEALTH AND U. S. PUBLIC HEALTH
SERVICE COOPERATING WITH TUSKEGEE INSTITUTE

Dear Sir:

Some time ago you were given a thorough examination and since that time we hope you have gotten a great deal of treatment for bad blood. You will now be given your last chance to get a second examination. This examination is a very special one and after it is finished you will be given a special treatment if it is believed you are in a condition to stand it.

If you want this special examination and treatment you must meet the nurse at _____ on

_____ _____ at _____ M. She will bring you to the Tuskegee Institute Hospital for this free treatment. We will be very busy when these examinations and treatments are being given, and will have lots of people to wait on. You will remember that you had to wait for some time when you had your last good examination, and we wish to let you know that because we expect to be so busy it may be necessary for you to remain in the hospital over one night. If this is necessary you will be furnished your meals and a bed, as well the examination and treatment without cost.

REMEMBER THIS IS YOUR LAST CHANCE FOR SPECIAL FREE TREATMENT. BE SURE TO MEET THE NURSE.

Macon County Health Department

Letter to the "subjects," 1933. This letter was sent to the study's "participants" to entice them to continue to be examined when there was no treatment provided.

(United States Public Health Service, Division of Venereal Diseases, Record Group 90 [1918–36], Box 239, Folder 2, Macon County, undated letter attached to letter from Dr. Clark to Dr. Vonderlehr, 21 April 1933, National Archives)

U. S. PUBLIC HEALTH SERVICE

This certificate is awarded to

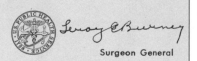

In grateful recognition of 25 years

of active participation in the

Tuskegee medical research study.

Awarded 1958

Surgeon General

Twenty-five-year participation certificate. In 1958, along with $25.00 for each year they had been in the study, this certificate was sent by name to the remaining study "subjects" by the Public Health Service, signed by Dr. Leroy E. Burney, the U.S. surgeon general.

(Centers for Disease Control Papers, Tuskegee Syphilis Study Administrative Records, 1930–80, Box 16, Folder Alabama-Miscellaneous, National Archives– Southeast Region, East Point, Georgia)

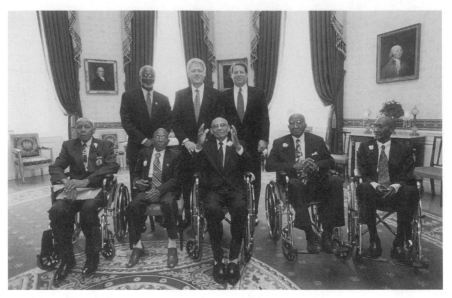

White House apology ceremony, 16 May 1997. Participants and survivors of the study (first row): Herman Shaw, Fred Simmons, Charles Pollard, Frederick Moss, Carter Howard. White House officials (back row): U.S. Surgeon General David Satcher, President William J. Clinton, Vice-President Albert Gore.
(White House Photography Office)

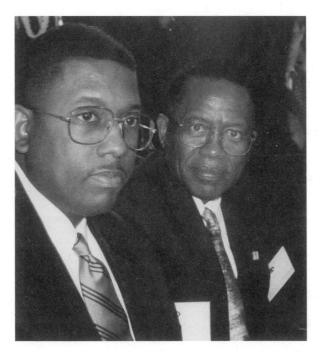

Attorneys Fred Gray Jr. and Fred Gray Sr. at the White House.
(Susan M. Reverby)

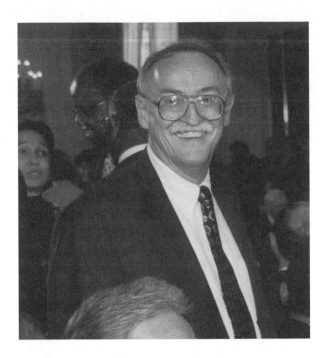

Historian James H. Jones, author of Bad Blood, *at the White House.*
(Susan M. Reverby)

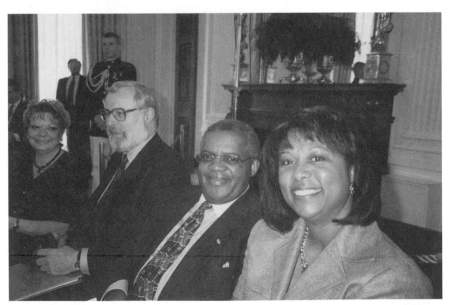

Joan Echtenkamp Klein (medical archivist/Legacy Committee member), Peter Buxton (Tuskegee Study whistleblower), Dr. Henry Foster (former surgeon general nominee), and Patricia Clay (administrator, Macon County Health Care Authority and Legacy Committee member) at the White House.
(Susan M. Reverby)

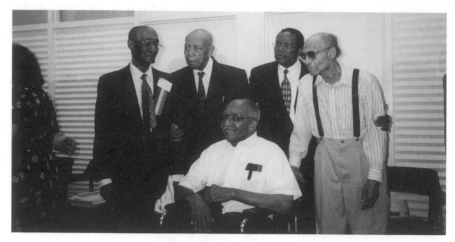

Survivors and attorney Fred Gray at the dedication of the Tuskegee Multicultural Center for Human and Civil Rights, Tuskegee, Alabama, 15 May 1998. Standing: Carter Haywood, Herman Shaw, Fred Gray, Charles Pollard. Seated: Frederick Moss.
(Susan M. Reverby)

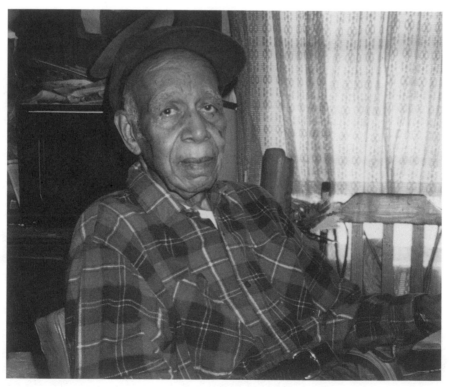

Herman Shaw in his home, Tallassee, Alabama, 10 November 1998.
(Susan M. Reverby)

iv

The Question of Treatment

THE TUSKEGEE STUDY OF
UNTREATED SYPHILIS

R. H. KAMPMEIER

The news media recently raised a great hue and cry following revelation of the study of a group of untreated syphilitics which was begun now 40 years ago and came to be known as the Tuskegee Study. Accounts and editorials in the printed news media stated outright or implied that treatment was purposefully withheld to evaluate the course of untreated disease. Only two will be quoted. *Time*[1] stated, "people with syphilis were *induced* to go without treatment. . . . For the past 25 years, the service has had a proven remedy available and *neglected* to use it on its select test cases." Even the AMA News[2] was trapped into writing, "None of the men in the study received treatment for syphilis, even after the *effectiveness* of penicillin became known." (The italics are the Editor's.)

In complete disregard of their abysmal ignorance, members of the fourth estate bang out anything on their typewriters which will make headlines. Small wonder William Osler wrote more than half a century ago,

> Believe nothing that you see in the newspapers—they have done more to create dissatisfaction than all other agencies. If you see anything in them that you know is true, begin to doubt it at once.

An exposition of the quarter-truth publicized will not reach the eyes of newsmen. It is just as well for it would be over their heads; furthermore they live to write today and to forget tomorrow, irresponsible in the "dissatisfaction" they create. Only a handful of us are left, who had much experience in the management of syphilis at about the time of the inception of the Tuskegee Study and who thus might put this recent "tempest in a teapot" into proper historical perspective. Therefore, I have elected to review the setting of the study in 1932 and its continuation as a text for the education of the younger generation of physicians, the majority of whom have little knowledge of the venereal diseases.[3] I have reviewed the papers upon the Tuskegee Study published over three decades to refresh my

Dr. R. H. Kampmeier was a noted syphilis specialist and taught at the Vanderbilt University School of Medicine.
Originally published in the Southern Medical Journal *65 (1972): 1247–51. Reprinted by permission from the* Southern Medical Journal.

memory of their content. Certain facts need emphasis as background to understand the initiation of the Study and its continuance.

The only acceptable study of the natural course of untreated syphilis in medical history was begun by Professor Boeck, of Oslo, who withheld treatment from 1,978 patients between 1891 and 1910, since the inadequacy of mercury and even its hazard in the management of acute syphilis was obvious to all experienced observers of that day. Of course, these patients could only be diagnosed *clinically* because the infectious agent was not to be identified until 1905 and the Wassermann test to be described until 1906. Boeck's pupil and successor, Bruusgaard,[4] in 1929, reported a follow-up study of 473 of these patients, 309 living and 164 dead with necropsy in 40. In summary, he reported that: 9.5% of the patients had developed neurosyphilis, 12.8% cardiovascular syphilis, 12.2% late benign syphilis, 23.6% had had clinical relapse, and 22.6% had died of other causes. This then was the state of knowledge regarding the prognosis of untreated syphilis at the time the Tuskegee Study was begun in 1932. (Two elegant reviews of Boeck's material appeared a quarter of a century later, in 1955, by Gjestland and by Clark and Danbolt.)

In 1910, Paul Ehrlich announced arsphenamine. His dream of a single sterilizing dose was quickly shattered by the appearance of infectious relapse and neuro-relapse. Several years later some of the complexities and hazards attending the use of arsphenamine were ameliorated to a degree by the development of neoarsphenamine which could be given by syringe. Nevertheless, the use of arseno-therapy was erratic, and generally without rhyme or reason,—an injection now and then, possibly for a symptom, some skin lesion, or when the patient had a ten dollar bill. The initial cost of the arsphenamines was fantastic.* Few doctors in the "teens" had need to become adept in venipuncture and intravenous treatment, other than in university clinics or public health clinics. The painful and often serious reactions to the arsphenamines, and later the painful effects of inept intramuscular injections of bismuth led to very irregular treatment and a high rate of clinical relapse in early syphilis.

Macon County, Alabama, the location of the Tuskegee Study, was a poor rural county. In the initial paper it was stated that "adequate treatment has not been freely available to most indigent citizens for a period longer than a decade," and "In connection with the administration of adequate treatment, the tendency of all patients, whether white or colored, is to become dilatory in returning to the attending physician during the observation period."[5]**

---

*When the German cargo submarine *Deutschland* popped up in Chesapeake Bay in 1916, much of its 1.5 million dollar payload was in arsphenamines. After our entry into the war, 1917, patent rights were forfeited and manufacturing was begun in the United States.

**Under the most sophisticated and intensive follow-up even in an urban community having a stable population, the completion of 60 weeks of treatment for *infectious syphilis* was discouraging in the days of chemotherapy. The Medical L Clinic of Vanderbilt University Hospital, with

As a sidelight, an experience is worth relating. In 1945, a colleague and I spent some days with a VD mobile unit in the State of Mississippi, visiting plantations and crossroads communities in the delta region of the State. I learned of the method of financing medical care among sharecroppers. Following a positive serologic test found upon the mobile unit's visit to a plantation, its owner might write on a scrap of paper to be taken to the doctor, "Give one treatment to. . . ." The injection could then be given, be charged to the planter, who in turn charged it against the sharecropper's account. I examined examples of such slips both in planters' and in doctors' offices. This was 13 years after the initiation of the Tuskegee Study!

The finding that continuous treatment of *early syphilis* (4 or more courses of an arsenical with interim mercury—at least 21 injections of an arsphenamine) reduced clinical or sero relapse to 21%, as against 89.2% in patients receiving 1 to 8 injections of arsenic, was described by Moore and Keidel,[6] in 1926 (just 6 years before the Tuskegee Study). These findings were verified and established by the Cooperative Clinical Studies* of 1932, the year of the inception of the Study.

In June of 1943, a preliminary report suggested the curative effect of penicillin in acute syphilis. Promptly under the auspices of the war-time Office of Scientific Research and Development, a cooperative program was organized to include certain Army, Navy and USPHS installations and selected civilian clinics for the study of the effectiveness of penicillin in the treatment of *acute* syphilis. Though this laid the foundation for today's treatment, a number of years were to pass during which several forms of penicillin and the results of their use could be evaluated and before treatment schedules could be recommended for general use. An authoritative report finally was made in 1948 by NIH to the AMA Council on Pharmacy and Chemistry (16 years after the inception of the Tuskegee Study). Early, because of limited supplies of penicillin, all of us involved in this study were not permitted to experiment in the treatment of late syphilis. However, by 1945, such permission was granted to the leaders in this study,—Drs. Wile, Moore and Stokes. Gradually, the efficacy of penicillin was established for some forms of late syphilis. The immediate results of penicillin treatment of late benign syphilis could be identified quickly. A collaborative study of the results of the treatment of paresis with pen-

---

Miss Anne Sweeney as director of social service, had an unmatched record of efficiency. But even here only 56% of Negro patients and 76% of white patients completed an acceptable course of treatment for *early* syphilis.

*Because of the heterogeneity of programs of antisyphilitic treatment in the 15 to 20 years after the introduction of arsenotherapy, and a decade's replacement of mercury by bismuth, medicine's first cooperative study came into being. It was to consist of a series of publications over a half dozen years following the first in 1932. These studies consisted of pooled clinical and therapeutic data from some 5 university hospital clinics and the USPHS.

icillin and an obviously necessary 5 year follow-up was ready for publication in 1958 (a quarter of a century after the beginning of the Tuskegee Study). Reference to cardiovascular syphilis is postponed at this point.

Hence the historical background for the Tuskegee Study begun in 1932 may be summarized as follows: (a) One study of the unmodified natural history of syphilis was extant, based on clinical diagnosis. (b) Within a half dozen years *Treponema pallidum* was identified, a not highly sensitive serologic test was developed, and a treponemicidal drug was produced. (c) After almost a decade of dependence upon a costly foreign supply or arsenicals, neoarsphenamine became available for general use by doctors unskilled in intravenous therapy and without guidelines as to what constituted adequate treatment, hence with frequent untoward effects and with results *commonly worse than no treatment* in terms of relapse resulting from interference with the development of natural immunity. (d) Only in the year of the initiation of the Study did become apparent as to what might constitute adequate treatment of *early* syphilis, with no inkling of the effect of arsenotherapy in later years of the disease. (e) And, finally, at that time it would have been a rare circumstance that an indigent person in a rural southern county would have received adequately weekly metal therapy for 60 and more weeks.

A Review of the Tuskegee Study. This was conceived in 1932 following a serologic survey of 1,782 male Negroes over age 25 in Macon County in 1931–33. Among these were 472 with at least 2 positive tests and 275 who had had treatment during the first 2 years of the disease. In 1933, the initial examinations were recorded for 399 untreated Negro syphilitic men, 201 presumed nonsyphilitic men, and the 275 syphilitic men who had had variable amounts of antisyphilitic treatment.[5] "The patients who had syphilis were all in the latent stage: any acute cases requiring treatment were carefully screened out for standard therapy."[7] The subjects thus had latent syphilis and were grouped as having become infected 3 years, 6 years, and 9 years previously—a highly significant fact (i.e., syphilis of 19, 22, and 25 years' duration before the penicillin, which the news media[1,2] think should have been used, became generally available). It is clear that the subjects were not deterred from obtaining treatment if they desired it or bothered to get what was available, the news media to the contrary. The report of the study at the 12 year point states that during these years a "considerable proportion of the syphilitics had received small amounts of treatment (usually 1 or 2 injections) although 12 had received as many as 10 injections." (These now needed to be excluded from the study.[8]) The fifth paper in 1954 comments that most of the study group remained untreated although "after careful questioning, it was found that 34 of 133 patients with syphilis had received injections or oral medication which might possibly have been penicillin; 11 of the 34 received more than 3 injections."[9] It was commented that general medical care had not improved in 20 years, and although there are excellent medical facilities in the county, costs are prohibitive or patients are unaware of them.

One paper is of especial interest because of the implications by news media of dishonesty and bribery in carrying out the study.[7] One of its authors is the black public health nurse who provided the continuity over years of study as examining physicians came and went. Stories of the rural roads so poor that in rainy seasons the subjects spent hours getting the nurse's car out of the mud, the reunion annually of the subjects as they met on the bus which picked them up at the crossroads, and the socializing, point up her rapport and empathy proven by the fact that she obtained 145 autopsies in 20 years and was refused only one. (The burial assistance mentioned by newspapers was through private philanthropy, the Milbank Memorial Fund.)

In preparation of this editorial I have reviewed all the papers of the study. I have alluded to those which are significant in view of the publicity given by the news media. The remaining papers detailing clinical studies and morbidity,[10–12] life expectancy,[13] and pathologic findings[14] are not basic to this editorial review. The final paper, in 1964, the 30th year of observation, summarized much of what had appeared in the papers which had appeared periodically.[15] Thus, the mortality during the first 12 years was 25% for the syphilitics and 14% for controls of about the same age. By the 20th year follow-up, 40% of the syphilitics and 27% of the controls had died. By the time of the 30th year evaluation, 59% of the syphilitics were dead, 21% alive and 20% lost to follow-up; for the control group, 45% were dead, 34% were living and 20% could not be traced. By now 96% of those examined had had treatment, as many as 33% having had "curative" therapy. Among the 90 living syphilitics 12% were said to have evidence of late syphilis—two-thirds of these of cardiovascular nature and known in most instances since 1948. (The results of pathologic studies were described better in 1955.[14]) Sixty-six percent continued to have a positive VDRL test, 91% an active TPI test and 97% were reactive to the FTA-ABS test.

This editorial was undertaken and completed after many hours of "library research" to clarify details surrounding the Tuskegee Study. The primary purpose is to expose the deleterious ramifications of an irresponsible press in its criticisms of the ethics and actions of the medical profession in its constant age-long efforts to improve the health of the human race. Secondly, it has the purpose of emphasizing Osler's aphorism concerning the press and to put the profession always on guard in this respect and to urge disbelief of the press until proven facts appear. Thirdly, by putting the Tuskegee Study in historical perspective, hopefully the reader will have learned that syphilitic disease acquired in 1921, 1924, and 1929 would have benefited not at all from the antisyphilitic treatment as used in those days or in 1932, the time of setting the Study, in terms of the *unlikelihood* of continuous adequate therapy. Additionally, it should be clear that treatment was *not* withheld, and though no treatment was forced upon men of the Study, they had the freedom of taking what treatment they found convenient or could afford as did their brethren in the community. (That some availed themselves of this is documented, both as regards metal therapy and penicillin.)

That the untreated as well as treated syphilitics had both a greater rate of mortality and morbidity than the untreated matched controls was documented to be somewhat of the order found by Bruusgaard[4] and others. This is not surprising. No one has ever implied that syphilis is a benign infection. Since the major cause of morbidity and mortality was related to cardiovascular disease, a final word must be directed to this problem.

Since it is obvious that a deformed aortic valve leaflet or a saccular aortic aneurysm can not be altered by medical treatment, the remaining questions are: (a) can aortic disease be prevented, and (b) if present, will treatment alter the course of cardiovascular disease—or in terms of the Tuskegee Study—would antisyphilitic treatment, if adequate in 1932, have prevented morbidity and mortality, ie, treatment after existence of latent disease 3, 6 or 9 years after infection or, even more, treatment with penicillin 19, 22 or 25 years after infection!

Basic to this question is whether uncomplicated syphilitic aortitis can be diagnosed—a question shrouded in controversy for four decades. In 1932, Moore and associates[16] suggested seven criteria for the diagnosis of uncomplicated aortitis on the basis of findings in 105 cases shown at autopsy. Unfortunately, they left numerous gaps in the clinical and pathologic evaluations. However, the Cooperative Clinical Group accepted these criteria in 1936, and they were applied in the earlier papers of the Tuskegee Study. Kampmeier and colleagues[17] reviewed this subject, documented disagreements by others of these criteria, and from their own necropsy studies concluded "that the clinical diagnosis of uncomplicated aortitis is, for practical purposes, impossible." Since this diagnosis is open to question, the evaluation of antisyphilitic treatment as a prophylactic against cardiovascular syphilis can be determined only indirectly. The best data were provided by the Clinical Cooperative Group, which evaluated the outcome of treatment of 1,936 patients having latent syphilis treated adequately, and in only 31 patients could the diagnosis of cardiovascular syphilis be made at a later date. Moore and his associates[18] published figures purportedly showing that treatment of patients having the *complications* of aortitis lived longer if given antisyphilitic treatment. (This and several other similar studies gave no consideration to the presence or absence of congestive failure as related to extension of life.) Kampmeier and Combs,[19] in a study of 163 patients having syphilitic aortic insufficiency, concluded that their "study does not indicate that adequate antisyphilitic treatment influences favorably the prognosis of syphilitic aortic insufficiency."

The implications for the Tuskegee Study are that if the men having latent syphilis of 3, 6 or 9 years' duration had been *forced* to take adequate treatment (60 or more weekly doses of a metal), cardiovascular syphilis might have been avoided in most. In our free society, antisyphilitic treatment has never been forced. Since these men did not elect to obtain treatment available to them, the development of aortic disease lay at the subject's door and not in the Study's protocol. As for the failure to exhibit penicillin in the treatment of these patients the same statements apply—in fact it has been indicated above that 34 patients had received treatment with penicillin. Such treatment was, of course, of little significance, since syphilis generally takes its toll in mortality and/or morbidity by a quarter of a century after infection. Obviously much literature has accumulated in the area of syphilitic cardiovascular disease since the papers quoted in the thirties and early forties. However, attention to them would be inappropriate in a discussion of continuing evaluations of the Tuskegee Study which were based on concepts of diagnosis and treatment as practiced in the days of arsenotherapy.

Though the "curative" effect of 60 injections of a metal in *continuous* order, and later a few injections of penicillin in the treatment of early syphilis became firmly established, the effectiveness of treatment of late, and especially late latent syphilis has never been so well proven. The Tuskegee Study was undertaken to shed some light on this, but added little to Bruusgaard's data. That these questions still remain is suggested by a recommendation of the National Commission on Venereal Disease,

That studies be undertaken to determine the effectiveness of current treatment of syphilis and gonorrhea, particularly of late latent and tertiary syphilis.[20]

Finally, in *recapitulation*, certain facts evolve. (a) At no time in the 40 year Tuskegee Study is there a hint that treatment desired by a subject was denied him; in fact all the periodic reviews reveal that more and more of the subjects had chosen to be treated *under the same circumstances as others in their community*, albeit inadequately, but as elected by the patient and/or his doctor. (The report* of 40 years stated all but one of the syphilitic group still living had had antisyphilitic treatment.) (b) The prognosis therefore in patients having late latent syphilis in the Study group was no better or no worse than that of many hundreds of thousands of other syphilitic US citizens of their generation bearing the diagnosis of late latent syphilis. (c) The most important manifestations of late syphilis, aortitis, as diagnosed in the uncomplicated state during the earlier years of the Study was *on dubious, or at best* upon controversial grounds. (d) The lethal complications of aortitis (coronary ostial stenosis, and especially aortic insufficiency or aneurysm) had never been proven indubitably to be altered by antisyphilitic treatment.

*Read at the Annual Meeting of the American Venereal Disease Association, June 1971—unpublished.

(e) Granted *adequate* treatment of late latent syphilis might have delayed or avoided the complications of aortitis, but accepting the clinical experience that these complications develop by about a quarter of a century after infection, it becomes obvious that the institution of penicillin treatment at 19, 22, and 25 years after infection would raise questions. Firstly, why should these men be singled out over their fellows in the community for treatment not forced upon others, and secondly, would it alter the prognosis at all!* (f) The Study has shown that untreated syphilis is accompanied by morbidity, mortality and pathologic findings as described by others in the past.

This editorial should point up Osler's accusations directed to an irresponsible press, and the irrelevancy of certain Congressmen's emotional reaction to the Tuskegee Study.

R. H. K.

REFERENCES

1. A matter of mortality. *Time* (Aug. 7) 1972.

2. Tuskegee study wouldn't happen today, PHS says. *AMA News* (Aug 18) 1972.

3. Greenburg JH (Editorial): Young physicians' knowledge of venereal disease. *JAMA* 220: 1736–1737, 1972.

4. Bruusgaard E: Uber das Schicksal der nicht spezifisch behandelten Leutiker. *Arch t Dermat u Syph* 157:309.

5. Vonderlehr RA, Clark T, Wenger OC, Heller JR Jr: Untreated syphilis in the male Negro: a comparative study of treated and untreated cases. *JAMA* 107:856–859, 1936.

6. Moore JE, Keidel A: The treatment of early syphilis. I. A plan of treatment for routine use. *Bull Johns Hopkins Hosp* 39:1–55, 1926. (Quoted in Moore JE: *The Modern Treatment of Syphilis*. Springfield, Ill, Charles C. Thomas, Publisher 1933)

7. Rivers E, Schuman SH, Simpson L, et al: Twenty years of followup experience in a long range medical study. *Pub Health Rep* 68:391–395, 1953.

8. Deibert AV, Bruyere MC: Untreated syphilis in the male Negro: III Evidence of cardiovascular abnormalities and other forms of morbidity. *J Ven Dis Inform* 27:301–314, 1946.

9. Olansky S, Simpson L, Schuman SH: Environmental factors in the Tuskegee study of untreated syphilis. *Pub Health Rep* 69:691–698, 1954.

10. Heller JR, Bruyere PT: Untreated syphilis in the male Negro: II Mortality during 12 years of observation. *J Ven Dis Inform* 27:34–38, 1946.

11. Shuman SH, Olansky S, Rivers E, et al: Untreated syphilis in the male Negro: background and current status of patients in the Tuskegee study. *J Chronic Dis* 2:543–558, 1955.

12. Olansky S, Schuman SH, Peters JJ, et al: Untreated syphilis in the male Negro. X Twenty years of clinical observation of untreated and presumably nonsyphilitic groups. *J Chronic Dis* 4:177–185, 1956.

13. Shafer JK, Usilton L, Gleeson G: Untreated syphilis in the Negro male: a prospective study of the effect on life expectancy. *Pub Health Rep* 69:684–690, 1954.

*In the days of the hazards of metal therapy, one well known syphilologist used to comment, "If the patient has had syphilis for 25 years without clinical disease, he is to be congratulated and not treated." I followed this advice, with exceptions, of course.

14. Peters JJ, Peers JH, Olansky S, et al: Untreated syphilis in the male Negro: pathologic findings in syphilitic and nonsyphilitic patients. *J Chronic Dis* 1:127–148, 1955.

15. Rockwell DH, Yobs AR, Moore MB Jr: The Tuskegee study of untreated syphilis: the 30th year of observation. *Arch Intern Med* (Chicago) 114:792–798, 1964.

16. Moore JE, Danglade JH, Reissinger JC: Diagnosis of syphilitic aortitis uncomplicated by aortic regurgitation or aneurysm: comparison of clinical and necropsy observations in 105 patients. *Arch Int Med* 49:753–766, 1932.

17. Kampmeier RH, Glass RM, Fleming FE: Uncomplicated syphilitic aortitis—can it be diagnosed? *Ven Dis inform* 23:254–262, 1942.

18. Moore JE, Danglade JH, Reissinger JC: Treatment of cardiovascular syphilis. Results obtained in 53 patients with aortic aneurysm and in 112 with aortic regurgitation. *Arch Int Med* 49:879–924, 1932.

19. Kampmeier RH, Combs SR: The prognosis in syphilitic aortic insufficiency. An evaluation of factors other than antisyphilitic treatment. *Am J Syph Gonor & Ven Dis* 24:578–589, 1940.

20. Report of the National Commission on Venereal Disease, DHEW Publication No. (HSM) 72-8125. Washington, DC, US Government Printing Office, 1972.

THE CONTRIBUTION OF THE TUSKEGEE STUDY TO MEDICAL KNOWLEDGE

CHARLES J. MCDONALD

When invited by Dr. Vernal Cave, local chairman for the Dermatology section of the National Medical Association, to outline the contribution of the "Tuskegee Study" to medical knowledge, I accepted his invitation with some enthusiasm, and a great deal of reluctance. Enthusiasm because I felt that acceptance of his invitation would serve as a stimulus to me as a physician, scientist, and educator to look at the accumulated data that have risen from the study and then draw my own conclusions as to the scientific importance of this long-term study of untreated syphilis. Reluctance because I felt that it would be difficult for me as a black physician to dissociate in my mind the scientific merits of the study from my emotional or gut responses to it, and that it would be difficult for me to present clearly the facts as I see them, in an unbiased manner, such that other black physicians would be able to draw their own conclusions when my material is presented to them. Because I was committed, though reluctantly, I plunged forth-rightly into the task and will present to you the facts as I see them.

My approach to the topic "The Contribution of the Tuskegee Study to Medical Knowledge" is that of a physician-investigator who has been actively engaged, for over 10 years, in experimentation on human subjects. My interpretations and conclusions, I trust, will be as unemotional and unbiased as is humanly possible.

To place my remarks in perspective, the reader should be given some insight into the extent of my perusal of the literature. I have reviewed all of the reports published from 1936–1963 which pertain to the "Tuskegee Study."[1-12] I have also reviewed several written reports on the Oslo Study by Bruusgaard,[13-16] the "Oslo Study" of Gjestland,[17] and the reports of Rosahn[18-20] and others which were considered by syphilologists as being of importance in establishing the scientific necessity and merits of the "Tuskegee Study." I have also attempted to consider the merits of the design of the "Tuskegee Study" in light of the scientific standards of the early 20th century and those established in the latter half of the same century.

What was the medical justification for the study? Was it necessary to study the

Dr. Charles J. McDonald was professor and head, Division of Dermatology, Roger Williams General Hospital, Brown University, Providence, R.I., when this article was written.
Originally published in the Journal of the National Medical Association 66 (1974): 1–7. Reprinted by permission of the National Medical Association.

natural course of syphilis in 1932 in the light of available data? The stated purpose of the "Tuskegee Study" was to compare health and longevity of an untreated syphilis population with an otherwise similar nonsyphilitic population. One may cite the lack of good immediate therapy such as penicillin when the study was initiated. There were questions as to the severity of untreated syphilis, particularly in view of the hazards of syphilis therapy as practiced in 1930. There were also controversies over the successfulness of syphilis treatment in the 1930's.

Kampmeier in 1943 stated that "it would be of great value if the prognosis in untreated syphilis were accurately known."[21] Stokes in 1944, 12 years after the initiation of the "Tuskegee Study" states that "the great ailment of modern syphilological practice is a lack of comprehension of the why and wherefore, rather than the what to do."[22] Clark and Danbolt, in 1955, in an interpretation of Stokes' quotation, 22 years after the initiation of the "Tuskegee Study," state that "comprehension of the 'why' and 'wherefore' lay in a better understanding of the prognosis of untreated syphilis. The beneficial effects of treatment in modifying the biological course of syphilis infections is well known. . . . lacking is quantitative information on what happens to those who go untreated. The reason for this lack lay in the absence of studies of large groups of untreated patients, thoroughly diagnosed and observed over sufficient periods of time." The Boeck material (and the Tuskegee material) provided such a group of patients.[23]

Gjestland in his monograph on a re-study of the Boeck-Bruusgaard material indicates that there are "three (basic) methods or techniques by which information on the outcome of untreated syphilis may be obtained":[17] these are;

1. From anamnestic data obtained from patients seen for the first time in late stages of syphilis. Many contributions to the literature present such groups of patients and attempt to draw sweeping conclusions as to effects of various amounts of treatment or no treatment.
2. From a specific group of untreated patients studied in retrospect such as the Bruusgaard study.
3. From a retrospective plus a prospective ⟨⟨no treatment⟩⟩ study such as the ⟨⟨Alabama (Tuskegee)⟩⟩ studies.
4. To these may be added a fourth technique, that used by Rosahn (1947) in his interesting ⟨⟨Autopsy Studies in Syphilis⟩⟩.

Shafter et al., reported in 1954 that in spite of the large number of reported studies on syphilis in the English and European literature there were, in 1930, no "accurate data relative to the effect of syphilis in shortening life span. There were no accurate data on the natural history of the disease leading up to the complications in the cardiovascular, and central nervous systems."[6] They go on to state that this information was necessary "to evaluate the effectiveness of programs of public health control with a reasonable degree of understanding of the natural history of the disease." Of those commenting on the need for such studies, only Shafter et al. were directly or indirectly involved in either the "Tuskegee or Oslo Study."

Why, in the light of the previously published Bruusgaard Study of the Boeck material, was it necessary to initiate the "Tuskegee Study?"

Before attempting to answer this question, one should become familiar with the Boeck-Bruusgaard material and the subsequent "Oslo Study" report[24] i.e., the completeness of the study, the conclusions drawn from the study, including some by Bruusgaard himself.

From 1890 to 1910, Caesar Boeck, chief of the Syphilis Clinic at the University Hospital, Oslo, Norway, and subsequently professor of venereology and dermatology, University of Oslo, hospitalized approximately 2,000 patients with primary and secondary syphilis until the lesions healed without specific treatment. These patients, by and large, came from the east side of Oslo and represented, in most instances, the lowest socioeconomic segment of society in Oslo. Cutaneous lesions were carefully described on admission to the hospital and regression and time of disappearance was noted in carefully kept records. Serological tests were not performed since none were available. Diagnosis rested purely on clinical observations. [Boeck did not treat his patients because, unlike his Norwegian contemporaries, he felt that ultimately the host defenses were sufficient to ward off the ravages of syphilitic infection. Treatment, he felt should be confined to the stimulation of the host's immune mechanisms.[17]]

Bruusgaard, Boeck's assistant, and successor, began in 1925 a follow up study of Boeck's former patients. The purpose of his study was to show "how syphilis progresses when little or no treatment is given and the patient's defense mechanisms were left to combat the disease alone."[24] This study culminated in the publication of the now famous "Oslo Study" which became available in 1929. Several conclusions were drawn from Bruusgaard's report of his study in 1929. The substance of these conclusions will be discussed and contrasted with findings in the "Tuskegee Study."

In spite of many criticisms of Bruusgaard's Oslo Study by eminent syphilologists of the day, his data were accepted as the best available material on untreated syphilis. Clark and Danbolt's comments in 1954 regarding the Bruusgaard study reads as follows: "As these estimates of prognosis have passed from textbook to textbook and from one scientific paper to another, they have taken on a significance entirely unwarranted by the nature of Bruusgaard's data."[23] Bruusgaard himself warned that acceptance of his data should be made "with the reservation which the nature of his material makes necessary."[17]

Among many defects cited in Bruusgaard's study that invalidated or limited its usefulness are: a) The study was a retrospective study and as such could not support or refute an hypothesis. It could only provide clues to the directions a well-planned prospective study should take. b) Only 20% of Boeck's original group of patients were located. This group of 473 patients formed the basis of the often quoted Oslo Study. c) Only a portion of the 473 patients were seen and examined by Bruusgaard. Most of the patients' information came from records of subsequent hospitalizations, autopsy records, etc. d) Since most of his material related to hospitalized patients, his sample was highly selected and was not representative of Boeck's original group. In fact, Sowder wrote in 1940 that "the direction of (Bruusgaard's) selection has been to exaggerate the seriousness of the disease rather than to minimize it."[16] For example, Bruusgaard is accused of searching out only those patients in Boeck's group who may have had central nervous system disease of sufficient severity to warrant hospitalization or institutional care. e) Since all of Boeck's patients were selected on the basis of clinical findings (serological tests were performed on none, and dark field examinations were performed in only a phase of the original study), it is not possible to determine the accuracy of the original diagnosis in many cases. f) Was the course of the disease in those examined the same as in those who were lost from observation? g) The study was too liberal in attributing a physical or pathological abnormality to syphilis.

Venereologists cited these defects in the "Oslo Study" as making for misinterpretation of the natural course of untreated syphilis. Therefore, a well planned prospective study, such as the "Tuskegee Study" could have been, was sorely needed.

It may be well to mention here that the "Oslo Study" and the "Tuskegee Study" patient populations represent the only two groups of patients who have been deliberately denied treatment for active syphilis. They differ, however, in a) the composition of their patient population; i.e., the "Tuskegee Study" was concerned with the late effects of untreated syphilis in a black male population; and the "Oslo Study" was concerned with the late effects of syphilis in a white male and female population. b) The stage of disease at the initiation of the study differed; i.e., the "Tuskegee Study" involved black males with latent untreated syphilis (all persons examined and having early syphilis were treated and excluded from the study); the "Oslo Study" involved persons with early (primary and secondary) untreated syphilis.

To my knowledge there were no other significant studies on the effects of untreated syphilis until Rosahn's 1947 "Autopsy Studies in Syphilis,"[18] and Gjestland's 1955 "Oslo Study of Untreated Syphilis."[17]

What are some of the major scientific criticisms of the "Tuskegee Study?"

A. The absence of a clearly defined protocol in a scientific study of such importance. I cannot write with authority regarding medical-scientific practices of the early part of the 20th century, however, after scanning the medical-scientific literature of the early half of the century, I became impressed with the absence in most respects of well-planned scientific methodology. The "Tuskegee Study" reports, by and large, fall into this category. Based on my observations, I think it would be safe to say that true scientific medicine did not have its birth until the mid 20th century.

B. The lack of informed consent. Informed consent, as a dominant legal doctrine is a product of the latter half of the 20th century, and even now the extent to which patients are truly informed is questionable. Many well established investigators are being accused of deliberately misleading patient volunteers, often taking advantage of their (patients') ignorance, economic status or the emergency nature of their disease.

Some critics of present day practices, who, by the way, agree that human experimentation is a worthwhile endeavor, and that human experimentation has contributed greatly to the advancement of modern medicine, feel that in order for the concept of informed consent to be a valid concept, socially and/or economically impoverished and uneducated persons should not be selected as subjects for research, since only the most educated in a population are capable of giving their informed consent.

Given these criteria for the selection of patient material in the 1930's, the "Tuskegee Study" would never have taken place.

C. Changes in key personnel over the years in a long range project, without a clearly defined protocol and standardization procedures, seriously weakened the continuity and thus the contribution of the study to medical knowledge. Dr. J. J. Peters, radiologist and pathologist, was to my knowledge, the only physician to remain a continuing member of the study group for a meaningful period of time.

D. The "Tuskegee Study" group consisted of black males only. In order for the study to be valid, not only should there have been an additional study involving black females, but white males and females also. This criticism is strengthened by the fact that in the 1930's there were thought to be great differences in the outcome of untreated syphilis in whites versus blacks, and males versus females.

E. The study may have been biased in favor of the cardiovascular examination from the second examination on. This bias was thought to be related to the purported high incidence of cardiovascular syphilis in blacks with latent syphilis, and the envisioned need to clarify the clinical diagnosis of early uncomplicated syphilitic aortitis.

F. Since all of the patients in the "Tuskegee Study" were culled from a population of latent syphilitics, the duration of their infection was not known.

What did the "Tuskegee Study" contribute to medical knowledge?

In contrast to the opinions of many physicians and syphilologists, it is my opinion that the "Tuskegee Study," in spite of its many weaknesses, did make significant contributions to medical knowledge as it pertains to syphilology. In order to appreciate this fact, one has to contrast the findings reported in this study with those reported in the more famous, but probably less contributory, Bruusgaard "Oslo Study,"[24] the 1947 "Autopsy Studies of Rosahn,"[18] and Gjestland's 1955 "Restudy of the Boeck-Bruusgaard material."[17]

I will begin this contrast with the Bruusgaard "Oslo Study." The significant findings in that study are as follows: (This study included 473 of Boeck's original group of patients. Three hundred and nine were living and 164 were dead, 40 of whom were autopsied.)

1. 28% of the patients were clinically free from symptoms and were serologically negative.
2. 14.8% had no clinical symptoms of systemic infection but were serologically positive.
3. 23% had clinical or autopsy evidence of syphilitic pathology of a serious nature. Among these:
   14% had cardiovascular disease
   2.8% had general paresis
   1.3% had tabes dorsalis

Bruusgaard's conclusions from these data are as follows:[17]

Syphilis is a disease which is accompanied by severe complications as early as in its secondary stage. Eye and ear affections are here the most frequent; there are often symptoms of a meningeal disease.

Far more important, however, are the late syphilitic diseases. First among these are affections of the heart and blood vessels . . . parenchymatous syphilis of the central nervous system lies far behind.

Neither do tertiary eruptions of the skin, mucous membranes and bones give particularly high figures . . . (in latent infection).

In summary, Bruusgaard's study suggested: a) a probability of spontaneous cure; b) continued latency; and c) the potential for a serious fatal outcome in a number of untreated syphilitics.

Let us contrast the significance of these findings with those reported in a series of articles entitled "Untreated Syphilis in the Male Negro."[1-12] The case material in these reports comprised the Tuskegee Study Group. Four hundred and twelve black male residents of Macon County, Alabama were found to have latent syphilis on serological examination. Anti-syphilis treatment was withheld, if at all possible, from these subjects from 1932. One hundred and ninety-two black males without serological evidence of syphilis were used as controls.

The data from these reports may be summarized as follows:

1. Vonderlehr et al. in the first report dated September 1936, or four years after initiation of the study, noted that the morbidity or rate of illness of a nonspecific nature experienced in the untreated population approached 84%. In the control

group, a figure of 39% was given.[1] The effect of syphilis in producing morbidity in early life was especially noted. In patients under 40, only 20% showed no evidence of morbidity in either the cardiovascular and central nervous systems, in the bones, eyes, gastrointestinal, respiratory and genito-urinary systems.

Of particular interest was the finding of some form of central nervous system disease in 26% of the untreated syphilitics, 7.8% of whom had definite clinical evidence of disease. This, in spite of previously held beliefs that neurosyphilis was almost nonexistent in blacks.

Eleven and a half % of the group was found to have disease in the bones, joints and skin.

2. Approximately 10 years later, in 1946, Heller, Bruyere, Smith and Usilton reported on the mortality rate in untreated versus treated syphilis, and in the group of control black males.[2–25,26] They reported "it will be seen at once that there was a much greater mortality among the syphilitics than among the controls," 24.6% versus 13.9%. The syphilitic individual had a much shorter life expectancy than the normal controls. The critical periods appeared to occur between the ages of 27–34 and 45–55. At age 25 syphilis shortened the life of its hosts by almost 40 percent. Overall life expectancy was 20% less than in the control populations.

In a study of treated syphilis and life expectancy, Smith et al. noted that "the average life span of persons under routine therapy for syphilis is shorter than that of the uninfected persons."[25]

3. In 1946, Deibert reported on the cardiovascular findings in the untreated versus control group.[3] He noted that there was a set of definite clinical findings that may be obtained by history, physical and fluoroscopic examination which when correlated could result in an earlier diagnosis of cardiovascular syphilis, especially uncomplicated syphilitic aortitis.

He noted that syphilitics showed more dilatation of the aorta than controls. Both the systolic and diastolic blood pressures were higher than in controls. (Syphilis had not previously been implicated as a significant etiological factor in hypertension.) The percentage of syphilitics in which evidence of arteriosclerosis could be detected was significantly greater than in the controls. An additional finding in every age group examined was the increased numbers of syphilitics showing pathological changes in the lymph nodes.

4. Peters et al. in 1954 reported on some of the most significant data obtained in the "Tuskegee Study."[8] Significant, because all of the examination data accumulated for this report, which included fluoroscopic examinations, gross autopsy examinations, and examination of all histological specimens, were performed by one physician. In the period from 1932 to 1952, 40% of the syphilitics versus 20% of the controls had died. It was noted that most of the lesions that could be attributed to syphilitic involvement were found in the cardiovascular system. Grossly, syphilitic aortitis was diagnosed in 40% of those autopsied. Of 24 patients spontane-

ously returning to a negative serological examination, only two had macro- and microscopic evidence of aortitis. Peters felt that his findings suggested that a "black" male with syphilis of more than 10 years duration, for which he has received no therapy and has a sustained seropositivity prior to death, would have roughly a 50–50 chance of demonstrating syphilitic cardiovascular involvement at autopsy.

He also noted that clinical evidence of aortitis was not confirmed on gross examination and histopathology in 19 patients, indicating that clinical efforts at that time were inadequate to some degree in aiding in determining etiology of aortitis.

Peters and his associates believed that the primary cause of death in 30% of the infected, untreated group could be attributed to syphilitic involvement of the cardiovascular or central nervous system.

5. Olansky and co-workers, in 1954, reported on the environmental factors in untreated syphilitics.[7] In this study, Olansky reported that the family status, community activities, housing status, work status, dietary status, and relative economic status of the untreated syphilitic population and the control were clearly the same. The results of this study clearly implied that in this population group excess mortality and morbidity could not be attributed to differences in socioeconomic status. Prior to this report it had been noted that there were socioeconomic differences in prevalence of syphilis and thus it was concluded that syphilis morbidity and mortality were directly related to socioeconomic factors rather than to nonspecific factors in disease; i.e., the same conditions that foster high prevalence rates for syphilis, foster high mortality rates from all causes.[27] It may be of interest to note that Rosahn reported in 1952 his findings on longevity in a group of white mice infected with Treponema pallidum.[20] It was his impression that a group of infected mice reared under the same circumstances as an uninfected group of mice suffered an adverse effect on longevity that could be directly related to nonspecific factors in the treponemal disease.

6. In another report Olansky and co-workers reported that even a small amount of treatment, if given to syphilitic patients whose disease duration was less than 15 years, would influence the outcome of the serological tests for syphilis.[11] They also noted that 27% of the patients with spontaneous serological reversal had some clinical manifestations of late syphilis.

7. Thirty years after the initiation of the study, Rockwell and associates reported that after age 55 "it appears that the process of aging emerges as a significant factor in causes of death in the syphilitics as well as the control group."[12]

They also reported that by 1939, 42% of the surviving untreated group had received some form of treatment, making continuation of the study questionable in at least a portion of the group. By 1963, 30 years after the initiation of the study, 77% of the survivors had received some form of therapy. The fact that 77% of the surviving members of the group had received some form of therapy, indicates to me that some form of treatment, no matter how little, is better than none.

Some of the most significant information coming from the Rockwell study relates to the comparative reliability of the various serologic tests for syphilis in detecting latent syphilis:

- 65% of the surviving group of 93 has positive VDRL's.
- 52% were reactive by the Kolmer Reiter Protein test.
- 89% were reactive by the TPI test, and
- 94.5% were reactive by the FTA-ABS test.

The FTA-ABS test was positive in four cases in which the TPI was negative, and reactive 12 times when the VDRL was negative. Thus indicating the superior reliability of the FTA-ABS test.

Space does not permit me to contrast fully the findings of the "Tuskegee Study" with those of Gjestland's 1955, "Re-study of the Boeck-Bruusgaard Material" or Rosahn's 1947 "Autopsy Studies of Untreated Syphilis."[17,18] However, I believe I am correct in stating that there are just as many criticisms of the scientific methodology in these studies as there are of the "Tuskegee Study." By and large these studies merely corroborate the findings in the earlier "Tuskegee Study."

In my opinion the greatest contribution of the "Tuskegee Study" lies not in the scientific merit of the publications that have emanated from it, but in the anguish and concern its revelation has provoked in the minds of lay persons, physicians, medical investigators and others. The degree of anguish and concern has been such that our entire nation has been stimulated to rethink and redefine our present day positions and practices as they relate to human experimentation.

In closing, it is apparent that in spite of its sociological, moral and scientific shortcomings, when compared with the more often quoted studies of a similar nature, the "Tuskegee Study did contribute a considerable amount of information to medical knowledge." I will not go so far as to agree entirely with Gjestland's 1955 comments, that "there is little doubt that the 〈 〈Alabama Study〉 〉 is the best controlled experiment ever undertaken in this particular field."[17] However, I do feel that as we should not let our concern for the immorality of this study die, we should not let our present sensitivities obscure the fact that this study has contributed and can continue to contribute a great deal to our knowledge of syphilology.

Black physicians, in particular should be determined to see to it that the contributions made by our black brothers in Macon County, Alabama, not be permitted to lie dormant, but be revived, reassessed and used in a meaningful way to aid in combatting the ravages of syphilis and related diseases as yaws, bejel, etc. which continue to have a high degree of prevalence throughout the continent of Africa and many of the underdeveloped equatorial countries.

LITERATURE CITED

1. Vonderlehr, R. A., et al. "Untreated Syphilis in the Male Negro." *J. Vener. Dis. Inform.*, 17:260–265, 1936.

2. Heller, J. R., Jr., and P. T. Bruyere. "Untreated Syphilis in Male Negro: II. Mortality During 12 Years of Observation." *J. Vener. Dis. Inform.*, 27:34–38, 1946.

3. Diebert, A. V., and M. C. Bruyere. "Untreated Syphilis in Male Negro: III. Evidence of Cardiovascular Abnormalities and Other Forms of Morbidity." *J. Vener. Dis. Inform.*, 27:301, 1946.

4. Pesare, P. J., and T. J. Bauer and G. A. Gleeson. "Untreated Syphilis in Male Negro: Observations of Abnormalities over 16 Years." *Amer. J. Syph.*, 34:201–213, 1950.

5. Rivers, F., et al. "Twenty Years of Follow-up Experience in Long-range Medical Study." *Pub. Health Rep.*, 68:391–395, 1953.

6. Shafter, J. K., and L. J. Usilton and G. A. Gleeson. "Untreated Syphilis in Male Negro: Perspective Study of Effect on Life Expectancy." *Pub. Health Rep.*, 69:684–690, 1954. *Milbank Mem. Fun. Quart.*, 32:262–274, 1954.

7. Olansky, S., and L. Simpson and S. H. Schuman. "Untreated Syphilis in Male Negro: Environmental Factors in Tuskegee Study." *Pub. Health Rep.*, 69:691–698, 1954.

8. Peters, J. J., et al. "Untreated Syphilis in Male Negro: Pathologic Findings in Syphilitic and Nonsyphilitic Patients." *J. Chronic Dis.*, 1:127–148, 1955.

9. Schuman, S. H., et al. "Untreated Syphilis in Male Negro: Background and Current Status of Patients in Tuskegee Study." *J. Chronic Dis.*, 2:543–558, 1955.

10. Olansky, S., et al. "Untreated Syphilis in Male Negro: Twenty-two Years of Serologic Observation in Selected Syphilis Study Group." *AMA Arch. Derm.*, 73:516–522, 1956.

11. Olansky, S., et al. "Untreated Syphilis in Male Negro: X. Twenty Years of Clinical Observations of Untreated Syphilitic and Presumably Non-syphilitic Groups." *J. Chronic Dis.*, 4:177–185, 1956.

12. Rockwell, D. H., and A. R. Yobs and M. B. Moore. "The Tuskegee Study of Untreated Syphilis. The 30th Year of Observation." *Arch. Int. Med.*, 111:792–798, 1961.

13. Harrison, L. W. *Bull. Hyg.*, 7:223, 1932.

14. Harrison, L. W. *Bull. Hyg.*, 16:458, 1941.

15. Harrison, L. W. "Venereal Diseases and Life Assurance." *Brit. J. Ven. Dis.*, 16:1, 1940.

16. Sowder, W. T. "An Interpretation of Bruusgaard's Paper on the Fate of Untreated Syphilitics." *Am. J. Syph. Gon. and V.D.*, 24:684–691, 1940.

17. Gjestland, T. "The Oslo Study of Untreated Syphilis. An Epidemiologic Investigation of the Natural Course of the Syphilitic Infection Based Upon a Re-study of the Boeck-Bruusgaard Material." *Acto Dermato. Vener.*, (Suppl. 34) 15:1–368, 1955.

18. Rosahn, P. D. "Autopsy Studies in Syphilis." *J. Vener. Dis. Inform.*, (Suppl. 21) 28:1–67, 1947.

19. Rosahn, P. D. "The Inadequate Treatment of Early Syphilis. Clinical Results in 409 Patients." *Am. J. Med. Sci.*, 193:534–543, 1937.

20. Rosahn, P. D. "The Adverse Influence of Syphilitic Infection on the Longevity of Mice and Men." *Arch. Dermat. Syph.*, 66:547–569, 1952.

21. Kampeier, R. H. *Essentials of Syphilology*. J. B. Lippincott Co., Philadelphia, 1943.

22. Stokes, J. H., and H. Beerman and N. R. Ingraham, Jr. *Modern Clinical Syphilology*, 3rd Edition, W. B. Saunders Co., Philadelphia, 1944.

23. Clark, E. G., and N. Danbolt. "The Oslo Study of the Natural History of Untreated Syphilis. An Epidemiological Investigation Based on a Re-study of the Boeck-Bruusgaard Material. A Review and Appraisal." *J. Chronic Dis.*, 2:311–344, 1955.

24. Bruusgaard, E. "Fate of Syphilitics Who Are Not Given Specific Treatment." *Arch. Dem. Syph.* (Berlin), 157:309–332, 1929.

25. Smith, D. C., and M. C. Bruyere. "The Effect of Treated Acquired Syphilis on Life Expectancy." *J. Ven. Dis. Inform.*, 27:7–13, 1946.

26. Usilton, L. J. "Mortality Trends for Syphilis." *J. Vener. Dis. Inform.*, 27:15–20, 1946.

27. Schamberg, I. L. "The Prognosis of Syphilis: A Critical Review of Clinical, Autopsy and Life Insurance Studies." *Am. J. Syph.*, 29:529, 1945.

THE "TUSKEGEE STUDY" OF SYPHILIS

Analysis of Moral versus Methodologic Aspects

THOMAS BENEDEK

On July 26, 1972, an article was published in the *New York Times* entitled "Syphilis victims in U.S. study went untreated for 40 years" [1]. Thirteen articles had been published since 1936 in seven major American medical journals about various aspects of this investigation, and the reporter did not imply that it had been conducted in secret [2–13]. However, her article was the instrument which began to focus attention on it outside of a rather small scientific community. Criticisms of the investigation were quickly aroused, particularly concerning ethical questions inherent in its conduct. Two weeks after the newspaper article appeared *TIME* magazine stated:

> At the time the test began, treatment for syphilis was uncertain at best ... but in the years following World War II, the PHS's test became a matter of medical morality. Penicillin had been found to be almost totally effective against syphilis. ... But the PHS did not use the drug on those participating in the study unless the patients asked for it. Such a failure seems almost beyond belief or human compassion [14].

In a publication of the National Association for the Advancement of Colored People we read 8 months later:

> Some 41 deliberately untreated victims of a carefully planned episode in human experimentation, together with a like number of heirs of those who failed to survive, have filed a complaint for 1.8 billion dollars in Alabama Federal Court. The plaintiffs were the survivors of the Tuskegee, Alabama syphilis experiment, in which 399 victims of the disease were left untreated and uninformed of the nature of their illness as part of a government-sponsored program [15].

A more general article about human experimentation stated that:

> The wound to be avoided is human experimentation that offends the public's sense of decency, such as the now notorious Tuskegee study, in which over 400

Dr. Thomas Benedek is a medical historian and professor of medicine at the University of Pittsburgh School of Medicine.
Originally published in the Journal of Chronic Diseases *31 (1978): 35–50. Reprinted by permission of Elsevier Science.*

black men with syphilis went untreated for up to 40 years so that experimenters could study the natural course of the illness [16].

These examples from the flurry of attacks on this investigation pertain entirely to its ethical implications and not to its scientific validity or value. This has been true of most of the criticisms. To review so protracted a medical undertaking fairly we must consider not only the research methodology that was prevalent at the inception of the investigation, but also the extent and reliability of the information about the subject to be investigated, as well as factual, methodologic and attitudinal changes which came about during its course.

Ethical and Methodologic Background

The clinical description of diseases was revolutionized in 1820–30 by Pierre C. A. Louis (1787–1872) in Paris when he introduced "the numerical method" to approach objectivity. Among the important principles of clinical investigation to which he called attention was that "we ought to know the natural progress of the disease, in all its degrees, when it is abandoned to itself" [17]. David W. Cheever (1831–1915), a Boston surgeon and a disciple of Louis in an essay on the applicability of statistics to the observation of diseases in 1860 formulated some of the philosophic problems which are central to the present article:

> By the natural history of disease we mean the succession of phases which it exhibits when left to itself, uncomplicated by other morbid processes, and unmolested by active treatment.
>
> Such knowledge (of the natural history) is, from the very nature of things, very difficult to acquire. The accumulated errors of the past, and the ever present obstacles of interest, prejudice and partiality, constantly impede our progress. . . . Most diseases are subjected to so active treatment, as must at once vitiate the result. The practitioner's own conscientious scruples against leaving any cases to the care of Nature alone, from the fear, magnified by his previous teaching, that he might be injuring his patients: the non-perception of the utility of the knowledge to be so acquired, and the dread of being exposed to the charge of malpractice all operate against obtaining a knowledge of the natural history of disease [18].

Philosophically, Cheever proved to be nearly a century ahead of his time. With the possible exception of an earlier decline in treatment that is "so active" as to be more injurious than the disease, his cautions remained unheeded until the 1940s, when the importance of careful planning of clinical experiments so as to maximize the yield of interpretable results began to be recognized [19]. This resulted in the common use of "control groups" of subjects who received either nothing or a substance known to the investigator to be inert. The control groups permitted at least brief periods of the natural history of diseases to be observed in detail. However, one may conclude that the uninfluenced course of diseases has more often been recognized in retrospect, when it was realized that various treatments had been both innocuous and ineffective. The urge to treat and its potentially counterproductive consequences were first considered in some detail by Eugene Bleuler (1857–1939), a Swiss psychiatrist [20]. However, he also did not analyze the ethical implications of withholding therapy.

Recognition that there are ethical corollaries to the use of "control" subjects was not simultaneous with this advance in clinical experimentation. According to the report of the Judiciary Council of the American Medical Association of Dec. 10, 1946, experiments on human subjects, in order to conform to the ethics of the Association, must satisfy three requirements: (1) the voluntary consent of the person on whom the experiment is to be performed must be obtained, (2) the danger of each experiment must be previously investigated by animal experimentation, (3) the experiment must be performed under proper medical protection and management [21]. The implications of non-treatment were not considered.

The code of permissible medical experiments which was published in 1947 as an outcome of the Nuremberg war crimes trial states in the third of its ten paragraphs that "The experiment should be based upon . . . a knowledge of the natural history of the disease or other problem under study" [22]. It also fails to concern itself with problems inherent in learning that natural history.

In 1948 A. C. Ivy reviewed the history and ethics of the use of human subjects in medical experiments [23]. He neither alluded to the Tuskegee Study or cited concepts that are more closely relevant to it than the foregoing opinion of the A.M.A. Judicial Council.

The notion that withholding treatment for the sake of the design of an experiment has ethical connotations was novel when A. B. Hill, a pioneer English biostatistician, discussed it in 1951. In commenting about the allocation of subjects to experimental groups, he stated that:

> It should be noted that by non-treatment is not implied no treatment. Almost always, the question at issue is, does this particular form of treatment offer more than the usual orthodox treatment. The contrast is not, and usually cannot ethically be with no treatment [24].

Immediate Background of the Tuskegee Study

The foregoing brief citations demonstrate that there were virtually no philosophic guidelines in 1930 to influence the formulation of a prospective study of patients with an untreated chronic disease. Only one example existed. The history of this, including recognition of some of its shortcomings, was the theoretical basis from which the Public Health Service investigators began.

The story of this model started in 1890, not with an investigation, but with a policy change by Dr. Caesar Boeck (1845–1917), the professor of dermatology at the University of Oslo. He stopped using the mercury treatment of syphilis that had been employed since the 16th century. According to J. E. Bruusgaard (1869–1934), who then was one of the Boeck's assistants, and eventually succeeded him, his attitude toward the treatment of syphilis had become that:

> The specific measures, potassium iodide and mercury, have a good effect on the clinical symptoms. They are, however, unable to fully cure the disease, and disturb the regulating effect of the body as well as its own healing power. The disease takes an atypical course, which frequently has the consequence of serious visceral manifestations, especially in the central nervous system. Only when the patient is overcome in the battle against the syphilitic virus are the specific measures indicated and must then be given in "powerful" doses [25].

Thus, Boeck did not act on a premise that mercury is entirely ineffective, but rather that it is undesirable because it interferes with what we would call immune mechanisms to a greater extent than it affects the pathogen. He continued to administer iron and quinine, which were employed as non-specific tonics for a host of complaints. Between January 1891 and December 1910, 2181 patients were diagnosed in Boeck's department to have syphilis and were not given the standard treatment of the time. Ninety % of the patients were hospitalized, usually for several months. Most of the 20 yr collection period had passed before 1906, when the two principal methods of laboratory diagnosis, dark field microscopy to prove the etiology of the primary lesion, and the Wassermann reaction to identify the disease after the primary lesion had resolved, were discovered. In view of the vast experience of the physicians this defect probably invalidated very few of the records. The policy of non-treatment was ended a few months after arsphenamine was introduced, because Boeck quickly became convinced that a really effective therapeutic agent now was at hand.

The clinical records that were generated during those 20 yr constituted a resource in which the natural history of syphilis could be studied, particularly because the patient population was rather homogeneous and not very mobile. The potential research value of these records was recognized by Bruusgaard after he had succeeded Boeck. Between 1925 and '27, 473 patients (21.6%) were selected for review. The selection tended to be weighted in favor of inclusion of the more severely affected, because they were more likely to have remained under medical care and therefore were easier to locate [26]. 164 patients had died (40 autopsies), and in 70% of these syphilis was *not* causally implicated in the deaths. Three

TABLE 1. *Sex and Race Related Manifestations in 6,420 Cases of Late Syphilis*

Race/Sex	W.M.	W.F.	N.M.	N.F.	Male	Female	White	Negro
Cases	1,318	780	1,704	2,618	3,022	3,398	2,098	4,322
Central nervous								
Cases	519	174	272	183	791	357	693	455
%	39.3	22.3	15.9	7.0	26.1	10.5	33.0	10.5
Cardiovascular								
Cases	115	38	306	190	421	228	153	496
%	8.7	4.8	17.9	7.2	13.9	6.7	7.2	11.4

Adapted from Table 6. [26].

hundred and nine patients were re-examined. It was particularly remarkable in view of the probable bias in the case selection that 65% of these, and 73% of the subgroup who had had syphilis for at least 20 yr, were free of symptoms. Furthermore, 66% of the asymptomatic cases had a negative Wassermann reaction. If the symptom-free, sero-negative cases are defined as having undergone "spontaneous cures," then 43% of the 309 fell into this category [25].

One other relevant piece of information about the natural history of syphilis was that there are definite sex-related and probable race-related differences in the occurrence of involvement of the central nervous and cardiovascular systems. Both kinds of tertiary manifestations occur more frequently in men than in women. However, syphilis of the central nervous system appears to be more prevalent among white than among Negro patients, while the opposite is true of cardiovascular involvement [27] (Table 1).

What was the state of anti-syphilitic therapy in the late 1920s? Arsphenamine had been introduced in 1910 [28], soon followed by related arsenical compounds which were hoped to be more stable and safer. In 1922 compounds of bismuth were introduced to supplement the arsenicals as well as the mercurials which, after more than four centuries of use, were not easily discarded [29,30]. Most therapeutic regimens consisted of alternating periods of administration of an arsenical and a bismuth preparation, often also still using a mercurial. An expert opinion in 1926 was that:

> The optimal amount of treatment for early syphilis with the plan advocated appears to be a full year of treatment after the serology of blood and spinal fluid have become and have remained negative, excepting only seronegative primary syphilis, in which a three course treatment, lasting 9 months, apparently produces satisfactory results [31].

In 1939, 60 weeks of uninterrupted metallotherapy was recommended for early syphilis, and more complicated regimens to treat the tertiary manifestations [32].

TABLE 2. *Outcome of Syphilitic Patients Observed for 5 + Yr in Relation to Number of Arsenical Injections Received**

Patients	Injections	Satisfactory Outcome	Cardiovascular Syphilis	Neuro Syphilis
54	None	87.0%	5.5%	3.7%
179	1–9	87.0%	5.0%	2.2%
195	10–19	87.7%	2.0%	1.0%
203	20–29	96.6%	2.0%	1.0%
161	30–39	97.5%	0.6%	1.9%
134	40 +	99.3%	0.0%	0.7%

*Diagnosed as latent syphilis at Johns Hopkins Hospital, 1914–1934. Adapted from Tables 9 and 10. [33].

Table 2 presents data which indicate that a shorter course of treatment would serve about as effectively and supports the opinion that was widely held that twenty injections of an arsenical provide the minimum amount of medication to affect the prognosis.

It also shows that only one syphilitic patient out of eight who was observed for 5 yr or more was healthier with "adequate" treatment than with little or no treatment [33].

Adverse reactions to the medications were the most commonly stated reason for failure to complete a course of treatment, followed by the inconvenience of the frequent visits that were required [34]. Toxic reactions occurred in about 15% of the patients, and the fatality rate from arsphenamine and neoarsphenamine was as high as 1% (12 of 1160 cases) [35,36].

In 1930, when the decision was made in the U.S. Public Health Service to initiate another investigation of untreated syphilis, the paper Bruusgaard had published in 1929 constituted the only pertinent literature. It suggested that syphilis tends to run a rather benign course, but suffered from the lack of laboratory confirmation of the initial diagnosis and lack of randomisation of the patient sample that was traced. In view of the expense, hazards, and poor completion rate of treatment, a prospective investigation of the natural course of syphilis was determined to be desirable, in particular to develop a standard against which results of new forms of treatment could be compared.

Coincidentally, the Julius Rosenwald Fund in 1930 selected one rural county in each of six southern States in which to conduct demonstration venereal disease control projects. The highest prevalence of positive tests for syphilis among these six was found in Macon County, AL. Of 3684 Black inhabitants tested, 39.8% had a positive Wassermann reaction. Only 2% of the positive reactors gave a history of having received anti-syphilitic treatment, and as a result of the survey 95% were begun on therapy with neoarsphenamine and mercury [37].

The Tuskegee Study

The following review is based on the published reports of the investigators and on correspondence which is now preserved in the National Library of Medicine. NO comprehensive report has been published either by the sponsoring agency (Public Health Service) or by any of the participating investigators. Statistical information as published is not entirely consistent because of "different interpretations by various clinicians and analysis in regard to the criteria set up for the selection of study patients," [10] and, therefore, a few compromise figures are used. The two principal events which occurred while the investigation was in progress that might have resulted in its revision or termination: the report of the Cooperating Clinical Group in 1934 and the discovery of the efficacy of penicillin in 1943, will be considered in their chronologic sequence.

The following factors, at least, need to be considered in planning a chronic investigation, and should be kept in mind in regard to the study under review.

(1) Are we certain that information we propose to seek does not already exist? (2) Are the questions posed in such a way that the results are likely to answer them? In other words, will the design of the experiment yield a maximum amount of information? (3) Can generalizations be made from information obtained from the experimental subjects, or do we know in advance that the data will largely be group specific? (4) Is new information likely to be obtained efficiently, and is it likely to be sufficiently important to justify the expenditures? (5) Is the proposed mechanism—availability of suitable subjects, staffing and funding—adequate to accomplish the experiment as it has been designed? (6) Has adequate consideration been given to potential hazards to the subjects and/or staff and have they been made aware of these and of their option not to participate in advance?

Because of the results of the Rosenwald Fund study, the Public Health Service chose Macon County, AL, in which to conduct a similar survey in 1931. This time 4400 Black residents who were at least 18 yr of age were tested. Two positive serologic tests for syphilis (Kolmer and Kahn) were found in 22.5% of the entire group and in 26.5% of the 1782 men who were at least 25 yr of age [8]. The difference between 39.8% and 22.5% probably is mainly explained by the exclusion from the second survey of a large number of children with congenital syphilis. According to the report of the Rosenwald Fund, the mean prevalence of congenital syphilis among those surveyed in the six counties was 28% with the unexplained greatest prevalence in Macon County—62%! Of the population of this county 82% was Black, and most were tenant farmers who were not likely to leave the area [8,38]. In 1930 there were fifteen white physicians practicing medicine privately in the county [38], and in 1932 there were only nine [8], but at both times there was only one Black physician. The major landmark of the region was the Tuskegee Institute (founded in 1881), and this is why the investigation came to be called the Tuskegee study.

The starting date of the investigation was Jan. 1933. The subjects had been selected during that and the previous winter. All that can be concluded from the publications in regard to case selection is that 84.5% of the potential subjects who met the required criteria were entered into the Study. They initially comprised 399 men who were at least 25 yr of age, had two positive serologic tests for syphilis but no primary lesion, and gave no history of having received treatment. Tertiary syphilis was diagnosed in 11.5% of these subjects. Men who were found during the case selection process to have primary syphilis were begun on treatment and were excluded from the Study. The exclusion of women was not explained, but presumably was decided upon to avoid abetting the occurrence of congenital syphilis. Two series of control subjects were selected: 201 age-matched non-syphilitic men and 275 men who had received an inadequate number of arsphenamine injections during the first 2 yr after the diagnosis of syphilis had been made [2, 2a].

The only comment about the rationale of the investigation which the investigation ever published is the following:

> As the result of surveys made a few years ago in southern rural areas it was learned that a considerable portion of the infected Negro population remained untreated during the entire course of syphilis. Such individuals seemed to offer an unusual opportunity to study the untreated syphilitic patients from the beginning of the disease to the death of the infected person. An opportunity was also offered to compare the syphilitic process uninfluenced by modern treatment with the results attained when treatment has been given [2, 2a].

A letter from the first director of the Study, Assistant Surgeon General R. A. Vonderlehr (1897–1973) to Dr. A. V. Deibert, to whom had been assigned the task of adding subjects to the Study, dated Dec. 5, 1938, reveals four attitudinal and factual elements about the Tuskegee Study which have not been published: that it was initiated without a long range plan, that the gathering of partially treated subjects had been fortuitous, why there had been more of these than untreated subjects, and why they were not deemed important to the Study:

> when the study was started in the fall of 1932 no plans had been made for its continuation and a few patients were treated before we fully realized the need for continuing the project on a permanent basis. Second, it was difficult to hold the interest of the group of Negroes in Macon County unless some treatment was given. This was particularly true in the patients with early syphilis. In consequence, we treated practically all of the patients with early manifestations and many of the patients with latent syphilis. . . . I doubt the wisdom of bothering to examine the treated individuals carefully because we already have in the clinic of the Cooperative Clinical Group a considerable number of Negro

males in the proper age groups who have received inadequate treatment and who are under observation [39].

Thus, the partially treated group of 275 men was not reported on after 1936. Whether an effort was made to have them complete their courses of treatment is unknown. It also is not clear when the decision was made to convert the data collection of 1932–33 into a chronic investigation. According to a report in 1953, "each of the patients was followed up with an annual blood test and, whenever the Public Health Service physicians came to Tuskegee, physical examinations were repeated" [6]. Twenty years later, another of the investigators construed that "At approximately 5-yr intervals, follow-up clinical and laboratory evaluations of these men have been conducted" [40]. Actually, clinical reexaminations, some of which were spread over 2 yr, were completed in 1939, '48, '52, '54, '63 and '70. In 1956 it was stated that "since 1939 annual serologic examinations have been attempted" [11]. Data on the number of serologic examinations that were conducted are not available, but it is known that improved methods were introduced periodically, such as the T. pallidum immobilization test which the investigators began to use in 1952 [11]. Autopsies were performed at the Tuskegee Veterans Administration Hospital and the tissues were sent to the Public Health Service laboratories in Washington, D.C. (later in Bethesda, MD) for microscopic examination.

The investigators never commented in a publication about budgetary constraints on their work. However, their correspondence reveals some of the consequences which must inevitably have resulted from the woefully inadequate total budgets of the Venereal Diseases Division of the Public Health Service. This deteriorated from its pre-1939 high of $1,000,000 in fiscal 1920 to a nadir of $58,808 in fiscal 1935, followed by an appropriation of $80,000 in each of the next 3 yr [41]. The more important of two examples pertains to the performance of autopsies. Whether or not an administrative procedure had been sought, none was found whereby the P.H.S. would pay for autopsies, which were a very important component of the total investigation. Therefore, financial support was requested at the outset from a private philanthropic organization, the Milbank Memorial fund, which then subsidized this segment of the Study throughout its course. Until 1952 the grant was $50 per autopsy, of which the pathologist,* at the Tuskegee Veterans Administration Hospital received $15. The remainder largely went to the undertaker [42]. For the next 13 yr the grant was increased to $100, of which the pathologist received $25. As recently as 1965 the chief of the Venereal Disease Division again begged that "Although I hesitate to presume on your generosity, I wonder if Milbank would consider increasing its allocation of $100.00 per autopsy to $175.00" [43].

*Dr. J. J. Peters performed the autopsies until 1963, when he retired. He was a diplomate of the American Board of Radiology.

Evidence that even expenditures of petty cash caused concern is shown in a letter in 1938 about the cost of mailing serum specimens from AL to the P.H.S. laboratory in New York:

> Dr. Mahoney informs me that the blood sera is (sic) arriving in New York in a satisfactory condition. I was rather shocked at the cost involved in sending the sera by airmail and special delivery, this averaging about $1.50 per mailing tube containing the sera of 7 or 8 patients [44].

The only adjustment in the composition of the two groups of men who remained under observation was made in 1938, during the first reevaluation. At that time 43% of the syphilitic patients who were reexamined had received at least one injection of an anti-syphilitic drug. Twelve had received ten or more injections and were therefore removed from the Study [4]. Fourteen men who had latent syphilis and had not been examined before 1933 were added.

How many control subjects contracted syphilis during the course of the investigation, or even before its inception, never was clarified. In August 1942 Deibert wrote to Dr. M. Smith, another P.H.S. Physician:

> During the reevaluation of the study in 1939 there were approximately fifteen of the control cases who were found to have either clinical or serologic evidence of a syphilitic infection. The discovery of these cases was largely due to the increased sensitivity of laboratory tests performed at that time. I would prefer that these cases remain untreated. Patients in the control group who were infected after 1939 should be treated [45].

In the preceding week Vonderlehr had in part overruled Deibert, having instructed Smith that all control subjects who had acquired syphilis since the Study began should be given appropriate treatment [46]. The number of these cases was not revealed. The only published statement was that "Also, a small number of patients who were included in the original non-syphilitic control group acquired syphilis during the period between the two examinations," (i.e. 1938 and 1946) [4].

The Relation of the Cooperating Clinical Group Report to the Tuskegee Study

In 1934, the year after the Tuskegee Study was begun, a group of American syphilologists organized as the 'Cooperating Clinical Group,' published their findings from a multicenter study of the effectiveness of the treatment of early syphilis. The data of Bruusgaard were used for comparisons. Only 20% of this composite group of patients remained under observation for as long as 2 yr, and only 4%

Years Observed	Norwegian Cases	Bruusgaard [25] Asymptomatic, Sero-Negative	American Cases	Stokes [47] Asymptomatic, Sero-Negative
3–10	79	24%	821	77%
10–20	66	36%	86	63%
3–20	145	30%	907	76%

were available 5–10 yr after the diagnosis had been made. Even though the regimens of metallo-therapy that were employed by the several participants varied considerably, Table 3 shows clearly that the cure rate exceeded the rate of spontaneous resolutions among the Oslo cases. The greater proportion of "satisfactory outcome" without adequate treatment shown in Table 2 (87%), than in the untreated (24%, or treated cases 77%), in Table 3 is attributable to differences in criteria. The former study required absence of clinical progression of symptoms for at least 5 yr and normal spinal fluid, but not necessarily a negative serologic status of the blood [33], while the latter two required negative serologic blood tests. Clinical findings of syphilitic involvement of the nervous system were about three times as frequent, and skin or skeletal involvement were twenty times as common in the untreated subjects in Oslo as in the treated American patients, albeit after a much longer time. No difference was found in the occurrence of heart disease, which was infrequent in both groups. The authors concluded that

> While the relative benignity of many aspects of untreated syphilis is conceded, the results . . . fully justify adequate and systematic modern treatment for early syphilis [47].

The Tuskegee investigators only once alluded to any of the data that were published by the Cooperating Clinical Group [3]. They did not discuss whether the therapeutic results bore any relevance to the ethical question of withholding therapy. However, it must be remembered that the C.C.G. demonstrated that various treatment programs were superior to no treatment specifically when they were initiated during an early phase of the disease, preferably within the first month, and at least in the first half year. That investigation was not designed to determine the effect of treatment when it is begun as late in the course of syphilis as all of the Tuskegee subjects were. Based on the reevaluation of 534 patients at least 5 yr after the completion of some form of metallo-therapy (mean follow-up 10.8 yr) at one of the Cooperating Clinics (Johns Hopkins Hospital), P. Padget in 1940 partially disagreed with the conclusion of the C.C.G. report. He concluded that "The palpable inferiority of irregular and intermittent treatment strongly suggests that, if continuous treatment cannot be given, no treatment is the desideratum" [48].

A study of the mortality of syphilitic patients, based on data from the C.C.G. study was published in 1937 [49]. The Tuskegee investigators could also have cited this to support the continuation of their project, but did not. In the five clinics whose patients had been under treatment or observation for at least 6 months there was a mean decrease of life expectancy between the ages of 30–60 yr of 7.1 yr for Negroes and 4.8 yr for white men with syphilis, equivalent to 30.5% and 17.3% of their respective life expectancies. The mortality data of the Tuskegee Study during its first 12 yr showed a decrease of the life expectancy in the same age group of Negro men with syphilis of only 4.6 yr or 20% [3]. Thus, a smaller detrimental effect was found in the presumptively untreated Tuskegee subjects than in a similar group of patients who had been at least partially treated.

The Tuskegee Study: Social and Legal Aspects

The most persistently made criticism of the Tuskegee Study has been that the subjects did not consent to participate on the basis of having been provided with adequate information. This attitude is expressed twice in the report of the panel which was appointed by the Secretary of the Department of Health, Education and Welfare in 1972 to evaluate the project. To wit:

The most fundamental reason for condemning the Tuskegee Study at its inception and throughout its continuation is not that all the subjects should have been treated, but rather that they were never fairly consulted about the research project, its consequences for them, and the alternatives available to them. Those who for reasons of intellectual incapacity could not have been so consulted should not have been invited to participate in the study [50a].

If the requirement of informed consent is to be taken seriously, should impoverished and uneducated Blacks from rural Alabama have been selected as subjects in the first place? Or should a concerted effort have been made to find subjects from among the most educated within the population at large, or at least to select from the given subgroup those subjects most capable of giving "informed consent?" Put more generally . . . One should look for subjects among the most highly motivated; the most highly educated, and the least 'captive' members of the community [50b].

The investigators made only two brief comments about effects of the psychosocial status of the subjects on the Study. In the first publication it was mentioned that

We had considerable difficulty in taking the histories of syphilitic Negro males. The average Negro is a most congenial person and he has a tendency to agree with almost anything that one wishes him to agree with. We spent an hour or more getting each one of these histories [2a].

The attempt to please someone who is perceived as an authoritarian figure is a common reaction under most circumstances. I doubt that the responses would have differed much had the interviews been conducted by Black physicians, since they too would have appeared as figures of authority. However, the rather good success in maintaining contact with the subjects during the first two decades of the Study has been credited to the work of one Black nurse, a graduate of the Tuskegee Institute [6]. In this social context the problem of obtaining a reliable history was the same as the problem of obtaining a considered decision whether to participate in a program which promised little inconvenience and some rewards. While these may appear pathetically modest to us, they were significant in this society.

Because of the low educational status of the majority of the patients, it was impossible to appeal to them from a purely scientific approach. Therefore, various methods were used to maintain and stimulate their interest. Free medicines,* burial assistance or insurance, free hot meals on the days of examination, transportation to and from the hospital, and an opportunity to stop in town on the return trip . . . all helped [6].

The investigators sought to take advantage of a deprived socio-economic situation, which included a paucity of medical care. They did not attempt to take from the subjects of their investigation any medical care of which they might *ordinarily* avail themselves. However, in order to preserve the investigation so far as possible they did take one step to prevent the systematic provision of anti-syphilitic therapy. This is documented in correspondence which was exchanged between local officials and P.H.S. physicians from April 27 until August 11, 1942. In the first of these letters Assistant Surgeon General Vonderlehr was informed that some of the syphilitic subjects were being called for examination for induction into the Armed Forces and were rejected because of a positive serologic test for syphilis. They were then directed to undergo treatment. Vonderlehr, who 10 yr earlier had no plans for a chronic investigation, now was of the opinion that:

The present study of untreated syphilis is of great importance from a scientific standpoint. It represents one of the last opportunities which the science of medicine will have to conduct an investigation of this kind [52].

*The subjects were denied surgery at the expense of the Public Health Service. (Letter from Vonderlehr to subject [51].)

Therefore, the Macon County Selective Service Board was furnished "a list containing 256 names of men under 45 yr of age who are to be excluded from their list of draftees needing treatment" [53]. In June the Board agreed to exclude these men. Two months later it was found that:

Some of the *Control* cases who have developed syphilis are getting notices from the draft boards to take treatment. So far, we are keeping the known positive patients from getting treatment. Is a control case of any value to the study if he has contracted syphilis? Shall we withhold treatment from a control case who has developed syphilis? (M. Smith to Vonderlehr, [54]).

Vonderlehr responded to this inquiry by recommending that the infected control subjects should receive "appropriate treatment," as cited before [46].

Since the minimum age for admission to the Study was 25 yr in 1932, all except the fourteen subjects who were added in 1938 must have been at least 35 yr of age at the time of this correspondence. Since men who were more than 38 yr of age ordinarily were not inducted, it is unlikely that many of the subjects would have been directed to treatment as a consequence of contact with the Selective Service Board. However, the officials who were responsible for the Study chose to prevent the loss from the Study of that portion.

The Alabama legislature in 1927 enacted a venereal disease control law which stated that:

The county health officer shall require persons infected with venereal disease to report for treatment to a reputable physician and continue treatment until such disease, in the judgement of the attending physician is no longer communicable [55].

Consequently, for the Study to be carried out in AL one of its laws had to be ignored by officials of a Federal agency, the Public Health Service. In 1942 officials of a second Federal agency, Selective Service, cooperated in the circumvention.

Despite the published acknowledgement that "a small number" of control subjects contracted syphilis during the first 5 yr of the Study [4, 45] and the unpublished comment on this matter after another 5 yr [54], the control subjects were presumed to remain non-syphilitic and, therefore, suitable for comparisons. Even without evidence to the contrary, such a supposition would be quite unlikely in a society which is known to have a high prevalence of this infectious disease. One of the investigators also informed me that some men did develop syphilis, but that since the policy had always been to treat primary syphilis, such infections did not affect the Study [56]. This assessment is not realistic either, because the clinical surveys were conducted far too infrequently for the investigators to routinely detect the primary or even the secondary lesions. Such cases would have had to be

TABLE 4. *Survival of Participants in Tuskegee Syphilis Study*

Observation from 1/33	410 Syphilitics		201 Controls		Ref.
	Known Dead	Unknown	Known Dead	Unknown	
12 yr	101 24.6%		28 13.9%		3
16 yr	140 34.1%	14.7%	40 20.8%	33.3%	5
20 yr	165 40.4%	10.0%	51 26.6%	9.4%	10
30 yr	242 58.7%	20.6%	87 45.5%	20.3%	13

detected by serologic testing. This was said to have been carried out at each examination, but results have not been published.

The family status of the subjects was commented on only as it was found in the reevaluation of 1951–'52. Virtually all subjects were or had been married. A larger proportion of the subjects who had had syphilis was widowed (9.8% versus 5.8%). They had had an average of 5.2 children, of whom 57.3% were living, while the control subjects had an average of 6.3 children, of whom 70.1% were alive [8]. No information was reported as to whether the difference in the survival of wives or of children was attributable to syphilis. Indeed, it was concluded that "the syphilitic and non-syphilitic groups interviewed are quite similar according to family status" [8].

Up to about 55 yr of age the subjects who initially had syphilis exceeded the control subjects in the number of their ailments, not necessarily related to syphilis. Thereafter, symptoms of ageing supervened in both groups and differences in symptomatology diminished. On Table 4 the mortality rates of the two groups are compared from the 12th to 30th yr of the Study. The mortality rate of the diseased subjects persistently was greater, but this difference also diminished with age. The extent to which treatment of syphilis was a factor in the reduction of the disparity is uncertain.

The Tuskegee Study and the Introduction of Penicillin Therapy

The modern era of anti-syphilitic therapy began in 1943, when penicillin was first administered to patients with primary syphilis [57]. The great efficiency of penicillin in this stage of the disease was recognized at once, but reliance on it alone to treat later stages took a decade to be fully accepted. This brings us to the question whether, indeed, the syphilitic subjects are likely to have been harmed, as has been alleged, because they were not systematically given a therapeutic course of penicillin soon after this drug became available. Secondly, to what extent was the Study affected by the non-systematic administration of penicillin?

Syphilologists in the 1940s had difficulty in drawing conclusions about the effectiveness of penicillin in late syphilis for two main reasons: (1) optimal dosage schedules had to be established and this was complicated by the successful efforts to produce new preparations which are excreted more slowly. When several penicillin products became available before a dosage schedule was established for one, it took longer to gather sufficient results to evaluate any one regimen. (2) Despite the optimism that was engendered by the response to penicillin of primary syphilis, there was no rapid way to determine whether the long term effect of penicillin on tertiary forms of the disease would be superior to that of metallo-therapy. Optimal penicillin dosages to treat the various phases of syphilis had at last become standardized by 1960, the 27th yr of the Tuskegee Study, when a Public Health Service guide stated that "Arsenicals have no place in modern syphilis therapy. There is also little, if any, indication for the use of bismuth" [58].

A typical comment about the treatment of visceral lesions in 1948 was:

There is no good evidence that the rate of healing is more or less rapid following penicillin (than metallotherapy). . . . Sufficient evidence is at hand to show that a single course of penicillin therapy will not induce prompt healing or prevent gummatous recurrence in all patients with cutaneous and/or mucous membrane gummas [59].

The organs which are most commonly affected in advanced syphilis are the central nervous system and the proximal portion of the aorta. In an uncontrolled study published in 1948 the results of penicillin treatment of 274 patients with general paresis who were observed for at least 1 yr following the treatment showed improvement in 62% [60]. A more recent investigation of 100 patients with central nervous system syphilis who were observed for an average of 21 yr after treatment failed to show superiority of penicillin therapy. Seventeen per cent of 36 patients who had received treatment other than penicillin, 56% of 34 patients who had received both penicillin and other treatment, and 20% of 30 patients who had been treated with penicillin alone suffered progressive deterioration of the nervous system. Of those who received penicillin, irrespective of the dosage, 39% were at least partial treatment failures [61].

Syphilitic involvement of the heart or aorta can not be diagnosed until an anatomic deformity of the aortic valve or adjacent structures has occurred. On the average, this takes place in about 10% of persons with untreated syphilis and begins 15–20 yr after the primary infection. By then the fundamental structural damage has taken place and further deterioration results from abnormalities of the heart action and blood flow, irrespective of the presence of absence of the pathogen [62]. At the time the subjects entered the Tuskegee Study they had had syphilis for from 3 to more than 30 yr. Thus, the 70 subjects who were examined in 1948 already had been diseased for at least 18 yr. At that examination 10% of the syphilitic and 2.4% of the control subjects had findings which could have been due to syphilitic cardiovascular disease [5]. The medical literature gave little impetus to the initiation of penicillin therapy in this circumstance. According to C. K. Friedberg in 1949: "The dosage of penicillin has not yet been standardized and its usefulness in cardiovascular syphilis cannot be properly evaluated until many years have elapsed" [63]. At last examination, in 1969, 2 of 76 syphilitic and 2 of 51 control subjects had findings consistent with those of cardiovascular syphilis [40].

Aside from the episode in 1942 when exemption from pre-military examinations was obtained for a minority of the subjects, the repeated assertion of the investigators that no efforts were made to prevent them from obtaining treatment probably was accurate. This might have been treatment specifically for syphilis, or since the advent of penicillin, also treatment for other infections which could incidentally have been anti-syphilitic. Of 160 diseased men who were examined in the 20th yr of the Study 64.0% had received some anti-syphilitic therapy. 27.5% of these 160, and 32.6% of 105 control subjects had received penicillin. Only 7.5% of the originally syphilitic subjects were considered to have received adequate treatment, all with penicillin [10]. At the 30 yr mark 96% of the 90 subjects who were examined had been treated, and treatment was considered "probably adequate" in 22% [13].

Aftermath and Analysis

On Nov. 16, 1972, 4 months after the Tuskegee Study began to become notorious, C. Weinberger, Secretary of Health, Education and Welfare, officially terminated it. Eight months after this a class action suit against the Public Health Service and some of the individual investigators was filed. Indemnity of 3 million dollars per participant was asked because of deaths, mental and physical suffering, and abnormalities in children of subjects due to congenital syphilis [15].

Let us look at the probability of survival to the time of the suit. At the inception of the Study 44% of the subjects were 25–39 yr of age and 56% were between the ages of 40–78 yr [2, 2a]. The life expectancy of a non-syphilitic Negro male in the Study area was such in 1933 that someone who was 30 yr old could expect to live until 1971, and if he were 50 yr of age in 1933 he could anticipate living until 1954 [7, 64]. The survivors who were examined in 1968 had a mean age of 69 yr and a maximum of 91 yr [40]. Consequently, virtually all subjects who were alive in 1973 had outlived the life expectancy of their non-syphilitic peers!

A tentative out-of-court settlement of the suit was reached on Dec. 13, 1974 and this was finalized with minor modifications on Sept. 18, 1975. It was agreed that U.S.A. would pay $37,500 to each surviving participant who initially had syphilis and $15,000 to each surviving control subject. The estate of a "syphilitic" who died before July 23, 1973, the date the suit was filed, shall receive $16,000 and the estate of control subjects who died before that date shall receive $5000. The sum to be paid to 36 "syphilitics" and to 8 "controls" who could not be located at the time of the adjudication or to their estates, shall depend on documentation whether or not they were living on July 23, 1973 [65].

Now that most of the principal facts have been presented, how does the Study stand up against the general principles of research which were outlined at the beginning?

(1) I believe that knowledge of the natural course of syphilis was sufficiently uncertain in 1930 and therapeutic problems were great enough that the undertaking of such an investigation was justified. The reports of the Cooperating Clinical Group [47–49] did not diminish the justification.

(2) We do not know to which specific questions answers were to be sought, either at the outset of the Study or at the uncertain time when it became longitudinal, because no protocol ever was published or alluded to. If, indeed, no comprehensive plan existed the probability that the quality of the information that would be obtained would justify the risks and expenses diminished greatly. We do know that two unknowns were being compared throughout the investigation: a diseased group which received uncertain amounts of treatment, and an originally unaffected group in whom the development of the disease under investigation was not adequately documented. While the investigators have been roundly criticized for having withheld treatment, their results were in part obscured by the fact that access to treatment was not restricted. From the available data we can only infer that many questions were not posed in a way whereby the maximum amount of information could be gathered.

(3) The limitation of the investigative subjects to Black men did not of itself diminish the potential general value of the data very much. Only syphilitic involvement of the central nervous system occurs less frequently in this racial group than in a Caucasian population, and one may therefore expect that a somewhat deficient amount of information about this group of manifestations could have been collected.

(4) The most glaring gap in the data is the lack of any investigation of the effect of syphilis on the family. What was the serologic status of the wives and children? How prevalent were signs of congenital syphilis? Blood could easily have been obtained to test for paternity at the time it was obtained to test for syphilis. What were the results of the serologic tests of the control subjects over the years? Other opportunities were missed as well. Since a group of inadequately treated syphilitic men was selected in the beginning, their course could profitably have been compared with that of the supposedly untreated subjects, the studies of the Cooperating Clinical Group not withstanding. The importance of some of the questions which were dominant in 1930 diminished when the much safer and more efficient

penicillin therapy became available. However, a new question could have been considered: What effect does penicillin have on late syphilis? This could have been addressed by randomly selecting a portion of the subjects and administering a presumably therapeutic course of penicillin to them, the others remaining as controls. It is unknown whether ethical, fiscal or other considerations prevented this course of action.

(5) Since the clinical ramifications of a disease are studied most efficiently in the environment in which it is prevalent, and the environment in this sense is both geographic and socio-economic, the site of the Study was appropriate. In view of the grossly inadequate budget of the Venereal Diseases Division of the P.H.S. during the early years of the Study one may question whether an investigation of this magnitude should have been attempted. It seems plausible that some aspects of the Tuskegee Study would have been improved by more adequate funding. The mean annual budget of the Venereal Diseases Division during the decade 1946–1955 had increased to $12,187,000 [41], and therefore the possibility for more adequate funding of the Study came to exist. Unfortunately, it is impossible to estimate how significant the improvements might have been since we lack knowledge of what procedural deficiencies the investigators recognized and considered remediable.

(6) Finally, was enough attention devoted to the hazards of the subjects? Criticisms of the lack of their informed consent are anachronistic, since this topic only began to receive much discussion following publication of the code for permissible medical experiments by the tribunal of the Nuremberg war crimes trial, some 16 yr after the Study had begun [22]. The P.H.S. did not adopt a policy definition of informed consent until 1966 [66]. The very critical report of the Advisory Panel which analyzed the Tuskegee Study referred to the cooperation of the local Selective Service Board with the Study director to exempt subjects from military conscription and thereby from one route to compulsory anti-syphilitic therapy [67]. Surprisingly, this report did not even mention the AL venereal disease control act. Because of their relatively high ages few subjects would have been lost from the Study had the Selective service procedure not been interfered with. In 1941 serologic evidence of syphilis was detected in 22.7% of the Black AL military recruits, a figure that is remarkably similar to the 26.5% found 10 yr earlier in the somewhat older Macon County population [68]. However, evidence that the Venereal Disease Control Act was having little impact can not be considered as justification to disregard it.

Virtually everyone would agree that it is unethical to withhold unequivocally efficacious treatment from patients who have a potentially fatal disease. One problem with which we have been struggling is whether the investigators absolved themselves from this conflict by restricting participation in their investigation to persons who were in a phase of the disease in which the treatment was much less efficaceous than when it is administered soon after the onset. The available treatment might have exerted a definitely beneficial effect on the prognosis of only 12.5% of the subjects [33]. While this is not negligible, it is the reason why I have emphasized the breach of law (legal ethics) over the breach of medical ethics, both as revealed in the conception of the investigation and in the negotiations with the Selective Service Board.

Conclusion

The importance to the practice of medicine of learning the natural history of diseases had been propounded for a century when the Tuskegee Study of the natural history of syphilis was undertaken. However, methodology for efficient clinical investigation which took into account ethical concomitants which are now important had not been developed. The Tuskegee Study had been in progress for 12 yr when the possibility of a dramatic improvement of treatment appeared, for 16 yr when new insights into the ethical implications of research began to be advocated, and was 39 yr old when it abruptly became the subject of severe criticism for ethical deficiencies. The author's thesis has been that ethical and methodological attributes must be evaluated separately first and the consequences of their interactions thereafter. In reference to a chronic investigation changes in ethics and in methodology must be viewed in their historical contexts. The righteousness of the ethical critics fails to take into account that in the context of the 1930s thoughtful physicians could detect no ethical dilemma in an investigation such as the Tuskegee Study, and also refuses to accept the evidence that very little would have been accomplished therapeutically by initiating penicillin treatment in the 1950s. Actually, if the investigators did perceive an ethical problem when they began their investigation, the results of the treatment of late syphilis which were reported during the first decade of the Study could have reassured them (e.g. [48, 49]).

At the other extreme from the criticism of ethics, Gjestland, in the monograph in which he reevaluated the data of Boeck and Bruusgaard, commented that "there is little doubt that the 'Alabama Study' is the best controlled experiment ever undertaken in this particular field" [69]. Since the Tuskegee Study was initiated without a comprehensive plan, this view is difficult to support. What is most regrettable is that, while ethical problems may have been historically unavoidable, methodologic defects, many of which were probably surmountable, precluded as much knowledge from being obtained as the participants could have made available.

As it turned out, Vonderlehr was correct when he wrote in 1942 that "The present study of untreated syphilis . . . represents one of the last opportunities which the science of medicine will have to conduct an investigation of this kind" [52]. In 1970 W. J. Brown, a successor as chief of venereal disease control in the P.H.S., used almost the same words, changing only the tense:

Since today it is both undesirable and impossible to study the effects of untreated syphilis on a large and homogeneous population group, the Boeck-Bruusgaard and Tuskegee studies are possibly the best information on the long-term course of untreated syphilis we shall ever have [70].

For this reason, as well as in compensation for the participation of more than 600 citizens of Macon County, AL the Tuskegee Study deserves to be fully documented in a monograph which is based on all of the data which are in the files of the Public Health Service.

REFERENCES

1. Heller J: Syphilis victims in U.S. study went untreated for 40 yr. *New York Times* pp. 1, 8. July 26, 1972.

2. Vonderlehr RA, Clark T, Wenger OC *et al*.: Untreated syphilis in the male Negro. *Ven Dis Inform* 17:260–265, 1936.

2a. Same as 2, plus discussion: *JAMA* 107:856–860, 1936.

3. Heller JR, Bruyere PT: Untreated syphilis in the male Negro. II. Mortality during 12 yr of observation. *J Ven Dis Inform* 27:34–38, 1946.

4. Deibert AV, Bruyere MD: Untreated syphilis in the male Negro—3. Evidence of cardiovascular abnormalities and other forms of morbidity. *J Ven Dis Inform* 27:301–314, 1946.

5. Pesare PJ, Bauer TJ, Gleeson GA: Untreated syphilis in the male Negro. Observation of abnormalities over 16 yr. *Am J Syph* 34:201–213, 1950.

6. Rivers E, Schuman SH, Simpson L *et al*.: Twenty yr of follow-up experience in a long-range medical study. *Publ Hlth Rep* 68:391–395, 1953.

7. Shafer JK, Usilton LJ, Gleeson GA: Untreated syphilis in the male Negro: Prospective study of effect on life expectancy. *Publ Hlth Rep*, 684–690, 1954.

8. Olansky S, Simpson L, Schuman SH: Untreated syphilis in the male Negro: Environmental factors in the Tuskegee Study. *Publ Hlth Rep* 69:691–698, 1954.

9. Peters JJ, Peers JH, Olansky S *et al*.: Untreated syphilis in the male Negro: Pathologic findings in syphilitic and non-syphilitic patients. *J Chron Dis* 1:127–148, 1955.

10. Schuman SH, Olansky S, Rivers E *et al*.: Untreated syphilis in the male Negro: Background and current status of patients in the Tuskegee Study. *J Chron Dis* 2:543–558, 1955.

11. Olansky S, Cutler JC, Price EV: Untreated syphilis in the male Negro. Twenty-two yr of serologic observation in a selected syphilis study group. *Archs Dermal* 73:516–522, 1956.

12. Olansky S, Schuman SH, Peters JJ *et al*.: Untreated syphilis in the male Negro. X. Twenty yr of clinical observation of untreated syphilitic and presumably nonsyphilitic groups. *J Chron Dis* 4:177–185, 1956.

13. Rockwell DH, Yobs AR, Moore MB: The Tuskegee Study of untreated syphilis. The 30th year of observation. *Archs Int Med* 114:792–798, 1964.

14. Anonymous: A matter of morality. *Time*, p. 54. Aug 7, 1972.

15. Anonymous: Black victims of syphilis experiment file class action suit for $1.8 billion. Equal Justice (publication of NAACP), 3:2, 1972.

16. Anonymous: Weighing Medicine's need to know against the individual's rights and safety in 'human experimentation.' *Med Wld News* 37, Passim. June 8, 1973.

17. Louis PCA: *Essay on Clinical Instruction.* Trans. by P. Martin. London: S Highley 1834, p. 27. (Original publication, Paris 1831).

18. Cheever DW: *The value and the fallacy of statistics in the observation of disease.* Boston: D Clapp, 1861, pp. 415. Also in Boston *Med Surg J,* 63, 1861.

19. Hill AB: Medical ethics and controlled trials. *Brit Med J* 1:1043–1049, 1963.

20. Bleuler E: *Das autistisch-undisziplinierte Denken in der Medizin und seine Überwindung.* 3rd edition Berlin: J Springer, 72–82, 1922.

21. Anonymous: Supplementary report of the Judicial Council, *Am Med Ass JAMA* 132:1090, 1946.

22. Nuremberg Military Tribunals: Trials of war criminals (The medical case). US Gov Printing Office 2:181–184, 1974. Reprinted in Shimkin MB: The problem of experimentation on human beings—I. The research worker's point of view. *Science NY* 117:205–207, 1953.

23. Ivy AC: The history and ethics of the use of human subjects in medical experiments. *Science NY* 108:1–5, 1948.

24. Hill AB: The clinical trial. *Brit Med Bull* 7:278–282, 1951.

25. Bruusgaard JE: Über das Schicksal der nicht spezifisch behandelten Luetiker. *Archs f Dermat u Syph* 157:309–322, 1929.

26. Sowder WT: An interpretation of Bruusgaard's paper on the fate of untreated syphilitics. *Am J Syph* 24:684–691, 1940.

27. Turner TB: The race and sex distribution of the lesions of syphilis in 10,000 cases. *Bull J Hopkins Hosp* 46:159–184, 1930.

28. Ehrlich P. Ueber die Behandlung der Syphilis mit Dioxydiamido arsenobenzol. *Klin-ther Wchnschr Berlin* 17:1005–1018, 1910.

29. Sazerac R, Levaditi C: Emploi du bismuth dans la prophylaxie de la syphilis. *Comp rendu Acad Sci Paris* 174:128–131, 1922.

30. Wright CS: Mercury in the treatment of syphilis. *Am J Syph* 20:660–680, 1936.

31. Moore JE, Kemp JE: The treatment of early syphilis—2. Clinical results in 402 patients. *Bull J Hopkins Hosp* 39:16–35, 1926.

32. Stokes JH: Some problems in the control of syphilis as a disease. *Am J Syph* 23:549–576, 1939.

33. Diseker TH, Clark EG, Moore JE: Long-term results in the treatment of latent syphilis. *Am J Syph* 28:1–26, 1944.

34. Pugh JH, Stokes JH, Brown LA *et al.*: A study based on personal follow-up results in a syphilis clinic of the patient's reasons for lapse of treatment. *Am J Syph* 14:438–450, 1930.

35. Cole HN, DeWolf H, McCluskey JM *et al.*: Toxic effects following use of arsphenamines. *JAMA* 97:897–904, 1931.

36. Clark T: *The control of syphilis in southern rural areas* p. 44 Chicago: Julius Rosenwald Fund, 1932.

37. *Op cit* No. 36, pp. 27–35.

38. *Op cit* No. 36, pp. 17–19.

39. Letter from Vonderlehr RA to Deibert AV, Dec. 5, 1938.

40. Caldwell JG, Price EV, Schroeter AL *et al.*: Aortic regurgitation in the Tuskegee Study of untreated syphilis. *J Chron Dis* 26:187–194, 1973.

41. Anderson OW: *Syphilis and society. Problems of control in the United States 1912–1964.* Chicago: *Hlth Inf Fdn, Res Ser* 22, 6, 53, 1965.

42. Letter from Isaacs L (Treasurer, Milbank Memorial Fund) to Vonderlehr RA, Apr 23, 1940.

43. Letter from Brown WJ to Robertson A (Executive Director, Milbank Memorial Fund), Aug 18, 1965.

44. Letter from Deibert AV to Vonderlehr RA, Nov. 7, 1938.

45. Letter from Deibert AV to Smith M, Aug 22, 1942.

46. Letter from Vonderlehr RA to Smith M, Aug 11, 1942.

47. Stokes JH, Usilton LJ, Cole HN *et al.*: What treatment in early syphilis accomplishes. *Am J Med Sci* 188:660–684, 1934.

48. Padget P: Long-term results in the treatment of early syphilis. *Am J Syph* 24:692–731, 1940.

49. Usilton LJ, Miner JR: A tentative death curve for acquired syphilis in white and colored males in the United States. *J Ven Dis Inf* 18:231–239, 1937.

50. Butler BN, Chairman, Tuskegee Syphilis Study *ad hoc* Advisory Panel: *Final Report*. US Dep't of HEW, PHS, (a) p. 14; (b) p. 29, Apr 28, 1973.

51. Letter from Vonderlehr RA to subject of Tuskegee Study, Apr 11, 1941.

52. Letter from Vonderlehr RA to Smith M, Apr 30, 1942.

53. Letter from Smith M to Vonderlehr RA, June 8, 1942.

54. Letter from Smith M to Vonderlehr RA, Aug 6, 1942.

55. *General laws of the legislature of Alabama*. Session of 1927. Montgomery: Brown p. 716, 1927.

56. Olansky S: Personal communication, Nov. 19, 1973.

57. Mahoney JF, Arnold RC, Harris A: Penicillin treatment of early syphilis: a preliminary report. *Am J Publ Hlth* 33:1387–1391, 1943.

58. Publ Hlth Ser Publ No. 743: *Syphilis. Modern diagnosis and management*. Washington: US Gov Printing Office, p. 12, 1960.

59. Tucker HA: Penicillin in benign late and visceral syphilis. *Am J Med* 5:702–708, 1948.

60. Kopp I, Rose AS, Solomon HC: The treatment of late symptomatic neurosyphilis at the Boston Psychopathic Hospital. *Am J Syph* 32:509–520, 1948.

61. Wilner E, Brody JA: Prognosis of general paresis after treatment. *Lancet* 2:1370–1371, 1968.

62. Webster B, Rich C, Densen PM *et al.*: Studies in cardiovascular syphilis. III. The natural history of syphilitic aortic insufficiency. *Am Heart J* 46:117–145, 1953.

63. Friedberg CK: *Diseases of the Heart*. Philadelphia: W B Saunders Co, p. 830, 1949.

64. Linder FE, Grove RD: *Vital statistics in the U.S.A. 1900–1940*. Washington: Gov Printing Office p. 150, 1943.

65. USDC, Mid Dist AL, Civil Action No 4126-N, Sept 18, 1975.

66. Epstein LC, Lasagna L: Obtaining informed consent. *Archs Int Med* 123:682–688, 1969.

67. *Op cit* No. 50, pp. 9–10.

68. Vonderlehr RA, Usilton LJ: Syphilis among men of draft age in the U.S.A. *JAMA* 120:1369–1371, 1942.

69. Gjestland T: *The Oslo study of untreated syphilis. Acta Derm-Ven*, 35, suppl 34, p. 31, 1955.

70. Brown WJ, Donohue JF, Axnick NW *et al.*: *Syphilis and other venereal diseases*. Cambridge: Harvard Univ Press, pp. 20–21, 1970.

NON-RANDOM EVENTS

BARBARA ROSENKRANTZ

James H. Jones's book about the Tuskegee Study of untreated syphilis in poor blacks (1923–1972) adds significantly to public knowledge of past events that are relatively close at hand. Many readers of the book will recall that the Associated Press broke the story of an experiment involving 412 black men whose advanced disease was followed clinically but not treated. The wire service story appeared in the long hot summer of 1972, and in the following months reporters and newspaper editors, the Tuskegee Syphilis Ad Hoc Panel of nine citizens appointed by an Assistant Secretary of HEW, the state of Alabama through Governor George Wallace's office, Ted Kennedy's Subcommittee on Health of the Senate Committee on Labor and Welfare, and the U.S. District Court of the Middle District of Alabama examined evidence and attempted to grasp the implications of what had occurred over a forty-year period. Initial disbelief and indignation gave way in time, leaving largely unanswered the two questions that investigators had locked together: "How did it happen?" and "How could it happen?" Jones addresses both these questions independently of and in relation to each other.

The book is divided into twelve short chapters each headed by a quotation that figures in the closely focused accounting of developments. Jones cannot be accused of understating the drama of the story: he sounds out the essential deception that implicated everyone who furthered this medical research based on deliberately withholding treatment of syphilis in diseased individuals. Jones first describes the historical background and the immediate circumstances preceding selection of the subjects and a control population for the "natural experiment" that was conceived by an officer of the Public Health Service. Then came the makeshift research protocol that passed scientific muster and government regulations in 1932 and acquired local cooperation. Jones located a rich archival lode in the official records of the Tuskegee Study that confirmed routine published "progress" reports appearing with some regularity beginning in 1936. This historical research and a number of personal interviews are the foundations for a scenario reminiscent of Walter Cronkite's most compelling reenactments. But Jones intends a grander

Barbara Rosenkrantz is emeritus professor of the history of medicine and science at Harvard University.
Originally published in the Yale Review 72 *(1983): 284–96. Reprinted by permission of Blackwell Publishers.*

purpose than titillating indignation, because he wants both to uncover the roots of this evil and to expose the tentacles connecting medical science and the "moral astigmatism" he associates with persistent refusal to question the procedures and purpose of the experiment.

Reference to inertia does not explain why the Tuskegee Study was carried past each barrier raised by scientists who were asked to evaluate or who volunteered their critical opinions. Limited funds for medical care of the poor and the uncertainties of treatment for elderly chronic syphilitics cannot justify this low-cost and low-visibility research. Jones is not about to trim the indictment by allowing authorities to hide behind claims of limited powers. Some HEW officials argued in 1972 that before penicillin became available in the late 1940s there was little that could have been done to improve the health of these victims of chronic disease, leaving only the charge of neglect to weigh heavily on professional conscience. In the final chapters Jones firmly rejects this most recent effort to temper guilt by restricting culpability to responsibility for assuring effective treatment—when it is available. These efforts to establish innocence had practical consequences, and Jones is at his best driving home this stubborn reality. "Had the subjects of the Tuskegee Study been taken advantage of?" he asks, and allows the customary room for shuffling around with explanations of how the best of intentions can, inadvertently, lead to harm. Ambiguities played a role, but when the chips are down, the powerful cannot be allowed to hide behind such shadows. In the first place, compensating the subjects and their families depended on accurate assessment of damages that dated from the beginning of the experiment. Second, Jones rolls out the disturbing record of official justification and denial of wrongdoing that tagged every inquiry about the experiment. He casts doubt upon Dr. Merlin K. Duval's sincerity when, as Assistant Secretary of HEW in 1972, he expressed sentiments of shock that "the study was permitted to continue past the time when penicillin became the effective drug of choice." This restricted view masked science's underlying hubris by focusing attention on the ordinary human potential for error through negligence. Accounts that attempt to share guilt by reference to the contexts limiting individual responsibility Jones finds particularly disingenuous. These explanations may lighten the burden but they also prevent confidence that similar harm will be averted in the future.

Jones is not simply another reporter reflecting after the fact. He first came across mention of the Tuskegee Study in 1965 while a graduate student doing research in the National Archives. After the AP story he went back to the records. Subsequently he worked closely with Fred Gray, the lawyer who handled the legal claims of living subjects and their families against the government. In the Epilogue, Jones uses the third person to describe the circumstances of his association with this distinguished and experienced civil rights lawyer. When Gray, a well-known figure in Macon County and the attorney for the Tuskegee Institute, sought legal assistance preparing for the trial, "Unexpected aid also came from . . . Jim Jones, a young historian who was preparing a book on the Tuskegee Study . . . and turned over mounds of materials he had uncovered on the experiment." The government settled out of court in December 1974 with payment of about 10 million dollars to be distributed among the plaintiffs and survivors of participants, leaving the sad task of locating these families to Gray and his assistants. The historian's research and sensibilities were valued in these efforts to redress personal injury.

In this book, on the other hand, the historian comes to terms with the social injuries inflicted by the Tuskegee Study. Jones identifies medical arrogance as the main culprit, and racism and bureaucratic callousness are the conditions which provided protection for this malpractice. Although the author cannot be held responsible for dust-cover blurbs, Jones should be satisfied with the front cover, which describes the book as "The scandalous story of . . . when government doctors played God and science went mad." On the back cover, advance reviews highlight this "bold report of scientific cruelty and moral idiocy" that shows "how the educated deliberately deceived and betrayed the uneducated . . . through a government agency," and "what can happen when bureaucratic indifference and malicious medical malpractice converge 'in the name of scientific inquiry.' " These advertisements reflect the book's argument that the victims of the Tuskegee Study suffered because of science's peculiar and relentless lust for information. This perverse and senseless behavior comes across as somehow characteristic of physicians, especially those protected from ordinary scruples by government employment. Nothing rescues the white Public Health Service doctors who directed the Study from disgrace (their reproduced photographs seem to reveal a tentative self-satisfaction), and nothing except their skin color relieves the distrust that eventually overwhelms incredulity at the cooperation of Tuskegee Institute's Andrews Hospital medical staff. Still, in the first half of the book, an abbreviated history of medicine, philanthropy, and social hygiene provides the backdrop against which these perpetrators of crime can be studied.

There is nothing mysterious about the Tuskegee Study's origins. It began when funds for six southern rural VD clinics dried up. In the decades after World War I the association of bad health with poverty and neglect was obvious to more Americans than it had been at any time in the past, although this connection had been made frequently before. Undoubtedly success in controlling well-known contagious diseases inspired confidence in medicine as the therapy of choice. Immunization against diphtheria all but eliminated that threat to children's lives, and there was hope that research with the microorganisms causing killers such as tuberculosis, pneumonia, and syphilis would lead to vaccines that could prevent or provide "magic bullets" to cure these diseases. The magnitude of the social and scientific tangles uncovered in campaigns against these scourges did not seem to dim conviction that vulnerability to disease—no matter what its origins—could be combatted. The possibility of conflict between broadly gauged programs to prevent sickness through improving the physical and social environment and more narrowly conceived emphases on immunizing susceptible individuals or isolating carriers of contagious disease did not appear significant. Where the cause of disease was unknown as in pellagra, or exposure to the causal organism was pervasive as in tuberculosis, thoughtful men and women, even those who lacked expert scientific knowledge, suggested the need for a sober long-term strategy.

The health of all classes of society would benefit from this insight; no conceivable antitoxin against venereal disease, for instance, was a more promising preventative than the Volstead Act since, as Harvard's Charles W. Eliot had reminded social hygienists, "in the white race the connection between drinking alcohol and prostitution is intimate." This suggested a social prophylaxis more powerful than any chemical agent known to science. Meanwhile, "demonstration projects" established in rural communities focused on the health of special populations such as children in Fargo, North Dakota, Murfreesboro, Tennessee, Salem, Oregon, and Tupelo, Mississippi, where the Commonwealth Fund put Harkness money to work through cooperation with the New York City–based Child Health Association in the 1920s. Small foundations were particularly keen to connect their special missions with the prestige of scientific medicine; as with the four Commonwealth Fund child health demonstration projects, where established plans were promptly made to "give them back" to local management within a fixed period, emphasizing the necessity of community initiative. The trustees of the Julius Rosenwald Fund came to the conclusion that their support of Negro education in the South would go further if medical training and care were also underwritten.

For this new venture the trustees turned to the Columbia University–trained sociologist Michael M. Davis, whose reorganization of the Boston Dispensary exemplified the desired symbiosis of medicine and social work. With Davis heading their medical department in 1929 and 1930, the Rosenwald trustees contributed first $10,000 and then $30,000 for treatment of syphilis by six county health departments in five southern states: Mississippi, Georgia, Alabama, North Carolina, and Tennessee. The sites were identified after Davis consulted Surgeon General Hugh S. Cumming and was told about the prevalence of VD in rural Mississippi, and how the Public Health Service was trying to maintain surveillance of contagious cases after direct federal support to the states for VD control had ended. Although PHS data confirmed popular wisdom about widespread syphilis among blacks, treatment was expensive and required a long course of unpleasant injections of highly toxic drugs. Contributions from the Rosenwald Fund would assist county health departments to demonstrate to white employers the efficacy of treatment of rural blacks, encouraging legislatures to make necessary appropriations.

Jones describes the negotiations with representatives of the Public Health Service through which Michael Davis also promoted the Fund's concerns. In the first place, support from the Fund was predicated on participation of black doctors and nurses wherever feasible. The Fund's role was to be distinct—a catalyst to activity rather than a substitute for local responsibility. Davis insisted on the principle of community involvement, even though plans for the project were inaugurated in 1928, so that timing was not auspicious and from the beginning state financial support was precarious. The demonstration clinics in Macon County, Alabama, were forced to close six months before the Rosenwald trustees reluctantly ended subvention to the entire VD control program in 1932 even though Macon County met the criteria of black participation and local effort admirably, for the State Board of Health agreed to employ a black doctor and nurse and the County Health Department was unusually forthcoming. The presence of the Tuskegee Institute must have particularly gratified old-timers at the Rosenwald Fund whose main commitment was to Negro education. As Jones shows, two other questions plagued Davis: the potential for exacerbating racial tensions implicit in statistics revealing a far higher rate of venereal infection among blacks than among whites in the same counties; and less openly, ambiguities about the role of personal behavior— particularly but not exclusively sexual behavior—and biological differences in blacks that could produce their dismal health profile, amply documented in Macon County.

The Rosenwald Fund's presence acted as a goad, Jones seems to suggest, to the otherwise dulled consciences of physicians employed by the Public Health Service. Before the Macon County demonstration clinics closed prematurely, the Fund "monitored" their function with special attention to negative impact on the black population. Davis hired a young black northern physician to investigate and evaluate everything from techniques used to collect blood samples and inject neoarsphenamine to the general epidemiological picture. Dr. Harris's criticism irked the experienced doctors on the scene, and the quotations from his reports to Davis, placed alongside letters from Dr. Wenger, the senior USPHS officer in Macon County to Dr. Taliaferro Clark, the physician who became Director of the Venereal Diseases Division at the end of a long PHS career, do not reflect well on the white government doctors. Dr. Harris observed poor clinical judgment in prescribing treatment, which was particularly invidious since, he wrote Davis, "the people were entirely ignorant of the character of the disease for which they were being treated, the reports submitted stated that one's blood was bad, in which case he should report to treatment." Because "bad blood" did not refer to a specific disease, there were many complaints when treatment seemed to be withheld in the face of symptoms. Jones describes Dr. Wenger as "disturbed" by Dr. Harris's evaluation; with some justification Wenger observed that the people of Macon County were "foreign" to Harris, "as if they came from Mars." From Wenger's perspective Harris was an outsider who failed to appreciate the six county clinics in which 1,271 persons had been treated in less than two years. But Harris's ultimate conclusions were really of a different order when he wrote, "It is useless to attempt to cure syphilis in the rural Negro population . . . until and unless some way is found to treat the large number of cases of tuberculosis, malnutrition and pellagra, and also to give some fundamental training in living habits." Michael Davis moved for further evaluation by sociologist Dr. Charles Johnson of Fisk University and syphilologists associated with the American Social Hygiene Association. The details of these events are pivotal to Jones's analysis. In chapters 5, 6, and 7 the impression of two opposing camps emerges despite the cooperation which Davis elicited from all parties concerned with the outcome of the Johnson and ASHA assessments. The Rosenwald trustees' decision to pull out of the syphilis control program stemmed from the economic crunch of the Depression rather than these evaluations. Jones records that regrets were expressed all around, and the Surgeon General predicted the demonstrations would serve as models for the future. But in *Bad Blood*, following after the paired Wenger-Clark and Harris-Davis correspondence, these sentiments seem ceremonial, barely covering racist and sexual innuendoes. Jones implicates these attitudes in the narrative that follows, setting the stage for the Tuskegee Study with the somewhat confusing inference that significant differences between the Rosenwald staff and the government doctors involved in Macon County demonstrations were throttled at the moment of conception. The charge is direct: although a national campaign against VD was launched by Surgeon General Thomas Parran in the late 1930s, it "never reached a select group of men in Macon County, Alabama. Years before . . . the PHS had sealed them . . . from all treatment programs for syphilis. . . . PHS officers returned to Tuskegee and converted the treatment program into a nontherapeutic human experiment."

According to Jones, everyone actually involved in the Alabama program would have preferred to treat and alleviate disease, but when this proved impossible the logic for the observation of untreated disease was already well established. Although this unanimous preference for treatment doesn't jolt our sensibilities as does the implacable agreement to withhold treatment, by contemporary standards it was surprising. In the 1930s, treatment of venereal diseases, including syphilis, was controversial. The foundations of this controversy were partly among nineteenth-century defenders of "purity" who, as Jones explains, "reformed" themselves to emphasize a single code of sexual responsibility for both men and women in the formation of the American Social Hygiene Association (1914). Jones writes that belief in the intransigent sexual promiscuity of blacks (and lower classes) led to "neglect of blacks by social hygienists," but that nonetheless "all races benefited from the social hygiene movement because of the emphasis these reformers placed on treatment." During World War I Congress provided funds for more treatment, but when this money dried up in the 1920s public health agencies and the ASHA returned to less expensive educational projects.

Jones's account smooths over conflicts about treatment. To pick up the story after Paul Ehrlich's discovery of chemical therapy (Salvarsan) in 1910, in the next year a predecessor of the ASHA enunciated criteria for its support of VD clinics which were based on assuring that education in "hygiene" accompanied treatment. Twenty out of twenty-seven clinics were shut when they failed to meet these standards. PHS doctors, especially those connected with the armed services, disputed the efficacy (although not the ethics) of this position, citing case statistics to support the treatment of VD like other contagious diseases. During the war there was disagreement over the effect of educational films and pamphlets that were handed out with prophylactics, although there was no remonstrance when "colored troops" in the AEF were required to receive preventive treatments after each leave from base camp and white men needed to report only after "exposure." If, as Jones says, after the war the PHS "functioned as little more than an appendage" of the ASHA, it was a contentious connection, typically marred by PHS physicians' criticism of ASHA refusal to endorse chemical prophylaxis in the 1920s. When Michael Davis asked physicians associated with the ASHA to join Parran from the PHS in evaluating the syphilis control demonstrations in 1932, he could not have been certain that Drs. Snow and Keyes would necessarily favor treatment. Four years later, at the start of the federal program from which Tuskegee Study participants were excluded, Davis wrote Parran, "If after the war the ASHA had only had the courage to deal with the problem boldly, as you have, instead of always treading softly, we should have been a lot further along."

Treatment was controversial in the 1930s for other reasons as well. Despite a better likelihood of cure when arsphenamines were combined with older therapies, there remained onerous costs and requirements associated with treatments over a prolonged period. Physicians who consulted William A. Hinton's standard text *Syphilis and Its Treatment* (1936) would have learned that abbreviate treatment might leave the patient asymptomatic but contagious, an outcome that others noted was particularly likely with uneducated and indigent patients. But Jones cites two articles published in 1932 where Michael Davis wrote that 80 percent of Americans could not afford the recommended therapy. Unfortunately, since this important statement is in a footnote for the chapter highlighting differences between PHS doctors and Rosenwald staff, it is too easy to get the impression that the impetus for nontreatment came from costs that were associated with racism and poverty in the South.

The book fails to note that the reliability of the Wassermann diagnosis for syphilis was also debated. Two dimensions were involved: first, sensitivity, so that negative results could be depended on to represent the absence of disease; second, specificity, which would eliminate false positive reactions. Although the Wassermann text was in general use, its specificity was not well regarded for malaria, and infection by other treponemal diseases such as pinta and yaws was known to produce misleading results. When Jones quotes doctors who noted that a "positive Wassermann" "reversed" after an abbreviated course of treatment, this may well be simply an acknowledgment of the instability of the Wassermann reagent or the unreliability of serological tests in the absence of distinct physical symptoms—a situation that was common in latent syphilis or in tertiary syphilis where cardiovascular and neurological involvement was undetected. When Hinton's book was published it included the most up-to-date medical knowledge, though there is no way to know whether practicing physicians took notice of this work by a black doctor in a Harvard laboratory who received little recognition from his own institution. But Hinton reflected the accepted view that syphilis was not transmissible in its late tertiary stage, and that treatment in these cases could not reverse the injury of disease, although under favorable conditions arsphenamine and bismuth combined might abort progressive deterioration. Although Hinton obviously did not write in the language common after penicillin therapy was introduced during World War II, he probably believed the blood-brain barrier was impenetrable, excluding the possibility of treatment reaching disease of the central nervous system. But there is no doubt that Hinton endorsed arsphenamine treatment for primary and secondary syphilis. In this cautious, systematic, and exhaustive text, observation of untreated disease is never mentioned. It seems unlikely that Dr. Hinton would have conceived any possible scientific or clinical value could have resulted, and he certainly believed that nothing less than intensive therapy over at least two years could improve the health of chronic syphilitic patients.

Although Hinton's work is not mentioned in *Bad Blood*, Jones discusses extensively the views of other medical contemporaries who commented directly and even critically on the Tuskegee Study to its sponsors. The government doctors' selective response to these scientific evaluations in the 1930s and 1940s was not a peculiar and inexplicable disregard of epidemiological, clinical, and laboratory evidence because syphilology left them plenty of opportunity to ignore chronic patients. Nonetheless, something is needed to explain why the men who initiated the study and the Tuskegee Institute, Veteran's Administration, and PHS doctors who made it possible seemed, in Jones's words, "to equate the absence of obstacles with a mandate." Because this passes ordinary human understanding, it is explained by Jones with reference to the arrogance and single-mindedness of the medical profession.

There is no reason to believe that any patients or potential patients were consulted when they became subjects in the Tuskegee Study of untreated syphilis. Nonetheless, before the Study began, Dr. Harris, the young physician who reported to Michael Davis on Macon County syphilis control, questioned the misleading implication of the term "bad blood" used by physicians in the clinics. Harris criticized the consequences of this deception, and when Professor Charles Johnson "analyzed" the meaning these words had for the 612 families he interviewed, it was abundantly clear that they did not refer to a specific disease, syphilis. Perhaps because Johnson was interested in documenting the extent of black poverty and ignorance, he did not zero in on the way that medical treatment was being used to impoverish blacks socially and psychologically, and he praised the demonstration clinics in his book. For his part, James Jones appears surprised and shocked at the physicians' failure to distinguish between patients and subjects, their neglect to inform participants of the Study's purpose, and the casual manner in which black men were deliberately misinformed throughout in order to secure their cooperation. Doctors felt free to behave in this way, Jones writes, because of "the insular position physicians had fashioned for themselves within American society. By the 1930s, medicine had emerged as an autonomous, self-regulating profession whose members were in firm control of the terms, conditions, content, and goals of their work." This understanding of the profession's position in the 1930s is essential to Jones's explanation of how it was possible for the Tuskegee Study to begin and continue in public view but veiled from responsibility for criticism.

There are many reasons why this seems wrong to me, but since in my view Jones is mistaken in his discovery of a central overriding explanation that accounts for the forty-year period, these disagreements should be disposed of briefly in this essay. Many obstacles to successful prevention and medical care of the venereal diseases remain to remind us of disputes over the diagnosis and treatment of syphilis. Furthermore, in the 1930s practicing physicians came from more varied social-class and educational backgrounds than today, were less secure economically, and more likely to be divided on the political questions of their day. These generalizations bear on the Tuskegee Study in one way that Jones does not address directly: public health doctors, especially PHS doctors, were "outsiders." Their behavior and social commitments were frequently at odds with those of local doctors, and they were sometimes viewed as competitors for patients who were not, to be sure, the most desirable patients. The origins of the public health doctors' ambiguous position is another subject, but among its consequences was a kind of isolation from local practitioners. This reality was reflected in attitudes and behavior of the government doctors. In the 1930s, when doctors who talked about "immunization trials" and "attack rates" were viewed with suspicion, when medical "autonomy" and "dominance" were less than obvious, when the rights of patients were not often recognized as potentially conflicting with doctors' interests, it is these "social contexts" of medicine that need analysis in order to grasp its practice.

The criteria Jones uses as standards of medicine in the 1930s are often inappropriate. At the same time I am simply astounded that after writing about "the patient's right to know as a matter of principle," and suggesting that "peer review was supposed to regulate medicine," Jones goes on to explain that in medical practice and medical research "there was no system of normative ethics on human experimentation . . . that compelled medical researchers to temper their scientific curiosity with respect for the patients' rights. . . . A formless relativism had settled over the profession." Patients' rights and peer review were primitive in the 1930s compared with the most inadequate formal regulations of the post–World War II, post-penicillin years, but the Hippocratic oath was a generally acknowledged system of "normative ethics." Not only Dr. Harris, but many other physicians in private practice and public health, as well as most informed laymen, were cognizant of its implications. The failure to consider the interests of black men involved in the Tuskegee Study (and the men *and* women excluded from the study for that matter), had many causes. Dr. Taliaferro Clark wrote Michael Davis that scientific research at other sites and the experience gained in the demonstration clinics led him to conclude that he had a "ready-made situation" for a study that would be scientifically valuable. Whether he was blind or deliberately unheeding of the tacit deception involved and the relevance of the Hippocratic oath, it was his failure. Davis also failed to recognize this deception when he read Clark's letter, as did other PHS, Andrews Hospital, and VA doctors, and Tuskegee Institute's principal. The flaw was probably not out of character in Clark any more than it was singular or insignificant. But it is wrong to read the next forty years' history as a tragedy prescribed by this intrinsic error.

An underlying determinism is, however, central to Jones's history. He is not swayed by the argument that the development of a relatively safe, economical, and effective treatment for syphilis altered the moral implications of nontreatment. Although most journalists covering the Tuskegee story in 1972 agreed that withholding penicillin marked a medical and moral rupture with the Study's subjects, a minority dissented and concluded with the *St. Louis Post-Dispatch* that "the immorality of the experiment was inherent in its premise." Early in the book *Bad Blood*, Jones writes that:

> Viewed in this light, it was predictable that penicillin would not be given to the men. . . . Having made the decision to withhold treatment at the outset, investigators were not likely to experience a moral crisis when a new and improved form of treatment was developed. Their failure to administer penicillin resulted from the initial decision to withhold all treatment. The only valid distinction that can be made between the two acts is that the denial of penicillin held more dire consequences for the men in the study.

This premise is protected throughout the book and leads Jones to see nothing new in the PHS and Tuskegee doctors' collusion to prevent men in the study from receiving any antibiotics for nonrelated illness. Committed to the interpretation that immorality was "inherent" from the outset, Jones is not overwhelmed by the turn of events when chemotherapy fundamentally altered the health prospects of the rest of the Macon County population. Certainly the contribution of bio-chemistry to the "conquest" of infectious diseases has different meanings for the physician, the epidemiologist, the ethicist, and the historian. In an important sense the historian writes from the perspective of the patient: the historian care-fully tells what happened because he wants to tell what difference it made. In this respect the historian "makes sense" of events by making clear what events were important. Lawrence Stone and Bernard Bailyn are among the historians who recently have praised "narrative" history that can convey these meanings.

Few historians today, it seems to me, set out with as good reason and as boldly as Jim Jones to teach a lesson. His archival research provides remarkable oppor-tunities for knowledge and even for understanding. The explanations of the Tuskegee Study that he uncovered appalled him because legitimate questions about its scientific merit were repeatedly smothered by pious references to the unfilled debt to subjects who had already suffered and died. Neither scientific nor historical analysis can allay the gnawing realization that the moral dilemmas man-ifest in the Tuskegee Study had irreversible consequences for powerless and vulner-able blacks. That stark reality, available to all who read Charles Johnson's *Shadow of the Plantation* when it was published in 1934, is foremost when we review the facts. As we, the privileged, ponder over their meaning, we should count our dulled senses as both accessory to those events and as a lesser casualty of our times. But the historian Jones's brief to redress these social injuries needs to be tested.

An historical study of conflict inevitably has normative implications, and in his study of Tuskegee Jones points the finger at deceitful doctors who personify the conceit of science. The few survivors who remained in 1977, when he conducted his last interviews, seem to have agreed with this and were understandably not satisfied with attempted justifications. Jones quotes one man who told him, "I don't know what they used us for." Nonetheless, the conclusion that the scientific errors and the social injustices evident in the Tuskegee Study have their origins and were sustained primarily by deception is not so clear. The history of medical knowledge and practice in America over the past century does not easily support that simple interpretation. If there is a strong thread in the events that marked the forty years the study endured, it must be somehow connected with the changing position of medicine; the efficacy of penicillin in curing syphilis and our belief in the right to be cured are consequences of the past as well as events that have themselves made history.

There is a particular irony in Jones's view that it was predictable that penicillin would be denied the Tuskegee subjects, because the therapeutic changes which penicillin heralded stimulated self-conscious research on the scientific and ethical hazards of clinical trials which inadequately accounted for non-randomized independent variables. In other words, experimental scientists and social scientists, especially those working on medical problems, have been concerned since mid-century to eliminate the self-fulfilling prophecy from experimental design. It cannot be denied that this is even more difficult for historians, but it is equally a desirable objective.

V

Historical Reconsideration

THE RHETORIC OF DEHUMANIZATION

An Analysis of Medical Reports of the Tuskegee Syphilis Project

MARTHA SOLOMON [WATSON]

An "inhuman experiment," "official inhumanity," and "an immoral study" were epithets the press used to describe the Tuskegee syphilis study when Jean Heller reported the details of it in July 1972.[1] The Tuskegee project was a forty-year longitudinal study conducted by The United States Public Health Service (PHS) to trace the "natural history" of untreated syphilis in the adult male Negro. PHS officials periodically conducted blood tests, physical examinations, X rays, and, finally, autopsies on 399 men with syphilis and 201 members of a control group who were free of the disease. Not only was no treatment administered to the men with syphilis, but they were discouraged and even prevented from seeking treatment outside the program (Jones 178). Since the disastrous consequences of untreated syphilis were well-known before the study began in 1932 and since satisfactory treatment was available even then, the ethical and moral ramifications of the study were profound. Public reaction to Heller's report forced a national investigation. An *ad hoc* committee appointed by the federal government to investigate the study concluded that such a longitudinal study was "ethically unjustified in 1932" and urged stronger restrictions on the use of human subjects. Senator Ted Kennedy's hearings on the study confirmed this view and resulted in the revamping of HEW guidelines for human experimentation (Jones 211, 214).

In his detailed study of the case, *Bad Blood: The Tuskegee Syphilis Experiment*, James H. Jones traces its history and examines the rationale provided by PHS officials and the individuals involved. Jones's thorough analysis indicates clearly the role of racial prejudice, confused medical thinking, and bureaucratic dynamics in instigating and continuing a passive observation of the devastating effects of syphilis on human subjects. His book highlights the "moral astigmatism" of the persons responsible (*Atlanta Constitution* 4A, quoted in Jones 14). However, despite the thoroughness of his analysis, Jones does not explore one very significant facet of the Tuskegee project: why the thirteen "progress reports" of it which appeared in major medical journals from 1936 to 1973 did not outrage the medical

Martha Solomon Watson is dean of the Greenspun College of Urban Affairs at the University of Nevada, Las Vegas.
Originally published in the Western Journal of Speech Communication *49 (1985): 233–47.*
Reprinted by permission of the Western States Communication Association.

community. Although these reports clearly delineated the nature of the study and its devastating consequences on the men involved, their publication generated virtually no criticism (Jones 257–58). In light of the vehement public reaction to Heller's 1972 report, the thirty-seven-year silence from the medical community is particularly striking.

My purpose is to examine the published reports of the Tuskegee study to determine the ways in which they obscured ethical issues. I contend that the published reports, reflecting the constraints of scientific writing, emphasized what Burke calls "the principle of discontinuity" (Burke 50). In Burke's terms, the reports encouraged readers to dissociate themselves from the subjects by highlighting the differences between the two groups and by dehumanizing the men involved. Rhetorically, the generic conventions of scientific writing not only encouraged neglect of ethical questions but also played an important role in the study's continuation. In brief, I argue that the reports of the study functioned rhetorically to diminish and obscure the moral issues involved. As a case study of scientific reporting, my analysis suggests that scientific writing employs rhetorical conventions which by their very nature tend to obscure or de-emphasize any ethical, "non-scientific" perspective.

A scholarly view of scientific reporting as rhetorical has become widespread. For example, Simons identifies specific factors such as the prestige of the journals and the "appearance of impersonal detachment and passivity" in the language of scientific articles as having a persuasive effect (*Persuasion* 33). With a similar perspective Kenneth Burke, contrasting the scientistic and dramatistic uses of language, avers that "even if any given terminology is a *reflection* of reality, by its very nature as a terminology it must be a *selection* of reality; and to this extent, it must function also as a *deflection* of reality" (45). Even "scientific" language is heavily rhetorical, for it necessarily obscures some aspects of the reality it reports. Paul Newell Campbell, probing the implications of one rhetorical feature, the author's *persona*, in scientific discourse, argues that scientists cannot escape revealing attitudes in their discourse, despite their claims for objectivity and neutrality, because the act of symbolizing entails the expression of "those attitudes, beliefs, biases, opinions" that constitute the *persona* of such discourse (404). Other scholars have explored additional dimensions of scientific rhetoric.[2]

Although the Tuskegee study provides a good case study of scientific reporting for several reasons,[3] enabling us to understand better how such writing functions rhetorically, the justification for the analysis derives ultimately from the suffering of the subjects themselves. Largely uneducated and seduced by small incentives offered by members of the medical community, the men unwittingly undermined their health and shortened their lives. Among the consequences of untreated syphilis were blindness, deep skin lesions, insanity, heart disease, and early death

(Jones 1–4). Using the euphemism "Bad Blood," the medical staff handling the study apparently tried to convey to the men that they were victims of syphilis (Jones 5–6). But the message was only partially understood. As one patient's widow notes, "I thought the doctors were trying to help him. I didn't know better."[4] A survivor reported, "I thought they was doing me good" (quoted in Jones 160). Unsuspecting patients labored under a terrible misconception while investigators periodically reported on health problems that developed because they remained untreated. As a consequence of this miscommunication and the silence of the more knowledgeable medical community, as many as 100 men may have died from syphilis-connected diseases (Jones 2).[5] Understanding the role scientific rhetoric played in this tragedy is, thus, the focus of this study.

The remainder of the essay falls into five sections: (1) a brief background of the Tuskegee study, (2) an analysis of the depiction of the disease in the research reports, (3) an examination of the description of the study itself in these same reports, (4) a discussion of the rhetorical function of (2) and (3), and (5) a consideration of rhetorical implications.

Background of the Tuskegee Study

To understand the Tuskegee study one must know something of its background. Concerned with the widespread incidence of syphilis among rural Southern Blacks, PHS officials in the late twenties began a treatment program funded by a private philanthropy. Unfortunately, the project lapsed in the early thirties when the private funding ceased. But by that time PHS officers had identified many Blacks suffering from syphilis and had established contacts in the Macon County area. Since a lack of outside support prohibited full treatment, the staff perceived an opportunity to take advantage of their groundwork in a new way—an observation of the course of untreated syphilis. As one doctor noted, "The thought came to me that the Alabama community offered an unparalleled opportunity for the study of the effect of untreated syphilis" (Jones 91).

The Tuskegee situation was ideal for several reasons. First, many of the cases had received no treatment and were, thus, in the terminology of the study, "pristine." Second, the victims were Black. Earlier controversy had developed over whether syphilis affected Blacks differently than Whites. Tuskegee provided an opportunity to explore that question. Third, Tuskegee offered the possibility of a prospective study, which could follow the course of the disease rather than simply catalog its effects after the fact. This was particularly significant since the only major study of the effects of untreated syphilis, by Bruusgaard in Oslo, cataloged the conditions of White patients at various stages of the disease who came to his clinic but were not treated (Jones 91–93). Bruusgaard did not trace the disease's course by following particular patients. Tuskegee could provide an effective contrast to his methodology.

From their perspective, PHS officials, constrained by funding from providing treatment, made a virtue of necessity. They instituted a nontherapeutic, longitudinal, prospective study of syphilis in adult male Blacks. Such studies, which withhold treatment beneficial to the individual patient, are usually justified on the grounds that they provide information which will enlarge medical knowledge. As Charles Fried explains in his essay "Human Experimentation: Philosophical Aspects," "In therapeutic experimentation a course of action . . . is undertaken in respect to the subject for the purpose of how best to procure a medical benefit to that subject. In nontherapeutic experimentation, by contrast, the sole end in view is the acquisition of new information" (699). Such studies, in yielding valuable information, can be condoned morally because they benefit the larger group although not the individual (Fried 701).

Officials who conducted and reported the Tuskegee project thus perceived their work as a legitimate and, indeed, beneficial undertaking. Unable to offer complete treatment, they tried to learn what they could about the ravages of syphilis. Kept from performing their job of treating disease, they assumed a new role: medical experimenters.

Even after Heller's exposé in the *New York Times*, there were those who defended the study. To vindicate the procedures used, they pointed to changed medical standards and the nature of the Tuskegee undertaking as a "study project" rather than a "treatment clinic."[6] Moreover, they supported the decision not to offer the highly effective penicillin when it became available because the major damage already had occurred in the subjects and the impact of the drug itself might have been harmful (Kampmeier 1251). Defenders also contended that the study's goal of tracing the results of untreated syphilis was appropriate and, from a broad view, even beneficial since the increased medical knowledge of the disease might have improved prevention and treatment (Kampmeier 1251; Jones 81–112; Vonderlehr et al. 260). Robert M. Veatch outlines the philosophical grounding for this approach in "Codes of Medical Ethics: Ethical Analysis" when he notes that medical practitioners may condone studies which are not beneficial to the individual patient if the information gained will "render service to humanity" (173). Clearly, from the first, some complex ethical issues surrounded the nature of the study, although the apparently unintentional misleading of the patients about the nature of their disease and its treatment was unacceptable (Wooten 18).

If we grant that the study did present difficult ethical issues, we must wonder why these were not even raised until it had been underway almost forty years. No attempt was made to conceal the study or to disguise it nature. Between 1936 and 1973 at least thirteen "progress reports" appeared in major medical journals with an estimated readership of 100,000.[7] One article, for example, spelled out the reduced life expectancy and increased disability of the untreated subjects (Pesare, Bauer, and Gleeson 201, 213). But, according to Jones, only one member of the medical profession or public objected to the study prior to the strenuous response of Peter Buxton, a PHS officer, which resulted in wide press coverage. That single letter dated June 1963, twenty-seven years after the first widely published report of the study, was filed at the Center for Disease Control in Atlanta with the notation, "This is the first letter of this type we have received." Moreover, Buxton contends that his objections met strong opposition and provoked heated defenses of the study but produced little immediate action (Jones 190). Apparently, the directors of the study did not perceive its ethical ramifications and depicted it in published reports so that its moral implications were not salient to most readers.

An examination of the reports suggests that the depiction of the patients in two contexts (in relation to the disease itself and as elements in the study) dehumanized them and helped the readers and authors dissociate themselves from the afflicted men. In describing the ravages of the disease, the reports highlighted the disease as a dynamic agent acting on and within the patients as scene. Explaining the study and its purposes, the journal accounts featured the doctors as noble agents pursuing knowledge and the afflicted patients as their agency for gaining information. The reports, then, offered a double-layered depiction: the study as a quest for scientific knowledge by impartial observers who note the activity of the disease on patients. Both depictions dehumanized the patients and highlighted the role of the experimenters as impartial observers and knowledge seekers. In so doing, the rhetoric obscured key ethical issues. Using Burke's pentad to explore these two depictions of the patients in greater detail can elucidate the rhetorical processes at work.

Depiction of the Disease: The Patient as Scene

The journal accounts of the study depict the disease as a dynamic agent bent on destroying its "host" through the cardiovascular and central nervous systems. The patient is the scene in and on which the disease operates. The emphasis is on the actions of syphilis and its results, particularly its contributions to early death and disability.

The initial report of the Tuskegee project, read at the 1936 AMA convention before appearing in the journal *Venereal Disease Information*, reveals a depiction of the disease which persists throughout the study. The agent is syphilis, whose effect is "the production of morbid processes involving the various systems of the body" and "disability in the early years of adult life" (Vonderlehr et al. 26). The study would, therefore, focus on the disease's particular effects: "Subsequently in more detailed analysis of the material attempts will be made to describe and evaluate specific changes brought about by the disease in the infected individual with particular reference to the cardiovascular system" (Heller and Bruyere 34). This act of disabling the victim is accomplished through impairment of the cardiovascular and central nervous systems: "Study of the untreated syphilitic and presumably non-syphilitic individuals under the age of forty indicates" that syphilis "tends greatly to increase the manifestations of cardiovascular disease. . . . Cardiovascular and central nervous system involvements were from two to three times as common in the untreated syphilis group as in a comparable group receiving even an inadequate treatment" (Vonderlehr et al. 261–65). Since the disease results in death, reports of increased morbidity among the untreated are not surprising. As the second report concludes, "The life expectancy of a Negro man with syphilis between the ages of 25 and 35 who is infected with syphilis and receives no treatment for his infection is on the average reduced by about 20 percent" (Heller and Bruyere 38). The reports catalog the ravages of syphilis in detail, furnishing frequent comparison to nonsyphilitic subjects. As the study progresses, details drawn from autopsies confirm the impact of the disease by describing its pathological signs (Peters et al. 127–48).

The scene of the disease's activities is, of course, the victim, but reports avoid such emotionally connotative language. The second article "deals particularly with the effect of the disease on the life span of the human host" (Heller and Bruyere 34). The first report of the study also contains the metaphor of victim as host or donor: "Such individuals seemed to offer an unusual opportunity to study the untreated syphilitic patient from the beginning of the disease to the death of the infected person" (Vonderlehr et al. 260). The more common designations of the victim as scene are "Male Negro" (which appears in the title of nine of the thirteen articles), "patients," "syphilitics," and "individuals." The third report of the study, published in 1946, clearly illustrates the depiction of the patient as scene. "Briefly, the study is a continuing attempt to follow the natural history of syphilis, uninfluenced by treatment, in adult male Negroes, with special attention to its effect on the cardiovascular system" (Deibert and Bruyere 301). As scene, the patient displays "manifestations," "presents evidence of," and "exhibits appreciably more morbidity" (Vonderlehr et al. 263; Deibert and Bruyere 313).

The reports, then, depict the disease as dynamic agent whose impairment of the central nervous system takes place in the "scene" of the patient. This emphasis on act is one with philosophical realism wherein "material objects exist externally to us and independently of our sense experience" (Hirst 77). One of the hallmarks of realism is that it minimizes the role and significance of the observer. Events, happening in an "out there," are recorded by a neutral, detached "observer" who sees them as they exist. A "realistic" attitude thus emphasizes the objectivity and detachment of the observer, while removing attention from his/her role or possible intervention in the events being reported.

Depiction of the Study: The Patient as Agency

The journal articles also characterize the study itself. The agents or actors are the PHS doctors whose credentials, affiliations with the Public Health Service, and usually prestigious titles are listed as author information in each article. Not only are their credentials explicitly listed, but they are depicted implicitly as members of a dedicated, self-sacrificing "team" (Rivers et al. 395). This view of the actors reveals itself in a 1955 report: "The contribution of time, thoughts, and energy of many individuals with the full knowledge that the fruits of their efforts would not mature until years later, and in other hands, has been vital. As in all such lifetime studies the devotion of these scientists and public health workers to the search for knowledge for the sake of knowledge and with selflessness must here be acknowledged" (Peters et al. 128).

The primary activity of these agents is observing, a passive act rather than a dynamic one. Articles are sometimes subtitled "observations" of various facets of the disease. They also "follow" and "survey the patients" (Deibert and Bruyere 301; Rivers et al. 391). The only dynamic acts of the doctors involve conducting tests or autopsies as part of the observational process. A 1950 report reveals the passivity and detachment of the directors in their recording of observations: "When the effect of differences in age distributions between the untreated syphilitics and the non-syphilitic controls was removed by a standardization procedure, significant differences in the combined mortality and morbidity could be demonstrated between the two groups" (Pesare et al. 213). One report praised the excellent, thorough care the doctors extended to the patients, noting its pragmatic impact. "The excellent care given these patients was important in creating in the family a favorable attitude which eventually would lead to permission to perform an autopsy" (Rivers et al. 394). The irony is striking: the "excellent" medical care, consisting in part of denying treatment, encouraged participation in a procedure to document syphilis's devastating effects.

The pupose guiding the doctors is clear—the pursuit of knowledge which may benefit mankind. As one early study notes, the primary problem in controlling syphilis is learning how treatment can prevent its transmission. But a secondary goal is understanding "the effect which treatment has in preventing late and crippling manifestations." Tuskegee provided a unique opportunity "to compare the syphilitic process *uninfluenced* by modern treatment, with the results obtained when treatment as been given" (Vonderlehr et al. 260, italics mine). A report eighteen years later in 1954 pinpoints the values and purposes of the study. It notes that in 1930 "no accurate data relative to the effect of syphilis in shortening of life" and "no accurate history of the disease leading up to these complications" were available. "This *information* was necessary in order to *evaluate* the effectiveness of programs of public health control with a *reasonable* degree of *understanding* of the natural history of the disease." The italics, which are mine, highlight the directors' focus on acquiring knowledge. The report documents shortcomings and gaps in the Bruusgaard study. Later, the authors assert that "such a study was needed to assist in the planning and execution of the national venereal disease control program which was then being planned for a later time" (Shafer et al. 685–87). A later report refers to the clear difference between the populations involved in the Tuskegee and Bruusgaard studies (race being primary), reaffirming implicitly the value of the project in filling out scientific knowledge. A "tabular listing" highlights the superiority of the Tuskegee project (Schuman et al. 544). Of special significance is the study's prospective, long-term nature. Unlike earlier work, the Tuskegee study's particular contribution is to trace the course of the disease across time. Clearly, the investigators feel the study is justified because it adds to scientific knowledge.

While no precise description of the scene within which the investigators work appears in reports of the study, the depictions of agents and purposes clearly imply its nature. Tuskegee is the geographical setting, but the larger medical and scientific communities are the scenes which provide the real context of the study. The doctors, observing the disease and examining the patients in Macon County, frame their activities as medical investigations. Thus, findings are reported in medical journals rather than popular periodicals, and a 1954 report presents a lengthy rationale that details the study's significance not only among other investigations of syphilis but also to public health programs (Shafer et al. 684–85). Another explicit reference to the scene as the medical community appears in the report entitled "Twenty Years of Followup Experience in a Long-Range Medical Study" (Rivers et al. 391–95). Even in a discussion of the "non-medical" aspects of the study, this essay claims that "the experiences recounted may be of value to those planning continuing studies in other fields." It concludes that "several points . . . may benefit anyone now engaged in planning or executing a long-range medical research study," finally observing that "the gains to medical knowledge derived from the horizontal, long-term study of illness and health are only just beginning to be realized" (Rivers et al. 391), 394–95). The report thus rhetorically sets the study's scene within a medical community which is just recognizing the significance of such projects.

The final pentadic element, agency, is clear: the patients suffering from syphilis are the instruments or means through which the doctors achieve their purpose. The initial report of the study notes, "The material included in this study consists of 399 syphilitic Negro males who had never received treatment, 201 presumably non-syphilitic Negro males, and approximately 275 male Negroes who had been given treatment during the first two years of the syphilitic process" (Vonderlehr et al. 260). While this perspective of patients-as-agency is inherent in the nature of such a medical project, regarding human subjects as agencies tends also to dehumanize them in a most literal sense: "The shortening of life expectancy observed in man" has "a counterpart in the white mouse, in which animal it has been shown by Rosahn that a syphilitic group has a significantly lessened life expectancy" (Olansky et al., "Untreated Syphilis" 177). Although the attitude toward the patients as agencies is usually detached, occasionally a hint of condescension appears. A 1954 report, for instance, examining the possibility that invironmental factors might be a confounding factor in the observed impact of syphilis, comments on the "nonchalant attitude of the patients toward calendars and time-reckonings." The description of their diet concludes "these men like relatively few dishes. As a rule they were interested only in meat (pork or chicken, never beef) and bread, and would select vegetables only upon the suggestion they do so" (Olansky et al., "Environmental Factors" 697). In a similar vein, the report in 1953 dealing with non-medical aspects of the study suggests the naïveté and limited perspectives of the patients: "Incentives for maximum cooperation of the patients must be kept in mind. What appears to be a real incentive to an outsider's way of thinking may have little appeal for the patient. In our case, free hot meals meant more to the men than $50 worth of free medical examination." Significantly, the researchers also note that "because of the low educational status of the majority of the patients, it was impossible to appeal to them from a purely scientific approach" (Rivers et al. 394, 393).

The central focus of these studies concerns purpose. While the results and analyses of the disease's course comprise the bulk of the articles, the discussions function solely to fulfill the objective in increasing "scientific" knowledge. This emphasis on purpose corresponds, as Burke notes, to philosophical mysticism, which is "the consciousness that everything we experience is an element and only an element in fact, i.e., that in being what it is, it is symbolic of something else" (50–51). This perspective deflects attention from actual human suffering to the function of the study in advancing medical knowledge. Implicit is a valuation of knowledge regardless of the human costs. By stressing the loftiness of the study's purpose, the depiction eclipses the agency used to achieve the goal. The study is more important than the individuals involved because it is a part or symbol of a larger and more significant scheme.

Rhetorical Function

These depictions of the disease and the study, reducing the Tuskegee patients to scene and agency, are common to reports of non-therapeutic projects, for the essence of such endeavors is the observation of a disease to catalog its effects and course. Moreover, they reflect the constraints of the genre of scientific writing, which prizes detachment and objectivity in the assessment and reporting of results. From the Tuskegee studies, we can identify four features of scientific investigation that impinge on the genre of scientific reporting: (1) the scientific method encourages the perception of distinctions and the investigation of their significance; (2) objectivity and detachment are desiderata; (3) science assumes knowledge as a primary value; and (4) the scientific approach is consistent across subject matter areas. In a culture which values the scientific method these elements are accepted almost without question. They become strategies enabling us to rise above our biases and predispositions when making observations.

However, while they may de-personalize our activities in many ways, these elements structure, constrain, and focus our perceptions. They can hamper our thinking if they distort our vision and obscure what should be salient features of reality. Within the reports of the Tuskegee project, these features of the scientific approach, acting as generic constraints, produce a malevolent, if unintended, distortion of reality. The generic constraints, working in concert with the perhaps unconscious racism of the experimenters, produce a powerful but unintentionally unethical rhetoric.

The realization of the generic features outlined above function to dehumanize the patients, to develop a powerful basis for communication within the medical community, and to play enthymematically on the reader's esteem for knowledge. In so doing, the rhetoric encourages myopia and insensitivity in both writers and readers in three broad ways.

First, the depictions deflect attention from the patients by casting them as scene and agency. The consequence is dehumanization and a process of division (as opposed to identification) between patients and the scientific community. A depiction focusing on the acts of the disease necessarily highlights the disease as a dynamic force, controlling and even crippling the "scene" it inhabits. While this view may be accurate, it associates a sense of inevitablity with the disease's progress which detracts from the patient's role and self-determination.

Also, stemming from an approach which prizes discriminatory powers and encourages categorization of phenomena on the basis of small distinctions, the reports highlight a relatively minor difference (skin color) between groups of subjects as it obscures their more numerous and significant resemblances. The scientific approach itself encourages investigators to assume the importance of the factor distinguishing one group of subjects from another and to rationalize the project on that basis. Not only are the subjects dehumanized by their status in the study, but also race (the primary factor distinguishing them from the subjects in Bruusgaard's earlier study and from most of the investigators) becomes a key variable in the Tuskegee project. Inherently, then, the study's avowed purpose of tracing the impact of syphilis on Blacks creates the basis for the dissociation between investigators and subjects. Instead of encouraging questions about the validity of racial stereotypes, the study implicitly justifies their significance. Science encourages the acquisition of knowledge to the point of becoming inadvertently a mechanism for encouraging racism.

Reporting the demographic background of the subjects further highlights the differences between them and the medical community. The use of "Male Negro" to designate the patients is significant. Without belaboring the racial elements in the study, one can still assume that this "Male Negro" title does little to establish common ground between the patients and the almost exclusively white readers of medical journals. Other terms used to refer to the victims are equally distancing. "Syphilitic," for instance, reduces the person involved to a simple manifestation of disease, or a "host" like the white rats mentioned earlier. Far from being led to identify and thus empathize with the subjects, readers of the journal articles are implicitly encouraged to distinguish themselves from the men studied.

Moreover, the use of these "scientific" terms for men suffering from syphilis plays into the scientific assumption that detachment is methodologically appropriate regardless of subject matter. The genre, in other words, encourages investigators to select such terms for the men and endorses their usage as appropriate for scientific reporting. Inherent in the genre, then, is a sometimes misleading and potentially destructive convention.

The terms and depictions employed in reports of the Tuskegee study, by highlighting the principle of discontinuity, obscure the moral and ethical implications of the materials being present (Burke 50–51). Interestingly, the organization of the study itself, which involved frequent rotation of doctors and little sustained contact with the subjects, reinforced this rhetorical distancing from the participants themselves (Jones 187).

Second, in direct contrast to the distancing between "Male Negroes" and the readership of the medical journals, the project directors establish a powerful basis for identification between themselves and the medical community by emphasizing the purposes of their study. Although the doctors are withholding treatment which could alleviate the suffering of victims, they re-define their activities as the observing of the consequences of the disease "uninfluenced" by treatment. Like medical scientists in research centers, they are pushing back the frontiers of knowledge. Knowledge becomes an absolute value: to learn is important, perhaps of paramount importance. Gaining knowledge fulfills one's professional roles and responsibilities. Thus, a commitment to research and the search for knowledge, powerful sources of identification between the doctors in Tuskegee and the larger medical community, enables the reports to cement professional bonds throughout the medical community.[8]

Third, on a more general level the focus on the study's purpose has powerful rhetorical impact because it plays enthymematically on the reader's esteem for knowledge. If knowing is a positive value, then efforts to gain knowledge are desirable. The Tuskegee study, therefore, is clearly a reasonable and even admirable activity. Moreover, in Burkeian terms, the focus on knowledge as a purpose rather than agency elevates it to an absolute value. Questions about the means used to gain the knowledge or even the value of the knowledge itself are eclipsed. Scientific inquiry becomes an activity beyond and above social critique. The depiction of the study as a scientific quest for knowledge thus not only gives it a mystical justification but also elevates it above mundane considerations of costs and effects. What is learned is important, regardless of the economic or human costs.[9]

Furthermore, by accentuating the distance between researchers and subjects while emphasizing lofty purposes, the study presents the medical community as an admirable elite. The process of disseminating information about the study through scientific medical journals enhances this image. Doctors talking to other doctors who share their attitudes and understand their professional commitments creates a closed communication network that reaffirms the bonds within the medical fraternity as it isolates the researchers from outside assessment. Society's respect for medical and scientific research further insulates the study. The process of communicating the results of the study, then, tends to obscure its ethical ramifications as it appeals subtly but forcefully to the shared values and self-image of the readers.

At the same time that the definition of and focus on the study's purpose helps create an almost mystical justification, its very longevity reinforces its value. Described in a 1953 report as "one of the longest continued medical surveys ever conducted," the study gains validation through its continuity (Rivers et al. 391). The periodicity of the reports and the reiterated references to earlier articles confer the presumption of value on it. The Tuskegee study as a continuing investigation becomes almost sacrosanct.

Rhetorical Implications

As a case study of the generic constraints of scientific reporting, the Tuskegee project suggests several observations. First, it reveals clearly that features inherent in the genre helped reinforce and even rationalize the latent racial prejudice of the investigators (Jones 60). The conventions of detachment and scientific discrimination accentuated the polarization between subjects and investigators. Significantly, there is no evidence that the authors manipulated the genre for their own ends. Rather, in this case, the genre itself encouraged a continuation of societal myopia and insensitivity.

Second, the study suggests that the genre of scientific reporting which deals with human subjects may be particularly prone to such problems because its very nature encourages detachment and divorces us from appropriate as well as inappropriate human reactions. In this respect, the fact that scienific rhetoric makes no distinction in its approach among inanimate objects, animals, and human beings is noteworthy. A genre which is in many ways insensitive to significant differences in content has severe limitations as a medium of communication. Clearly, a rhetor has some control over any genre, but generic conventions may be so powerful, pervasive, and esteemed by society that they severely restrict rhetorical choice. Rhetors inculcated with those generic conventions may become insensitive to alternatives and blind to the limitations and assumptions inherent in them.

Third, the study clearly indicates that the posture of much scientific reporting as objective and value-free is misleading. The scientific process itself structures and skews our perceptions. What emerges from our observations and appears in our reports is, at best, one slice of reality. If the perspective distorts our observations significantly, as it did in the Tuskegee project, the result is unethical, even if unintentionally so. Such reports are particularly malevolent because they wear the mask of objectivity and truth.

Finally, the broadest rhetorical ramification of the type of scientific reporting discussed here is the creation of a discontinuity between scientific inquiry and more concrete and specific human concerns. All the factors mentioned above contribute to the process: the creation of a discontinuity between subjects and observers, the identification of observers with a larger medical community, and the elevation of the quest for knowledge to an absolute value. In concert, these rhetorical strategies suggest and implicitly reinforce an "in-out" group attitude which isolates scientists from the larger community. Such reporting, by emphasizing the principle of discontinuity discussed by Burke, encourages readers to dissociate themselves from other human beings and to regard the subjects as "scenes" or "agencies" in their endeavors. The possible consequences of such depictions are vividly evident in the Tuskegee study.

The Tuskegee study reveals how rhetorical conventions can obscure the vision and perceptions of rhetors and their audiences. The features distinctive to scientific reporting, "objectivity" and "detachment," can encourage our neglect of crucial human concerns. Rhetorical conventions can become not mere shapers of discourse, but perceptual blinders. Such conventions, when they facilitate stereotypical thinking and distorted vision, become dangerous intellectual straitjackets.

In essence, the Tuskegee study reveals the hollowness of claims that scientific language is always neutral, objective, and value-free. Detachment from the content being discussed can be valuable in helping us exercise our reason and monitor our judgments. But such detachment or objectivity assumes that reason must always dominate human activities. It urges the preeminent value of rationality in the conduct of our lives and in our research. While all of us appreciate the importance of reason in human affairs, we also recognize the value of human emotion in tempering our behavior. Insistence on objectivity and detachment is a great asset in the pursuit of knowledge, but this stance reflects only one aspect of a broad spectrum of human concerns. These qualities embody one beneficial perspective, one set of values. As the Tuskegee study shows, this perspective and the language which conveys it can mislead even well-intentioned people. If allegiance to objectivity and detachment blinds us to other values, it produces neither humane behavior nor sound science.

NOTES

Ms. Solomon would like to thank Miller Solomon who first drew her attention to the Tuskegee project and whose editorial assistance on early drafts of the essay was extremely helpful.

1. "Inhuman Experiment" 16, "Official Inhumanity" II 6, "An Immoral Study" 2D, Jones 221.

2. Wander 226–35, Kelso 17–29, Simons 115–30, J. A. Campbell 375–90, and Mechling and Mechling 19–32.

3. For example, the diversity of authors involved abrogate questions of individual idiosyncracies in report writing. Second, the lack of reaction in the medical community indicates clearly the impact of the reports in obscuring ethical questions. Finally, the thirteen progress reports provide a complete and manageable corpus.

4. Carrie Foote quoted in Brown 12. Jones also reports that the men thought they were being "doctored" for a disease rather than merely observed to trace its course (5–6).

5. Brown estimates the number at 250 (13).

6. Seabrook 2A, "The Forty Year Death Watch" 16. Cf. Capron 692–94 for a discussion of "beneficial" versus "non-beneficial" research.

7. Jones 257–58, estimate of Dr. Donald Printz quoted in Seabrook 2A.

8. One may speculate that public health officers assigned to rural Alabama did not enjoy the most prestigious of assignments. Participation in a large-scale study which was reported periodically in national medical journals undoubtedly made the assignment more attractive. As Jones notes, the study provided not only a relief from the tedium of clinic treatments, but also "the intellectual excitement of becoming researchers on a scientific experiment, one that their superiors regarded as very important." Moreover, for physicians with scientific ambitions, the Tuskegee study afforded opportunities "to publish and advance their careers" (Jones 186).

9. Significantly, the discovery of penicillin's great efficacy in treating syphilis encouraged continuation of the study, although the information the study yielded had little practical value. That penicillin could obliterate the ravages of syphilis made learning about its consequences more urgent, for they would soon become part of medical history. Reports after penicillin's discovery argued that it "can never be duplicated since penicillin and other antibiotics are being so widely used in the treatment of other diseases thereby affording a definite treatment for syphilis" (Jones 179). The focus on the study's purpose thus provided a justification for its continuation regardless of its practical value.

REFERENCES

"An Immoral Study." *St. Louis Post-Dispatch* 30 July 1972: 2D.

Brown, Warren. "A Shocking New Report on Black Syphilis Victims." *JET* 9 Nov. 1972: 12–17.

Burke, Kenneth. *Language as Symbolic Action.* Berkeley: University of California Press, 1966.

Campbell, John Angus. "The Polemical Mr. Darwin." *Quarterly Journal of Speech* 61 (1975): 375–90.

Campbell, Paul Newell. "The *Personae* of Scientific Discourse." *Quarterly Journal of Speech* 61 (1975): 391–405.

Capron, Alexander Morgan. "Human Experimentation: Basic Issues." Ed. Warren T. Reich. 4 vols. *Encyclopedia of Bioethics.* New York: Free Press, 1972. 2:692–97.

Deibert, Austin V. and Martha C. Bruyere. "Untreated Syphilis in the Male Negro: III. Evidence of Cardiovascular Abnormalities and Other Forms of Morbidity." *Journal of Venereal Disease Information* 27 (1946). 301–14.

Fried, Charles. "Human Experimentation: Philosophical Aspects." *Encyclopedia of Bioethics.* Ed. Warren T. Reich. 4 vols. New York: Free Press, 1978. 2: 698–702.

Heller, J. R. and P. T. Bruyere. "Untreated Syphilis in the Male Negro: Mortality During 12 Years of Observation." *Journal of Venereal Disease Information* 27 (1946): 34–38.

Hirst, R. J. "Realism." *The Encyclopedia of Philosophy.* Ed. Paul Edwards. 8 vols. New York: Macmillan, 1967. 7:77–83.

"Inhuman Experiment." *Oregonian* 31 July 1972: 16.

Jones, James H. *Bad Blood: The Tuskegee Syphilis Experiment.* New York: Free Press, 1981.

Kampmeier, R. H. "The Tuskegee Study of Untreated Syphilis." *Southern Medical Journal* 65 (1972): 1247–51.

Kelso, James A. "Science and the Rhetoric of Reality." *Central States Speech Journal* 31 (1980): 17–29.

Mechling, Elizabeth Walker and Jay Mechling. "Sweet Talk: The Moral Rhetoric against Sugar." *Central States Speech Journal* 34 (1983): 19–32.

"Official Inhumanity." Editorial. *Los Angeles Times* 27 July 1972: II6.

Olansky, Sidney, Stanley Schuman, Jesse J. Peters, C. A. Smith, and Dorothy Rambo. "Untreated Syphilis in the Male Negro." *Journal of Chronic Diseases* 4 (1956): 177–85.

Olansky, Sidney, Lloyd Simpson, and Stanley H. Schuman. "Environmental Factors in the Tuskegee Study of Untreated Syphilis." *Public Health Reports* 69 (1954): 691–98.

Pesare, Pasquale J., Theodore J. Bauer, and Geraldine Gleeson. "Untreated Syphilis in the Male Negro." *American Journal of Syphilis, Gonorrhea, and Venereal Disease* 34 (1950): 201–12.

Peters, Jesse J., James H. Peters, Sidney Olansky, and Geraldine A. Gleeson. "Untreated Syphilis in the Male Negro: Pathologic Findings in Syphilitic and Nonsyphilitic Patients." *Journal of Chronic Disease* 1 (1955): 127–48.

Rivers, Eunice, Stanley H. Schuman, Lloyd Simpson, and Sidney Olansky. "Twenty Years of Followup Experience in an Long-Range Medical Study." *Public Health Reports* 68 (1953): 391–95.

Schuman, Stanley H., Sidney Olansky, Eunice Rivers, C. A. Smith, and Dorothy S. Rambo. "Untreated Syphilis in the Male Negro." *Journal of Chronic Disease* 2 (1955): 543–58.

Seabrook Charles. "Study Genocidal—CDC Doctor." *Atlanta Journal* 27 July 1972: 2A.

Shafer, J. K., Lida J. Usilton, and Geraldine A. Gleeson. "Untreated Syphilis in the Male Negro." *Public Health Reports* 69 (1954): 684–90.

Simons, Herbert W. "Are Scientists Rhetors in Disguise?: An Analysis of Dissuasive Processes within Scientific Communities." *Rhetoric in Transition: Studies in the Nature and Uses of Rhetoric.* Ed. Eugene E. White. University Park: Pennsylvania State University Press, 1980, 115–30.

———. *Persuasion: Understanding, Practice, and Analysis.* Reading, Mass.: Addison-Wesley, 1976.

Smart, Ninian. "History of Mysticism." *Encyclopedia of Philosophy.* Ed. Paul Edwards. 8 vols. New York: Macmillan, 1967. 5:420.

"The Forty Year Death Watch." *Medical World News* 18 Aug. 1972: 15–17.

Veatch, Robert M. "Codes of Medical Ethics: Ethical Analysis." *Encyclopedia of Bioethics.* Ed. Warren T. Reich. 4 vols. New York: Free Press, 1978. 1:172–79.

Vonderlehr, R. A., Taliaferro Clark, O. C. Wegner, and J. R. Heller, Jr. "Untreated Syphilis in the Male Negro." *Venereal Disease Information* 17 (1936): 260–65.

Wander, Philip C. "The Rhetoric of Science." *Western Journal of Speech Communication* 40 (1976): 226–35.

Wooten, John T. "Survivor of '32 Syphilis Study Recalls a Diagnosis." *New York Times* 27 July 1972: 18.

THE TUSKEGEE SYPHILIS STUDY IN THE
CONTEXT OF AMERICAN MEDICAL RESEARCH

SUSAN LEDERER

The Tuskegee Syphilis Study dominates discussions of racism and American medical research. There are compelling reasons for this; a forty-year, government-sponsored study of untreated syphilis in African American men is unique in the history of medical research. But racism has not been unique in American medicine, nor has the research exploitation of men, women, and children of color. Looking at investigations beyond the no-treatment syphilis study in which African Americans participated as research subjects is one way to enlarge our understanding of the ways in which racism structured the interactions of American medical researchers and black subjects.

Research and the Tuskegee Syphilis Study

The Tuskegee Syphilis Study is an infamous event in the history of American medical research. There are good reasons, however, to question whether research is, in fact, the most appropriate lens for viewing the study. I argue that the conduct of the white government physicians may be better understood in the context of the history of human dissection, a history in which racism figured prominently. The Public Health Service investigators who staffed the study over four decades regarded their African American subjects neither as patients, nor as experimental subjects, but as cadavers, who had been identified while still alive.

As historian James Jones has noted, the Tuskegee Syphilis Study did not originate as a fully developed research plan with clearly identified objectives or end points. The study began when the Julius Rosenwald Fund, citing the adverse economic effects of the Great Depression, withdrew its funds for treating African Americans diagnosed with syphilis. At this point, Dr. Taliaferro Clark of the Public Health Service identified "a ready-made situation" in which to study the effects of untreated syphilis in Macon County. He proposed a short-term study, six months or one year, to follow a group of men infected with syphilis who had received no

Susan Lederer is assistant professor in the Section of the History of Medicine in the Yale School of Medicine.
Printed by permission of Susan Lederer.

treatment. But when this initial assessment period ended in 1933 and Dr. Raymond Vonderlehr, the acting director of the Division of Venereal Diseases at the Public Health Service, assumed control, the study took a dramatic new course. Rather than ending as planned, Vonderlehr dictated that investigators would follow the men until their deaths.

Critical to the revamping of the Tuskegee Study was provision for postmortem examination to confirm the effects of untreated syphilis. In 1933, Vonderlehr noted that "the proper procedure is the continuance of the observation of the Negro men used in the study with the idea of eventually bringing them to autopsy."[1] Like a twentieth-century version of Burke and Hare, the notorious nineteenth-century Edinburgh resurrectionists, Vonderlehr and his PHS colleagues identified bodies for dissection while the individuals were still alive.[2] In so doing, the PHS investigators adopted a variety of methods to preserve the integrity of the bodies; in order to avoid contaminating the data, they prevented the men from gaining access to medical treatment for syphilis. They forged links with physicians in Macon and the surrounding counties to get the dead to the autopsy table as quickly as possible. Unlike Burke and Hare, the PHS doctors did not smother or strangle their subjects; instead they allowed syphilis to take its toll.

At the same time, investigators devoted considerable effort to obtaining legal permission for performing an autopsy on study participants from surviving family members. In order to obtain consent for postmortem examinations, PHS investigators offered strong, even coercive incentives. After 1935, families who gave permission for autopsy received a $50 burial stipend. The $35 families received ($15 went to the pathologist) enabled them to bury their loved one. Made possible by funds from the Milbank Memorial Fund, the stipends were withheld if families refused to authorize an autopsy. To facilitate further the consent process, Vonderlehr assigned black nurse Eunice Rivers the delicate task of approaching families to obtain consent for autopsy. She proved extraordinarily successful in obtaining familial permission. In a 1953 *Public Health Reports* paper, Rivers noted "only one refusal in 20 years and 145 autopsies obtained."[3] Even one refusal, however, is noteworthy. Some families chose to exercise the right to refuse an autopsy, even in the face of such powerful inducements as the "burial insurance."

Why did these investigators who were willing to withhold treatment for syphilis, to deceive the men about the nature of their participation, to mislabel diagnostic tests as therapy, go to such lengths to insure that families gave consent for postmortems? In part, investigators found working with families served their interests. Not only did burial insurance serve as incentive for gaining permission, but Rivers explained how community knowledge of the cash payments encouraged individuals to report deaths of participants: "They would let me know when somebody died because in those days $50 was a whole heap of money for a funeral."[4]

Placing the Tuskegee Study in the context of human dissection may also explain the investigators' extraordinary compliance with rules regarding autopsy and the simultaneous breach of the operative rules regarding human experimentation. Even before the American Medical Association adopted its first formal principles regarding human experimentation in 1946, leading American medical researchers had identified by the early twentieth century several necessary conditions for ethical human experimentation. These included prior animal studies, consent of the patient/subject, and responsibility for harm to the subjects. The PHS investigators breached these conditions in the conduct of the Tuskegee Study, but they had apparently not violated any laws. Although federal and state legislatures had considered proposals for regulating human experimentation in the first two decades of the twentieth century, no laws governing the conduct of human research were enacted until 1974 (on the heels of public disclosures about the Tuskegee Syphilis Study).[5]

Unlike the case of human experimentation, state laws regulated access to dead human bodies for dissection and autopsy. By 1932, when the Tuskegee Study began, many American state legislatures had enacted statutes regulating the disposition and use of dead human bodies. Some of the laws explicitly noted the physician's responsibility to obtain consent from family members before a postmortem examination.[6] As attorney George Weinmann noted in 1929, "the general rule is that the unauthorized autopsy of a dead human body is a tort, giving rise to a cause of action for damages."[7] An increasing number of Americans pursued lawsuits against hospitals and physicians for performing unauthorized autopsies on family members. Successful suits with monetary damages prompted pathologists and hospital administrators to urge more attention to the methods of obtaining written consent for autopsy as a protection against both individuals and institutions. There is some indication that African Americans and other ethnic groups were asked for permission. Explaining how Memorial Hospital improved a higher rate of cooperation with requests for autopsy, New York physician William Hoffman noted that doctors approached the family in business suits rather than white uniforms and avoided such words with "gruesome connotations" as *autopsy*, *inquest*, or *necropsy*. Using this new approach, Hoffman reported for the six months between July and December 1932 that of the seventy-one deaths in the hospital, the families of "All Germans, Danes, Irish, Negroes and all Italians but one consented to autopsy."[8]

In the state of Alabama, an anatomical practice act permitted the distribution of unclaimed dead human bodies to medical schools for "the advancement of medical science." The law included provisions to allow surviving friends and family members to claim the body, so long as they could provide the money for burial. Although anatomical acts did not materially alter the social origins of the dead bodies available for dissection (in the 1920s, for example, interstate shipment of dead black bodies to northern medical schools continued), the law protected (at least, in theory) both whites and African Americans with money for burial from being turned over to medical schools.[9] Intent on getting postmortem evidence for the syphilis study, PHS investigators scrupulously complied with the legal requirements for family permission for the autopsy. For Vonderlehr and his colleagues at the Public Health Service, the dead took precedence over the living.

African Americans as Research Subjects

In the thirteen papers from the Tuskegee Syphilis Study published between 1936 and 1973, investigators identified the study participants as "syphilitics," "patients," or "syphilitic Negro males." In no published paper did investigators characterize the men as research subjects, but in 1955 the men were, for the first time, described as "volunteers with social incentives."[10] Once the study had ended amid a flurry of news reports and congressional hearings, some of the survivors of the study recalled being used as "guinea pigs" by government doctors. The equation of African Americans with laboratory animals has a history nearly as long as the term *human guinea pig* (introduced in 1906 by British writer George Bernard Shaw).

In the 1940s a University of Pennsylvania researcher elaborated a number of parallels between his Negro research subjects and laboratory animals. In an after-dinner speech intended to divert his colleagues, William Osler Abbott described some of his problems using "professional guinea pigs." In 1931 Abbott and his coworker T. Grier Miller had developed a new technique for rapidly intubating the human intestine from mouth to rectum.[11] Although advised to try the new device on animals, Miller and Abbott apparently never performed the animal studies. After numerous self-experiments, they attempted to locate subjects in the hospital wards, and finally turned to healthy men and women who would agree to the procedure. During the height of the depression, Abbott and Miller approached a young relief administrator, hoping to gain cooperation in using unemployed men as subjects. Unlike her counterpart in Chicago who sent men on relief to laboratories to participate in research for payment, the Philadelphia administrator refused to send men to Abbott's laboratory, especially when she learned that they would be required to swallow a flexible twelve-foot tube to which a rubber balloon was attached and inflated once inside the intestine.[12]

Frustrated by the employment bureau, Abbott asked the wives of his colleagues to distribute slips of paper instructing beggars to come to the hospital for a job paying $2 a day. He also used the bridge over the Schuylkill River as a "hunting ground" for potential participants, to no avail. Finally, his secretary suggested that the doctors call in their black janitor; they eventually promised Harry fifty cents for every healthy human subject who appeared at the laboratory door at 8:30 A.M. in a sober and fasting state.

Abbott's first subject, Flip Lawall, "tall, broad-shouldered, black as the ace of spades, and by profession a light-weight prize fighter," was joined by several other young black men.[13] Employing this population as research subjects, Abbott insisted, was not without problems. Alluding in a stereotypical fashion to the men's penchant for thievery, Abbott complained that his "animals" also enjoyed a larger intake of corn liquor, pork chops, and chewing tobacco than the white rats in the medical school. He described how, on one occasion, he had attempted to insert a flexible rubber tube into one man's duodenum using fluoroscopic guidance, when he noticed a small piece of metal. Recognizing the tip of a .38 caliber revolver bullet, Abbott confronted his subject who admitted that the previous night his jealous "sweetheart" had shot him after seeing him with another woman earlier in the evening. Such events, Abbott explained, "led me to wish at times I could keep my animals in metabolism cages."[14]

Abbott encountered more serious problems in the spring of 1935 when he scheduled an exhibit on intestinal intubation for the American Medical Association meeting in Atlantic City. Arranging for the men to be intubated at a local hospital before their appearance at the convention, Abbott was stunned when his "guinea pigs" threatened to walk out at the last minute unless they received double pay. Only an impassioned eleventh-hour appeal to the third-year medical school class and the offer of the same pay received by the "striking blackamoors" enabled Abbott to continue the demonstration using student volunteers. He fired all the black subjects and refused to have anything more to do with them.

After several months, Abbott reconsidered his position. "Those boys may have been short on morals but they were long in gut," he remarked, "and in the end I went to Harry once again to throw out a feeler." He discovered that his "boys" had "graduated from stealing inkwells to house furnishings;" all but two had been convicted of burglary, and his first subject, Flip Lawall, was serving a ten-year sentence in the state penitentiary for a rape conviction.

An advertisement in a local newspaper brought a fresh group of potential subjects to Abbott's laboratory. Some of the men and women who answered the ad winced at the description of swallowing the tubes, and many others apparently quailed at Abbott's insistence that they sign a statement prepared by the university attorney outlining every step of the experiment and stating that subjects recognized and accepted any risks associated with the procedure. (The document was more of an indemnification agreement than a consent form.) Abbott ended up with a roster of subjects, young and old, white and black, male and female, although he noted that his "clientele" generally dwindled down to hefty, older women, the human counterpart of the "big, lazy, overweight bitch [from the animal house] that could be counted upon to lie and wag her tail while being worked over."[15]

Abbott's intubation experiments differed in a number of important ways from the Tuskegee Syphilis Study. His initial black subjects were all ostensibly healthy men, who knew that they were receiving payment for their participation in research. They were not patients. What the men actually understood about the risks associated with swallowing the tubes and the frequent X rays is impossible to know. Abbott did refer to his own efforts to safeguard them from the effects of "overfrequent" radiation, but, given his instrumental attitude toward the men, it seems unlikely that he explained the risks in any detail. Assumptions about race informed the investigator's attitudes toward the men, their reliability, and their level of comprehension.

Abbott jokingly equated his professional guinea pigs with laboratory animals, but reliance on Harry the janitor to arrange for the men to come to the lab bears remarkable similarity to the ways in which laboratories obtained both animals and human cadavers for study. Black technicians, janitors, and caretakers routinely located and supplied these materials—alive and dead. At Johns Hopkins University, for example, the surgeon Willis Gatch recalled how each January William Halsted would call him into his office to inform him that he was ready to start his experimental work in the Hunterian Laboratory. Gatch would then hire a Negro boy to procure dogs and instruct him on how to etherize them.[16] In similar fashion, Nurse Rivers functioned as a conduit for the bodies of black men needed for postmortem examinations.

A year after Abbott recounted his problems with professional guinea pigs, novelist Richard Wright used his own experience as a porter in a medical research facility to make a larger point about racism and American society. In a 1942 *Harper's Magazine* article, Wright described how he had spent the winter of 1932 working in a laboratory at the Michael Reese Hospital in Chicago. In addition to scrubbing floors, cleaning up after diabetic dogs, shaving rabbits, and feeding guinea pigs and mice, Wright recalled how he and the other Negro porters "would gape in wonder at doctors examining animals" and ponder the "indecipherable scientific jargon" on the cage labels. Curious about one of the experiments, he asked a doctor about one of the animals, only to be rebuffed. On another occasion in the laboratory, two of Wright's fellow porters began to fight; in the process they knocked over many of the animal cages, killing some animals and freeing others. Anxious to save their jobs, the porters attempted to restore order in the lab. Relying on memory and guesswork, they filled cages with the same numbers of animals, replacing dead stock with live animals, and waited for the doctors to notice. To their surprise, no questions were ever raised about the incident, prompting Wright to speculate:

We often wondered what went on in the laboratories after that secret disaster. Was some scientific hypothesis, well on its way to validation and ultimate public use, discarded because of unexpected findings on that cold winter morning? Was some tested principle given a new and strange refinement because of fresh, remarkable evidence? Did some brooding researcher get a wild, if brief, glimpse of a new scientific truth? At any rate we never heard.[17]

Wright's conclusion belied the title he gave the story: "What You Don't Know Won't Hurt You: A Belated Report on the Progress of Medical Research." Not knowing was neither a benefit to the porters kept in ignorance about the experiments, nor a boon to the medical researchers who were uninformed about the wholesale switching of the laboratory animals.

In an autobiographical account, *Black Boy*, first published in 1944, Wright included a number of incidents from his stay at the Michael Reese Hospital absent from the magazine article. Noting "the sharp line of racial division drawn by the hospital authorities," he recalled how one of his jobs was to restrain dogs until they received an injection of Nembutal, after which a "young Jewish doctor" would slit their vocal chords, so that the animal howls would not disturb patients in other parts of the hospital. The sight of the dogs lifting their heads and soundlessly wailing made a powerful impression upon him. In his autobiography, Wright recorded how he considered going to the director's office and telling him about the exchange of animals. Loyalty to his coworkers and dislike for the man led him to keep his silence.

> The hospital kept us four Negroes, as though we were close kin to the animals we tended, huddled together down in the underworld corridors of the hospital, separated by a vast psychological distance from the significant processes of the rest of the hospital—just as America had kept us locked in the dark underworld of American life for three hundred years—and we had made our own code of ethics, values, loyalty.[18]

Litigating Medical Research

Professional codes of ethics did not always protect human subjects—white or black—from researchers. In rare cases, Americans, including African Americans, sought redress from the courts when physicians overstepped the bounds of experimentation. In the 1940s the mother of a young African American man sued a white physician in the District of Columbia whose surgical experiments caused severe injury to her son. Before the suit was eventually settled out of court, newspaper publicity about the case raised a number of questions about experiments on African Americans.

In 1940 John Bonner, a junior high school student, donated skin to a badly burned cousin for an experimental skin-grafting procedure. Although Bonner was only fifteen at the time, surgeon Robert Moran did not obtain parental consent before undertaking the surgical experiment in the charity clinic of Episcopal Hospital. In an effort to treat the burned woman, Moran surgically removed a flap of skin and formed a "tube of flesh" from the boy's armpit to his waist, which he attached to the boy's cousin. The two remained surgically joined for four days, when Bonner began to experience shock and anemia. The boy lost so much blood that he required several transfusions, and he spent nearly two months in the hospital recovering from his experience.[19]

In 1941 Margaret Moore, the boy's mother, brought suit against the physician for assault and battery. Even though Bonner's mother had not given her consent, the trial court ruled in favor of the physician, noting that a minor's permission for the operation was sufficient in this case. Appealed to the District of Columbia Court of Appeals, the higher court ruled that although children could consent to medical therapy in exceptional cases, the Bonner case did not involve a therapeutic benefit for the boy.

> Here the operation was entirely for the benefit of another and involved sacrifice on the part of the infant of fully two months of schooling, in addition to serious pain and possible results affecting his future life. This immature colored boy was subjected several times to treatment involving anesthesia, blood letting, and the removal of skin from his body, with at least some permanent marks of disfigurement.[20]

Although the appeals court instructed the lower court to retry the case, the parties reached an out-of-court settlement.[21]

The case of *Bonner v. Moran* has been discussed in the bioethics literature in the context of legal precedents for allowing healthy children to donate kidneys. But the suit may be important for other reasons as well. The ruling of the appellate court suggests that there were in fact some legal (and financial) constraints on white physicians whose experiments on black subjects ended in injury or harm to the participants. Less tangibly, the "newspaper notoriety" surrounding the boy's heroism, which apparently resulted in public contributions of money for his future education, suggests a wider public appreciation for both the costs and benefits of human experimentation.

The Bonner case, Abbott's intestinal intubations, and the Tuskegee Syphilis Study illustrate different aspects of race and research in American medicine. Differences in study design, investigators, and subjects influenced the research experience, and race informed the conduct of these experiments as it did other aspects of American life. In the case of an "experiment in nature," as investigators termed the no-treatment syphilis study, investigators actively deceived their "patients" to retain them in their studies. In such explicitly nontherapeutic studies as the intestinal intubations, white investigators needed cooperation from their subjects; they reserved their contempt for their "guinea pigs" even as they supplied the financial compensation required to recruit them. But Abbott's experience also illustrates how research subjects attempted to negotiate the terms of their participation in research. Like the men in Abbott's studies, John Bonner's mother contested the terms of her son's participation in medical research. Unlike Flip Lawall and the other men who lost their bid for higher wages, Margaret Moore proved successful in obtaining financial compensation for the injuries her son incurred at the hands of a surgical innovator. Looking at researchers and research subjects in the case of the Tuskegee Study and other experiments provides a broader context in which to view the ways in which racism structured what Richard Wright labeled "the dark underworld of American life."[22]

NOTES

1. Quoted in James H. Jones, *Bad Blood* (New York: Free Press, 1993), p. 132.

2. For Burke and Hare, see Ruth Richardson, *Death Dissection and the Destitute* (London: Routledge and Kegan Paul, 1987).

3. E. Rivers, S. Schuman, L. Simpson, and S. Olansky, "Twenty Years of Followup Experience in a Long-Range Medical Study," *Public Health Reports* 68 (1953): 391–95 (quotation on p. 394).

4. Jones, *Bad Blood*, p. 154.

5. See Susan E. Lederer, *Subjected to Science: Human Experimentation in America before the Second World War* (Baltimore: Johns Hopkins University Press, 1995).

6. Autopsies undertaken for forensic purposes did not require familial consent. See George H. Weinmann, "A Survey of the Law Concerning Dead Human Bodies," *Bulletin of the National Research Council* 73 (1929): 58.

7. Ibid., p. 58.

8. William J. Hoffman, "Postmortem Examinations: Method of Obtaining Permission," *Journal of the American Medical Association* 101 (1933): 1199–1205.

9. There were some notable differences, however, in state laws. In 1913, for example, North Carolina's statutes exempted the bodies of Confederate soldiers and their wives from dissection, and they further provided that no white body could be sent to a Negro medical college. See George B. Jenkins, "The Legal Status of Dissecting," *Anatomical Record* 7 (1913): 387–99. See also D. C. Humphrey, "Dissection and Discrimination: The Social Origins of Cadavers in America, 1760–1915," *Bulletin of the New York Academy of Medicine* 49 (1973): 819–27.

10. The words *volunteers with social incentives* appear on a chart comparing the Tuskegee Study with the all-European Norway (or Oslo) Study; see Stanley Schuman, Sidney Olansky, Eunice Rivers, C. A. Smith, and Dorothy S. Rambo, "Untreated Syphilis in the Male Negro," *Journal of Chronic Diseases* 2 (1955): 545.

11. Abbott (1902–1943) received his M.D. from the University of Pennsylvania in 1928, where he also served as an instructor (1931–37), associate (1937–41), and assistant professor (1941–43). Abbott's mother, Georgina Osler, was a niece of Sir William Osler. See William C. Stadie, "William Osler Abbott," *Transactions of the Association of American Physicians* 58 (1944): 7–9. For the technique, see T. Grier Miller and W. Osler Abbott, "Intestinal Intubation: A Practical Technique," *American Journal of the Medical Sciences* 187 (1934): 595–99.

12. In 1930, the Department of Pathology at the University of Illinois College of Medicine used 80 unemployed men ages 20–76 from the state employment bureau in studies of skin reactions and other procedures; see William F. Petersen and Samuel A. Levinson, "General Correlations in One Hundred So-Called Normal Men," *Archives of Pathology* 9 (1930): 151–82.

13. See W. Osler Abbott, "The Problem of the Professional Guinea Pig," *Proceedings of the Charaka Club* 10 (1941): 249–60.

14. Petersen and Levinson, "General Correlations."

15. Abbott, "Problem of the Professional Guinea Pig," p. 259.

16. Willis D. Gatch, "My Experiences with Dr. Halsted," *Surgery* 32 (1952): 466–68.

17. Richard Wright, "What You Don't Know Won't Hurt You: A Belated Report on the Progress of Medical Research," *Harper's Magazine* 186 (1942): 58–61.

18. Richard Wright, *Black Boy* (New York: HarperPerennial, 1993), p. 370.

19. See "Use of Fifteen Year Old Boy as Skin Donor without Consent of Parents as Constituting Assault and Battery," *JAMA* 120 (1942): 562–63.

20. *Bonner v. Moran*, 75 U.S. App. D.C. 156, 126 F.2d 121 (1941). See Sharon Romm, "Robert Emmet "Pete" Moran: Washington's Myth and Master," *Aesthetic Plastic Surgery* 14 (1990): 43–51.

21. See George J. Annas and Michael A. Grodin, *The Nazi Doctors and the Nuremberg Code* (New York: Oxford University Press, 1992), pp. 202–3.

22. Wright, *Black Boy*, p. 370.

A CASE STUDY IN HISTORICAL RELATIVISM

The Tuskegee (Public Health Service) Syphilis Study

JOHN C. FLETCHER

Introduction

This paper discusses the problem of making transhistorical moral judgments using the case of the *so-called** Tuskegee Syphilis Study as an example. Can a later generation validly place moral blame on Public Health Service (PHS) physicians who began the study in 1932? Are past decisions and actions morally relative only to the standards of the times and within the social circumstances in which these standards apply? What reasons count for and against a retrospective moral judgment? Some personal and historical comments are followed by an overview of an approach to these questions.

Personal and Historical Comments

Not then a reader of the venereal disease literature, I learned of the PHS syphilis study through Jean Heller's 1972 news story.[1] In 1966, Peter Buxton, then a PHS venereal disease investigator, courageously tried to stop it. After six years of PHS resistance to his efforts, he turned to a journalist friend and the news broke to an incredulous public. Ironically, in 1966 the PHS reformed policy to protect human subjects of research. In July 1966, Surgeon General William H. Stewart mandated prior group review of human-subjects research.[2] The same month I began a two-year study of the ethics of medical research at the National Institutes of Health's (NIH) Clinical Center. Thereafter, research proposals to the NIH's extramural program that involved human beings had to undergo local review of the rights and welfare of subjects, the appropriateness of methods for informed consent, and relation of risks to benefits.[3] How could both events—resistance to the Buxton

---

*I say "so-called" because a more accurate name is "The Public Health Study (PHS) of Partially Treated Syphilis in Macon County, Alabama." The PHS was morally responsible for the study in its entirety. The misnaming of the study is an illustration of how racism works against black persons. Tuskegee University and the townspeople are touched by a legacy of shame, each time the name is used. Changing popular usage is a lost cause, but one must protest the usage.

John C. Fletcher is Emeritus Cornfield Professor of Religious Studies and former director of the Center for Biomedical Ethics, University of Virginia.
Printed by permission of John C. Fletcher.

protest and policy on prior group review—have occurred virtually side by side in the same agency? I later learned from James Jones's 1981 classic history of the experiment that in 1965 a Detroit physician had written a letter of moral protest to a scientist at the Centers for Disease Control (CDC) who had written an article on thirty years of observation of the subjects.[4] The letter went unanswered. As a bioethicist at the NIH's Clinical Center from 1977 to 1987, I learned personally how a large and complex scientific bureaucracy can house the best and the worst on a moral spectrum.

My interest in the PHS syphilis study and its legacy has several sources. Alabama was my home until early adulthood. There I idealistically entered the Episcopal ministry in 1956.* Encouraged by a then-liberal religious tradition to engage in issues of social justice, I worked with others of like mind for a "new South" to emerge out of poverty and segregation. Since southern reformers looked to the federal government as an ally in the 1950s and 1960s, it was a harsh blow to learn that government physicians and agencies did research "on" rather than "with" uninformed black Alabama sharecroppers.**

At the NIH from 1966 to 1968, I must have come close to learning about the experiment. I assembled ten meetings, now called "focus groups," of leaders from each institute to discuss a question: "What are the most important ethical issues that your institute's research poses for society in the next five to ten years?" Although the question was future oriented, some participants commented about past research activities that were "beyond the pale" of research ethics in 1968. The NIH received and analyzed spinal fluids and autopsy specimens of the Alabama subjects, but none of dozens of officials mentioned the study.[5]

Later, I taught biomedical ethics at the University of Virginia's School of Medicine for ten years (1987–97). The three PHS officers who led the study until 1943 graduated from this medical school. Dr. Taliaferro Clark had the idea for a study of untreated syphilis for a brief period. The occasion for his idea was the loss of income to the Julius Rosenwald Fund caused by the Great Depression. The fund had no more resources to continue support for a PHS project of syphilis detection and treatment demonstration in six sites in the South, including Macon County, Alabama. At an impasse, Clark salvaged a convenient sample of infected and untreated black subjects to study. He wanted to compare the outcomes of black persons with untreated syphilis with those of whites, because such a study had

---

*I found the profession rewarding for its proximity to life's most important questions and passages but requiring loyalty to a theistic worldview which I cannot accept with intellectual honesty or bring to bear on the most important issues in bioethics. After many years of struggling with these issues and myself, I resigned from the Episcopal ministry in 1990.

**Mortimer Lipsett, director of the Clinical Center, NIH (1976–81) discussed the change in the ethos of clinical research in his lifetime by the use of these prepositions. Dr. Lipsett employed me as his assistant for bioethics in 1977.

been done with all-white Norwegians with syphilis in Oslo in the early twentieth century.[6]

Dr. Hugh Smith Cumming (1869–1948), surgeon general of the United States, made the official decision to approve the study. Dr. Raymond Vonderlehr succeeded Dr. Clark when he retired in 1933. Vonderlehr's dedication to continue the study as director of the PHS's Division of Venereal Diseases (1933–43) in large part explains the study's longevity.* He was succeeded by Dr. John R. Heller, a PHS officer (but not a Virginia-trained physician) with extensive field experience in Alabama. I met Dr. Heller at the NIH in the late 1970s. He adamantly denied that any moral wrongdoing had occurred in 1932 or on his watch.[7] Dr. Heller became director of the National Cancer Institute in 1948.

I also cochaired the Tuskegee Syphilis Study Legacy Committee with Dr. Vanessa Northington Gamble. With funding from the CDC, the committee met at Tuskegee University in January 1996. I was invited, due to my lobbying the PHS from early 1994, to make an official apology for the study.[8] The committee's mission was to alter the study's destructive legacy. We discussed the social wound left by the study, which is large and fresh in the collective memory of African Americans who associate the study to conspiracy and genocide aimed at people of color. Even further, the committee recognized, this legacy seriously impedes participation of African Americans in AIDS prevention and research.[9]

We pressed our cause that President Clinton should apologize to the survivors, their families, and the community of Tuskegee, which unfairly bears the shame of the study's name. To his administration's credit, President Clinton made an apology at a ceremony held at the White House on 16 May 1997. The apology was certainly apropos, but it was offered at the wrong place. The committee had strongly urged the site of Tuskegee itself to enhance the symbolism of the event, to promote racial healing, and to make it feasible for more family members of the subjects to attend.[10] I conclude these comments with two questions: How many black persons, even now, remember an apology for the experiment that was given at the "White House"? How many would remember an apology given by a president who journeyed to Tuskegee?

Overview of the Approach

This four-part paper addresses the question of the validity of transhistorical moral judgments about the PHS syphilis study. Part One describes a method to assess the validity of a transhistorical moral judgment. Part Two uses this method to evaluate the validity of moral judgments made by an official body and others in 1973 that the study was unethical at its inception, due to lack of informed consent

*The key figures and their many colleagues are hereinafter referred to as Clark and Vonderlehr et al.

to research. This part includes a section pointing to two bodies of moral guidance in 1932 by which Clark and Vonderlehr et al. could have been challenged.

Part Three argues for a graded approach to moral blame, focusing on PHS researchers and officials in the 1950s and 1960s for their moral blindness to the most objectionable features of the study. Part Four examines two concluding questions: Why did the PHS study endure so long without serious internal moral challenge, and what lessons can be learned from the experiment about protection of human subjects in our own era and in the future?

Part One. A Method to Judge Past Standards and Conduct

This paper originated as a response to a question posed to me by the Advisory Committee on Human Radiation Experiments in 1994: "Can we judge the standards and conduct of those who preceded us?"[11]

We plainly can and do make transhistorical moral judgments. Indeed, we *must* make such judgments to be loyal to moral norms and to transmit moral evolution to a new generation. The task of transmitting moral evolution also requires accuracy and truthfulness about the history of reform of social practices, which must document the most serious moral lapses and errors. The history of the morality of human experimentation and the role of the PHS syphilis study is a significant case in point. The United States is considered a world leader in innovation in the ethics of research; however, the PHS leaders who began a public process of reform were among those who condoned the syphilis study.

If we fail to judge the past, however measured our judgments, we will lose in our collective memory the harm and suffering caused by older practices. We will lose, too, in our moral evolution the ability to change those harmful practices. Making such judgments is risky; it invites the fallacy of misplaced moralism, caused by imposing present-day judgments onto the past, but it is not necessary to commit this fallacy. To avoid doing so, valid transhistorical judgments require two tasks. The first, with the aid of historical research, is to put ourselves as much as possible in the moral position of those who are under scrutiny. Were they morally culpable in their own time?

To pursue this task, one must examine both the practice of wrongdoing and any movement to abolish it by law or to reform it in social practice. The challenge is to identify the moral norms of the day, as well as any social movements aimed at shifting those norms to abolish certain practices. For example, we now cast moral blame on past practices of slavery, racial segregation, and economic exploitation of child labor, and we object to the conduct of those who defended such institutions and practices by the standards of their times. However, each of these practices and the movements to reform them have long and complex histories which were prefaced by the moral witness of gifted individuals. Slavery required three centuries to abolish in the United States; racial segregation is illegal in its overt forms but still embedded in our social practice; although children are legally protected in this nation from exploitative labor practices, multinational corporations operate today in countries where child labor is cheap and loosely regulated, if at all.

Every reform movement has a moral dimension, and we find reformers appealing to moral ideals that did not prevail *at the time* of the objectionable practices because the majority of people were loyal to competing moral standards. Abolitionists and reformers in these movements mainly appealed to the supremacy of moral ideals of equality and respect for persons, whether these ideals emanated from religious tradition or a theory of natural rights. The ideals required specification and reforms of morally discredited practices to penetrate society and win the loyalty of larger numbers.

The second task is one of historical comparison with a moral aim: comparing present to past practices and the standards that undergird them. The moral aim is to view the past as a negative "paradigm case," to enhance moral education for future decisions and to prevent reoccurrences.

Part Two. Was the PHS Study "Ethically Unjustified in 1932"?

Did the Study Violate the Norm of Informed Consent?
When the PHS syphilis study was reported in the press, the assistant secretary for health appointed the Tuskegee Syphilis Study Ad Hoc Advisory Panel in 1973 to review the study. The panel concluded that the study was "ethically unjustified in 1932," that is, at the study's inception.[12] Also, Senator Edward Kennedy stated that the study "was an outrageous and intolerable situation in which this Government never should have been involved. . . ."[13] Are these moral judgments valid?

The panel's judgment was based on a premise that the subjects had been deprived of informed consent to a study of a disease with a known risk to human life.[14] But in 1932 the norm of voluntary informed consent when based on a concept of respect for the individual's autonomy that *outweighs* the beneficence of medical treatment or research was not a part of the ethos of American researchers. Thus the panel's judgment is flawed because informed consent was not an intact norm of researchers at the time. It is true that a few exceptional investigators, like William Beaumont and Walter Reed in the nineteenth and early twentieth centuries, sought the voluntary informed consent of their subjects for dangerous studies. But Beaumont and Reed were exceptions to the norm in nontherapeutic research.[15]

Notwithstanding, it is a historical fact that no one protested the PHS study of untreated syphilis at the time on the basis of informed consent. Not until the 1960s was there any organized movement to reform human experimentation motivated by loyalty to any particular moral norm. Moreover, the PHS study was not cited in Henry Beecher's famous article of 1966 naming twenty-two unethical or marginally ethical studies.[16] Beecher may have known of the study but omitted it due to its inception in a much earlier era.

The original study design was a six- to eight-month investigation of the natural history of untreated syphilis, using comprehensive physical examinations and X rays, lumbar puncture, and specimens from autopsies. There was never an intent to seek informed consent for this study. On the contrary, the intent was to disguise the study as treatment to make it acceptable. Dr. Clark's own words were: "To secure the cooperation of the planters . . . it was necessary to carry on this study under the guise of a demonstration and provide treatment for those cases uncovered . . . in need of treatment."[17]

Notably, the decision to give some treatment resulted from an objection to the original design. When Dr. Clark presented the plan to Alabama public health officials and local physicians, they insisted that the subjects should receive some treatment. An agreement was reached that subjects who tested positive for syphilis were to receive eight doses of neoarsphenamine and some additional treatment with mercury pills, unless contraindicated on medical grounds.[18] All of the men in the study received one or the other drug or both, which were known at the time to be inadequate to treat syphilis.[19] The standard of care for treatment of syphilis at the time was a one-year treatment regimen of arsphenamine and bismuth of mercury.[20]

In *Bad Blood*, Jones saw the objection as political, arising from concern that the landowners for whom the subjects worked would not cooperate with a plan that lacked treatment.[21] However, the physicians and officials may have operated with a degree of medical beneficence. Clark and Vonderlehr and the others were physicians who quickly compromised to give therapy. Also, state public-health officials could have been trying to stay within reach of an Alabama public health law passed in 1927. This and later laws were probably violated by the experiment.[22]

The compromise in study design had two morally relevant consequences. First, it brought a "fatal flaw" into the original scientific plan to study untreated syphilis.[23] Due to partial treatment, all information was basically uninterpretable. Despite the scientific idealism (mixed with concepts of racial medicine) that inspired it, the study has to be viewed as a scientific failure that exploited and then wasted the sacrifice and suffering of the subjects. PHS officials through the years worried about the same issue. Dr. Austin Deibert discussed the contamination of results by partial treatment in 1938.[24] Dr. Albert Iskrant, chief statistician of the Division of Venereal Diseases, sounded the same alarm in 1948 and also asked whether the study was in accord with Alabama law.[25] His concluding comment about the study was: "Perhaps the most that can be salvaged is a study of inadequately treated syphilis."[26] The PHS took no action in 1948 but in 1951 expended a significant effort under Dr. Sidney Olansky to strengthen and overhaul the structure and efficiency of the experiment. No one proposed to stop it for either scientific or humanitarian reasons.

Secondly, even partial treatment provides a valid context within which to discuss the issue of informed consent and the ethics of Clark and Vonderlehr et al. as physicians. Did they violate the *medical* ethics of the time since some treatment was involved and they failed to obtain consent to it?

Scholars' Views on the History of Informed Consent in Medicine

Scholars of history and ethics are divided about the prevalence and force of a norm of informed consent in nineteenth- and early to middle twentieth-century medicine. In a fine review of this question, Faden and Beauchamp compare the widely divergent views of Martin Pernick, a social historian, and Jay Katz, a psychiatrist member of the Yale law faculty.[27] They write: "Where Katz sees no informed consent, Pernick finds it in abundance."[28] Pernick acknowledged differences between historical practices and the modern concept of "informed consent," but his study of nineteenth-century materials and cases concluded that "truth-telling and consent-seeking have long been part of an indigenous medical tradition."[29] He found that the concept and practice were prompted by efforts to benefit patients therapeutically, rather than by any theory of individual rights or self-determination. Katz, on the other hand, while accepting the historical existence of such concepts and their role in early-twentieth-century legal cases, wrote of the "history of silence with respect to patient participation in decision making. . . . When I speak of silence I do not mean to suggest that physicians have not talked to their patients at all. . . . They have not, except inadvertently, employed words to invite patients' participation in sharing the burden of making joint decisions."[30] Katz's main point is that up until the 1970s, physicians did not have meaningful discussions with patients about their choices and alternatives in treatment and research. Faden and Beauchamp concede more to Katz than to Pernick as to the lack of a pervasive practice of informed consent in medicine.

Faden and Beauchamp compared these two views from a perspective on models of ethical justification. They argued that the earlier practices that Pernick found in abundance were defended by a "model of beneficence" that used disclosure and consent seeking to further the aim of therapeutic benefits for the patient. Education and motivation improved patients' chances for a better response to therapy. Both Pernick and Katz acknowledge the influence of this view. Thus, there is a real historical link between treatment given in the PHS study and a paternalistic practice of informed consent in medicine in the early twentieth century. Disclosure and seeking the consent of patients for the patient's welfare but not participation was a familiar practice in medicine at the time.

The primary aim of Clark and Vonderlehr et al. was not treatment of syphilis.

Two ideas, one scientific and one ethical, motivated them. First, Clark saw an "unparalleled opportunity for the study of the effect of untreated syphilis."[31] A theory of a different natural history of syphilis in blacks, compared to whites, was commonly held but unproven among Clark's physician contemporaries. Dr. Joseph Earl Moore, a well-respected expert on syphilis, gave a favorable peer review of the proposed study. He was convinced that the course of syphilis in blacks was different than in whites. The common view, shared by Moore, was that the disease attacked the cardiovascular functions in blacks and the neurological functions in whites. Moore's review carried great weight in moving the study forward. A large element of racial bias was thus embedded in the study's hypothesis. The Norwegian study, published in 1929, showed that cardiovascular complications were common and neurologic damage was rare. As Jones put it, "Anyone who was not predisposed to find differences might have looked at these facts and concluded that the disease was affecting both races in the same way."[32] Nonetheless, at its inception, a reasonable scientific argument could have been made for a six-month to one-year study of untreated syphilis in blacks and whites along with following those who died to autopsy.

The other imperative was one of medical beneficence. The investigators and other central characters in this unfolding tragedy, like Nurse Eunice Rivers and the physicians at Tuskegee's John A. Andrew Hospital, believed that the benefits of bringing the subjects into the orbit of "government medicine" with its complete physical examinations, detection of co-morbidities like tuberculosis and other problems, was so preferable to the status quo, that the attention the subjects would receive more than justified the effort.

However, if research was the overriding goal, Clark and Vonderlehr et al. deceived themselves as scientists by adding therapy. The Oslo study had investigated the natural history of totally untreated syphilis. Now the two studies would not be comparable. In the ethos of the time, Clark and Vonderlehr et al. are more blameworthy at the outset for flawed science than as physicians who failed to seek informed consent. A short-term study of untreated syphilis would likely have refuted the racial hypothesis. Nonetheless, Clark and others lacked the courage to defend a nontherapeutic study to the end. If they had stood this ground and failed, the nation would have been spared the legacy of the study. However, they successfully compromised to start the study, which from the outset was a scientific mistake leading down a true ethical "slippery slope" and resulting in an eventual avalanche of moral problems. When Dr. Vonderlehr and others extended the study, especially into the 1950s, the risks of death due to withholding effective treatment were vastly higher, as well as violations of other ascending norms of research, like informed consent.

My conclusion is that the ad hoc committee inappropriately placed moral blame on Clark and Vonderlehr et al. by using a contemporary ethical understanding of participatory informed consent. Faden and Beauchamp describe this understanding as defensible on the basis of an "autonomy model," within which respect for the principle of autonomy and the value of self-determination had a higher societal value than the beneficence principle. These scholars find no evidence for any version of this understanding until the 1950s. Also, the record shows no debate about consent whatsoever among Clark and Vonderlehr et al. or any other interested parties at the time.

The history of the gradual ascendancy of an autonomy model over a beneficence model in research is marked by controversy and resistance to the full practice of informed consent from within government agencies charged with regulatory oversight, such as the Food and Drug Administration in the 1960s and the NIH itself.[33] This hierarchy of values was still not firmly in place in American medicine and research even in the early 1980s, when a president's commission affirmed "shared decision making" in health care, a term that clearly reflects Katz's view of the order of values at stake.[34] Indeed, as the concluding part of this paper will show, there are significant weaknesses in the current system to protect human subjects by prior group review and informed consent of subjects or their legal representatives.

The Ethos in 1932: "Formless Relativism"?

James Jones viewed the ethos of research in the United States in the early 1930s as follows:

> In medical research, as with medical practice, work was evaluated by peer review. The scientific method provided the yardstick for measuring the validity of investigations, and the assessments of fellow workers determined which researchers received kudos. Results were what counted. Many investigators whose work involved nontherapeutic research on human beings no doubt were enlightened souls who viewed their patients as people and thought in terms of "informed consent" decades before the term was coined, but there was no system of normative ethics on human experimentation during the 1930s that compelled medical researchers to temper their scientific curiosity with respect for the patients' rights. Here, as in private practice, a formless relativism had settled over the profession, holding that one investigator's methods of conducting an experiment were about as ethical as another's.[35]

It is true that "there was no system of normative ethics on human experimentation during the 1930s." However, there were two contemporary ethical resources that could have challenged the study. One was specific to human experimentation in Germany and the other was the common morality.

German physicians prompted substantial debate about the ethics of clinical drug trials by a powerful German pharmaceutical industry. In 1930, after bitter debate about exploitation of subjects in drug trials, including prisoners, the Berlin Medical Board appealed for prior group review of research, that is, that there should be "an official regulatory body to which proposals for experiments on man should be submitted."[36] This body would have been similar to a National Human Investigation Board that Jay Katz recommended for the United States in the 1973 ad hoc panel review of the PHS study and on several other occasions.[37] This idea has not been implemented except in the form of ad hoc national reviews of specific research as required by federal regulations.

The idea of national prior group review was easily defeated in Germany due to opposition from leading researchers and the drug industry. However, out of this debate came a remarkable set of guidelines on new therapies and human experimentation, released by the German minister of the interior in February 1931.[38] One guideline held that it was contrary to medical ethics to take advantage of social distress and deprivation. Clearly it was relevant to the PHS syphilis study but was not applied; in the realm of medical research ethics America was isolated in these years.[39] Surgeon General Cumming was doubtless unaware of these guidelines and their relevance to the Alabama project. In much the same way, the Nazi doctors' cruel research made a mockery of the 1931 guidelines, which, in my view, were more comprehensive and insightful than the Nuremberg Code itself. But the Nuremberg Tribunal did not use them to judge the Nazi experiments. Their legal status in Germany during the 1930s and 1940s was questioned during the trial.[40]

The 1931 guidelines did not mention prior group review. In 1932, Clark conducted a conventional peer review of the proposed study, selecting his own reviewers from peers in syphilology.[41] The earliest practice of prior group review was probably at the NIH's Clinical Center in 1953. It was a form of partially disinterested peer review in a group deliberately designed for the purpose.[42] It was not until after the revelation of the PHS syphilis study that Congress in 1974 required local prior group review by disinterested parties of all federally funded human subjects research. The NIH's intramural program was not covered by the law until 1993, thus showing how slowly the process of reform of research ethics works in relation to federal agencies. Prior group review is still not legally mandated for privately funded studies involving human subjects. This problem will be discussed further in Part Four.[43]

Another source of moral challenge could have been from the common morality of the time. There one could find a prima facie moral rule that persons ought to be honest, not deceive others without justification, and be truthful with those who have a moral claim on the truth. How does one access the common morality of past times? Ronald M. Green, a Dartmouth College philosopher, adapts the strategy of the "reasonable person" rule in law to morality. Such a person should have a good grasp of the facts of the case and be well informed as to the prevailing moral standards of that time.[44]

In 1932, how would a reasonable person have answered this question: do these black men with syphilis, and the planters for whom they work, have a just moral claim to know that the men are being recruited for a study in which the best known treatment for syphilis (a one-year program of treatment with arsenicals and mercury) will be withheld in order to study the natural history of syphilis? One can easily imagine a challenge.

Clark and Vonderlehr et al. labored hard to be deceitful. Their effort is indirect proof of some level of awareness of violating a commonsense standard of honesty. Believing that the subjects could not understand the truth, they carried out a systematic program of planned deceit mainly to secure cooperation. When approaching potential subjects, they did not discuss a medical diagnosis of syphilis but used the local colloquialism of "bad blood." In doing so, they exploited the economic and social distress of their subjects to facilitate their research.[45] They did not disclose the experiment but deliberately disguised research activities as treatment. A dramatic example was the presentation of a required spinal tap performed in John A. Andrew Hospital at Tuskegee, the site of a former treatment center, as a "special treatment."[46] Spinal taps at the time had much greater risk of serious complications of paralysis and blinding headaches than the procedure as we know it today. Dr. Clark's discussed deceit in a memo to Dr. Vonderlehr: "I agree with you that the treatment work should continue during the period of spinal fluid testing in order to minimize the amount of attention that will be given to this activity by the people of the community.[47] Clark later explained his beneficent deceit to his consultant, Dr. James Earle Moore of Johns Hopkins: "These negroes [sic] are very ignorant and easily influenced by things that would be of minor significance in a more intelligent group."[48]

Would a reasonable person, well-informed and motivated in 1932, have excused Clark and Vonderlehr et al. from the ordinary moral duty of honesty? One can certainly imagine a plausible challenge from this source. The argument here is simply that ordinary moral challenges *could* have been made in 1932. However, one cannot with historical confidence go on to judge that these *ought* to have been made or that Clark and Vonderlehr et al. were morally deficient by not considering the likelihood of such a challenge. The system of human experimentation then was virtually closed to the common morality and to external oversight, especially from nonscientists. It is doubtful that the trustees of the Rosenwald Fund or the Milbank Fund, which later supported the study, knew of the deception used in recruitment. The point here is that the lack of a "system of normative ethics on human experimentation" in 1932 does not imply that there were no moral norms at all from which to measure the morality of the motives and actions of Clark and Vonderlehr et al. It is implausible that they would have been held personally or professionally accountable in terms of these norms. At the time there was no specific moral context of accountability for researchers whose activities breached common morality or lagged behind advanced German thought in research ethics. Bodies of ethical guidance have to be created from actual historical experience and reflection on moral error.

Part Three: A Graded Approach to Moral Judgment

Placing Moral Blame Accurately

The two major core values that compete and conflict in the tragic history of this case are: 1) society's interests in research to understand disease and to alleviate or prevent human suffering and untimely death, and 2) the protection owed by society and physician-investigators to human subjects of research, whose individual welfare and rights, as well as their autonomous and informed choices to participate in research, deserve the highest respect regardless of their condition or rank in society. The argument thus far blames Clark and Vonderlehr et al. more for disloyalty to the first value than to the second, which was barely visible in American research ethics in the 1930s.

Where does the locus of moral blame, in the name of the second value, truly belong in this infamous case? An accurate transhistorical judgment must be made to transmit a reliable account of moral evolution to future generations. Using the approach demonstrated above on the informed-consent question, it is now appropriate to ask: were the leaders of the PHS study in the post–World War II period until 1966 morally culpable according to contemporary standards?

Protests of the Study

One looks in vain for moral protests on behalf of the well-being of the subjects before 1965. As described above, there were several protests from within the PHS in the name of the first value, but none for the second. An external protest came in a June 1965 letter from Dr. Irwin Schatz of the Henry Ford Hospital in Detroit. After reading a report on the study, he wrote to the primary author, Donald H. Rockwell:

> I am utterly astounded by the fact that physicians allow patients with a potentially fatal disease to remain untreated when effective treatment is available. I assume you feel that the information which is extracted from observations of this untreated group is worth their sacrifice. If this is the case, then I suggest that the United States Public Health Service and those physicians associated with it need to reevaluate their moral judgments in this regard.[49]

Dr. Anne Yobs, coauthor of the report, received the letter and filed it with this attached comment: "This is the first letter of this type we have received. I do not plan to answer this letter."[50] Dr. Schatz's lone voice must be heard in a context of moral silence from the thousands of readers of the thirteen published articles (1936–73) about the study.[51]

The next protest was Peter Buxton's. He was more informed than Dr. Schatz about the moral features of the whole study. His protest was wide-ranging. His strategy gradually alerted officials to the risks of remaining passive in the face of moral questions about lack of treatment and racial implications. Finally in 1969, a panel of outside experts (all physicians) were assembled by the PHS to review the study. Only one, Dr. Gene Stollerman of the University of Tennessee, raised moral questions about the study and the obligation to treat the subjects maximally.[52] His lone view did not prevail and the study continued until it was exposed.

The Ethos of Human Experimentation (1947–1966)

Turning to the evolving ethos of medical research in the period from 1947 to 1966, there is historical evidence of slow but progressive advocacy for the second value. Some major benchmarks of this progress are the Nuremberg Code (1947), the Helsinki Code of the World Medical Association (1964), and the PHS human subjects policy itself (1966). However, the ascendancy of the second value in research practice and of socialization of researchers in loyalty to a new hierarchy of values was painfully slow; it met with deep resistance, and is still controversial in some respects today. The history of the ethics of human experimentation in the twentieth century is an ongoing struggle for a hierarchy of values placing the second above the first value. The evolution of a "system of normative ethics on human experientation"* has in retrospect taken half a century and is still evolving.

For valid transhistorical judgments, there must be a relevant moral context *at the time* within which decision makers would have been morally accountable. Due to the slow and gradual change in the ethos over this period, and the resistance to moral insights from within government itself, it is wise to take a *graded* approach to moral blame for the worst features of the PHS study. In effect, this would mean that Senator Kennedy's categorical judgment is far more fitting for the period of the 1960s than for the 1940s or 1950s. One can, however, find enough of a real moral context to assign some blame at this earlier time. The main criteria is that judgment must be proportionate to the degree to which loyalty to the second value had penetrated a previously closed system of human experimentation and begun to transcend the first value.

Others have described the tumultuous history of the reform of human experimentation in this period.[53] The events of these years dramatically posed progressively stronger claims of the second value, a score of crises and scandals depicted in

*This quotation is from Jones's description above of the ethos of the 1930s.

TABLE 1. *Research Ethics Scandals*

Thalidomide and FDA	1962
Jewish hospital cancer study	1963
Baboon-to-human heart transplant	1964
Willowbrook hepatitis study	1965
Beecher article	1966
"Tea Room Trade"	1967
Tuskegee (PHS-CDC) study	1932–72
Fetal research	1973

Table 1, and a government that had to overcome deep resistance among its own scientists to higher loyalty to the second value.

During this period the ethos of research did not lack for expressed moral obligations to benefit and heal the sick and to do the least harm possible in each endeavor. The Nuremberg Code in 1947 was a special point of entry of loyalty to the second value. Historically, we know that the moral claims of the code, especially in reference to informed consent, were more influential at the time and throughout the 1950s with researchers in the military than in the PHS or in academic medicine.[54] Many American researchers self-righteously viewed the code as promulgated for Nazi physicians but not for Americans. Dr. Heller said in interviews with James Jones that he made no association between the code and the syphilis study.[55] However, there were clinician-investigators at the NIH's Clinical Center who used the Nuremberg Code to shape policy for the institution in 1953 and as they innovated use of prior group review.[56] By 1964, the World Medical Association had adopted a very detailed code for researchers that distinguished between obligations in the contexts of therapeutic and nontherapeutic research.[57] The United States was a member of this body. A progressively different ethos from that in 1932 and in 1947 had begun to take shape. After 1964, there was a clear moral context of accountability very much like a point of no return on a long journey.

Dr. John Heller led the study from 1943 to 1948. Some moral blame must be assigned to him and others for totally ignoring the implications of the Nuremberg Code for the study. Although he and many American researchers viewed the code as only for Nazi barbarians, his colleagues at the NIH were already using the code to shape practices to protect human subjects. It is implausible that a reasonable person at the time could make a judgment that Dr. Heller *ought not* to have associated the content of the code to his study.

The next section ranks the most serious moral violations of continued support of the study, which began with Dr. Heller and increased in moral blameworthiness along a succession of PHS officials. They failed to recognize or remedy severe moral violations progressively blameworthy by the moral lights of the period.

Specific Moral Wrongs and Harms

Adding to Risks of Death and Ill Health. First, the PHS maintained a study for forty years that did great harm to the study's subjects who had syphilis and shortened their lives. Subjects from ages 25 to 45 when the study began had a 20 percent lower life expectancy than controls of the same age.[58] The subjects were also in a condition of poor health and in higher danger of death from other conditions than controls.[59]

Penicillin was available and effective to treat syphilis by 1943. In fact, the PHS began giving penicillin to patients with syphilis in some clinics across the nation.[60] The Alabama subjects were never informed of this development. In 1943, Dr. Heller became director of the Division of Venereal Diseases and could have given penicillin to the subjects and stopped the study. Dr. Heller and subsequent directors of the venereal disease division bear moral responsibility for deliberately shortening lifespans and inflicting remediable human suffering. They were: Dr. Theodore J. Bauer (1948–52), Dr. James K. Shafer (1953–54), Dr. Clarence A. Smith (1954–57), and Dr. William J. Brown (1957–71). All of the surgeons generals of this period were also morally responsible.

In 1951, when the PHS syphilis study was being reviewed after Dr. Iskrant's criticism, Dr. Heller acknowledged that the experiment shortened subjects' lives but defended it with a scientific duty to extend the study. His statement reveals two breathtaking realities: 1) he viewed the lives and health of socially and economically distressed human beings as expendable for the cause of science, and 2) he was morally blind to the central issue. He claimed:

> We have an investment of almost 20 years of Division interest, funds and personnel . . . as well as a responsibility to the survivors for their care and really to prove [to them] that their willingness to serve, even at risk of shortening life, as experimental subjects [has not been in vain]. And finally a responsibility to add what further we can to the natural history of syphilis.[61]

Heller elevated science as a moral cause over the welfare of human subjects. He also distorted reality by attributing motives of "service" and altruism to persons whom he knew were uninformed as to their role as subjects. When subjects died, Heller and others did not inform their survivors of the likelihood that death could be attributed to having been enrolled in this study.

As the study endured and became routinized in the bureaucracy, it became an end in itself, and the human beings it used became purely means to this end. The supporters of the study knew full well that subjects were dying sooner and were sicker than controls. The Helsinki Code states: "In the purely scientific application of clinical research carried out on a human being, it is the duty of the doctor to remain the protector of the life and health of that person on whom clinical research is carried out."[62] In the context of accountability to this code and their profession, the second generation of PHS officials must be viewed in the moral position of scientists who consciously condoned increased premature death and ill health to pursue flawed science.

The reflections of philosopher Hans Jonas in 1969 help to frame the major moral wrong done by the study. Contrary to Walsh McDermott, who argued for the moral priority of the first value, Jonas defended the dignity of the individual over the advancement of knowledge. McDermott had said in 1967:

> . . . the hard core of our moral dilemmas will not yield to the approaches of "Declarations" (i.e., Helsinki) or "Regulations" (i.e, the FDA's 1967 human subjects regulations); for as things stand today such statements must completely ignore the fact that society, too, has rights in human experimentation.[63]

In response, Jonas wrote that social progress through medical research

> is an optional goal, not an unconditional commitment. . . . Let us also remember that a slower progress in the conquest of disease would not threaten society, grievous as it is to those who have to deplore that their particular disease be not yet conquered, but that society would indeed be threatened by the erosion of those moral values whose loss, possibly caused by too ruthless a pursuit of scientific progress, would make its most dazzling triumphs not worth having.[64]

The PHS syphilis study was clearly a "ruthless" pursuit of knowledge but no "dazzling" triumph of knowledge. To appreciate the contrast, one should measure the costs in human suffering and death with the fact that no joint article was ever published comparing outcomes of the Oslo study and the PHS syphilis study.

Racial Bias and Unfairness. A second moral violation of the study was to the standard of justice or fairness by the racial bias involved in selection of subjects. A just research enterprise distributes the benefits and burdens of research as fairly as possible over a whole population. Even in the face of the 1960s civil rights movement, PHS authorities were unmoved by the unfairness and racial bias involved in selection of subjects. Each subject was a poor black male, the main point of Buxton's protest. The study would never have been done, especially with such deception, in a social context of white persons with syphilis. By 1966 or earlier, this thought certainly ought to have moved someone in the PHS to action.

Moral Inconsistency between PHS *Policy and Practice.* Leaders of the PHS in the mid-1960s were guilty of a glaring and unfair moral contradiction, as well as hypocrisy. They made PHS policy to protect human subjects of research and were morally blind to violations long since done to the subjects' health, autonomy, and dignity as persons. From 1966 to 1972, PHS leaders protected the Alabama study from Buxton's criticism with one hand and with the other effected reforms provoked primarily by loyalty to the second value. Loyalty to this value would clearly condemn the PHS for violating the norm of informed consent and for deception.

Condoning Deception in Research Activities. Fourth, significant moral harm was done to the dignity and autonomy of the subjects by deliberately masking the real purpose of the study to facilitate recruitment. Subjects were also deliberately deceived into believing that tools of research were "treatment." Moral debate about the justification for deception in experimentation began in earnest in the early to mid-1960s around the Milgram authority experiments[65] and Humphreys' "Tearoom Trade" study of homosexuality.[66] A practice of poststudy debriefing subjects about the use of deception gradually became normative in research in this period. This development shows how far loyalty to the second value had progressed.

Philosopher Robert Nozick argued in 1968 that, even if justified, when a prima facie moral obligation must be infringed upon, the infringement leaves "moral traces"[67] and cannot simply be set aside.[68] Debriefing of deceived subjects responds to the "moral traces" of infringing on the claims of informed consent to seek knowledge that could not have been otherwise gained. There were hosts of scientists in the PHS at the time aware of the massive degree of deception involved in the syphilis study. Moral blame for the indignities suffered due to this cause must fall on them. No review of this feature of the experiment occurred until the ad hoc panel did so in 1973.

Part Four: Final Questions

This discussion would be incomplete without addressing two final questions. First, how could the study have endured so long without serious internal moral challenge? Second, what moral lessons from the study are vital to carry into the future?

Moral blindness and racism do not adequately explain why the PHS study endured. Other main causes had to be chronically poor communication and systematic avoidance of ethical issues within particular branches of the PHS. It is also difficult to understand how reform efforts at the NIH did not motivate more attention to the syphilis study in the PHS. These efforts from 1953 to 1977 to innovate in methods of prior group review are described elsewhere.[69] As in the wider research community, the norms of the NIH culture permitted wide latitude with regard to informed consent and did not require prior group review of each research project with patients or of a single experiment involving one or a few patients.[70] Nonetheless, the insulation of the syphilis study from criticism could not have occurred if communication between branches of the PHS had been better.

There may well have been a contribution to the failure of dialogue from the NIH side, as well, because the NIH was involved scientifically in the syphilis study. In the 1950s and 1960s, the NIH was a relatively new agency where streams from two research cultures and one research bureaucracy met but with apparently little creative or critical interaction. The first was an older prewar research culture marked by a few general moral norms and a large degree of ethical relativism, as noted by Jones. It was this culture that created and supported the PHS syphilis study from 1932 to the 1960s. The second was a post-Nuremberg research culture. It was marked by high commitment to the best science, to informed consent (tinctured heavily with flexibility and the therapeutic privilege), and to new forms of prior peer review of proposed research. The founders of the NIH's intramural program were largely members of this second culture. A third stream, a research bureaucracy with written ethical requirements on human subjects of research, grew up around the NIH's extramural grants and contracts program in the 1960s. The 1966 and 1971 PHS-NIH policies requiring local institutional review boards and prior group review were required of grantees and contractors in this program.

More historical research is needed about whether the principals in these three arenas ever discussed ethical issues among themselves. If they did so, it was without much perspective on the implications that strong commitments to post-Nuremberg research ethics within the intramural program had for the extramural program or for earlier research like the PHS syphilis study. Did the right hand (PHS-CDC) know what the left hand (NIH–extramural/intramural) was doing? If great spaces of social distance between these three arenas could be demonstrated, it would help greatly to explain how the syphilis study endured.

In conclusion, what are the main lessons of the experiment for the task of protecting human subjects of research now and in the future? The first is clear, namely, to be vigilant about social and economic vulnerability to research exploitation. Vulnerable groups that come to mind are among the stigmatized and legally vulnerable citizens or strangers in our midst, e.g., substance abusers, illegal aliens, persons with HIV-AIDS, the homeless, or the poor who lack health care of any type.

Also, private-sector research, rather than research conducted by government, may pose greater risks of exploitation because there is an unfinished task in extending the legal protections of informed consent and prior group review to all citizens equally. Current U.S. law and regulations extend only to subjects in certain federally funded or regulated projects. Universalizing the scope of legal protection to research subjects regardless of source of funding, as has now been done by the 21 member countries of the Council of Europe, is a moral imperative for the U.S. Congress.[71] A large and unknown number of human subjects are at risk in research projects funded through the private sector. Once the world's leader in initiatives to protect human subjects, the United States has fallen behind.

A second lesson is that reliance on one main ethical resource, e.g., the professional ethics of individual investigators, the major ethical resource of previous eras, did not prevent the PHS study from occurring. The relevance of the lesson is that overreliance on the major resource of prior group review will not be adequate to prevent research projects that, on reflection, should have never been done. We need a plurality of resources to protect human subjects: a strong body of ethical guidance for researchers, effective institutional review boards (IRBS), and enlightened federal and state policies about human experimentation.

Today IRBS have authority to approve, alter, or deny proposed human-subject research projects. However, all is far from well with IRBS. According to a recent investigation of the Office of Inspector General (OIG), "the effectiveness of IRBS is now in jeopardy."[72] The report cites these escalating pressures on IRBS: expansion of managed care leading to pressure to accommodate research sponsors for income, increased commercialization of research, proliferation of multicenter trials, new types of research such as genetic testing, an increased number of proposals, and increased consumer demand for access to research.

According to the report, the main problems of today's IRBS are: 1) IRBS review too much, too quickly, with too little expertise, 2) IRBS conduct minimal continuing review of approved research, 3) IRBS face conflicts that threaten their independence (e.g., locating IRBS in offices of grants and contracts that bring in research dollars), 4) institutions provide little training for investigators and board members, 5) institutions make little effort to evaluate IRB effectiveness, and 6) there are an alarming number of violations of informed consent and unethical advertisements for subjects. The report warns about the potential for self-serving motives in the emergence of for-profit independent IRBS that contract with pharmaceutical firms and hospitals to review research. Vigilance is especially required on this front. The OIG report makes several important recommendations for reform, which include relaxation of requirements of time-consuming routine review to enable more time to focus on projects with significant risks, federal requirements for education and training of investigators and IRB members, mandatory registration of all IRBS with the government, and insulation of IRBS from conflicts of interest.

A third lesson from the study is about the human potential for moral and institutional blindness. Moral sensitivity can be overwhelmed by excessive loyalty to the welfare of an institution and one's role within it. Strong and uncritical loyalty to an institution and role impair independence of observation, judgment, and action, especially to prevent or moderate conflicts of loyalty and conflicts of interest. The syphilis study became an institution unto itself, and loyalty to it desensitized PHS officials and scientists to their conflicts of loyalty and conflicts of interest. They were appointed by society to protect the public health, yet they were officially charged with supporting a study that did great harm to subjects and to the public interest.

Some professions are better prepared and trained than others to detect and prevent conflicts of loyalties and conflicts of interests. Physicians and biomedical researchers do not receive the same degree of education and training about such issues as attorneys and behavioral scientists. For this reason, "because physicians are not trained to look for conflicts of interest, they often find themselves enmeshed in them without recognizing the problem."[73] The challenge for moral education about research ethics lies in a critical view of the contemporary consumer and market-place driven research environment. Large research organizations and enterprises, rather than individually funded researchers, have the momentum and resources in today's environment. If the moral focus ought to be on large organizations, conflicts of loyalty, and conflicts of interest, then there will be a place for the PHS syphilis study in moral education. Discernment can be aided by accurate judgments of how and why the Public Health Service of the United States once abandoned its moral compass in the name of science.

REFERENCES CITED

1. Jean Heller, "Syphilis Victims in U.S. Study Went Untreated for Years," *New York Times*, 26 July 1972, A1, A8.

2. Surgeon General, PHS, DHEW. "Investigations Involving Human Subjects, Including Clinical Research: Requirements for Review to Insure the Rights and Welfare of Individuals." PPO 129, Revised Policy, 1 July 1966.

3. Robert Levine, *Ethics and Regulation of Clinical Research*, 2d ed. (New Haven: Yale University Press, 1986), p. 323.

4. James H. Jones. *Bad Blood*. 2d ed. (New York: Free Press, 1993), p. 190.

5. Ibid., pp. 124, 149.

6. E. Bruusgaard. "Uber das Schicksal der nich spezifisch behaldelten Lueticker" (The Fate of Syphilitics Who Are Not Given Specific Treatment), *Archive fur Dermotologie und Syphilis* 157 (1929): 309–22.

7. After an interview with Dr. Heller, James Jones wrote: "Had Dr. Heller wished to end the experiment by giving the men penicillin, he could have done so. Yet penicillin presented no more of an ethical issue to Dr. Heller than earlier treatment had. When asked to comment years later (1976), he could not recall a single discussion about giving the subjects penicillin. It was withheld for the same reason that other drugs had been held back since the beginning of the experiment: Treatment would have ended the Tuskegee study. Dr. Heller asserted: 'The longer the study, the better the ultimate information we would derive.'" Jones concludes: "The men's status did not warrant ethical debate. They were subjects, not patients; clinical material, not sick people." See Jones, *Bad Blood*, p. 179.

8. With others, including Dr. Gamble, I was a speaker at a 23 February 1994 symposium on the study and its legacy held at the University of Virginia. The audience saw a film, *Bad Blood*, produced in 1992, in which a Dr. Sidney Olansky, a high-ranking PHS officer involved in the later stages of the study was interviewed. He completely denied any moral wrongdoing, defending the study in terms of medical beneficence. He showed no moral regret or reflection on the criticism that had been leveled at the study. Dismayed and appalled by the denial and self-righteousness in his face, I set aside my prepared text and gave an impromptu talk about the basic need to face moral errors and why an official apology for the study was appropriate. For more than a year, I campaigned with the help of others to PHS officials. Their decision was that an apology alone, without any other positive plan of action, would be "gratuitous." The committee's task was to flesh out a fuller response to the study's legacy, which included funding from the Department of Health and Human Services for education of research trainees in ethics, assistance with participa-

tion of minorities in research activities, and a grant to Tuskegee University to preserve important papers, photographs, and artifacts from the study.

9. Jones, *Bad Blood*, especially chapter 14, for his excellent discussion of this point.

10. I declined to attend the ceremony to protest its being held at the White House rather than at Tuskegee and still feel strongly that President Clinton was ill-advised in a decision not to travel to Tuskegee. Nonetheless, for the first time, the government did accept its moral responsibility in the president's apology. A great deal of credit for encouraging this event and for the collateral program to fund education in bioethics for researchers and assist minority participation in research should go to Dr. David Satcher, director of the Centers for Disease Control, and to Dr. Donna Shalala, secretary of the Department Health and Human Services.

11. I wrote this paper concurrently with the Advisory Committee's completion of its official report. The report has a systematic ethical framework for making transhistorical moral judgments; see Advisory Committee on Human Radiation Experiments, *Final Report* (Washington, D.C.: U.S. Government Printing Office, 1995), pp. 196–223.

I believe the discussion that follows is compatible with the committee's view of the task. For an extensive discussion of the committee's framework and implementation of it, see Tom L. Beauchamp, "Looking Back and Judging Our Predecessors," *Kennedy Institute of Ethics Journal* 6 (1996): 251–70.

12. Tuskegee Syphilis Study Ad Hoc Advisory Panel. "Final Report," in *Ethics in Medicine*, ed. Stanley J. Reiser, Arthur J. Dyck, and William J. Curran (Cambridge: MIT Press, 1977), pp. 316–21.

13. Jones, *Bad Blood*, p. 214.

14. Ibid., p. 211.

15. Albert R. Jonsen, *The Birth of Bioethics* (New York: Oxford University Press, 1998), pp. 127–28.

16. Henry K. Beecher, "Ethics and Clinical Research," *New England Journal of Medicine* 274 (1966): 1354–60.

17. Jones, *Bad Blood*, p. 100.

18. Ibid., p. 99.

19. Ibid., p. 119.

20. Ibid., p. 207.

21. Ibid., p. 99.

22. Ibid., p. 212.

23. Ibid., p. 131.

24. Ibid., p. 173.

25. Ibid., p. 181.

26. Ibid.

27. Ruth R. Faden and Tom L. Beauchamp, *A History and Theory of Informed Consent* (New York: Oxford University Press, 1986), pp. 56–60.

28. Faden and Beauchamp, *Informed Consent*, p. 57.

29. Martin S. Pernick, "The Patient's Role in Medical Decisionmaking: A Social History of Informed Consent in Medical Therapy," in the President's Commission for the Study of Ethical Problems in Medicine and Biomedical and Behavioral Research, *Making Health Care Decisions* (Washington, D.C.: GPO, 1982), 3:3.

30. Jay Katz, *The Silent World of Doctor and Patient* (New York: Free Press, 1984), pp. 3–4.

31. Jones, *Bad Blood*, p. 95.

32. Ibid., p. 93.

33. See an excellent discussion of the debate, in the Drug Amendments Act of 1962, over informed consent and the exception in the law, i.e., physicians were not required to obtain the consent of subjects if they deemed it "not feasible or, in their professional judgment, contrary to the best interests of such human beings"; in William J. Curran, "Governmental regulation of the

use of human subjects in medical research: the approach of two federal agencies," *Daedalus* 98 (1969): 542–94.

34. President's Commission for the Study of Ethical Problems in Medicine and Biomedical and Behavioral Research, *Making Health Care Decisions*. Vol. 1. (Washington, D.C.: GPO, 1983).

35. Jones, *Bad Blood*, pp. 98–99.

36. Norman Howard-Jones. "Human experimentation in historical and ethical perspective." *Social Science in Medicine* 16 (1982): 1436. See also Paul M. McNeill, *The Ethics and Politics of Human Experimentation* (New York: Cambridge University Press, 1993), p. 42.

37. Jay Katz, "Human Experimentation and Human Rights." *St. Louis University Law Journal* 38 (1993): 7–54.

38. P. M. McNeil, *The Ethics and Politics of Human Experimentation* (New York: Cambridge University Press, 1993), pp. 40–41; see also H. M. Sass, "Reichsrundschreiben 1931: Pre-Nuremberg German Regulations Concerning New Therapy and Human Experimentation." *Journal of Medicine and Philosophy* 8 (1983): 99–111.

39. Jay Katz might have cited this guideline in support of his point about exploitation in his minority report. It would have been a fine rhetorical point, i.e., that the danger of exploitation of distressed human subjects in order to carry out research was a living moral idea in Germany at the very time the PHS study was being conceived.

40. See George J. Annas and Michael Grodin, *The Nazi Doctors and the Nuremberg Code*. (New York: Oxford University Press, 1992). There is some dispute about whether the guidelines were legally binding in Germany before and during the Second World War. McNeil argues that they were "legally binding" (Katz, "Human Experimentation," p. 41). He followed Sass's claim (see note 38 above) that they were legally binding throughout the Nazi period. At best, there seems to be confusion about the legal status of the guidelines.

41. Jones, *Bad Blood*, p. 103.

42. The first meeting of the Medical Board of the Clinical Center was on 16 January 1952. No mention of a Clinical Research Committee (CRC) appeared in subsequent minutes until 3 March 1953.

A document describing this committee and the NIH policy on the ethics of clinical research, "Group Consideration of Clinical Research Procedures Deviating from Accepted Medical Practice or Involving Unusual Hazard," was issued in 1954. The Medical Board established a CRC in the same year. The document begins by noting that primary responsibility for the "formulation and conduct of clinical research and medical care is on the principal investigators designated by each Institute Director, in conformity with standards and principles of legal, ethical, and administrative propriety established by the Director, NIH." The document then describes a two-level practice of "group consideration," one by committees of each institute, and a second by the CRC. It states that the role of the CRC is to "serve as an expert body to advise on problems concerning clinical research involving unestablished or potentially hazardous procedures referred to it by the Director, NIH, institute or clinical directors, or the Director of the Clinical Center." The practice of using this committee is later described in Stuart M. Sessoms, "Guiding Principles in Medical Research Involving Humans," *Hospitals*, 1 Jan. 1958, p. 44. Another early document (12 March 1954), "Use of Human Volunteers in Medical Research," was produced by the surgeon general's office. The document noted that prior group review was "non-mandatory."

43. The National Institutes of Health Revitalization Act of 1993, Public Law 103–43, 10 June 1993, Section 492A.

44. Ronald M. Green, personal communication, 21 June 1994.

45. Jay Katz made this point eloquently in his minority report which is appended to the 1973 panel, p. 320, and in this volume.

46. Jones, *Bad Blood*, especially chapter 8.

47. Ibid., p. 123.

48. Ibid.

49. Ibid., p. 190.

50. Ibid.

51. These articles are listed by Jones in ibid., pp. 281–82.

52. Ibid., p. 195.

53. David Rothman, *Strangers at the Bedside* (New York: Free Press, 1991); Albert Jonsen, *The Birth of Bioethics* (New York: Oxford University Press, 1998), pp. 125–65.

54. Jonathan D. Moreno, "Reassessing the Influence of the Nuremberg Code on American Medical Ethics," *The Journal of Contemporary Health Law and Policy* 13 (1997): 347–60.

55. Jones, *Bad Blood*, p. 180.

56. Sessoms, "Guiding Principles in Medical Research."

57. The Helsinki Code, amended as of 1975, is reprinted in Levine, *Ethics and Regulation*, pp. 427–29.

58. J. R. Heller and P. T. Bruyere, "Untreated Syphilis in the Male Negro: II. Mortality during Twelve Years of Observation," *Journal of Venereal Disease Information* 27 (1946): 39.

59. J. K. Shafer et al. "Untreated Syphilis in the Male Negro: A Prospective Study of the Effect on Life Expectancy," *Public Health Reports* 69 (1954): 88.

60. Jones, *Bad Blood*, p. 178.

61. Ibid., p. 182.

62. Levine, *Ethics and Regulation*, p. 429.

63. Walsh McDermott, "Opening Comments—The Changing Mores of Biomedical Research: A Colloquium on Ethical Dilemmas from Medical Advances," *Annals of Internal Medicine* 67, Supp. 7, No. 3, Part II (1967): 39–42. Quote is from p. 42.

64. Hans Jonas, "Philosophical Reflections on Human Experimentation," *Daedalus* 98 (Spring 1969): 245.

65. Stanley Milgram, "Issues in the Study of Obedience: A Reply to Baumrind," *American Psychologist* 19 (1964): 848–52.

66. Laud Humphreys, *Tearoom Trade: Impersonal Sex in Public Places* (Chicago: Aldine Publishing Co., 1970).

67. Robert Nozick, "Moral Complications and Moral Structures," *Natural Law Forum* 13 (1968): 1–50.

68. For a discussion of the "moral traces" concept in biomedical ethics, see Tom L. Beauchamp and James F. Childress, *Principles of Biomedical Ethics*, 4th ed. (New York: Oxford University Press, 1995), p. 105.

69. J. C. Fletcher and F. G. Miller, "The Promise and Perils of Public Bioethics," in *The Ethics of Research Involving Human Subjects: Facing the Twenty-First Century*, ed. H. Y. Vanderpool (Frederick, Md.: University Publishing Group, 1996), pp. 155–84.

70. Advisory Committee on Human Radiation Experiments, "Research Ethics and the Medical Profession," *Journal of the American Medical Association* 276 (1996): 403–9.

71. F. William Dommel and Duane Alexander, "The Convention on Human Rights and Biomedicine of the Council of Europe," *Kennedy Institute of Ethics Journal* 7 (1997): 259–76.

72. Department of Health and Human Services, Office of Inspector General, Institutional Review Boards: A Time for Reform, June 1998. OEI-01-97-00193.

73. Roy G. Spece, David S. Shimm, and Allen E. Buchanan, Preface to *Conflicts of Interest in Clinical Practice and Research* (New York: Oxford University Press, 1996).

THE TUSKEGEE SYPHILIS EXPERIMENT
Biotechnology and the Administrative State

BENJAMIN ROY

Beginning in 1932, the Public Health Service (PHS) conducted a project at the Tuskegee Institute that withheld treatment from a group of black men who had contracted syphilis. Ostensibly, its purpose was to further the understanding of the natural course of the disease. The study continued for 40 years until its exposure in 1972. The US Department of Health, Education, and Welfare convened an ad hoc panel on the Tuskegee Syphilis Study.[1] The panel did not formulate questions, but investigated questions assigned to it by the government using documents indicated to be *directly* related to the Tuskegee Syphilis Study, thereby excluding documents judged to be *indirectly* related to the study. On this basis, all reviews to date have examined narrow aspects of the administration of the study and concluded that the Tuskegee Experiment was a *clinical* study by well-intentioned but scientifically naive investigators whose decisions, against the historical background, were not overtly racist.[1,2] This portrays an effort to benefit the many by unraveling fundamental questions of disease process. This is a primary reason that the government puts forward to engage in human experimentation with its citizens.

This article rejects these conclusions and maintains that the Tuskegee Syphilis Study was instead the economic exploitation of humans as a natural resource of a disease that could not be cultivated in culture or animals in order to establish and sustain US superiority in patented commercial biotechnology. Its use was for the applied science of syphilis serology. Initially, the Tuskegee Experiment served to evaluate and standardize the nontreponemal syphilis tests. Later, the Tuskegee Experiment was a resource to develop and commercialize specific treponemal tests. Furthermore, by the 12th year of the study, there was evidence that many subjects did not have syphilis at all. The Tuskegee serological and clinical studies did not address any basic science questions of the pathogenesis or immunology of syphilis other than the practical applied science of serologic testing. The basis of these conclusions are the documents considered to be *indirectly* related to the study.

In the late 1920s, the PHS pursued three avenues of syphilis research. The first was the Clinical Cooperative Study initiated in 1928. The second study was a

Dr. Benjamin Roy is in the Department of Psychiatry, Albany Medical College, Albany, N.Y.
Originally published in the Journal of the National Medical Association *87 (1995): 56–67.*
Reprinted by permission of the National Medical Association.

"serological dragnet" funded by the Julius Rosenwald Fund that began in 1930; it was restricted to African Americans of six southern counties. The third was a 1934 evaluation of serological tests for syphilis developed by US researchers. These lines of investigation conformed to an outline that divided the labor of research across several specialized groups.[3]

Untreated Syphilis and Drug Evaluation

The principal standard against which to measure the value of therapeutic innovations was untreated disease.[3] This was one purpose of the Tuskegee Syphilis Experiment that, although portrayed as an isolated study, was a member of a constellation with several clinical functions. It provided the general knowledge (ie, untreated disease) against which to check the results of diagnostic, therapeutic, and other research procedures.

The Clinical Cooperative study was a spin-off of a League of Nations study that coordinated observation of syphilis treatment at US and European clinics. Five US sites were under the direction of the PHS Division of Venereal Diseases. These sites included Johns Hopkins University, Baltimore, Maryland; the Mayo Clinic, Rochester, Minnesota; the University of Pennsylvania, Philadelphia, Pennsylvania; Case Western Reserve University, Cleveland, Ohio; and the University of Michigan, Ann Arbor, Michigan.[4–9] This study began in 1928, 4 years before the Tuskegee Study. The presence of Udo J. Wile of the University of Michigan gives some insight to the experimental philosophy of this panel. Wile bored holes in the skulls of mentally ill patients with general paresis at Michigan's Pontiac State Hospital. Then, he aspirated brain tissue to show that this tissue could transmit syphilis to rabbits.[10] This was an important finding for basic science, but it had no therapeutic or diagnostic benefit, and the patients were incompetent to give consent. Wile did not approach the families for consent. In response to public outcry, Wile was unapologetic— "You may quote me as having absolutely no interest in the matter, whatever people may wish to think regarding the experiments."[11]

The first series of papers examined 3244 cases of early syphilis. Most of the patients received arsphenamine, while 350 received neoarsphenamine. In August 1930, the study group presented the initial results at the International Congress of Dermatology and Syphilology at Copenhagen.[12] The study addressed the comparative effects of different chemotherapies and the response to treatment of clinical manifestations and syphilis serology (Wassermann reaction). From this framework, the group planned to formulate a standard treatment for syphilis.[13]

The study had a major shortcoming, however. There was no control group of untreated syphilitic patients against which to measure the worthiness of the treatments, nor could one assess the usefulness of reversions in serologic testing. The only existing body of data on untreated syphilis was the 1929 report by Bruusgaard of the clinical status of syphilitic Norwegians who remained untreated for more than 30 years.[14,15] In 1890, Caesar P. M. Boeck, Chief of the Syphilis Clinic at University Hospital, Oslo, deliberately withheld mercurials from 1404 people with syphilis. When arsphenamine became available in 1910, all patients at the Oslo clinic received arsphenamine. The Bruusgaard material was the collection of patients who did not return for follow-up and therefore did not receive arsphenamine.

The Cooperative Clinical Study reformulated its data to exploit the Bruusgaard data as an untreated control group.[13] The contrast was dramatic: neurosyphilis was four times more frequent, and bone and skin lesions were up to 26 times greater in untreated patients, while 77% of treated patients had negative serology and remission of symptoms. The Cooperative Group concluded that the clinical efficacy of arsphenamine was incontrovertible. Yet in 1972, to defend the decision to withhold treatment from the Tuskegee subjects, the PHS claimed that arsphenamine was ineffective and would have been of little value to the men of the Tuskegee Experiment.

The use of the Bruusgaard material points to the usefulness of the Tuskegee Syphilis Study as a reliable control group. The Clinical Cooperative Group complained that small numbers, lack of spinal fluid studies, and uncertainty regarding previous treatments made the Bruusgaard material inadequate. The PHS boasted that the existence of controls, serologic examinations, and spinal fluid examinations made the Tuskegee Syphilis Experiment superior to the methodological weaknesses of the Bruusgaard material. Additionally, whereas the Bruusgaard patients were untreated, early syphilis patients lost for a considerable period to follow-up, the Tuskegee Study included untreated late and latent syphilis subjects followed continuously over time.[15] Norwegian scientists later disputed this claim.[16]

The Development of Nontreponemal Tests

The major utility of the Tuskegee Syphilis Experiment was its provision of sera to develop and standardize serological tests for syphilis. Diagnostic tests and therapeutics had considerable commercial value. Intense international competition for the production and marketing of diagnostics and therapeutics shaped the research policies of several nations.

A series of studies conducted by the PHS had two components: the first concerned the comparison and standardization of existing US serologic tests; the second was the development of new tests. At the request of the American Society of Clinical Pathologists, the PHS organized the Committee on Evaluation and Serodiagnostic Tests for Syphilis to assess the value of existing serological tests for syphilis. Because of the expressly economic intent to support improvement of US tests, competitive British and German tests were excluded from analysis. The protocol for the serological survey was made known in 1934.[17] The sensitivity and specificity of a range of tests were compared using known syphilitic sera (positive controls) and known nonsyphilitic sera (negative controls). Absolute positive sera establish the sensitivity of a test, ie, the ability to detect disease in people who have the disease. Negative sera establish the specificity of the test, ie, the absence of reactivity in people who do not have the disease. There could be no question of prior treatment in positive controls nor any question of syphilis in negative controls to accomplish these ends. During the Tuskegee study, presumed positives who turned out to be negative either by incidental treatment or by seroconversion were deleted from the study, and presumed negatives who tested positive were moved to the syphilitic group. Alterations of diagnostic groups in this way could never be tolerated in a clinical study. However, in retrospect, these maneuvers maintained the credibility of the Tuskegee positive and negative control groups for the purposes of the applied science of serological testing.

The first survey was published in 1935.[18] The numbers of late syphilis, syphilitic spinal fluids, and nonsyphilitic controls corresponded to the numbers in the Tuskegee Syphilis Experiment. This study did not explicitly state that it used Tuskegee sera. The first clinical report on the Tuskegee Syphilis Study in 1936 confirmed that Tuskegee sera comprised the testing sera for the serodiagnostic test evaluation of 1935.[19] The sequence of publication and authorship establish the priority of studies and the utility of the Tuskegee patients. The author for the serological study was Hugh S. Cumming, Surgeon General of the United States. In contrast, Raymond Vonderlehr, author of the clinical paper, was an assistant surgeon. The usefulness of the Tuskegee group was their sera. Their clinical status was only important to establish them as credible positive controls. Treponema could not be grown in culture and it could not be produced artificially. *Treponema pallidum* only grew in living humans or animals (rabbits and monkeys). The PHS repeatedly complained that it was not possible to extrapolate the findings with animals to humans. This was the driving argument for human experimentation. The Tuskegee subjects were a renewable culture source of *T pallidum* and antitreponemal antibodies. Tuskegee sera defined the use of existing serological tests and new ones for the next 40 years.

Joseph E. Moore, MD, chief syphilologist at Johns Hopkins University, was the clinical consultant to the Tuskegee Syphilis Study and a principal architect of the Clinical Cooperative Study.[20] Moore criticized the methodology of the 1935 evaluation of serodiagnostic tests for syphilis. He complained that the evaluation assessed serological tests under ideal conditions in the laboratories of the inventors. In his opinion, it was best to evaluate the usefulness or performance of these tests under general laboratory conditions. The need to evaluate serological tests in general laboratory circumstances meant a need to return to the Tuskegee well.

Serological testing was a cornerstone of syphilis control. The second survey, published in 1937, assessed serological tests in the hands of 30 state and private laboratories.[21-23] It recommended annual surveys for state laboratories using positive and negative controls provided by the PHS. The need for serodiagnostic evaluation was clearly put as a need for the PHS to regulate and license laboratories that performed syphilis tests.[24] Therefore, the Tuskegee sera also enabled the PHS to exercise its lawmaking power to regulate the industry of syphilis serodiagnosis. The PHS used its police power to create the Tuskegee Syphilis Study, which in turn was used as an instrument to further expand the borders of its administrative lawmaking domain. Once a year, the Tuskegee subjects were sampled daily over several weeks for the sole purpose of providing sera for regulatory and standardization purposes unrelated to research.

Useful tests demonstrated specificity equal to 99%; sensitivity was problematic and varied from 65% to 88%. A major drawback for all tests was the false-positive rates in leprosy and malaria of 59% and 15%, respectively. In other words, the nontreponemal tests could not distinguish syphilis from leprosy. Similar conclusions were drawn for the use of these tests on cerebrospinal fluid.[25,26] These observations directed research to develop tests with greater specificity for syphilis diagnosis after 1936.

The market for syphilis serodiagnosis was considerable. The PHS wanted free tests, but was aware of the opposition that would ensue. The committee recommended that state laboratories perform the cheaper flocculation tests, and that Social Security be used to pay private laboratories to perform the more expensive complement fixation tests.[26]

The National Venereal Disease Act of 1938 further extended and centralized the administrative law and police power of the PHS. It also granted greater latitude to pursue human research. If there had been any question of the study's lawfulness, apart from its ethics, the legislation of 1938 provided legal shelter for its continuance. The Tuskegee Syphilis Study was legal. No one was ever indicted or charged with violating the law. The first studies following this act exploited human experimentation to investigate the problem of false-positive reactions in malaria. The PHS inoculated psychiatric patients with *Plasmodium vivax*-infected blood from other psychotic patients, while others were exposed to bites of malaria-infected mosquitoes (similar to the Walter Reed yellow fever experiments).[27,28]

Research continued for improved antigens and better techniques of detecting antibodies. The introduction of cardiolipin improved the sensitivity of the non-treponemal antigen tests.[29] A cocktail of cardiolipin combined with lecithin and cholesterol created a nontreponemal antigen that enhanced reactivity. The NY State Department of Health patented and licensed the use of cardiolipin to companies that marketed syphilis tests.

Movement toward tests that measured specific reaction for treponemal antigens accelerated with the demonstration of high reactivity for Palligen, a commercial suspension of killed noninfectious Reiter strain spirochete manufactured by Sachsische Serumwerk of Dresden, Germany. To ascertain its purity, investigators inoculated animals with the preparation expecting it to induce syphilis. However, Palligen did not induce infection. This raised concern that the preparation did not contain true *T pallidum* but some other treponemal organism. Despite this shortcoming, the Germans clearly made an advance. Scientists in the United States predicted that improved treponemal tests would become the method of choice by reducing the false-positive reactions associated with beef heart lipoidal antigens.[30,31]

The third survey was the Washington Serology Conference of October 1941.[32] From 1936 to 1946, there were no further clinical reports on the Tuskegee patients. The Venereal Disease Research Laboratory (VDRL) implied that the study was abandoned and then resumed in 1939.[33] However, internal memos show that the study was delayed further until a new field physician was properly trained at Johns Hopkins (Vonderlehr R. October 1937. Unpublished data). The critical role of positive sera to the serodiagnostic study more clearly explains the anxiety that some patients had received treatment (Diebert AV. November 1938. Unpublished data). Moore suggested that new untreated syphilitics be added to the group to correct this problem (Diebert AV. March 1939. Unpublished data).

This maneuver remedied the needs of the serodiagnostic study, but it was a violation if it was a clinical study. Patients cannot be added and deleted as desired from clinical studies without undermining the assumptions of the statistical analyses—randomness and equal variance. However, the Tuskegee Experiment was not a clinical study. Movement of subjects between groups enhanced the applied science of the Tuskegee Syphilis Experiment by the deliberate cultivation of positive and negative serum standards. The treated Tuskegee syphilitics were dispensable because it was not a clinical study; a separate clinical serodiagnostic study had more than sufficient numbers of partially treated syphilitics (Vonderlehr R. December 1938. Unpublished data).

The absolute need for the Tuskegee sera has no greater example than the PHS response to an unforeseen complication. One year before publication of the second serodiagnostic study, a change in the Tuskegee administration threatened access to Tuskegee sera. John Kenney, MD, former medical director of the Tuskegee Institute and adversary of certain PHS policies, returned to his position at Tuskegee (Smith M. November 1941. Unpublished data). The PHS moved its autopsies from Tuskegee to funeral homes, and curtailed burial payments directly to Tuskegee to escape detection by Kenney. These extraordinary maneuvers must have been political subterfuge intended to keep the study covert. This suggests fear that Kenney (who was at odds with the American Medical Association by his espousal of national health care and criticism of its exclusion of blacks) would oppose the Tuskegee Syphilis Experiment.

This period also corresponds to a pressing development in the competition for diagnosis and treatment of infectious diseases. German pharmacologists developed sulfonamides in 1908 and within a few years had synthesized a number of antibacterial compounds.[34] The most important of these was Prontosil, patented in 1932 in Germany, 1934 in France, and 1935 in England. The first reports of its activity against both experimental and clinical infections with streptococcus, staphylococcus, and pneumococcus appeared in the German literature in 1935.[35–37] These organisms were important causes of skin and wound infections during war. Animal experiments by French investigators in 1935[38] and English clinical trials in 1936[39] confirmed the activity of Prontosil.

The use of sulfonamides for syphilis was unknown. Because they proved to be beneficial treatment for gonorrhea, the sulfonamides cast a specter like arsphenamine before they were even tried in the treatment of syphilis. Until the sulfonamides, there had been no drug to treat gonorrhea. Like arsphenamine, Prontosil was metabolized to an active intermediate, leaving the door open for the patenting and marketing of the intermediate. A 1939 US publication summarized knowledge of the sulfonamides and presciently commented: "The welfare of the patient must not be sacrificed in the race for new and marketable chemotherapeutic compounds."[34]

Thus, before World War II, the PHS acquired financial muscle using the Social Security Act of 1936, added to its regulatory powers using the Venereal Disease Research Act of 1938, and responded to the economic pressures of German science, which introduced treponemal antigens and a new class of therapeutic medications. The United States entered World War II 5 weeks following the Washington Serology Conference. Hopeful to contain the spread of syphilis and gonorrhea, and to make US medicine independent of German advances, the military and the PHS put pressure on domestic researchers.

After 1942, the combination of cardiolipin, lecithin, and cholesterol displaced lipid antigens in the flocculation tests. The prime test of this period that is still used today is the VDRL test.[40] All Tuskegee sera were stored and used by the VDRL in Staten Island, New York, before its move to Chamblee, Georgia in the mid-1950s. The PHS used Tuskegee sera to develop the VDRL test.

The Credibility of Syphilis Diagnoses

One of the driving forces for improved serologic diagnosis may have been the Tuskegee Syphilis Experiment itself. There are indications that the serological surveys of 1935 and 1942 may have relied on dubious samples that were positive reactors in the Wassermann test, but that did not evidence clinical correlates of syphilis. The first clinical report appeared in 1936; it emphasized the incidence of cardiovascular disease.[19] It was an a priori conclusion that cardiovascular disease in blacks with positive Wassermann tests or a clinical diagnosis of syphilis was caused by syphilis. The second report appeared in February 1946 and focused on mortality and reduction in life expectancy.[41] It mentioned that of 129 subjects who had died, 93 came to autopsy. In December 1946, the third paper gave clinical cardiovascular measurements to present contentions of increased disease among the Tuskegee subjects, yet avoided claiming that the etiology was syphilis.[42] This paper followed, in order, in the same journal, an autopsy examination of untreated syphilis from Yale Medical School.[43] In 1950, the fourth paper stated that by 1948, investigators completed a total of 98 autopsies.[44] Finally, in 1955, the pathological study presented 124 autopsies performed from 1933 to 1952.[45]

Table 1 shows a contrast between these reports. The annual rate of deaths for the period 1948 to 1952 was twice that for the period 1933 to 1944. Yet, the rate of autopsies remained constant. Therefore, as the number of deaths rose, the ratio of autopsies to death declined to 47% of that from 1933 to 1944. The periods 1933 to 1944 and 1933 to 1952 showed a similar percentage of deaths that came to autopsy: 72% and 75%, respectively. Yet, the percentage of deaths, autopsied for the period 1948 to 1952 was only 34%; this is a 45% reduction.

If the percentage of deaths resulting in autopsies had remained constant, then the PHS would have had to perform at least 55 autopsies to match the doubled death rate. However, the PHS conducted only 26 autopsies. World War II did not interfere in these statistics because an arrangement with the Selective Service Commission excluded both syphilitic and nonsyphilitic control subjects from military service. By conservative and generous estimates, these numbers suggest that between 1948 and 1952, the Tuskegee investigators deliberately reduced the number of autopsies. Because the clinical reports did not state the specific numbers of syphilitics and controls autopsied, an accurate distribution of the autopsies between groups is not possible. However, the inference is that from 1948 to 1952, autopsies of syphilitic subjects dropped 49%, while that of controls decreased by 60%. Alternatively, the PHS might not have been able to keep pace with the accelerated rate of death. This is an unlikely explanation; the PHS was too efficient. Examiner bias is offered unwittingly in the pathological report by a preamble of excuses that the subjects were black and autopsies were performed "under inconceivably adverse circumstances."[45] These considerations do not alter the conclusion that the PHS manipulated the autopsies of syphilitics to diminish findings that contradicted laboratory and clinical diagnoses of syphilis.

Despite insistence by the PHS that the Tuskegee group displayed clinical evidence of syphilis, there were discrepancies in the clinical reports. Although there

Variable	1933 to 1944[41]	1933 to 1948[44]	Time Period 1944 to 1952	1948 to 1952	1933 to 1952[45]
Years	12	16	8	4	20
Total deaths	129	140	87	76	216
Syphilitic	101	(109)†	64	(56)	165
Controls	28	(31)	23	(20)	51
Death rate	10.75	8.75	10.87	19	10.8
Syphilitic	8.4	(6.81)	8	(14)	8.25
Controls	2.33	(1.94)	2.87	(5)	2.55
Total autopsy	93	98	31	26	124
Syphilitic	(69)	(73)	(23)	(19)	92
Controls	(24)	(25)	(8)	(7)	32
Autopsy rate	7.75	6.13	3.88‡	6.5	6.2
Syphilitic	(5.75)	(4.56)	(2.87)	(4.75)	4.6
Controls	(2.0)	(1.56)	(1.0)	(1.75)	1.6
Autopsy/death	0.72	0.7	0.36	0.34	0.57
Syphilitic	(0.68)	(0.67)	(0.36)	(0.33)	0.56
Controls	(0.86)	(0.81)	(0.35)	(0.35)	0.63

*These data are compiled from two clinical reports, Heller[41] and Pesare,[44] that made mention of autopsies up to 1944 and 1948, respectively, and the pathological report of Peters.[45] Peters presents data for all autopsies performed from 1933 to 1952. The difference between information from Peters and Heller was taken as the number autopsied between 1944 and 1952, whereas, the difference between data from Peters 1955 and Pesare 1950 represents the number autopsied between 1948 and 1952. The Heller and Pesare reports did not state the specific numbers of syphilitics and controls autopsied. These data are inferred by using the fraction of the total number of autopsies to the total number of deaths for the period 1933 to 1952 as a conservative estimate of the missing data for syphilitics and controls that were autopsied from 1944 to 1952 and 1948 to 1952. This is fair considering that the Public Health Service used this method to make assumptions about the incidence of clinical disease in subjects it was unable to examine.
†The interpolated figures appear in parentheses.
‡Comparing Heller with Pesare, there were just 11 deaths and 5 autopsies between 1944 and 1948. These numbers were too low to analyze separately, but they may contribute to an artifactual reduction of the autopsy rate for the period 1944 to 1952.

was significantly greater cardiovascular disease, there was no evidence that this was syphilitic in nature. The papers avoided stating that syphilis accounted for cardiovascular disease. This conclusion was inferred from the assumption that blacks were syphilitic; therefore, any findings presumably were due to syphilis. Despite clinical evidence of neurologic impairment in some patients, no subject developed tabes dorsalis, general paresis, or other pathognomonic complications or neurosyphilis. The rate for neurosyphilis was inferior to the Cooperative Clinical Study. The Tuskegee patients did not develop neurosyphilis. Furthermore, the clinical reports found reasons not to make comparisons with the Bruusgaard data or earlier Tuskegee reports. These discrepancies did not go unnoticed and met with criticism by Norwegian researchers before publication of the pathological reports.[16] The PHS continued to stand behind the claim that the disease complications noted in the Tuskegee patients were syphilitic. Only one paper that reported titers for 65 syphilitic subjects gives any insight into the criteria for positive syphilis serology: in 1939, 31% were negative, 42% were positive on *undiluted* serum or had titers 1:4 and 14% were doubtful.[44] Only pathologic diagnosis would resolve the issue of the presence or absence of syphilis.

The pathologic report that appeared 10 years later, in 1955, did not support these assertions.[45] This is important because the pathological examination was the only part of the Tuskegee clinical study that followed a protocol. The pathologist was blind to the history or diagnosis before autopsy and followed strict criteria for gross and microscopic examination to establish a pathologic diagnosis of syphilis. The Yale autopsy study of 1946 compared its findings against the Bruusgaard material. However, the Tuskegee pathologic report avoided any comparisons. Table 2 compares data from the three studies. The Yale study reported summary data not differentiated by race for 150 whites and 48 blacks. The Bruusgaard data was interpolated for comparison.[46] The Tuskegee Experiment had six criteria for gross examination, but only one criteria—linear striations of aortitis—distinguished syphilitics from the controls. A histological diagnosis of syphilis had to meet seven criteria. By microscopic examination, only 24 (27%) had definite syphilis; if the assessment excludes 5 doubtfuls and includes 12 minimal reports, this percentage rises to 40%. Eight cases with arteriosclerosis were attributed incorrectly to syphilis. Microscopic and gross examinations agreed on a diagnosis of syphilis in only 25 (28%) subjects; they excluded syphilis in 37 (42%).

Although the clinical reports of Tuskegee assumed an increase of syphilitic cardiovascular disease in blacks over whites, the pathologic report shows an equivalent incidence compared with the Yale study. Positive syphilis serology did not correlate with a pathologic diagnosis of syphilis. Sixty-nine percent had positive serological tests, but only 38% of these met criteria for syphilitic aortitis. The rate of positive syphilis serology equaled that of the Yale study, which also showed an unreliable relationship between the serologic test for syphilis and pathological diagnosis of syphilis. This relationship was even more tenuous for Tuskegee blacks than for whites.

There also was no correlation between clinical and pathological diagnoses of aortitis. Thirty-six of 62 autopsies had clinical diagnoses of aortitis, but only 16 were confirmed: eight of the negative autopsies had arteriosclerosis with fusiform dilatation—an equally common finding in the controls. The most provocative findings were the equivalent presence of bronchopneumonia and pleural effusions in both syphilitics (48% and 54%, respectively) and controls (34% and 63%,

	Tuskegee[45]		Yale[43]	Bruusgaard[14]
	Untreated	Control		
Number	89	32	198	473
CNS examined	46	13	116	
Positive STS	60 (67%)		137 (69%)	
Negative STS	29 (33%)		61 (31%)	
Normal autopsy			121 (61%)	307 (65%)
Positive STS	23 (25%)		80 (40%)	68 (14%)
Negative STS	14 (16%)		35 (18%)	132 (28%)
Doubtful			6 (3%)	107 (23%)
Anatomic lesions	18 (20%)		77 (39%)	166 (35%)
Cardiovascular				
Aortitis	19 (21%)	2 (6%)	55 (28%)	
Aneurysm arch	7 (8%)	0	9 (5%)	
Coronary disease			4 (2%)	
Ruptured aneurysm			9 (5%)	
CNS (total)	2 (4%)		7 (6%)	36 (8%)
Tabes dorsalis	0		3 (3%)	
Neurosyphilis	1 (2%)		2 (2%)	
Meningitis	1 (2%)		2 (2%)	
Other organs				
Liver cirrhosis	14 (16%)	6 (3%)	1 (0.5%)	
Bronchopneumonia	43 (48%)	11 (34%)		
Pleural effusion	48 (54%)	20 (63%)		

Abbreviations: CNS=central nervous system and STS=serologic test for syphilis.
*These are methodologically different studies. The Bruusgaard study[14] was a retrospective clinical study, the Yale study (Rosahn)[43] was a retrospective autopsy study, and Tuskegee (Peters)[45] was a prospective autopsy study. Rosahn did not include patients with doubtful or minimal changes as syphilitic, whereas Peters included even doubtful cases, which may have inflated the findings. Peters stated that "some degree of subjective variation is unavoidable." Twenty-five subjects (28%) had anatomical lesions by both gross and microscopic examination, but 7 of these were "minimal"; therefore, 18 subjects are considered to have had definite syphilis. In comparison, Rosahn had 77 patients with definite syphilis. The presence of aortitis was most pathognomonic of syphilis. Rosahn did not report whether the diagnosis of aortitis was based on gross or microscopic examination. Peters reported 29 aortitis based on the presence of linear striations on gross examination. However, microscopic examination showed only 19/89 (21%) syphilitic subjects that met definite histologic criteria for aortitis (12 with gross thickening of the aortic wall and 7 with medical necrosis). Syphilitic gumma were reported for 9/168 (5.4%) Yale subjects, whereas none were reported for Tuskegee subjects.

respectively). Coupled with the high incidence of cirrhosis of the liver that was 32 times greater in Tuskegee syphilitics than Yale syphilitics, these conditions raise the consideration that environmental and nutritional factors, shared by both syphilitics and controls, interfered in clinical diagnosis, pathological diagnosis, and serological testing. None of these conditions were reported for the Yale or the Bruusgaard studies.

The clinical and pathological papers of the Tuskegee study were worthless but tolerated because shortcomings of this kind were explained on the basis of biological differences between blacks and whites that supposedly led to different biological outcomes in the presence of disease. The a priori principle that explained the presence of disease also explained its absence. Because of biological differences, blacks were more syphilitic than whites; because of biological differences, the absence of findings meant that blacks had syphilis that escaped detection until better means of diagnosis were available.

Unlike the serological reports and the initial clinical report, the pathological report, which was to be the most important, was not published in JAMA. The report stopped at 1952. Yet for 3 years, it remained unpublished and did not appear until 1955 in the first issue of the *Journal of Chronic Diseases*, a new journal edited by Joseph E. Moore, clinical consultant to the Tuskegee Syphilis Experiment. Moore was also editor of the *American Journal of Syphilis, Gonorrhea and Venereal Diseases*, the more appropriate venue for a report of this kind. However, it was not published there. This raises the consideration that established journals rejected the paper on scientific merit and that it was published finally through political influence. Its style avoided presenting data directly. Lack of syphilis at autopsy corroborated the lack of syphilis in the clinical study. Negative studies receive low priority for publication. The shortcomings in clinicopathologic correlation also may account for the limitation of the use of Tuskegee samples to 82 of 410 presumed syphilitics after 1946. This is 20% of the total number of syphilitics, which corresponds to indications that only 20% of those autopsied had true syphilis. It is unlikely that this is a random occurrence. There is no doubt that some of the Tuskegee subjects had syphilis. However, the PHS could not establish syphilis in the majority. It fell prey to its prejudice, to a priori reasoning, and to its own advances in syphilis diagnosis based on those Tuskegee subjects who had syphilis.

The PHS marketed the Tuskegee subjects as the most syphilitic subjects in the United States. Yet the percentage of subjects with definite anatomical lesions of syphilis was 49% and 43% that of the Yale and Bruusgaard studies, respectively. It took scientific fraud to reach this percentage. The PHS did not inoculate the Tuskegee subjects with the syphilis organism, but it did give them the diagnosis of syphilis, and it seems that it did what it could to make it stick. Although one consequence of these actions was to further entrench biologically deterministic conventions regarding African Americans and venereal disease, its prime motivations were the potentially damaging economic consequences for US serological tests; an industry relied on and was regulated by PHS research at Tuskegee. The negative clinical and pathological studies undermined the credibility of serological standards that the PHS used to elevate and enhance the competitive stance and profitability of American tests. Any revelation that the sera were not syphilitic would have caused irreparable damage to the commercialization of US serological tests. The PHS restricted its future studies, particularly the development of treponemal tests, to unequivocally syphilitic Tuskegee sera. Despite having collected sera from 410 syphilitic subjects, the next series of studies employed only 82 sera.

The Development of Treponemal Tests

In 1948, Robert Nelson of Johns Hopkins University successfully maintained infectious *pallidum* (Nichols strain) isolated from rabbit testicular syphiloma in culture for several days.[47] In 1949, Nelson and Mayer[48] used cultured *T pallidum* to demonstrate several things. First, antibody from syphilitic human serum immobilized virulent *T pallidum* in vitro. Second, the antibody bound complement to kill the organism. The cultures became noninfectious. Antitreponemal antibody was distinct from Wassermann reagin.[48] This became known as the *T pallidum* Immobilization (TPI) test. The TPI was highly specific. It had an exceptionally low incidence of false-positive reactions in leprosy and malaria, while being highly sensitive. Moreover, it allowed quantitative titration of antitreponemal antibody. It became the standard measure of all newly developed tests. However, because of its technical difficulty and requirement for rabbit colonies, it was an impractical and expensive test for diagnostic purposes (as much as $100 per test in the 1950s).

Despite these shortcomings, the TPI was a pivotal invention in syphilology. The PHS recognized its importance immediately.[49] In 1952, the PHS convened a meeting of all laboratories under the Division of Venereal Disease for the sole purpose of standardizing the TPI within and across laboratories—including laboratories in other countries. The initial studies used antibodies from rabbits with experimental syphilis. Subsequent studies examined the TPI in humans.

Collaborative studies performed with sera from the VDRL in Staten Island, New York, in the early 1950s used Tuskegee sera.[50,51] The VDRL examined the TPI in treated and untreated patients with syphilis.[52,53] The sera for untreated late syphilis included "Macon County Health Department, Tuskegee, Alabama" from the Tuskegee Syphilis Study. The publication of pilot serological studies based on Tuskegee sera preceded a publication confirming the continued credibility of their syphilitic status.[54] There was preparation for yet another serologic evaluation survey. The new serodiagnostic survey was the Serology Evaluation Research Assembly (SERA) Study of 1956–1957.[55] This publication did not state explicitly the use of Tuskegee sera. However, subsequent publications from the PHS mentioned that Tuskegee sera from the VDRL serum bank comprised sera used in the SERA study.[56] Tuskegee sera also were used to assess the worth of additional tests: the Reiter protein complement fixation test[57,58] and the Treponema complement fixation test-50.[59]

Tuskegee sera ushered in the most important diagnostic test since the TPI—the fluorescent treponemal antibody absorption test (FTA-ABS). The FTA-ABS is the present standard for syphilis diagnosis. The introduction of the TPI test in 1949 also provided a method to extract crude treponemal antigen from infected rabbit testicles. The initial fluorescent conjugate to detect antibacterial antibody used fluorescein isocyanate. In 1957, the VDRL used unimpeachable positive human syphilis sera from "laboratory stocks," ie, Tuskegee sera, to develop a fluorescent antibody test that would demonstrate antibodies for *Treponema*.[60]

The fluorescent treponemal antibody (FTA) test was tested in the SERA study. It was more sensitive than treponemal pallidum complement fixation. However, the original FTA detected antibodies for both group and specific antigen. This was overcome in two ways. In 1958, an alternative fluorescein conjugate was introduced, fluorescein isothiocyanate (FITC).[61,62] The VDRL immediately tested FITC as an alternative to fluorescein isocyanate "by examining well-documented serum specimens." Fluorescein isothiocyanate was an improvement over the original FTA test that used fluorescein isocyanate.[60] Preabsorption of sera with sonicates of Reiter strain Treponema eliminated the antibodies for group antigen. Subsequent testing for specific antibody to *pallidum* demonstrated increased sensitivity and specificity. "Eighty-two specimens were included from the 1962 Tuskegee study" to develop the FTA-ABS.[61] The FTA-ABS may have benefited in another way. It could distinguish false-positive serology from true syphilis, a fact of no small importance in a group in which some subjects may have been incorrectly considered to have syphilis for 30 years. The FTA-ABS was commercialized. Internal memos from the Venereal Disease Branch of the PHS were explicit: "the development and our endorsement of the FTA-ABS test rested on Tuskegee sera" (Lucas JB. February 1970. Unpublished data).[68]

The FTA-ABS quickly became and remains the standard diagnostic test for syphilis. It replaced the TPI. A 2-year study of the World Health Organization (WHO) globalized the FTA and FTA-ABS tests.[63] The VDRL distributed control sera to Japan, Italy, Denmark, England, and France for use in serological surveys. The Tuskegee patients were a likely source of control sera distributed to state and private laboratories in the United States and, through the WHO, to laboratories throughout the world.[64] The WHO was a market for syphilis serology. Other nations were dependent on the PHS for standardization and application of a US test. From the myriad national tests of the 1920s, the world came to use two US tests, the VDRL slide test and the FTA-ABS, both rooted in the Tuskegee Syphilis Experiment.

Serological tests for syphilis were commercially lucrative. In the United States, syphilis testing increased from 2 million in 1936 to 28 million in 1943 and remained steady at 12 million annually into the 1960s.[65] The predictability of this market was assured by laws requiring syphilis testing for marriage certificates, newborns, military recruits, industrial physical examinations, and admissions to hospitals.

United States hegemony in syphilis serology lapsed following the demise of the Tuskegee Syphilis Experiment. Whether there is a causative relationship is uncertain. However, it would appear that technological developments in other countries that usurped US tests preceded the undoing of the Tuskegee Syphilis Experiment. In 1965, a test using smaller volumes of serum detected antitreponemal antibodies by hemagglutination of sheep red blood cells; use of an absorbent eliminated group-specific antibodies.[66] This test became known as microhemagglutination. The test is easier to perform than the FTA-ABS and does not require fluorescent microscopy. Variations of this test slowly replaced the FTA-ABS and are marketed in the United States by Japanese companies. Another test by British manufacturers is the hemagglutination of turkey red blood cells without the use of an absorbent.[67] Microhemagglutination tests dominate syphilis serology outside the United States. It is unclear to what extent the development of these tests exploited positive syphilitic control sera (Tuskegee sera) provided by the VDRL through the WHO program for standardization.

Comment

The Tuskegee Syphilis Study became an instrument of PHS international health politics. It must be recalled that the PHS initiated the Clinical Cooperative Study as part of a League of Nations study. In 1920, the Supreme Court distinguished authority of the United States from authority of the Constitution (*Missouri v Holland*, 252 US 416). International agreements fell under authority of the United States, outside of the reach of constitutional questions or interpretation. This granted unlimited power to the government regarding activities falling under international agreements. Therefore, with regard to its use for international health, the Tuskegee Syphilis Experiment may potentially have been at the discretion of the absolute power of the state. From 1932 to the 1970s, the Tuskegee Syphilis Experiment allowed US investigators and biotechnology to wrest control from German researchers to dominate and maintain leadership in syphilis serology. The monopoly of syphilis technology contributed to a superior position in the WHO. The PHS dominated the World Forum on Syphilis and Other Treponematoses in 1962. Its utility to biotechnological competitiveness in diagnosis and treatment of venereal diseases is a hidden but more plausible reason that the Tuskegee experiment was not terminated.

The utilitarian economic advantages of the Tuskegee Experiment prejudiced the science. The Tuskegee Experiment progressed within concepts of science and scientific method that had an analytical philosophical basis in positivism. Positivism ignores data that contradicts a convention. Positivism considers that established conventions remain true, but that contradictory data point to different relationships between conventions. Consequently, the scientist reorders the relationship between accepted conventions to fit the data. Syphilology established several conventions, and it became the function of experimentation to verify these conventions. The most important convention was that the positive serological test for syphilis was infallible and was a certain demonstration of syphilis. The next convention was that African Americans had more syphilis and suffered less from it. This evolved from 19th century US ethnological descriptions of Africans as biologically inferior and insentient beings comparable to animals; this justified their use in experimentation and was also the basis of social and educational policy regarding blacks. The potentially fraudulent behavior of PHS scientists not only protected conventions in syphilology, but also more importantly sustained the integrity of biological determinism.

The discrimination between documents *directly* and *indirectly* related to the Tuskegee Syphilis Experiment was a deception that continues to protect biological determinism and contributed to a lopsided ethical examination and legal regulation fo the commercialization of human products. This device protected two unexplained issues. First, there was no clinical protocol because the purpose of the study was not clinical; however, there were strict protocols for the serological studies. Second, although never mentioned by historians or the ad hoc panel, the original contract between the PHS and the Alabama Department of Health to initiate the Tuskegee Experiment contained a patent agreement that made any invention sole property of the United States.

LITERATURE CITED

The author thanks the New York State Library, the History of Medicine Division of the National Library of Medicine for access to *Historical Documents Directly Related to the Tuskegee Syphilis Study*, and Reginald Peniston, MD, Warren Mebane, MD, and Irwin Hassenfeld, MD, for advice and discussions.

1. Tuskegee Syphilis Study Ad Hoc Advisory Study Panel, *Final Report*. Washington, DC: US Department of Health, Education, and Welfare; 1973.

2. Jones JH. *Bad Blood: The Tuskegee Syphilis Experiment—A Tragedy of Race and Medicine*. New York, NY: Free Press; 1981.

3. Stokes JH. The clinical approach to syphilis, with suggestions for its revival and development. *Archives of Dermatology and Syphilology*, 1920;2:473–492.

4. Clark T, Parran T, Cole HN, Moore JE, O'Leary PA, Stokes JH, et al. Cooperative clinical studies in the treatment of syphilis, I: introduction. *Venereal Disease Information*. 1932;13:135–138.

5. Stokes JH, Cole HN, Moore JE, O'Leary PA, Wile UJ, Clark T, et al. Cooperative clinical studies in the treatment of syphilis. Early syphilis. *Venereal Disease Information*. 1932;13:165–183.

6. Stokes JH, Cole HN, Moore JE, O'Leary PA, Wile UJ, Clark T, et al. Cooperative clinical studies in the treatment of syphilis. Early Syphilis. Section II. Results of treatment in early syphilis. *Venereal Disease Information*. 1932;13:207–231.

7. Stokes JH, Cole HN, Moore JE, O'Leary PA, Wile UJ, Clark T, et al. Cooperative clinical studies in the treatment of syphilis. Early syphilis. Section III. Results of treatment in early syphilis. *Venereal Disease Information*. 1932;13:253–293.

8. Moore JE, Cole HN, O'Leary PA, Stokes JH, Wile UJ, Clark T, et al. Cooperative clinical studies in the treatment of syphilis. Latent syphilis. The treatment of latent syphilis. *Venereal Disease Information*. 1932;13:407–412.

9. O'Leary PA, Cole HN, Moore JE, Stokes JH, Wile UJ, Clark T, et al. Cooperative clinical studies in the treatment of syphilis. Asymptomatic neurosyphilis. *Venereal Disease Information*. 1937;18:45–65.

10. Wile UJ. Experimental syphilis in the rabbit produced by the brain substance of the living paretic. *J Exp Med*. 1916;23:199–202.

11. Lederer SE. The right and wrong of making experiments on human beings: Udo J. Wile and syphilis. *Bull Hist Med*. 1984;58:380–397.

12. Stokes JH, Cole HN, Moore JE, O'Leary PA, Parran T, Wile UJ. Cutaneous and mucosal relapse in early syphilis and its differentiation from reinfection. *Venereal Disease Information*. 1931;12:55–66.

13. Stokes JH, Usilton LJ, Cole HN, Moore JE, O'Leary PA, Wile UJ, et al. What treatment in early syphilis accomplishes. *Venereal Disease Information*. 1934;15:341–363.

14. Bruusgaard E. Uber das Schicksal der nicht spezifen behandelten Luetiker. *Archiv fur Dermatologie und Syphilis*. 1929;157:309.

15. Schuman SH, Olansky S, Rivers E, Smith CA, Rambo DS. Untreated syphilis in the male Negro. Background and current status of patients in the Tuskegee Study. *Journal of Chronic Diseases*. 1955;5:543–558.

16. Gjestland T. The Oslo study of untreated syphilis. An epidemiologic investigation of the natural course of the syphilitic infection based upon a re-study of the Boeck-Bruusgaard material. *Acta Derm Venereol (Stockh)*. 1955;35(suppl 34):1–368.

17. Cumming HS, Hazen HH, Sanford AH, Senear FE, Simpson WM, Vonderlehr RA. The evaluation of serodiagnostic tests for syphilis in the United States. *JAMA*. 1934;103:1705–1707.

18. Cumming HS, Hazen HH, Sanford AH, Senear FE, Simpson WM, Vonderlehr RA. The evaluation of serodiagnostic tests for syphilis in the United States. *JAMA*. 1935;104:2083–2087.

19. Vonderlehr RA, Clark T, Wenger OC, Heller JR. Untreated syphilis in the male negro. A comparative study of treated and untreated cases. *JAMA*. 1936;107:856–860.

20. Moore JE. The American evaluation of serodiagnostic tests for syphilis from a clinician's standpoint. *American Journal of Syphilis, Gonorrhea and Venereal Diseases*. 1936;20:207–213.

21. Parran T, Hazen HH, Sanford AH, Senear FE, Simpson WM, Vonderlehr RA. The efficiency of state and local laboratories in the performance of serodiagnostic tests for syphilis. *Venereal Disease Information*. 1937;18:4–11.

22. Parran T, Hazen HH, Sanford AH, Senear FE, Simpson WM, Vonderlehr RA. Efficiency of state and local laboratories in the performance of serodiagnostic tests for syphilis. *Am J Clin Pathol*. 1937;7:20–32.

23. Parran T, Hazen HH, Sanford AH, Senear FE, Simpson WM, Vonderlehr RA. Efficiency of state and local laboratories in the performance of serodiagnostic tests for syphilis. *Am J Public Health*. 1937;27:15–23.

24. Hazen HH, Parran T, Sanford AH, Senar FE, Simpson WM, Vonderlehr RA. The evaluation of serodiagnostic tests for syphilis upon the spinal fluid. *Venereal Disease Information*. 1937;18:132–142.

25. Hazen HH, Parran T, Sanford AH, Senear FE, Simpson WM, Vonderlehr RA. The evaluation of serodiagnostic tests for syphilis upon the spinal fluid. *South Med J.* 1937;30:465–471.

26. Hazen HH. The serodiagnosis of syphilis. *JAMA.* 1937;108:785–788.

27. Burney LE, Mays JRS, Iskrant AP. Results of serologic tests for syphilis in non-syphilitic persons inoculated with malaria. *Am J Public Health.* 1942;32:39–47.

28. Olansky S, Harris A, Hill JH. A preliminary study of apparent biological false positive reactions in four serological tests for syphilis and the treponemal immobilization test. *American Journal of Syphilis, Gonorrhea and Venereal Diseases.* 1953;37:23–28.

29. Pangborn MC. A new serologically active phospholipid from beef heart. *Proc Soc Exp Biol Med.* 1941;48:484–486.

30. Erickson PT, Eagle H. Evaluation of spirochete complement fixation reaction in comparison with the Eagle flocculation and Wassermann procedures. *Venereal Disease Information.* 1940;21:31–37.

31. Kolmer JA, Kast CC, Lynch EK. Studies on the role of Spirocheta pallida in the Wassermann reaction: complement fixation in syphilis, leprosy and malaria with spirochetal antigens. *American Journal of Syphilis, Gonorrhea and Venereal Diseases.* 1941;25:300–318.

32. Parran T, Hazen HH, Mahoney JF, Sanford AH, Senear FE, Simpson WM, et al. Preliminary report on the Washington Serology Conference. *Venereal Disease Information.* 1942;23:161–194.

33. Olansky S, Harris A, Cutler JC, Price EV. Untreated syphilis in the male negro. *Arch Dermatol.* 1956;73:516–522.

34. Long PH, Bliss EA. *The Clinical Use of Sulfanilamide, Sulfpyridine and Allied Compounds.* New York, NY: MacMillan Co; 1939:1–13.

35. Domagk G. Ein beitrag zur chemotherapie der bakteriellen infektionen. *Dtsch Med Wochenschr.* 1935;61:250–253.

36. Klee P, Rohmer H. Prontosil bei streptokokkenerkrankungen. *Dtsch Med Wochenschr.* 1935;61:253–255.

37. Anselm E. Unsere erfahrungen mit Prontosil bei puerperalfieber. *Dtsch Med Wochenschr.* 1935;61:264.

38. Levaditi C, Vaisman A. Action curative et preventive du chlorhydrate de 4'-sulfamido-2,4-diamino-azobenzene dans l'infection streptococcique experimentale. *Comptes Rendu Hebdomadaires des séances de l'Academiedes Sciences.* 1935; 200:1694–1896.

39. Colebrook L, Kenny M. Treatment of human puerperal infections and of experimental infections in mice with prontosil. *Lancet.* 1936; 1:1279.

40. Harrié A, Rosenberg AA, Riedel LM. A microflocculation test for syphilis using cardiolpin antigen. *J Venereal Disease Information.* 1948; 29:72–75.

41. Heller JR, Bruyere PT. Untreated syphilis in the male Negro, II: mortality during 12 years of observation. *J. Ven Dis Inform.* 1948; 27:34–38.

42. Delbert AV, Bruyere MC. Untreated syphilis in the male Negro, III: evidence of cardiovascular abnormalities and other forms of morbidity. *j Venereal Disease Information.* 1948; 27:301–314.

43. Hosahn PD. Studies in syphilis, VII: the end results of untreated syphilis. *J. Ven Dis Inform.* 1946; 27:293–301.

44. Pesare PJ, Bauer TJ, Gleeson GA. Untreated syphilis in the male Negro. *American Journal of Syphilis, Gonorrhea and Venereal Diseases.* 1950; 34: 201–213.

45. Peters JJ, Peters JH, Olansky S, Cutler JC, Gleeson GA. Untreated syphilis in the male Negro. Pathology findings in syphilitic and nonsyphilitic patients. *Journal of Chronic Diseases.* 1955; 1:127–148.

46. Sowder WT. An inpterpretation of Bruusgaard's paper on the fate of untreated syphilitics. *American Journal of Syphilis, Gonorrhea and Venereal Diseases.* 1940; 24:884–891.

47. Nelson RA. Factors affecting the survival of *Treponema palidum* in vitro. *American Journal of Hygiene.* 1948; 48:120–132.

48. Nelson RA, Mayer MM. Immobilization of *Treponema Palidum* in vitro by antibody produced in syphilitic infection. *J Exp Med.* 1949; 89:389–393.

49. Magnuson HJ, Thompson PA. Treponemal immobilization text of normal and syphilitic serums. *Venereal Disease Information.* 1948; 30:302–320.

50. Miller JL, Slatkin MH, Feiner RR, Portnoy J, Cannon AB. Treponemal immobilization text. Reliability of results for the diagnosis of syphilis. *JAMA.* 1952; 149:987–991.

51. Shafer JK et al. Untreated syphilis in the male Negro—a prospective study of the effect on life expectancy. *Public Health Rep.* 1954; 59:684–690.

52. Edmundson WF, Kamp M., Olansky S. Study of the TPI test in clinical syphilis, II: comparison with the VDRL slide test in treated early symptomatic syphilis. *Archives of Dermatology and Syphilology.* 1955; 71:381–386.

53. Edmundson WF, Olansky S., Wood CE, Kamp M. Study of the TPI test in clinical syphilis, III: late syphilis. *Archives of Dermatology and Syphilology.* 1955; 71:387–390.

54. Olansky S, Harris A, Cutler JC, Price EV. Untreated syphilis in the male Negro. *Arch Dermatol.* 1950; 78: 516–522.

55. United States Public Health Service. Serology evaluation and research assembly (SERA) study, 1956–1957. Washington, DC: US Government Printing Office; 1959. PHS publication 650.

56. Hunter EF, Deacon WE, Meyer PE. An improved FTA text for syphilis, the absorption procedure (FTA-ABS). *Public Health Rep.* 1964; 79:410–412.

57. Brown WJ, Price EV, Simpson WG. The Relter protein antigen test compared with the TPI and other treponemal and nontreponemal antigen techniques in the diagnosis of syphilis. *J Invest Dermatol.* 1960; 34: 223– 227.

58. Brown WJ, Bunch WL. How good is the Relter protein complement fixation test for syphilis. *Crom Med J.* 1959; 52:783–787.

59. Portnoy J. Complement fixation with small volumes of reagents. Application to a *Treponema pallidum* complement-fixation test for syphilis (TPCF 50). *Am J. Clin Pathol.* 1959; 31:316–322.

60. Deacon WE, Falcone VH, Harris A. A fluorescent test for treponemal antibodies. *Proc Soc Exp Biol Med.* 1957; 98:477–480.

61. Riggs JL, Selwald RJ, Burckhalter JH, Downs CM, Metcalf TG. Isothiocyanate compounds as fluorescent labeling agents for immune serum. *Am J. Pathol.* 1958; 34:1001–1038.

62. Deacon WE, Freeman EM, Harris A. Fluorescent treponemal antibody test. Modification based on quantitation (FTA-200). *Proc Soc Exp Biol Med.* 1960; 103; 827–839.

63. Deacon WE. Fluorescent treponemal antibody test. *In: Proceedings of World Forum on Syphilis and Other Treponemaloses.* Atlanta, Ga: US Department of Health, Education, and Welfare, Public Health Service, Communicable Disease Center; 1962:244–248.

64. Stout GW. Development of serologic standards. *In: Proceedings of World Forum on Syphilis and Other Treponemaloses.* Atlanta, Ga: US Department of Health, Education, and Welfare, Public Health Service, Communicable Disease Center; 1962:237–239.

65. Vonderlehr RA. Must we let it happen again? *In: Proceedings of World Forum on Syphilis and Other Treponemaloses.* Atlanta, Ga: US Department of Health, Education, and Welfare, Public Health Service, Communicable Disease Center; 1962:182–188.

66. Rathley T. Hemagglutination tests utilizing antigens from pathogenic and apathogenic *Treponema Pallidum.* WHO *Venereal Disease Research.* 1966; 40:242–248.

67. Sequeira PJL, Lidmago AD. Treponemal hemagglutination test. *British Journal of Venereal Diseases.* 1973; 49:242–248.

vi

Rethinking the Role of Nurse Rivers

AN INTERVIEW WITH NURSE RIVERS

HELEN DIBBLE & DANIEL WILLIAMS

ER = Eunice Rivers Laurie
HD = Helen Taylor Dibble
DW = Daniel Williams

ER: The Milbank Foundation was down here. And they were doing huge blood tests of everybody in the county. And they had their stations and they found that syphilis, that the county was saturated with syphilis and a Dr. Perry, you remember him, Miz Dibble

HD: a hah

ER: worked on doing the treatment of all of these patients. They had their clinics set up all over. After Dr. Perry left, ah, . . . I'm not so certain who started the second massive test but it was done through the state department. And they had this bus following, no this was then before the bus, um, this is when I came with them, went to work with the people cause to get there. And working in the clinics—yes, Wenger and Vondelehr started this. And, um, out of this came the patients. We treated, we went all over the county—made, survey in the whole county—and sometimes we would take two and three hundred blood tests a day. And out of that group came the treatment clinics. And out of the treatment clinics came this study. And, ah, the people, we had two hundred negatives and four hundred positives. I worked with both the treatment clinic and the survey.

Um, what the people are fussing so about now is that these people were not given treatment. Well, in the early days . . . mu . . . arsphenamine, bismuth, it was . . . the treatment was really worse than the disease if it was not early syphilis. Because we came up with so much syphilis. The people's dental hygiene was very, very poor. And we had people who were getting mercury rubs to come up with sore mouths and their teeth coming out. It was just ridiculous. We had . . .

HD: The cause of this [drugs you were using?]

ER: The cause of this was the mercury. And see, the mercury was a salve and they put it on the patient. They had a belt with a little rubber on the inside and we

Originally taped by Helen Dibble and Daniel Williams, 1977, Tuskegee University Archives, Tuskegee University, Tuskegee, Ala. Transcription by Susan M. Reverby with the assistance of Carmen Bryant. Reproduced by permission of Tuskegee University.

321

told the patients how to apply this mercury, one night on this side, on alternating sides, they wear this belt all the time, see. We had lot of people who came up, had this type of reaction.

Well, we also had people who got reaction from neoarsphenamine. This was intravenous drug. So that it was, uh, it was six of one and half a dozen of another as far as I was concerned. And this is one of the things that the medical profession said. If syphilis was *not* active, the treatment was worse than the disease. And then to repeat myself, that out of this came the people that were entered into the study. Originally they selected four hundred positives. They were brought in, examined, given complete examinations: X rays, whatever, eye examinations. Dr. Perry was living then at the hospital. We went to his office with these people for the eye examinations [clears throat].

HD: And you could go to the VA

ER: Yes, we went to the VA. We did the examinations at John Andrew Hospital and any case that they wanted some specialist to see like the ear man, or the throat man, or the eye man, we took them to the VA hospital where Dr. Perry and Dr. Peters worked with us. Because we go there, been over there many days till after five o'clock doing fluoroscopes and that kind of thing. So these people were given the physicals, but any special examinations they were referred to the hospital, to the VA hospital. And [clears throat] then those that they put in the study . . . now a lot of those patients that were in the study did get some treatment. There were very few who did not get any treatment at all, and they had trouble,

DW: 'Cause . . .

ER: We had trouble with people who were not in the study, wanting to come with our group because they didn't want to get the medicine, see. They felt that this medicine was bad, see, and they didn't want to get it. We had an awful time explaining to them why they couldn't be in on the study, see. Because I would tell them all about it, I'd tell 'em "Man you're not old enough to go into the study. These is old folks," [laughs] and you're young . . . and get them away like that. But they were concerned that they got all, that this group got all of this and they only went to the clinic and got the treatment and some of them were such bad reactions that they just didn't come back for their treatment. Umm, these patients, as I said before, were given these complete physical examinations.

DW: Now who gave them that?

ER: Well who, whatever, doctor that came. And in the early days Dr. Vonderlehr and Dr. Wenger. There were many, many doctors who came. Mr. Williams, now I don't remember their name, one doctor, if I could remember his name, he was very fond . . . Deibert, Dr. Deibert, came and he worked a long time with us.

And Dr. Heller and . . . we just had doctors, doctors, I don't know all of them who worked with the and did these examinations.

HD: And they were from the Public Health?

ER: Yeah, they were from Public Health in Atlanta and Washington at that time 'cause this was where they were. It was years, years after that they moved to Atlanta. Um . . . my ah, ah duties were to get the patients in to the clinic for the examination. I [clears throat] later, to begin with, I used my new Chevrolet with the rumble seat to bring these people in. And the roads were very, very poor then. We brought the patients in, ah, every morning we had a group schedule.Let's see, we'd schedule six patients to begin with and now we brought those six patients, three patients, in, however many we had scheduled, bring in as many as we possibly could that morning, and when I, my duties were to get blood, get the urine for the test, and whatever else the doctors wanted me to do. Then while they were examining, when I had finished, completed my work, they were continuing the examinations, I went back into the country and brought the others that were supposed to be in. While they were getting examined I would take that group back and come back and now make, oh maybe, when I was doing that with this group, the doctors would take the bloods and all and we'd go back with the patient to his home where we picked him up, see. And ahh [clears throat]

DW: How many trips a day did you make like this?

ER: How many?

DW: Em huh.

ER: That all depended. Now, ordinarily I would have to leave by seven o'clock in the morning to get back to go to Hurtsboro and get back 'cause many of the roads were wet and rainy. It was almost out of reason. But I would go, it never got too bad that I would tell the doctors I couldn't go. We'd go and pick the patients up and bring them back. I did at least two trips a day in the early days and sometimes it'd be three. I'd have to bring in somebody, and go back and pick them up, this kind of thing. 'Cause they were very anxious, and they were, they considered themselves somebody . . .

HD: Riding in the car?

ER: Yes, that the nurse . . . and you see we gave them dinner and the doctors prescribed for them. He didn't give medicine for syphilis, but if a man came in and he had a terrible cold or had something else he would prescribe for him, he'd give him something for that cold. And we always carried, we carried, we always carried, the iron tonic, ah and aspirin tablets and vitamin pills. This was a part of our medication that they got, and sometimes they, they really took it and enjoyed it very much. And these vitamins did them a lot of good. They just loved those and ah they enjoyed that very, very much.

HD: A lot of your patients were from Hurtsboro?

ER: Yeah, we had patients from Hurtsboro, we had patients who lived in Bullock County, Auburn, Notasulga, Shorter. We had some patients who lived in Columbus. And . . . we would send them a notice and they would come to their center and where they were, we originally picked them up or they would furnish their own transportation. We had in Columbus about six and we let them know when the doctor was coming so that they could arrange their trip, and all six of them would come up sometimes and they would furnish their own transportation to get their treatment and we had worked way into the night because we had scheduled, if we schedule six here and then six come in from Columbus you see what what you get into. You don't want them no-don't-come-back-ahh-we-can't-do-you thing. This is the type of work that was done. Ahh, and as I said, the patients were given their dinner. The patients themselves considered themselves, considered themselves being as very fortunate. Because in those days they didn't, see, they didn't know what Tuskegee was all about down at [unclear] and Hurtsboro. And they would come up here and be examined. And I'd take them to town, they just loved to go to town. Some go to town and believe it or not there were many men who had never been to Tuskegee. Well, then I would take, when I found that out, I'd take them, we'd tour Tuskegee Institute—while you getting your examination, these two over here we'd go through the Tuskegee Institute. And then when they had all the industry and trades and everything they just thought it was just something grand that they would see this. And when they'd go back home in the afternoons if you didn't get to see it and I'd got to see it I worked with you. That what Tuskegee had—if you missed it, man you missed it. You better get back up here and that person would try to come back up here to see. "Miss Rivers, when can you take me." I had gone down there many Saturdays and put them in my car and bring them up here to see Tuskegee, Tuskegee Institute . . .

HD: Was this . . . [unclear]?

ER: This was because they had never, as close as ahh Magnolia, I don't know where, you don't know anything much about that, but anyway, about seven, eight miles out. Really it was impossible they didn't know. And I had spent many Saturday mornings going down there and bringing them up here, taking them to the campus, taking them to town. Now I said, "You now, all do whatever you want to do 'cause we're going to leave at five o'clock." "All right, Miss Rivers." And this, this is the way they saw it, see, and this is what impressed them so much, and then from, those were in the early days, the very early days.

We had, they started out doing spinal punctures, but we got a lot of ahh poor, I mean a lot of reactions to the spinal punctures. For one thing they're supposed to lie flat at least six hours, but the patients would go back home and sometimes I'd say, "You can go to bed." But if he's feeling all right he wouldn't go to bed, see. So they had to rule out the spinal punctures as a regular thing. Now there were some special cases, something special or new symptoms, they would do it. And when they first started the work, I think it lasted about six months when we were getting all these positives, then they decided, um, we would, because I think when the project first started they then, it wasn't to carry on, see, it wasn't going to continue. It was just a short study, but after they got into the study and they found, Dr. Vonderlehr and Wenger said there was so much information that they wanted to continue and at that time they were comparing this study with the study in Norway with the white man, see.

DW: Em hm

ER: And this time didn't give them enough information. Now one of the things they found that, they said that syphilis affects the white man's central nervous system. It affects the Negro's cardiovascular system. This was some of their, their findings from what they said. So after they got into this they wanted to continue, and as I said we, when the study first started, I think they worked here about nine months, and as far as we were concerned the study was closed in that nine months. Well, the next year, maybe six or eight months, they decided to come back to Tuskegee and this is when that letter was written. I think it was to draw up of their contract that we would, they would continue and that it would be permanent and I would be the person to follow through. So this is the reason they called the thing Miss Rivers' study because, they called it Miss Rivers' [laughs] . . . [laughing] . . . [unclear] it was Alabama at that time and they called it Miss Rivers' project and Miss Rivers could make them do anything she wanted, they tell me, and I, I would go to the bat for them if one of them said that, that he was mistreated by some of the doctors. I said to him I went to that doctor and I told him what the patient had told me and I told him [voice gets stern] that I didn't expect, I expected them to be treated as human. Now when they couldn't do that, well, we *would* contact the office in Washington, so they calmed down and said, "Well, Miss Rivers, I didn't mean, is that the way they took it?" and I said, "Yeah, that's the way they took it." I says, "Oh no, be kind to them. Talk to them like they're people. Don't come in mistreating them, I don't care if they don't know A as big as he is, don't mistreat my patients. And so that carried from one group because we very seldom had the same group to come back. Well, when a new group would come, he had already been oriented to as what Nurse Rivers' expected [laughs] from him. And I would tell every one of them, "Don't mistreat my patients. You don't mistreat them. I said, now, 'cause they don't *have* to come. And if you mistreat I will *not* let them up here to be mistreated."

HD: Now you were taking them to doctors for treatment for other things?

ER: No, I wasn't taking them for other things. But if the doctor recommended . . . now he would have some patients, and he would tell them I think you ought to see your family doctor and he'd tell me, "Miss Rivers, you, I think you ought to follow through and see that this patient gets to a doctor," see. And I would tell the patient, I'd say to the patient, "Now, who is your doctor and you go to see your doctor." I said, "Now you can make your own arrangements to get to a doctor" because at that time we had doctors down in Shoreham, doctors in Hurtsboro and doctors up in Notasulga, and this kind of thing that we did. . . .

HD: Now let me ask you again about this spinal puncture that you were speaking about. Was that a form of treatment?

ER: No it was a getting someone's spinal fluid ah hah for tests. They do that to find out about central nervous system disease. This was very, very crude when it first started, you know, not developed. But this is what they were trying to do. And they got so many negatives and this group, and they just discontinued it after they were having so many problems.

So that the study continued. And then another feature of it was the autopsies. I had an awful time—now this was me, wasn't family, going to you asking you, when autopsy, knowing how you felt about it, because then people were not aware of what an autopsy was. And they were crude. So I, I had to learn because when I went to, to confirm autopsy I had to explain to them what the procedures were. I had to guarantee them that they would not mar that body. They didn't want the public to know that we had cut that body, the family didn't. OK. I had to get make Dr. Peters promise that we would not mar that body where it would be exposed. And he wouldn't. He was always very, very careful about it. If we did a, a, went into the heads, skull, we always did, you know, the incision in the back. We made *sure* that that face was not marred. We never marred any and when we finished we ourselves would take cream and rub over that face to make it pliable because if you had gotten one person who was not, the body was not, was misused, we always—and I just felt that that was my responsibility. I would not want somebody to do that to a member of my family. And this was the way I made, I felt about them. And this was the way they felt about me. What if ah they learned that, if there was anything, if they felt that they were mistreated, they came to Miss Rivers. And they would tell Miss Rivers, and as I said I would get on the doctors about it. And they were always, tell, promise me, about it, "Miss Rivers, I didn't know was that the way"—I said, "That's the way they took it so don't say that any more, don't do that anymore, see." And this is the way we carried on.

And as the study continued and during the time when they were not here, when the doctors were in between times, it was my responsibility to visit all of the patients and check on them to see how they were doing, and ah if they needed to go to a doctor I should recommend it because a lot of them felt they couldn't go to another doctor if they wanted to. They want Miss Rivers and the doctor, the government doctors had been—and they'd wait to see what Miss

Rivers say, see. And a lot of times I'd go to them and ah find that there was somebody that needed medical attention. I would recommend. Now I'd say, "Who's your family doctor? Who comes to see your wife and your children? Who do you take your wife and children to? And I had so many of them just say, "Ha ha, don't take them to nobody." "You get yourself on up there and take them to the doctor's and see what's *wrong* with them. That's what you need to do." So that, this is during the absence of the doctors, it was my responsibility to contact every patient. At least I did this about once every two or three months. I would make my rounds.

And at the same time I was part time, when they were not here, I was over doing part-time work with the county health department doing the maternity work in the clinics. Um, so that then I took, after that I took this part-time home visiting with the Macon County Health Department so this gave me an opportunity to, to see the family as a whole, too. I could go and see them and they always, it was, it is a funny thing about it. The confidence that they had in Miss Rivers. If a new doctor came and I gave him an expression that I didn't like him, they didn't like him either, and I had to be very, very careful [laughs]. "Miss Rivers, that man,"—and sometimes they would say about them—"Miss Rivers, that man don't know what he's doing, does he." And I'd say, "Ah hah, yeah." I'd say, "What did they do?" [laughing]. "Well, he did, well, I don't know. Well, you say he's all right." "Well, I said the government sent him down here, darling." You know, for me to say who is and who isn't [laughs,] that's the way they would react.

And as the times continued to grow we continued getting our autopsies, sending the specimens, again we sent specimens to Washington, and as the offices moved to Atlanta we sent the specimens there. That's where they were tested. If the ah something, we always got ah a copy of the autopsy and placed it with the patient's records, see, and this was the thing that was so disturbing to me was that somehow all of the records of this study and the health department has been destroyed.

HD: They have?

ER: Un huh.

DW: Do you know when this happened? . . .

ER: I think . . . I really don't know when it happened. But I had placed, and Mrs. Merce may have been there, he had gotten, you know, files. All the records were in the file in the health department, a copy of all the records, plus all of the clinic records, you know Perry's records, Dr. Perry's records. All of those people. When I went when this thing started to looming up and I went to look for the records and I could not find them. You can't find them, un huh. So I was told that the records were destroyed.

DW: Does the state health department in Montgomery keep any of these?

ER: I don't think so. I don't think they keep anything.

HD: What about the public health?

ER: Well, now the public health records in Atlanta. Their records are in Atlanta. July of last year, or a year ago, I went to Atlanta, they took me to Atlanta, to go over the records they had up there and give them information as far as I could remember on these records, getting the context of families and all this. They have them in Atlanta. But there's nothing in Macon County. Nothing in Macon County.

HD: But they have a complete file in Atlanta on each patient?

ER: Yeah. Yes.

DW: From the very beginning?

ER: Yes.

HD: So that is preserved, the records are preserved?

ER: Yes. They are preserved in Atlanta. I haven't talked with Dick? now in a good while. After I got sick they promised me that they wouldn't worry me anymore with it, see. So they don't bother me unless it is something unusual, then they call me. Because they have a nurse here now, Mrs. James, I believe whose working—

DW: What's this person do from Atlanta?

ER: Mrs. James?

DW: No, not James?

ER: Yeah he works in Atlanta. I don't know what Dick's last name is. I don't know whether I have it here. He's in the Atlanta office, um hum.

HD: Is this Mrs. James the nurse following through now?

ER: Um hum. She's working with all the patients and *now* they are getting all the Medicare, they're getting everything now. All of their, I don't know what's going to happen. I guess maybe they will, what they going to do when they pay them all off, the patients all are thinking now they're going to get money.

DW: You're still helping them find them and helping them right now, aren't you?

ER: Un huh. Yeah, I'm still working on it. Dick Bruce in Atlanta. He's the person in charge now. Yeah, they, they ah I think they're going to continue, I'm sure they are, I think that is what Miz James said, that she's doing nursing, I know, home visits and all this on the patients.

HD: Are they still working on this as a study?

ER: No. Uh huh. I don't think so. 'Cause who ever, they told me that, see, after they entered into this lawsuit. Now this is what Dick told me to begin with, I have to say. He said that the study, whoever we started with, if the study had been discontinued in the forties it would have been all right.

HD: That was before they got penicillin?

ER: Yeah, uh huh.

HD: And suppose they got the treatment penicillin?

ER: Penicillin, uh huh, that was often two penicillin days right there? This is what he told me that they said and I don't know who they were, I guess, but they told me, he said, "Miz Laurie, the mistake that we made is that we continued to look after, if we had started the treatment, no, if we had discontinued in the forties this, nothing would have happened, see. So this is what is going on now. So that the patients are getting complete medical care now for anything.

Do you want to ask me some questions. Whatever you ask I'll try to answer. I mean—

DW: Going back those persons that have treatment . . . I mean who came out positive. When they were treated well, it didn't help them? In other words, the treatment didn't register with them. Now I know you're the nurse [laughs]

ER: I know what you have reference to. Um what they said, that they had latent—

DW: Yes, that's right.

ER: Latent syphilis and the drug—

DW: [unclear]

ER: Un huh, the drug, say, what damages syphilis was going to do, already done, and this was uh huh that particular treatment did not help them. Syphilis had done already the damage that it was going to do so that I, I guess maybe I don't know how. And I don't know what the medical profession, what they saw, and how they, 'cause I do know they were very, very critical, see, and I understand Dr. James just pitched a fit—

HD: He didn't want a—

ER: Um hum, 'cause Dr. James—

HD: 'Cause Dr. James was here, wasn't he, when Dr. James was here?

ER: He worked, you know, the bus was here and I worked on the bus. And Dr. James told folks up there in Washington I would not let him see the patients, that I would not let them get treatment. And when they told me that, I said I can't, I hate to dispute it. I said we're supposed to respect the medical profession but Dr. James is lying, saying I, the only thing I would do, I would tell Dr. James this is one of the patients. Now it was up to him if he wanted to treat him. Yeah, Dr. James, he was tough. Dr. James was here.

HD: That was in the early . . .

ER: Dr. James was here in the late fifties, I believe, maybe early sixties. Anyway, he was here just before the fuss, ah ah, just before the fuss was discontinued. So this is, ah ah, I don't know, but nobody knows what I went through here, you'd have thought I was a doctor mistreating the patients. And I, 'cause a lot of them, I don't know, I think that there was a lot of the jealousy with the medical profession and me, see, because they felt that I was not letting the patients get the treatment. I never told anybody that you couldn't get treatment. I told them, "So, go get . . . So who's your doctor? If you want to go to the doctor, go and get your treatment." They didn't tell you you *couldn't* be treated.

And another incentive, one of the things, after, ah ah, several years in the treatment, as I said before, I took them back and forth to dinner, we fed them at the VA hospital, ah and in the early days I took them sightseeing—

[Interruption from outside]

—oh yeah and some of the doctors um, and the unfortunate thing about, it was felt that and this happened to be our doctors that I wouldn't let the patients get treatment, see, if they needed it. And I never, never did do that. They had to fall back on, this is my thinking, that they had to fall back on something, have an excuse, and maybe the medical profession was on them so they put it on me, that I wouldn't *let* the patients get the treatment. But I never told anybody not to take treatment. 'Cause I, but I always said this: that if I had a positive Wassermann and . . . I still say that it wasn't giving me any trouble, I would never take [unclear] and neosalvarsan. And when penicillin first came in, I wouldn't have taken it. We had two prenatals to die over there in John Andrew Hospital. In one of the clinics that had gave her some penicillin and sent her upstairs and she was dead before she got upstairs almost . . .

DW: You'd just gone so far . . .

ER: Um hum. And see a lot of people are allergic to penicillin. And you just don't go and and give penicillin and things like that without some test, without knowing anything. So another patient we had who was treated un un and she lived in Shorter or Milstead. We treated her that morning. Doctor Wendis was working that morning. The woman got her treatment and she walked on out. I didn't know she had a reaction to. She went out and sat in the square, waiting for twelve o'clock come so she could go home. And when that woman got home she took sick there and they didn't tell us, nobody told us, they took her on home. Well, she was dead before that night, before the night come. So we had, so Dr. Smith said don't bother those folks down there for nothing because they were fixing to sue us. And he said, "Miz Rivers, don't you go down there, hear, 'cause they were fixing to get me. Don't go down there." So these are a lot of the problems that we had and I don't think that the people, the lay people, didn't know. And they, well, folks just, they had to put it on somebody so I just on down here . . .

HD: Let me ask you this.

ER: Um hum.

HD: During the time that you were making the study, were any of these people who were in the study, did any of them really get very ill with syphilis and that they weren't treated for that at that time?

ER: That I don't know, Mrs. Dibble. We—and I forget to mention this Dr. Dibble was very, very liberal, any reactions that we had, any patient that was very sick after, as a result of the treatment, all I had to do was bring them over to the hospital and Dr. Dibble would admit that patient. And that never occurred, and that occurred very, very seldom. We had one man from down in Milstead who had an aneurysm; all of his chest was eroded and his great big win[?] was up like this and of course we, everybody thought that, that he was just, wouldn't live, but then he made two crops with this thing. But every time he would have or get sick or anything, he wasn't given any medications. We took him, it was understood that we would take him, to the hospital and that man, and we felt sure this aneurysm would rupture, you could see just the pulses [unclear] and he died and that thing never did erupt. Um hum. So that it is a very, very complicated situation. Nobody I don't think, not knowing it and listening to the theory could, would appreciate, what I am saying because it really is a storybook affair. All of this technical stuff that they would have. It was, it just didn't show. We got something else out there and all together different and nobody knew a thing about and uh Dr. Wenger used to say, 'cause we had people who were well up in their years and Dr. Wenger was cussing this man, laughs, it was so, he'd say, "Eunice, where the hell this man been." I said, "I don't know, Dr., I have no idea." Well [unclear], this thing and the other thing and he ain't got a pain and he's better off than I am [laughs], so that it was one of the things I hope whatever they do, they'll show, show something.

HD: [unclear] . . . If you gave the medication, would it interfere at all with the study.

ER: Oh, Mrs. Dibble, we ah quite often the patient came in and he had troubles that were *not* related to ah ah the study. Ah we have had doctors who would, who were ah the visiting doctors didn't do this very much because they did not have licenses. But they would suggest, ask Dr. Smith to give this man a prescription for the medicine. And um Dr. Smith kept all kinds of medicines in his office and these people did not have prescription finance at this time and, but they would refer them to Dr. Smith or to your husband. I had taken them to your husband, and he said, they tell me, they said, "Miss Rivers, can you find a doctor when he's having this pain, or something." I don't know what the exact cause or maybe blood pressure was up or somethin, and they'd give him somethin for his blood pressure and that kind of thing, you see. But now actually for syphilis I don't know, I don't remember, I don't know whether there were these things more related that I think were related to this disease, see, but we had—I was looking at somebody's record the other day. Man went to Birmingham, record treatment in Birmingham and he still in the study [laughs]. As I go through the records, I see where various ones had gone to Birmingham for rapid treatment, had treatment in Montgomery do rapid treatment and *still* in the study.

HD: They went for rapid treatment?

ER: Huh?

HD: Rapid treatment?

ER: Rapid treatment was this eight-hour, sixteen-hour thing they put in, they put the patient to bed and they give him a continuous drip of the medicines, see, for so many hours. They just lie down there instead of giving them one injection today and another day but they would give this continuous ah ah treatment right straight on through for, say, twenty-four hours and then begin again. And then they'd come home, you know. Send them home with that patient's and family reaction, see, to the stuff. That type of treatment didn't last too long, but some of our patients in the study did go to rapid treatment centers. One of them even now, why he's doing very fine. I know one, but there may be others.

HD: Do you think that they were satisfied? Now you said that they had made a similar study on whites in Norway. How long was that study, I wonder? In comparison to Tuskegee?

ER: Maybe if it, that study, isn't going on still they were following all of the descendants of the people of the trauma patients. Now I don't know whether this has been discontinued or not. But I know that when we were working the people from Norway came over here and they sat with us in the clinic and watched me bring the patients in and followed me through what I was doing and what the doctors did. And at that time their study started back in 1920 or something like that, maybe early, but they were following the descendants of these patients, see, and this was one of the things that Dr. Heller had suggested that we ought to do is follow the descendants, the children, and all the off-spring, but it never got off the board. So that this is what happened. But I don't know know whether we followed too much of the kids.

HD: How many are living of that original group that you started with in your study? You said there were 400?

ER: I was noticing on some records or some of the records that 80 some odd of the positives still living. I don't know about the controls, the 200 in that 200 group, I don't know. But ah they are concentrating on this 80, 87, or 80 something positives. And they may be taking care of the negatives. I'm not, I don't know about that. But this is . . .

HD: And they put in this lawsuit for the payment. . . .

ER: The patients who are living are supposed to get $37,000. The descendants of the ones who have died, their relatives will get $15,000.

DW: I keep forgetting so much that you've gotten so many awards and everything for such good service in the health profession. What is your philosophy of life? That you worked with people all these years, done so much for so many, what would you tell young people?

ER: I would, I feel about the situation, I think that ah you've got to have something within to make you see that person's position. In other words, put yourself in my place. Would you want, I'll say, would you want me to come up and, and ignore your desires or your feelings your opinions? You have opinions just like I do.

This is your privilege. And I just think that we should not judge a man for what he is. If he's got one shoe on and one boot or bare-footed, he's a human being. I said do for that man like you do for Rockefellers because he had money. Not for the dollar but for the human being. That's the way I see it. And I have, my husband used to get absent minded and sometimes my patients would call and they'd say Miz Laurie or Miss Rivers, they still call me oh, and I did this and general nursing too. "Miss Rivers my baby is sick. Wouldn't you come and see what's doing," and I have, have gotten up out of my bed cold and go to see what could I do for that child or for that person. If I didn't see that somethin and I didn't go the hospital just as big as though I had [laughs], Miz Dibble's husband used to have put up with me with so many things. But that person was in *need*. And if I'm able to help him a little bit, I think that is my duty, whatever the situation is. Don't care who he is, don't care where he came from, where he's going, I have nothing to do with that. But I want to help him or help her, whatever the situation was. He may be the worst drunk, maybe the worst, as we say, human being possible, I have nothing to do with that. That's what I, if what I can do to make him comfortable or make it better for him, this is what I did.

DW: Were you ever a midwife?

ER: No, I was never a midwife. I did everything but the . . . [laughs]

HD: You worked with the midwifery program, though, didn't you?

ER: No, I didn't work with the midwifery program as such. I worked with the maternity, you know, the clinics and all. But the midwifery program, I never did work with that, that was too slow for me. I couldn't go and sit up half a night or nothing [laughs]. I worked in the maternity clinics and with the county health department. I did, I worked with the venereal disease control thing. I worked with them. During World War II [unclear] I followed all the soldiers' contacts and everything and got them in for treatment, blood tests, and this kind of thing. And I worked with the mothers and the babies in the maternity and infant clinic but not midwifery, I couldn't do midwifery. That was too slow, woo.

HD: Back up a little bit. You didn't say how you got into this program to begin with, the study program. Where were you working and how did it get to you and—

ER: Well, that goes way back. When I came, when I came out of school, I worked with the state health department on the Moveable School under Mr. Tom Campbell, headquarters in Tuskegee. In '22. I came back, Mr. Monroe Work and Mrs. Work got me in this job with the Moveable School and the state health department. I was employed by the state health department, assigned to the extension department, see. And we worked and I worked there teaching home nursing in this Moveable School. I'm sure you know about that. But we went all over, and my part, we had the home economics worker, the farm agent, and the nurse. Well, I was responsible for the nursing, the health part of it. The sanitation, I was the sanitation officer and I always went. And in those days these kids would not do that now. It was a lot of pellag[r]a. I worked for the extension department for four years.

At that time Alabama was not in the registration area. Babies were being born and people were dying. So they called me from Mr. Campbell, the state department, gave me a car and about seven counties and midwives and undertakers. That was my job. And I went into . . . I did, my job was to go into each, wherever I went in whatever county, and I used to spend about two weeks there. And I had to make a birth certificate on every child under six years old. And then I brought this in, and any deaths that had occurred. I made a, a certificate on that. I went, when I came in from this county I went into the Bureau of Registrar of Vital Statistics, and I dumped all the lists that I had and sometimes I had stacks like this of birth certificates and death certificates that had occurred. Then the office, then the people in the office went through these birth certificates that *I* brought in. If they didn't find any birth certificates then they recorded what I brought in. And they tell me when I was down in south Alabama, Greene County and all those counties down there, that there were gobs and gobs of people certificates that I brought in.

DW: People owe you a whole lot for really recording their births.

ER: That's right.

DW: For their being here. For their coming and going.

ER: For the death certificates I went to the undertakers. I would go through his . . . records and sometimes they had no records and sometimes the people I lived with knew who died when and that kind of thing. I would ask the people that I lived with about who died, and how many people is dead, and who buried them and this kind of thing, see. And sometimes I'd have to go to the families to find out this information. Go to the undertaker to find out, to get all his reports, see, and this is how I got started. This is what I was doing when I first started. And I worked then with the Bureau of Vital Statistics, and then while I was out there they had started me as sort of general supervisor of the midwives and I told that lady I just didn't want that, not to be bothered with that, 'cause them women wasn't gonna do what you say and I never shall forget that I was teaching a class one day talking about the mommas and the babies and everything. So, I was telling about keeping them clean and keeping down there and everything and bathing them, so I said, one woman said, "Miss, Miss, I want to ask you a question." I said, "All right." She said, "Is you going to bathe that woman?" And I says, "Sure." "You're sure going to kill her too." [Laughs.] "Don't y'all listen to what that child said 'cause she don't know." Those are the kind of things that you had to . . . oh Lord. "You going to bathe, you going to bathe that woman?" I said, "Yes ma'am. I"m going to bathe her, I'm going to show how to bathe a bed patient," 'cause in those days a woman stayed in bed nine days and I was teaching them how to bathe the patient with the patient in bed. She said, "Let me ask you one question. Is you going to bathe that woman?" I said, "Yes." "You going to bathe that woman?" I said, "Yes ma'am sure am." I was showing her to protect this part, you know, and everything. "You're going to kill that woman. Let me tell you all something, that child don't know what she is doing. She doesn't know what she's talking about. She don't know what she is talking about."

DW: [laughing in background] Right then you said what's the use? [laughing]

ER: [mumbling but seems to be agreeing]

HD: Then you left that—

ER: Then I worked till '31, '31, and I came . . . then they discontinued that. They thought Alabama had gotten into the registration area, their doctor, I forgot what the man's name is, they were very, very proud of me. And I had, and they admitted that I had done a good job and worked very, very hard 'cause I, 'cause all the time I would go to church meeting, you'd see me in my little car, riding in it, writing up these babies, you know, writing up these children, getting them in. And when their folks found out what I was doing, so they kept me busy. So after they got Alabama in the registration area and they had learned what it was all about then that the depression came so there was out.

So I was getting ready to go to New York. Dr. Dibble said, "Miss Rivers, what's you going to do now?" I said, "I am to the Seaview Hospital." Dr. Dibble said [sounds horrified], "Oh no, Miss Rivers, oh no no." And I was the night supervisor and that was just as bad as working with the midwives [laughs]. So I said, "O.K." I didn't feel particular about going to New York, but I says I had been offered this job so he said, "No, you ain't going nowhere. We need a night supervisor here and personally you do it." So then I worked, I said, "Well, Dr. Dibble, I cannot go to work now." He said, "No, 'cause you're so run down you be dead before you get on there." And he gave me a month and I went on as night supervisor in January or February '31 and worked as night supervisor till '32.

And then, this, I worked until it came, the study came, they wanted somebody, was in July. Yeah, I worked for them until July. And they came down here. Dr. Dibble gave me a leave of absence to work with them, he felt I was the person that they needed to work with them. So then I worked there. And then when the work was discontinued, Dr. Dibble said ah, "Miss Rivers, whatch you going to do?" [unclear] "I don't know, Dr. Dibble." "You're going to work, come on, come on." And I went back down there and worked two months, and then they and then went back to the federal bureau . . . worked two months there as a night supervisor?

DW: Are you from Macon County?

ER: No, I'm a Georgian. I'm from Georgia.

DW: What part?

ER: Southwest Georgia, Jakin, Georgia.

HD: I've never heard of that, Jakin.

DW: Well, I've heard of many places because my mother and father was born there.

ER: Oh, is that right, what part?

DW: Pittsville.

ER: Oh, that's a good piece.

DW: [unclear]

ER: No, I was southwest Georgia, on the Georgia, Florida, Alabama line.

DW: Oh down there [unclear].

ER: But I knew Dothan, twenty-seven miles from Dothan. Used to be a big sawmill near—

DW: Near Blakely? That's the one?

ER: Yeah, ah huh

[unclear discussion back and forth about places]

HD: I said you been here so long that this is home.

ER: Yeah, after my mother and father passed and my sister living, there's just two of us, she's living in Tennessee. The only thing we have down there is the home.

HD: [unclear] If you had stayed there you never would have met Mr. Clarence.

ER: I sure wouldn't have, I sure wouldn't have. He didn't never ask me to marry him, he just told me he was going to marry me [laughs].

Is there anything else you can think of?

DW: Has life changed for you since all this stuff came out?

ER: Well, Mr. Williams, it upset me terribly to begin with. And I, I, I just, it was really beneath the belt. And plus I had so many agitators coming in. Nobody knows what a, a, what I'm going through with. And the people in Atlanta had said, "Mrs. Rivers, Ms. Laurie, so we know what you've done. You forget it." And I said, "Well, I won't forget it." And so I, but, people have just, they have just turned it. You couldn't—

DW: Turned it around—

ER: You can't tell 'em, you can't tell, you couldn't tell 'em and I—Miz Dibble, did you see that the TV folks gave me a thing [laughs] I was so mad that day I didn't know what to do and when I saw that thing I wanted to get a rock but another thing that provoked you. They wouldn't come and sit down here all over my house, you know, and that kind of thing. So I told them. I was trying to straighten, tell them how the thing got started and what we did and all of this at that particular way time back then. And then I found out I wasn't getting anywhere. The last group that came, the man came there to the door. He told me he was somebody from one of them broadcasting stations. I said, "You'd don't coming in here." I mean, just as ugly. I said . . . "I said no you're not coming in my house." He said, "We want ta—" I said, "Uh uh, you're not going to make no pictures of me." I said, "Don't you come back here anymore for anything." So they they intended to get me because they parked up there at the church and walk back up here. So Miz Cooks[?] came in here one day. And when I went to open the door for her she drove in the driveway where you are and then they were getting ready to take pictures. "Don't take my picture, don't take my picture." She says, "You do I'm going to call the police right now." [Laughs.] For, but, as I started to say, it got under my skin to begin with. And but afterwards, I just said, well this is one of those things. Every time I pick up the newspaper you find somebody and I guess I'm just a victim of it. I know personally that I am not guilty of *what* they says, see, and at that particular time those people were given good attention for that particular time. And plus ah all of their medications. Oh, this is another thing that they say, that we didn't tell them that they had syphilis. Well, in those days the word "syphilis," we didn't know what syphilis, I means the general people didn't know what syphilis was, see, and it was not used. 'Cause I had been to the conferences, some conferences where they spoke of it as bad blood. They spoke of gonorrhea as the running. They didn't, the syphilis, it was not, it was not until the late years that they started the word, certainly in the late '40s they started using the word "syphilis." So we were not hiding from them what they had, that they had bad blood, that they didn't have syphilis. We never told them that.

HD: You'd tell them that they had bad—

ER: Bad blood. This is what they knew that they had, bad blood. But you cannot get them to put those two together. Just like I told you something like the people who came here, I said well, now, in this day and time we say "syphilis" and "gonorrhea" and I said you think nothing about it. I said but you know in those days, the people, "claps," "the running," and "bad blood." That was it. I said you didn't get out and tell the folks he had running, or he had bad blood, or your name was mud, your name was mud. So this, they had, to me they had gotten the thing all out of proportion. And we treated them then for the same thing, but they had no name, they had a different name for them and they knew it. 'Cause they could get to the clinic, Mr. Williams, and you could hear them teasing each other about where they been and who, [laughs] they were just having a good time. Uh huh. Don't it catch up with ya. Uh huh. I know it catch up with ya. Uh huh, yes sir, uh huh. "What you done in the dark sure come to the light," ah ah. I sure loved the expressions of those folks [laughs]. So they knew. So they knew. But the word "syphilis" was not used.

HD: Was anything done to protect the families of the syphilitic persons in the house?

ER: Whatch you mean, is the—

HD: A person, a man who had syphilis.

DW: Anything done to protect his wife?

HD: Or his children or anyone.

ER: Well, ah ah, what we did was to get the entire family, try and get all of the family and do blood tests on them. And if they had, as long as they were negative, we just kept them—the only thing that we did was to tell them to be sure to have your blood checked, you know, every so often. And we kept them under surveillance so that if anybody in the family came up with a positive they started to treat them right off. Work them up and get them right off. But nothing said to prevent it . . . [unclear]

HD: Prevent the spreading of it?

ER: We just add and they would get the person. If the man, the patient had early lesions they gave him the medication. Because usually we would tell them that if they had a rash this first dose is going to clear that rash up. But don't you, you have relationships, you come back next week for your treatment and just treated them, keep them on the treatment, see, . . . [long silence] now this is what it was.

HD: Now, you said there were 400 in the initial—

ER: Four hundred in the positives, initial, we started off with these 400 positives in this study. The next year or maybe a year from that time, they decided that they needed some comparisons and so these 200 positives were classified into age groups and so many age groups so as to compare . . .

DW: Do you find nowadays that there are people who don't want to know what happened? People in their families who were in the study, people to know they were going?

ER: Ah ah, some of them. That's so. Now it was up until this money came up.

DW: Oh.

ER: [Laughs] Now I can say that. It was until they found out that wanted to get some money. Now they tell everything. [Laughs]

DW: I often wondered about that.

ER: Ah huh, this, the money proposition has made it a big change, a big change. But up until the money proposition came up, 'cause I know two men who would not have wanted anybody to know that they were ever even, even in the study. But now 'cause I had one, two, three tell me, "Miss Rivers, I will meet you in town, or where you all working, I will meet you." "At the veteran's hospital on such and such a day." "Well, I'll be there. That, don't you come to my house where these people are. Or I don't want to be seen talking to you too much, see." But now since the money proposition, it is altogether different. Because I had one man come in, to come in to tell me, this same man had come to the house, he had called me and asked me if he could talk with me. And I said yes. I wondered what in the world he was talking about. So he came up and he wanted to know about what he had been reading, was it true. I told him yes. So I said, anybody contacted you. He said no. I said, well, go down and talk with Fred Gray. He'll get this straightened out.

DW: You know, it is peculiar thing how all that you done for them and in a sense you're the cause of their getting all of this, you know.

ER: Well, this is the thing that really . . .

DW: What do you get?

ER: Nothing.

DW: [Laughs]

ER: This is true, this is true. But this is the way they feel about it. This is the way they feel about it. And I understand that some of them are a very, very critical towards me, *blaming* me for ah, 'cause one man, one lady was talking about—I said now stop blaming me when he's supposed to get the money. I ain't getting nothin. I said at least he's going to get $37,000. You ought to be happy that I did this. But this is what they said.

HD: That's right [unclear].

ER: No, it is supposed to be the 17th of February or something like that.

HD: Never heard of . . .

DW: Do you want to turn this off now?

ER: Yes, you can.

YOUR SILENCE WILL NOT PROTECT YOU

Nurse Rivers and the Tuskegee Syphilis Study[1]

EVELYNN M. HAMMONDS

I've been afraid to know more about this story. I sat in the library over an hour killing time—flipping through magazines, talking with a friend, making several trips to the water fountain. I stared at her picture on the poster from the Schlesinger Library's Black Women's Oral History Project.

Her face has always looked so familiar to me. The reddish-brown skin and the gray hair brushed back from her forehead in the style worn by many of the women from the central part of Georgia where she and my family were reared. Her hands were large and looked as if they were used to hard work. She had a shy smile on her face. When I could not postpone it any longer, I sat down to read the words of Eunice Rivers, the black woman who had been a major character in an ugly episode in American history, the Tuskegee Syphilis Study.

In July 1972, the world first learned that for forty years the United States Public Health Service had been conducting a study of untreated syphilis on almost four hundred black men in Macon County, Alabama. From 1932 to 1972, 399 men who had syphilis and another 201 who were free of the disease serving as controls, were a part of what became known as the Tuskegee Study. While whites reacted with shock at the exposure of such scientific abuse in their own country (which was for many of them comparable to the crimes of the Nazis against Jews during World War II), African Americans almost universally saw the study as just one of the more blatant acts of genocide long perpetrated against our communities by whites.

As the indifference of the medical and public health establishments has allowed the slow, steady increase of AIDS in African-American communities to continue unabated, many black people have likened the tragic AIDS epidemic to the Tuskegee Study. In the case of AIDS, many African Americans feel that we have little reason to trust public health experts, still largely white, who were part of an agency that used a group of poor black men as their guinea pigs for forty years. But there is

Evelynn M. Hammonds is associate professor of the History of Science in the Program in Science, Technology, and Society at the Massachusetts Institute of Technology.
Originally published in Evelyn C. White, The Black Women's Health Book: Speaking for Ourselves (Seattle: Seal Press, 1994): 323–31. Copyright © Evelynn M. Hammonds and reprinted by permission of Seal Press.

another lesson we need to learn from the Tuskegee Study as we enter the second decade of the AIDS epidemic, and that is about our own responsibilities as black women to speak about the ravages of this disease in our communities. The story of the Tuskegee Study and particularly Nurse Eunice Rivers' role in it, should remind us of the ways in which we can be made complicit in the suffering of our own people.

What's Done in the Dark Is Revealed in the Light

While historians have known the detailed story of the Tuskegee Study since 1981, when white male historian James H. Jones published his book, *Bad Blood: The Tuskegee Syphilis Experiment*[2], most people have only recently learned of the event from articles in *Essence* magazine. There have also been television programs about the study (a *Nova* special and a segment on the news show *PrimeTime Live*) and a play, *Miss Evers' Boys*, which was written by David Feldsuh, a white man. In the play, the character of Miss Evers is based on the black public health nurse who worked on the Tuskegee Study, Nurse Eunice Rivers. It was Nurse Rivers' job to serve as a liaison between the white doctors who designed and ran the Tuskegee Study and the black men who were its subjects. She kept track of the men in the study, visited with them and came to know their families. She tried to protect them from the racist behavior of the doctors and consoled their families when the men died of the disease. By all accounts, it was the men's trust in Nurse Rivers that kept them in the study. Yet, despite her performance of her duties and the care and concern she displayed toward the men in the study, Nurse Rivers has been depicted in Jones' book and Feldsuh's play as a problematic figure—carrying the weight of the questions: Did she knowingly participate in deceiving the men? Or was she herself a victim of the study?

Furthermore, while she was the only female officially involved in the study, Nurse Rivers was not the only woman who had to deal with its consequences. In addition to the above questions, we need to ponder: What of the wives of the men? How many of them were put at risk because of the failure to treat the men? And most importantly, what are we, as African-American women, to make of various attempts to cast Nurse Rivers as a collaborator in one of the most unethical medical studies of this century?

Eunice Verdell Rivers

Eunice Verdell Rivers was born in 1899 in Early County, Georgia.[3] With her father's encouragement and support, she decided to study nursing. She graduated from the nursing school at Tuskegee Institute in 1922. Her first job was with the Movable School, which was a specially built bus that traveled across Alabama providing hands-on demonstrations of canning, mattress-making, carpentry, animal husbandry and midwifery to black folks with no access to formal education. Following a short stint as a night nursing supervisor at the John A. Andrew Hospital on the Tuskegee Institute campus, Nurse Rivers was recruited in 1932 to join the public health project on the study of venereal disease in Macon County. She remained on the project for the next thirty-three years. In addition to her work on the syphilis study, she also collected information and recorded data on births and deaths in the black population. She often had to travel alone to do this work, going from planation to plantation in the southern part of the state. Nurse Rivers also taught midwifery for a number of years and worked on other issues related to infant and maternal health among the poorest blacks in Macon County.

In April 1958, Eunice Rivers became only the third recipient of the Oveta Culp Hobby Award, the highest commendation given to an employee of the Department of Health, Education and Welfare. The citation read, "for notable service covering 25 years during which through selfless devotion and skillful human relations she has sustained the interest and cooperation of the subjects of a venereal disease control program in Macon County, Alabama."[4] The irony of her receiving this award for her work on the Tuskegee Study would only become apparent more than a decade later when the details of the study were revealed to a wider public.

Always Mindful

Since the troubling details of the Tuskegee episode have come to light many people have asked the following question: How could a black woman, educated and trained as nurse, willfully participate in a study that ultimately harmed so many of her people? I believe that part of the answer lies in the way Jones depicted Nurse Rivers in *Bad Blood*, which is perhaps the most widely cited text on the study.

From the opening pages of the book, Jones displays a great deal of moral outrage about the study. Noting the pivotal role that Nurse Rivers played in the experiment, he writes, in the book's acknowledgements: "I owe an enormous debt to Eunice Rivers (Laurie) for spending several days with me and helping me to see the experiment through her eyes. More than any other principal of the Tuskegee Study, she increased my tolerance for ambiguity."[5] On the contrary, it is clear from the manner in which Jones renders the story that his vision was skewed. He did not understand nor convey the complexity of the study through Nurse Rivers' eyes.

Eunice Rivers knew firsthand the world of poor black people living in Alabama during the Depression. She could not fail to see how segregation sat like a heavy boot on the backs of all blacks in the South. Though she was an educated woman and one of the few black nurses in Alabama, Nurse Rivers too felt the weight of segregation and oppression on her back. She knew she had to be careful as she traveled around the state collecting birth and death records. She had to be mindful always that her job put her close to white people who were threatened by her professional status. At the same time, she had to consider and attend to the feelings of blacks who might have been disdainful toward her because of her close working relationships with whites. In short, she straddled two worlds.

Early in her career, white supervisors praised Nurse Rivers for her ability to win the trust of the black community, wherever she was dispatched. On one occasion, a white nurse suggested that she might follow Nurse Rivers to learn the secret of her success. But she would have none of that. "You tell me what you want me to do in the office and I'll go and do it," Nurse Rivers replied. "But you're not going to follow me there. The first thing the Negroes would say was that I had been framing them."[6] Nurse Rivers walked this line throughout her career.

Because of our national amnesia about the conditions black people lived under before the civil rights movement, it is difficult for us to remember the world of the segregated South. Black women nurses, social workers, teachers and the few clerks who worked in white-owned stores, played a much more central role in the lives of black people than they do today.

For example, I can remember as a small child, going on Saturday shopping trips with my mother and sister to a major department store in downtown Atlanta. My mother always took us to this particular store because she had a black women friend who worked as a clerk, not a saleslady (in those days the title "saleslady" was reserved for white women) in the girls' and women's department. My sister and I liked going to this store because my mother was always less tense and anxious when we shopped there. Her friend would help pick out clothes for us and then stand guard at the one dressing room we were allowed to use. She wouldn't let the white salesladies talk down to my mother and even at a young age, my sister and I understood the importance of her protection. And certainly, when our friend was home on the weekends, as a valued member of her church and community, the role she played was validated by all. These women were seen as muting the force of a system of apartheid that at any moment could turn a simple shopping trip — during which a black child might innocently touch a pretty dress on a rack—into an ugly and dangerous racial incident.

It is within this context that Nurse Rivers carried out the duties of her job. She had no ambitions to be a doctor, she wanted to be a nurse because she was, in her own words, "interested in the person, and it just never occurred to me that I wanted to be a doctor . . . the nurse plays an important part there. She's closer to the patient. Patients would get to the point where if they're not sure, they're going to ask you. They get you in the middle."[7]

"These Are Grown Men"

When Nurse Rivers became involved in the Tuskegee Study, she fiercely protected the men, making sure that the young, white doctors who gave them their yearly checkups understood that the men were human beings. "They're human," she told the doctors, who often treated the men insensitively. "You don't talk to them like that. . . . If anything happens that you can't get along; that you can't get it through their head, just call me. We'll straighten it out. But don't holler at them. These are grown men."[8]

To the white physicians conducting the study, the men were nothing more than experimental "subjects." To Nurse Rivers, men like Charles Pollard and Lester Scott (two in the study who are mentioned by name in Jones' book) were deserving of courtesy and respect. Her duties included keeping track of the men in the study, driving them to the hospital for their annual blood tests and checkups and providing them with medicine and tonic throughout the year. The most difficult part of her work was obtaining permission from the men's families to allow the government to perform autopsies after their deaths. She sat with the families and talked them through their fears about the autopsies and at the urging of the widow of the first man in the study to die, she requested that the Public Health Service provide burial stipends of fifty dollars for each family. The autopsies were difficult for her. She attended every funeral. "I was expected to be there," she said. "They were part of my family."[9]

At the Crossroads of Race and Gender

While Nurse Rivers was protective of the men in the study and provided care to them and their families, she also knew that they were being denied treatment for syphilis.[10] In her response to questions about this matter, she reiterated what the doctors had told her about the study: that its purpose was to make a comparison with a similar study that was being conducted on white men in order to determine if syphilis manifested itself differently in black people. The devastating nature of the late stages of syphilis was visible to all. It is a condition characterized by tumors and ulcers on the skin, bone deterioration and often severe damage to the cardiovascular and central nervous systems. Syphilis could cause blindness, progressive paralysis, and in those whose spinal cord nerves were affected, it impaired movement of legs, producing a stumbling gait.

As Jones noted, all these complications were known to medical science before the Tuskegee Study began. Eunice Rivers was not alone in accepting the Public Health Service physicians' view that a study of the late stages of syphilis in black people was needed. Dr. Eugene Dibble, the black medical director of the Tuskegee

Institute and head of its hospital, had given his approval to the study from its inception and had also performed some of the spinal punctures and autopsies on the men. Dr. William Perry, a black physician from the Harvard School of Public Health, sanctioned the study and participated in it. Dr. Jerome J. Peters, a staff physician at the Veterans Hospital in Tuskegee, likewise performed spinal punctures and autopsies on the men. In 1969, nearly thirty-seven years after the study began, most in the predominantly black medical establishment in Macon County had sanctioned the study.

Nurse Rivers perceived the study and its impact this way: While the men did not get treated for syphilis, they did get "good medical" care—care they would not have received otherwise because of their socioeconomic status. Neither Tuskegee Institute nor other local hospitals had provided adequate care for the poor black people in Macon County. As Nurse Rivers saw it, the fact that the men were given cardiograms and other expensive tests over the course of the study, meant they had access to quality care that few of their station ever received. Nurse Rivers consistently mentioned care when questioned about the ethics of the study. Nonetheless, she did not refrain from addressing the overriding problem of the research, "The doctors didn't tell the patients they had syphilis."[11]

Who Shall Be Called to Account?

While some might construe Nurse Rivers' response as a casting aside of her own responsibility and complicity in the study, I think her answer reflects the complexities in the experiment, the majority of which have been largely ignored. Jones devotes a major portion of *Bad Blood* to describing Nurse Rivers' work and the trusting relationships she established with the men in the study. He spends far too little time documenting her relationship with the black and white male physicians who supervised her. Castigating her for "ethical passivity," Jones seems almost personally aggrieved that Nurse Rivers was unable to stop the experiment. He does not call to account the male physicians who had much more power and authority than she.

Thus, in his rendering of the story, the black woman nurse becomes the center of the ethical dilemmas raised by the Tuskegee Study. The person who in fact had the least amount of power to resist or question the study is blamed. Eunice Rivers was in no position based on her education or her work to evaluate the scientific merits of the study. And to be sure, the white physicians who supervised her were extremely adept at masking the ethical issues raised by the study. Despite their approval of the study, neither the black male medical establishment nor the administrators (again black and male) of Tuskegee are depicted as central figures in Jones' book. All these men, both black and white, are spared the censure Eunice Rivers receives.

"We're Sick Too"

The Tuskegee Study is a story of the betrayal of poor black men and women. The men in the study and their mates were betrayed by both black and white male physicians who cared little about their lives because the people were black and poor. In the beginning of the study, the black physicians who lent their support to it, saw in the project a way to enhance their standing with the white medical establishment. These men knew full well the implications of the study and the system of racialized medical research from which it had emerged.

They put their professional interests above the medical needs of their people. They put their well-being above that of the fifty unnamed women and children who contracted syphilis because of the government's failure to treat the men.[12] We know nothing of the plight of these women or their children.

Eunice Rivers was also betrayed. Praised for her work with the men in the study by white physicians who noted her skill at warning the physicians of "eccentricities" of the patients, Nurse Rivers stood in the middle. She watched black male physicians cooperate with and validate a study controlled by white men.

She was called upon to console, but was powerless to advocate for the wives of the men who asked her why only men could be in the study. "We're sick too, Nurse Rivers," they said. As a middle-class, educated woman who interacted with both black physicians and the poor black men who were subjects in the study, Nurse Rivers lived in two communities. She saw herself as at least trying to do something for people others had forsaken.

Silent No More

Eunice Rivers died at age eighty-seven in Tuskegee, Alabama. Her obituary noted that she had been a member of the Greater St. Mark Missionary Baptist Church for forty years. She organized the church's nurses' guild, taught women's Bible classes, was a member of the sisterhood, Trustee Board, Women's Missionary Board and Religious Education Board.[13] She lived a life of service to her community, but no one was served by her silence.

I wish that Nurse Rivers had been able to see that the Tuskegee Study was wrong. I wish that she had been able to speak. But I will not ask her to carry the weight for what was a failure on the part of the entire black community. I will not ask a lone black woman to carry the moral obligations of our community by herself.

This is a burden we must all bear. Black people face the same dilemma today as AIDS continues to spread unchecked in our families and neighborhoods. The toll AIDS is taking on African-American women and children is as ignored as the plight of the women in the Tuskegee Study.

Too few black physicians, nurses and public health workers are talking about the multitudes of black men, women and children with AIDS who are languishing in hospital beds. Too few historians, social scientists, community activists, religious and political leaders are speaking out. Because of homophobia and shame, too few black families are revealing the cause of death of the many young men and women they are laying to rest.

But listen up. Our silence will not stop the AIDS epidemic. Nor will our acceptance of the medical establishment's inertia and racism exonerate us from our responsibility to our sisters and brothers. We must speak about the failures to stop AIDS. The African-American community must deal with the sensitive issues that are at the heart of this matter—all unsafe sexual practices, but especially unprotected homosexual and bisexual relations and intravenous drug use. If we do not speak out, then another generation will be perfectly justified in asking us, as we today ask those involved in the Tuskegee Study, why blacks stood silent while our people died.

NOTES

1. The title is taken from a line in Audre Lorde's essay, "The Transformation of Silence into Language and Action," in *Sister Outsider: Essays and Speeches*. (Freedom, CA: The Crossing Press, 1984).

2. James H. Jones, *Bad Blood: The Tuskegee Syphilis Experiment* (New York: The Free Press, 1981).

3. The biographical information on Nurse Rivers is taken from the interview conducted by Lillian A. Thompson for the Black Women's Oral History Project. It is published in *The Black Women's Oral History Project* (Westport: Meckler Publishing, 1991), volume 7, pp. 213–242. In 1952, Eunice Rivers married Julius Laurie and took his surname. However, in published works, she is most often cited as Nurse Eunice Rivers.

4. Jones, p. 169.

5. Jones, op. cit., p. xi.

6. *The Black Women's Oral History Project*, op. cit., p.230.

7. Ibid., pp. 240–241.

8. Ibid., p. 233.

9. Jones, op. cit., p. 154.

10. Eunice Rivers, Stanley Schuman, Lloyd Simpson and Sidney Olansky, "Twenty Years of Followup Experience in a Long-Range Medical Study," *Public Health Reports*. vol. 68, No. 4, April 1953, pp. 391–395. This paper, which lists Eunice Rivers as co-author, unabashedly opens with the statement, "One of the longest continued medical surveys ever conducted is the study of untreated syphilis in the male Negro."

11. Jones, op. cit., p. 219.

12. Jones, op. cit., p. 255.

13. Program from the funeral service of Eunice Verdell Rivers Laurie, September 1, 1986. Tuskegee University Archives. My thanks to Wellesley College Professor Susan Reverby for her assistance.

NEITHER VICTIM NOR VILLAIN
Eunice Rivers and Public Health Work

SUSAN L. SMITH

From 1932 to 1972 white physicians of the United States Public Health Service (USPHS) carried out an experiment on approximately 400 rural black men in Macon County, Alabama. The study, which historian James Jones has described as "the longest nontherapeutic experiment on human beings in medical history," was predicated on following the course of untreated syphilis until death.[1] Historians have focused on the study as scientifically unjustifiable and as an unethical experiment that highlights the racism of American medicine and the federal government. While affirming the validity of these assessments, I reexamined the experiment to return to the troubling question of why black professionals, such as nurse Eunice Rivers (Laurie), supported the project.

Black health workers and educators associated with Tuskegee Institute, a leading black educational institution founded by Booker T. Washington in Alabama, played a critical role in the experiment. Robert Moton, head of Tuskegee Institute in the 1930s, and Dr. Eugene Dibble, the Medical Doctor of Tuskegee's Hospital, both lent their endorsement and institutional resources to the government study. However, no one was more vital to the experiment than Eunice Rivers, a black public health nurse. Rivers acted as the liaison between the men in the study and the doctors of the USPHS. She worked in the public health field from 1923 until well after her retirement in 1965. She began her career with the Tuskegee Institute Movable School during the 1920s in rural Alabama. This traveling school for African Americans provided adult education programs in agriculture, home economics, and health. After a decade of service with the school, Rivers became involved in the infamous Tuskegee Syphilis Study in 1932. How could a nurse dedicated to preserving life participate in such a project?

Although historians have noted the key role that Rivers played in the experiment, they have presented her as a victim by virtue of her status as a woman, an African American, and a nurse. Groundbreaking work by James Jones, for example, interpreted much of Rivers's participation as driven by obedience to higher authority. A more satisfactory consideration of her role as an historical subject is

Susan L. Smith is associate professor of history at the University of Alberta.
Originally published in the Journal of Women's History 8 *(1996): 95–113. Reprinted by permission of Indiana University Press.*

in order; yet, examination of Rivers's role does not necessarily lead to an interpretation of her as an evil nurse. What does it mean, then, to talk about the historical agency of black women within racist and sexist social structures? Indeed, Rivers was neither a victim nor a villain but a complex figure who can only be understood within her historical context. She acted in ways she determined to be in her best interests and in the interests of promoting black health. Consistent with the responses of at least some black health professionals and educators at the time, Rivers did not question the experiment because she did not find it objectionable.

I became curious about the response of Rivers and other black professionals to the syphilis experiment during my work on the National Negro Health Movement, a black public health movement during the first half of the twentieth century. A small but active group of black professionals in medicine, dentistry, nursing, and education, along with community women, organized public health programs across the nation to improve the health of African Americans. By 1930 black nursing schools and medical institutions had produced some 5,000 black nurses and 3,700 black physicians, many of whom were involved in community health projects.[2]

Drawing on federal records from the USPHS, manuscript collections at Tuskegee University (the black college formerly known as Tuskegee Institute), and an oral history of Eunice Rivers, this article analyzes the meanings of the experiment from the perspective of black health professionals, especially Rivers. Her story raises important questions about the gendered nature of public health work, the constraints on black middle-class reform efforts, and the costs and benefits to the poor.

The actions of Eunice Rivers can best be understood when set within the context of twentieth-century public health work. In her capacity as a public health nurse, Rivers acted as the mediator between black clients and the government, implementing health policy at the local level. Indeed, she was the key to maintaining subject interest in the experiment for forty years.[3] Paradoxically, it is a "tribute" to her years of hard work at developing relationships with people in the surrounding countryside through her public health work with the Tuskegee Movable School that the men in the Tuskegee Syphilis Study continued to cooperate year after year.

In order to better understand the work of Eunice Rivers in the Tuskegee Syphilis Experiment, it is important to analyze her activities with the Tuskegee Movable School. When Tuskegee Institute established the Movable School in 1906, it marked the beginning of organized black agricultural extension work in the United States. Booker T. Washington referred to this form of rural schooling for adults as "A Farmer's College on Wheels." Washington and his assistants convinced government leaders to fund part of the costs of the Movable School and include it within the extension service work of the U.S. Department of Agriculture and the state of Alabama, although housed at Tuskegee Institute. The Movable School was one of the programs through which Washington attempted to secure government assistance and financial support during an era in which government neglect of the needs of African Americans was the norm.[4]

In the spirit of Washington's racial uplift philosophy, black extension agents from the Movable School tried to turn black tenant farmers into healthy, thrifty landowners. Landownership was a key to black freedom from white control. Extension agents wanted to liberate poor black people from the oppressive nature of the southern agricultural system, an economic arrangement which left many people trapped in a cycle of debt and poverty. Most African Americans in Alabama worked on white-owned cotton plantations where they rented their land and faced a losing financial battle. In 1925 in Macon County, home of Tuskegee Institute, 90 percent of the rural African Americans were tenant farmers.[5]

In the early twentieth century, many rural African Americans lived in unhealthy surroundings and faced a range of health problems including malaria, typhoid fever, hookworm disease, pellagra, and venereal disease, along with malnutrition and high infant and maternal mortality rates. Black extension agents and health workers throughout the South tried to address these problems in several ways. They launched programs to promote diversified farming, including vegetable gardens to improve the diet, to screen homes against insects that carried diseases, to build sanitary privies or toilets to minimize contact with human wastes, and to educate people about personal hygiene.[6]

Extension programs such as the Tuskegee Movable School tried to improve living conditions and reduce the migration of black farmworkers out of rural areas. The Movable School, a mule-drawn wagon later replaced by a truck, carried several Tuskegee graduates in agriculture, home economics, and nursing to work in the countryside among the rural poor. Initially the extension agents held teaching sessions in community institutions, such as churches, but by 1920 they decided that they could reach more people by going directly to their homes, either tenant houses on plantations or the homes of the few black landowners. The educational philosophy of the Movable School like that of all extension work was to teach by example and to win the trust of the farmworkers.[7]

The black educators from Tuskegee Institute who worked with the traveling school urged the rural black poor to participate in their programs. Based on previous experiences with local government and its history of upholding white supremacy, many poor African Americans initially were reluctant to participate in rural development programs for fear of being exploited. They were distrustful of the state and its representatives, given their mistreatment at the hands of landlords, the courts, railroads, and law enforcement agents.[8]

Health concerns were an integral part of the agenda of rural development programs, including the work of the Movable School. Although male farm agents and female home demonstration agents addressed health issues informally as part of their lessons in agriculture and home economics, the inclusion of a public health nurse with the Movable School in 1920 marked the beginning of formal health education work.

Throughout the early twentieth century the black nurse was a key figure in spreading the gospel of health or health education to African Americans. As the field of public health nursing expanded in the twentieth century and public health workers placed more emphasis on individual hygiene, nurses came to symbolize the ideal teachers. Public health nurses were especially important in rural areas where access to doctors was severely limited. They had more independence and autonomy than nurses in other fields. Despite discrimination in training, wages, and promotion, black nurses felt a sense of responsibility for the health needs of black communities. By 1930 there were 470 black public health nurses in the country, 180 of whom worked in the South where they constituted 20 percent of all public health nurses.[9]

The public health nurse was in an excellent position to assess the health needs of rural African Americans. Uva M. Hester, a Tuskegee graduate in nursing, became the first black public health nurse to work for the Movable School. She found the health conditions of rural families simply unbearable because of the unsanitary state of many homes. Hester stated that she was appalled by the flies, the dirt, and the small rooms in the cabins she visited. Her first week's report chronicled the inadequate health services available in rural Alabama.

> Tuesday: I visited a young woman who had been bedridden with tuberculosis for more than a year. There are two openings on her chest and one in the side from which pus constantly streams. In addition, there is a bedsore on the lower part of the back as large as one's hand. There were no sheets on her bed.... The sores had only a patch of cloth plastered over them. No effort was made to protect the patient from the flies that swarmed around her.[10]

These same themes of unhealthy conditions and inadequate bedside care recurred frequently in Hester's reports from her travels throughout the county. Public health nurses provided health education, comfort, and care where they could, but they usually operated with limited resources.

Eunice Rivers (1899–1986) joined the Movable School in January 1923, happy to have a job and also steeped in Tuskegee's philosophy of service to the rural poor. Like others who worked with the traveling school, Rivers attended Tuskegee Institute, graduating from the School of Nursing in 1922. Born in rural Georgia, she was the oldest of three daughters of a farming family. Rivers became a nurse because of parental encouragement. She remembered that, before her mother died when Rivers was only fifteen years old, her mother had told her to "get a good education, so that I wouldn't have to work in the fields so hard." Her father also promoted education for his daughters, working long hours in a sawmill to help finance it. Rivers eventually followed her father's advice to study nursing despite her protesting, "but Papa, I don't want to be no nurse, I don't want folks dying on me."[11]

Gender prescriptions influenced the shape of Rivers's public health work as she traveled from county to county. She directed most of her health education messages, including discussion of sanitation, ventilation, and cleanliness, to rural women. Public health programs focused on women because they were expected to be the ones most responsible for the health of their families. Rivers informed women about specific diseases, such as malaria and typhoid fever, and taught them how to make bandages from old clothes, care for bedridden patients, and take a temperature. Women often asked questions at these health meetings and seemed eager for information. In addition, Rivers gave dental hygiene lectures to children on how to brush their teeth, and she handed out tubes of Colgate toothpaste donated by the company. Her public health work with men focused on "social hygiene," which usually meant information about the dangers of venereal disease.[12]

In 1926 Rivers redirected some of the focus of her public health work. The state transferred her from the Alabama Bureau of Child Welfare, in which she performed her Movable School work, to the Bureau of Vital Statistics. Her new mandate was to assist the state in creating a system of registration for births and deaths, as well as aid efforts to regulate lay midwifery and lower infant mortality rates. She continued to travel throughout Alabama with the Movable School, but she focused her attention on pregnant women and midwives.[13]

Rivers was well liked by her clients who appreciated her visits. She reached many people through her Movable School position and worked in over twenty counties in her first year alone. She visited hundreds of people every month; during one particularly busy month she tended to 1,100 people. J. D. Barnes, a white extension agent in Greene County, reported to Tuskegee Institute in 1928 that rural women remembered Rivers's visits and the way she made people feel good in her company. He wrote, "one woman asked me when I was going to have that sweet little woman come back to the county again."[14]

Rivers, who grew up with a class background similar to that of the people she aided, attributed her successful relationships with rural people to her attitude toward them. "As far as I was concerned," she explained, "every individual was an individual of his own. He didn't come in a lump sum." She remembered that sometimes people would ask her how she ever received entry into certain homes where visitors were not welcomed. Rivers would reply:

Well, darling, I don't know. I was brought in there. They're people as far as I'm concerned. I don't go there dogging them about keeping the house clean. I go there and visit a while until I know when to make some suggestions. When I go to the house I accept the house as I find it. I bide my time.[15]

Her approach, she concluded, was nothing more than mutual respect between herself and those she assisted. The trust and close relationships that she developed with rural African Americans through her work with the Movable School proved to be a tremendous asset in her work for the USPHS.

In 1932 Eunice Rivers, along with leaders of Tuskegee Institute, became involved with a study by the USPHS that appears to contradict her efforts to improve black health. Rivers's need for employment, as well as her interest in black health conditions, influenced her decision to accept employment with the USPHS. During the early 1930s, financial cutbacks caused by the onset of the Depression ended her job with the Movable School. Facing unemployment, she accepted a job as night supervisor at the John A. Andrew Memorial Hospital at Tuskegee Institute and worked there eight months until she learned of the position with the federal government. When asked in later years why she went to work with the Syphilis Study she replied: "I was just interested. I mean I wanted to get into everything that I possibly could."[16] An equally compelling reason, no doubt, was her statement: "I was so glad to go off night duty that I would have done anything."[17] Thereafter, Rivers worked part-time for the USPHS and part-time in maternal and child health for Tuskegee's hospital and then later for the county health department.

In the early twentieth century, private foundations and the federal government focused attention on controlling venereal disease. The USPHS first addressed the topic of venereal disease during World War I when the federal government became concerned about the results of tests of military recruits that showed that many men, black and white, were infected with syphilis. The USPHS formed the Division of Venereal Disease to promote health education in black and white communities.[18] In the late 1920s the Julius Rosenwald Fund, a philanthropic foundation with strong interests in health care for African Americans, assisted the federal government in venereal disease control work. The foundation provided financial support to develop a demonstration control program for African Americans in the South. This project to detect and treat syphilis began in 1928 in Bolivar County, Mississippi, among thousands of black tenant farmers and sharecroppers, and it appeared to show that nearly 20 percent of the men and women had syphilis. The Rosenwald Fund next expanded the program from Mississippi to counties in other southern states, including Macon County in Alabama.[19] In 1932, when the Depression led the Rosenwald Fund to discontinue its financial support, leaders of the USPHS launched the Tuskegee Syphilis Study in Alabama. Initially, the study was to continue for about six to twelve months.

White assumptions about the health and sexuality of African Americans influenced the way medical authorities interpreted statistical data on venereal disease. Some black leaders criticized the high syphilitic rate always cited for African Americans as well as the expectation that syphilis was endemic to black populations because of sexual promiscuity. For example, Dr. Louis T. Wright, a leader of the National Association for the Advancement of Colored People (NAACP) and surgeon at Harlem Hospital in New York, wrote that even if there were high rates "this is not due to lack of morals, but more directly to lack of money, since with adequate funds these diseases can be controlled easily."[20]

Confident that racial differences affected health and disease, white physicians of the USPHS expected the Tuskegee study to provide a useful racial comparison to an Oslo study that traced untreated syphilis in Norway. However, the Oslo study was a retrospective study examining previous case records of white people whose syphilis went untreated, unlike the Tuskegee study, which was designed to deliberately withhold available treatment from black people. The development in 1910 of Salvarsan, a toxic arsenic compound that was the first effective treatment for syphilis, prompted the end of the Oslo study. Dr. Raymond Vonderlehr, an official at the USPHS, even proposed that they expand their investigation, suggesting that "similar studies of untreated syphilis in other racial groups might also be arranged." He suggested that they conduct a study of Native Americans with untreated syphilis.[21]

Black leaders at Tuskegee Institute endorsed the government study, to the relief of the federal officials, in the belief that it would help the school in its work for African Americans. The government doctors selected Macon County because they had identified it as having the highest rate of syphilis of all the Rosenwald study groups, with a rate of about 35 percent, and because they rightly concluded that Tuskegee Institute could provide valuable assistance. Dibble, the medical director of Tuskegee's hospital, supported the experiment on the grounds that it might demonstrate that costly treatment was unnecessary for people who had latent or third-stage syphilis, echoing the justifications provided by the USPHS. More importantly, Dibble urged Moton, head of Tuskegee Institute, to support the study because Tuskegee Institute "would get credit for this piece of research work," and the study would "add greatly to the educational advantages offered our interns and nurses as well as the added standing it will give the hospital." Moton agreed to allow the school's employees to examine the men in the study at Tuskegee's Andrew Hospital. Apparently, he believed that federal attention to the poor health conditions in the county would help the school get more funding for programs.[22]

Black educators and doctors at Tuskegee envisioned future financial benefits from cooperating with the federal government in the study. Such a belief grew out of Tuskegee's long history of lobbying the federal government for funding and assistance. Since the days of Booker T. Washington, black leaders at Tuskegee had witnessed evidence of at least limited government cooperation. For example, Washington and, later, Moton garnered government support for the Movable School and the National Negro Health Movement and succeeded in getting a black veterans' hospital located at Tuskegee, despite the absence of a black medical school.[23]

The experiment, officially known as "the Tuskegee Study of Untreated Syphilis in the Negro Male," was not a government secret, kept hidden from health professionals. It lasted for forty years and was publicized widely in the black and white medical community without evoking any protest. In the mid-1930s Dr. Roscoe C. Brown, the black leader of the Office of Negro Health Work at the USPHS, convinced the National Medical Association (the black medical organization) to display an exhibit on the study provided by the USPHS. Dr. Brown argued that it "would be an excellent opportunity for the use of this timely exhibit on one of our major health problems." Members of the black medical establishment knew the subjects of the experiment were poor black men, but they did not see this as problematic. Not until 1973, after a journalist broke the story to the general public, did the black medical establishment denounce the study as morally, ethically, and scientifically unjustified. By then, a modern black civil rights movement and a popular health movement critical of medicine resulted in an atmosphere of changed consciousness about rights and responsibilities.[24]

Why did black health professionals, including Rivers, not challenge the study? Dr. Paul B. Cornely of Howard University, a black public health leader since the 1930s, remembered with regret that he knew about the experiment from the beginning. He understood the nature of the study and had followed it all along, never questioning it. He explained in retrospect: "I was there and I didn't say a word. I saw it as an academician. It shows you how we looked at human beings, especially blacks who were expendable." Cornely taught about the study in his classes at the Medical School of Howard University, a black college in Washington, D.C., yet no student ever raised a challenge to what he now sees as its racist premise. Dr. Cornely asked himself why he did not see the full ramifications of the project. "I have guilt feelings about it, as I view it now," he explained, "because I considered myself to be an activist. I used to get hot and bothered about injustice and inequity, yet here right under my nose something is happening and I'm blind."[25]

No doubt a number of factors contributed to the response of black professionals, including class consciousness, professional status, and racial subordination. Historian Tom W. Shick argued that the black medical profession did not challenge the experiment because "black physicians were clearly subordinates, never co-equals, within the medical profession." Furthermore, he believed that the process of professionalization in medicine led them to defend the status quo. James Jones stated that class consciousness permitted black professionals to deny the racism of the experiment.[26]

Although subordinate status no doubt constrained the response of black professionals, they did not protest the syphilis study because they did not view it as unjust. Indeed, black educators and health professionals supported the study because they saw it directing federal attention toward black health problems—a primary goal of the black public health movement. As far as they were concerned, this was a study that focused the objective gaze of science on the health conditions of African Americans. It was one more way to increase the visibility of black needs to the federal government. Rivers shared the viewpoint of black health professionals and assisted with the experiment in the belief that the study was itself a sign of government interest in black health problems.

Why, despite a history of well-founded suspicion of government, did black tenant farmers take part in the government study? Large numbers of poor African-American men and women came to the government clinics because of the impact of the Tuskegee Movable School and Rivers. The experiment began in October 1932 as Rivers assisted the USPHS in recruiting and testing rural black people in Macon County for syphilis so physicians could identify candidates for the study. Rivers was familiar with this work because she had assisted with the earlier syphilis treatment project sponsored by the Rosenwald Fund. Most likely her presence contributed to local interest in the clinics; Rivers and the government physicians were overwhelmed by the number of people who showed up at the sites to have their blood tested.[27]

Equal numbers of women and men appeared at the clinic sites, which proved to be a problem because the government doctors had decided to study only men. Dr. Joseph Earle Moore of Johns Hopkins University School of Medicine suggested the study focus on men because, he argued, women's symptoms of syphilis at the early stage were usually mild, and it was more difficult for physicians to examine internal organs.[28] Yet, as much as the doctors and Rivers tried to test only men, women showed up at the clinics, too. Attempts to segregate the men led to new problems. According to Dr. Vonderlehr, "In trying to get a larger number of men in the primary surveys during December we were accused in one community of examining prospective recruits for the Army."[29] Rivers reported that some of the women, especially the wives of the men selected for the study, were mad that they were not included because "they were sick too." Some even told her, "Nurse Rivers, you just partial to the men."[30]

Jones cited Charles Johnson's 1934 investigation of African Americans in Macon County, *Shadow of the Plantation*, as evidence that poor African Americans participated in the study because of their tradition of dependence and obedience to authority.[31] Yet, Jones's own work suggests that poor African Americans in fact questioned authority, including that of white physicians. For example, Jones described one man who criticized the way a government doctor drew blood samples and recounted how "he lay our arm down like he guttin' a hog." The man reported: "I told him he hurt me. . . . He told me 'I'm the doctor.' I told him all right but this my arm."[32] Rivers remembered that sometimes the young white doctors would behave rudely toward the men and the men would ask her to intervene. A man told her once: "Mrs. Rivers, go in there and tell that white man to stop talking to us like that." So she went in and said: "Now, we don't talk to our patients like this. . . . They're human. You don't talk to them like that." The doctor even apologized.[33]

Rural African Americans cooperated not out of deference to white doctors but because they wanted medical attention and treatment for their ailments, and they had come to trust Nurse Rivers as someone who helped them. Even though the government doctors in the study changed over the years, Rivers provided the continuity. Without her assistance it is doubtful that the experiment would have been able to continue for so long with such cooperation from the subjects of the experiment. In addition, participating in the study gave these tenant farmers increased status as they gained an official association with both the prestigious Tuskegee Institute and the federal government, relationships typically unavailable to men of their class.

The men stayed with the study for forty years because they believed that they received something worthwhile. Rivers found that the men who joined the study "had all kinds of complaints" about what ailed them, and they continued with the study in order to get free treatments. However, the men joined under false pretenses because the health workers never informed the men that they had syphilis or that they would not receive treatment. Instead, the men were told they would be treated for "bad blood," a vague term that referred to a range of ailments, including general malaise. The men were not told that they could spread the disease to their sexual partners or that they were part of an experiment predicated on nontreatment of syphilis until death. What the USPHS provided was annual physical examinations, aspirin, free hot meals on the day the government physicians visited, and financial support for burial expenses. In a rural community where there was almost no formal health care available, and if poor black people could locate it they could not afford it, the study did provide certain types of limited benefits that convinced the men to stay with the study.[34]

As for Rivers, what motivated her to work for the experiment for so many years? Historians have argued that Rivers participated because, first, she could not have understood the full ramifications of the study, and second, as a black female nurse she was in no position to challenge the authority of the white male physicians.[35] Evidence suggests, however, that Rivers had sufficient knowledge of the study to know that the men were systematically denied treatment. Rivers was one of the authors, listed first, of a follow-up paper about the study published in 1953 in *Public Health Reports*. However, even if Rivers herself did not write the report, which read like a tribute to her role in the study, her actions made clear that she was well aware of the terms of the experiment. After all, she was one of the people who helped to implement the policy, designed by the leaders of the USPHS, to prohibit the subjects of the study from receiving treatments for syphilis from anyone else. This meant denying the treatment available during the 1930s, even if it was highly toxic mercury ointment and a long series of painful salvarsan injections, and after World War II when penicillin became available. At the same time that Rivers assisted with the treatment of syphilis in other public health programs, she helped carry out the experiment's plan to bar the men in the study from treatment.[36]

Finally, based upon how Rivers operated as a nurse, suggestions that she merely deferred to authority are not convincing. She no doubt knew how to tailor her comments and behavior to a given situation to preserve her position and dignity. However, despite the racial, gender, and medical hierarchies under which she operated, she saw herself as an advocate for her patients and acted accordingly. She did not hesitate to intervene on their behalf, even consulting one doctor when she questioned the procedures of another.

If ignorance and deference do not explain her behavior, what does? Her need for employment and the prestige of working for the federal government certainly contributed to her participation. She was proud of her work, and the federal government honored her for her assistance in the experiment. For example, in 1958 she received an award from the Department of Health, Education, and Welfare "for an outstanding contribution to health, through her participation in the long-term study of venereal disease control in Macon County, Alabama."[37]

Most importantly, Rivers considered her participation in the study merely a continuation of her previous public health work. Public health work was gendered to the extent that women, especially in their capacity as nurses, implemented health policy at the local level and had the most contact with people in the community. In Rivers's case, since the early 1920s her job had been to provide health education directly to people in the communities surrounding Tuskegee. Her duty as a nurse was to care for her clients, and she did. In her work with the experiment, she genuinely cared about the men with whom she worked. One of the government physicians even told her that she was too sympathetic with the men. As Rivers explained: "I was concerned about the patients 'cause I had to live here after he was gone." Indeed, she knew each man individually and, after he died, she attended the funeral service with the man's family. "I was expected to be there," she recalled, "they were part of my family."[38] In nominating Rivers for an award in 1972, Thelma P. Walker revealed that Rivers "has been my inspiration for her enthusiasm. . . . She inspired such confidence in her patients and they all seem so endeared to her." Walker discovered "how deeply loved she was by the men in her follow-up program. They felt that there just was no one like Mrs. Rivers."[39]

When the press exposed the study in 1972, it was confusing and heartbreaking for Rivers to hear the criticism after receiving so much praise. Rivers responded by defending her actions. "A lot of things that have been written have been unfair," she insisted. "A lot of things." First, Rivers argued that the effects of the experiment were benign. In her mind it was important that the study did not include people who had early syphilis because those with latent syphilis were potentially less infectious and would be less likely to transmit it to their sexual partners. As she explained, "syphilis had done its damage with most of the people."[40] Yet, as historian Allan Brandt noted, "every major textbook of syphilis at the time of the Tuskegee Study's inception strongly advocated treating syphilis even in its latent stages."[41] Furthermore, evidence suggests that not all of the men had latent syphilis, given that when men in the control group (about 200 black men without syphilis) developed syphilis, the physicians merely switched them over to the untreated syphilitic group.

Second, Rivers accounted for her participation by stating that the study had scientific merit. Even as she admitted, "I got with this syphilitic program that was sort of a hoodwink thing, I suppose," she offered justification. With great exaggeration, she depicted Macon County as "overrun with syphilis and gonorrhea. In fact, the rate of syphilis in the Negro was very, very high, something like eighty percent or something like this."[42] She recalled that the USPHS doctors planned to compare the results of the study with one in Norway on white people and that "the doctors themselves have said that the study has proven that syphilis did not affect the Negro as it did the white man."[43]

Finally, based on the available health care resources, Rivers believed that the benefits of the study to the men outweighed the risks. She knew the men received no treatment for syphilis, but she explained:

> Honestly, those people got all kinds of examinations and medical care that they never would have gotten. I've taken them over to the hospital and they'd have a GI series on them, the heart, the lung, just everything. It was just impossible for just an ordinary person to get that kind of examination.[44]

She continually asserted that the men received good medical care despite the fact that the men received mostly diagnostic, not curative, services. Yet she maintained

> they'd get all kinds of extra things, cardiograms and . . . some of the things that I had never heard of. This is the thing that really hurt me about the unfair publicity. Those people had been given better care than some of us who could afford it.[45]

What bothered Rivers was not the plight of the men in the study but that of the women and men who came to her begging to be included, even leading her occasionally to sneak in some additional men. As for the men in the experiment, Rivers concluded that they received more, not less, than those around them: "They didn't get treatment for syphilis, but they got so much else."[46]

Racism, extreme poverty, and health care deprivation in rural Alabama, where so little medical attention could mean so much, contributed to a situation in which white doctors from the federal government could carry out such an experiment. One of the legacies of the syphilis experiment is the reluctance of many

African Americans to cooperate with government public health authorities in HIV/AIDS health education and prevention programs out of the fear of a genocidal plot.[47]

The Tuskegee Syphilis Study also relied on the assistance of black professionals. Nurse Eunice Rivers, as well as health workers and educators from Tuskegee Institute, Howard University, and the National Medical Association, never challenged the study because they believed that it was an acceptable way to gather knowledge. Rivers and other black professionals shared the dominant vision of scientific research and medical practice and did not consider issues of informed consent or the deadly consequences of such an experiment. Perhaps professionalization and class consciousness blinded them to the high price paid by the poor, rural black men in the study.[48]

Yet, ironically, black professionals saw this experiment as consistent with their efforts to improve black health. After public censure forced the halt of the experiment, Rivers declared her innocence in the face of criticism, not on the grounds that she was a victim who was uniformed about the true nature of the experiment but rather because she insisted that she had acted on her convictions. She emphasized:

> I don't have any regrets. You can't regret doing what you did when you knew you were doing right. I know from my personal feelings how I felt. I feel I did good in working with the people. I know I didn't mislead anyone.[49]

Rivers remained convinced that she had acted in the best interests of poor black people.

Black professionals faced a dilemma imposed by American racism in how best to provide adequate health services to the poor within a segregated system. Furthermore, the gendered nature of public health work meant that the nurse, invariably a woman, was at the center of public provisions, both good and bad. Thus, the role of Eunice Rivers has drawn particular attention. As her actions show most starkly, black professionals demonstrated both resistance to and complicity with the government and the white medical establishment as they attempted to advance black rights and improve black health. Rivers and other black professionals counted on the benefits of public health work to outweigh the costs to the poor. In the case of the Tuskegee Movable School they were undoubtedly right, but as the Tuskegee Syphilis Experiment shows, there were dire consequences when they were wrong.

NOTES
This article is based on material drawn from my book, *Sick and Tired of Being Sick and Tired: Black Women's Health Activism in America, 1890–1950* (University of Pennsylvania Press, 1995).
I thank the following for their comments on earlier versions: Andrea Friedman, Vanessa

Northington Gamble, Linda Gordon, Susan Hamilton, Darlene Clark Hine, Judith Walzer Leavitt, Gerda Lerner, Donald Macnab, Leslie Reagan, Leslie Schwalm, the University of Wisconsin-Madison Women's History Dissertators' Group, the audience at the Ninth Berkshire Conference on the History of Women at Vassar College, New York, June 1993, and my students at the University of Alberta. This research was supported by a Women's Studies Research Grant and a Rural Policy Fellowship, both from the Woodrow Wilson National Fellowship Foundation. I also thank archivists Aloha South, at the National Archives in Washington, D.C., and Daniel T. Williams, at Tuskegee University, for their assistance. Finally, special thanks to Dr. Paul Cornely for sharing his memories with me.

1. James H. Jones, *Bad Blood: The Tuskegee Syphilis Experiment* (New York: Free Press, 1981; expanded edition 1993), 91 (page numbers refer to the 1981 edition). See also Allan Brandt, "Racism and Research: The Case of the Tuskegee Syphilis Study," in *Sickness and Health in America: Readings in the History of Medicine and Public Health*, ed. Judith Walzer Leavitt and Ronald L. Numbers (Madison: University of Wisconsin Press, 1985), 331–343; Tom W. Shick, "Race, Class, and Medicine: 'Bad Blood' in Twentieth-Century America," *Journal of Ethnic Studies* 10 (Summer 1982): 97–105; and Todd L. Savitt, "The Use of Blacks for Medical Experimentation and Demonstration in the Old South," *Journal of Southern History* 48 (August 1982): 331–348.

2. Herbert M. Morais, *The History of the Negro in Medicine* (New York: Publishers Company for the Association for the Study of Negro Life and History, 1967), 100–101.

3. Eunice Rivers Laurie, interview by A. Lillian Thompson, 10 October 1977, in *The Black Women Oral History Project*, vol. 7. ed. Ruth Edmonds Hill (New Providence, N.J.: K. G. Saur Verlag, A Reed Reference Publishing Company, 1992), 213–242, from the Arthur and Elizabeth Schlesinger Library, Radcliffe College. See also Jones, *Bad Blood*, 6, 158; Brandt, "Racism and Research," 337; Darlene Clark Hine, *Black Women in White: Racial Conflict and Cooperation in the Nursing Profession, 1890–1950* (Bloomington: Indiana University Press, 1989), 154–156.

4. M. M. Hubert to Thomas Campbell, May 26, 1922, Box 101, Correspondence 1922, Record Group 33, U.S. Extension Service, National Archives, Washington, D.C.; B. D. Mayberry, "The Role of Tuskegee University in the Origin, Growth and Development of the Negro Extension Service," unpublished manuscript (1988), 111, author's possession; Thomas Monroe Campbell, *The Movable School Goes to the Negro Farmer* (Tuskegee Institute: Tuskegee Institute Press, 1936; reprint, New York: Arno Press and the New York Times, 1969), 145.

5. Monroe Work, "Racial Factors and Economic Forces in Land Tenure in the South," *Social Forces* 15 (December 1936): 214–215; Charles S. Johnson, *Shadow of the Plantation* (Chicago: University of Chicago Press, 1934), 7, 104, 109, 112, 128; Pete Daniel, *Standing at the Crossroads: Southern Life Since 1900* (New York: Hill and Wang, 1986), 7.

6. Dr. Hildrus A. Poindexter, "Special Health Problems of Negroes in Rural Areas," *Journal of Negro Education* 6 (July 1937): 400, 403, 412; U.S. Public Health Service, "Report to Congress on the Extent and Circumstances of Cooperation by the Public Health Service with State and Local Authorities in the Drought Stricken Areas Under the Provisions of the Deficiency Act of February 6, 1931," March 1, 1931 to November 30, 1931, General Files, 1924–1935, Box 99, Record Group 90, United States Public Health Service (hereafter USPHS), National Archives, Washington, D.C.

7. Campbell, *The Movable School*, 118, 121, 126; Thomas Campbell, "Extension Work Among Negroes in the South," Correspondence 1935, Box 290, Record Group 33, U.S. Extension Service; *Rural Messenger* 1 (26 May 1920): 9; Thomas Campbell, Report of Movable School Work to Washington, D.C., August 1922, Box 6, Tuskegee Institute Extension Service Collection, Hollis Burke Frissell Library, Tuskegee University, Tuskegee, Ala.

8. Monroe N. Work, "The South's Labor Problem," *South Atlantic Quarterly* 19 (January 1920): 7–8 (located in finding aids folder, Monroe Nathan Work Papers, Hollis Burke Frissell

Library, Tuskegee University, Ala.). See also Pete Daniel, *The Shadow of Slavery: Peonage in the South, 1901–1969* (Urbana: University of Illinois Press, 1972, 1990); Daniel, *Standing at the Crossroads*, 54–58.

9. Stanley Rayfield, Marjory Stimson, and Louise M. Tattershall, "A Study of Negro Public Health Nursing," *Public Health Nurse* 22 (October 1930): 525; Karen Buhler-Wilkerson, "False Dawn: The Rise and Decline of Public Health Nursing in America, 1900–1930," in *Nursing History: New Perspectives, New Possibilities*, ed. Ellen Condliffe Lagemann (New York: Teachers College Press, 1983), 89–106; Barbara Melosh, *"The Physician's Hand": Work, Culture and Conflict in American Nursing* (Philadelphia: Temple University Press, 1982), chapter 4; Hine, *Black Women in White*, Introduction.

10. Uva M. Hester's report for her work in Montgomery County for the week of June 19, 1920 is reprinted in Campbell, *The Movable School*, 113–115, especially 113.

11. Eunice Rivers Laurie, interview, *The Black Women Oral History Project*, 220, 224; see also 216–219. See also Henry Howard, Report of Movable School, 1923, Extension Agents Reports, Alabama, microfilm reel 11, p. 2, Record Group 33, U.S. Extension Service; Jones, *Bad Blood*, 109–110; Hine, *Black Women in White*, 134, 154; Susan M. Reverby, "Laurie, Eunice Rivers (1899–1986)," in *Black Women in America: An Historical Encyclopedia*, ed. Darlene Clark Hine (New York: Carlson Publishing, 1993), 699–701.

12. Eunice Rivers, "Health Work with a Movable School," *Public Health Nurse* 18 (November 1926): 575–577; Eunice Rivers, reports on her Movable School work, monthly reports for 1924, Box 6, Tuskegee Institute Extension Service Collection; Eunice Rivers Laurie, interview, *The Black Women Oral History Project*, 228; Jones, *Bad Blood*, 110; Hine, *Black Women in White*, 154.

13. *Proceedings of Session on Negro Social Work at the Alabama Conference of Social Work*, Birmingham, April 9, 1929, Box 1, Work Papers, p. 15; T. J. Woofter, "Organization of Rural Negroes for Public Health Work," *National Conference of Social Work Proceedings*, fiftieth session (1923): 72.

14. J. D. Barnes, "Serving the Community," printed in *Southern Letter* 45 (March–April 1929): 2.

15. Eunice Rivers Laurie, interview, *The Black Women Oral History Project*, 234.

16. *Ibid.*, 230.

17. Rivers, quoted in Jones, *Bad Blood*, 111.

18. *Annual Report of the Surgeon General of the Public Health Service of the United States for the fiscal year 1918* [hereafter *Annual Report of the USPHS*] (Washington, D.C.: U.S. Government Printing Office, 1918), 97; *Annual Report of the USPHS* (1919), 281, 297; Allan M. Brandt, *No Magic Bullet: A Social History of Venereal Disease in the United States Since 1880* (New York: Oxford University Press, 1987), 56, 77.

19. Paul Carley and O. C. Wenger, "The Prevalence of Syphilis in Apparently Healthy Negroes in Mississippi," *Journal of the American Medical Association*, June 7, 1930, Box 356, Record Group 51, Mississippi Department of Health, Mississippi Department of Archives and History, Jackson, Miss.; *Annual Report of the USPHS* (1929), 273; "Recent Progress in the Program of the Julius Rosenwald Fund in Negro Health," [1938?], p. 9, Central File 1937–1940, Box 599, Record Group 102, Children's Bureau, National Archives, Washington, D.C.; Jones, *Bad Blood*, 54, 59–60.

20. Louis T. Wright, "Factors Controlling Negro Health," *Crisis* 42 (September 1935): 264. See also Jones, *Bad Blood*, 23; Brandt, *No Magic Bullet*, 157–158; Brandt, "Racism and Research," 332; Elizabeth Fee, "Sin vs. Science: Venereal Disease in Baltimore in the Twentieth Century," *Journal of the History of Medicine and Allied Sciences* 43 (April 1988): 141–164.

21. Report to the Public Health Service by Dr. Vonderlehr, July 10, 1933, Division of Venereal Diseases, general records 1918–1936, Box 182, Record Group 90, USPHS; Jones, *Bad Blood*, 27, 88, 92–95, 167. See also Brandt, *No Magic Bullet*, 40; Brandt, "Racism and Research," 333–334. My thanks to Vanessa Northington Gamble for clarifying the ways in which the Oslo study differed from the Tuskegee Syphilis Study.

22. Robert Moton to Hugh Cumming, October 10, 1932, general correspondence, Box 180, Robert Russa Moton Papers; Eugene Dibble to Robert Moton, September 17, 1932, general correspondence, Box 180, Moton Papers; Jones, *Bad Blood*, 74, 76.

23. Pete Daniel, "Black Power in the 1920s: The Case of Tuskegee Veterans Hospital," *Journal of Southern History* 36 (August 1970): 368–388; Vanessa Northington Gamble, "The Negro Hospital Renaissance: The Black Hospital Movement, 1920–1945," in *The American General Hospital: Communities and Social Contexts*, ed. Diana E. Long and Janet Golden (Ithaca: Cornell University Press, 1989), 101–2.

24. Roscoe C. Brown to W. Harry Barnes, president of the National Medical Association, May 27, 1936, and Roscoe C. Brown to Assistant Surgeon General Robert Olesen, September 2, 1936, Group IX, general records 1936–1944, Box 195, Record Group 90, USPHS; "Final Report of the National Medical Association Tuskegee Syphilis Study Ad Hoc Committee," August 1, 1973, p. 13, Moorland-Springarn Research Center, Howard University, Washington, D.C.; Jones, *Bad Blood*, 7; Brandt, *No Magic Bullet*, 158.

25. Dr. Paul B. Cornely, interview by the author, tape recording, Howard University, Washington, D.C., July 24, 1989.

26. Shick, "Race, Class and Medicine," 104–105; Jones, *Bad Blood*, 167–168.

27. Eugene Dibble to Monroe Work, September 9, 1933, general correspondence, Box 180, Moton Papers; *Annual Report of the USPHS* (1933), 96–97; Jones, *Bad Blood*, 68–69, 111, 114; Brandt, "Racism and Research," 335.

28. Jones, *Bad Blood*, 104.

29. Vonderlehr, quoted in Jones, *Bad Blood*, 120.

30. Eunice Rivers, quoted in Jones, *Bad Blood*, 165.

31. Jones, *Bad Blood*, 68.

32. Quoted in Jones, *Bad Blood*, 80.

33. Eunice Rivers Laurie, interview, *The Black Women Oral History Project*, 232.

34. Eunice Rivers, Stanley H. Schuman, Lloyd Simpson, and Sidney Olansky, "Twenty Years of Followup Experience In a Long-Range Medical Study," *Public Health Reports* 68 (April 1953): 393; Jones, *Bad Blood*, 6, 69, 71, 73, 114; Brandt, "Racism and Research," 335, 339; Hine, *Black Women in White*, 155–156.

35. Jones, *Bad Blood*, 163–164, 166; Brandt, "Racism and Research," 337 (note at bottom of page).

36. Eunice Rivers *et al.*, "Twenty Years of Followup," 391–395; Catherine Corley, Department of Public Health, Alabama, to Eunice Rivers Laurie, Macon County Health Department, May 26, 1953, Eunice Rivers Laurie folder, Biographical files, Hollis Burke Frissell Library, Tuskegee University, Tuskegee, Ala.; Jones, *Bad Blood*, 7, 46, 161–162, 178.

37. Eunice Rivers Laurie, interview, *The Black Women Oral History Project*, 237; Jones, *Bad Blood*, 169.

38. Jones, *Bad Blood*, 128, 155, 160–161.

39. Thelma P. Walker, nomination letter for Eunice Rivers Laurie, January 11, 1972, Eunice Rivers Laurie folder, Biographical Files.

40. Eunice Rivers Laurie, interview, *The Black Women Oral History Project*, 231. See also Jones, *Bad Blood*, 107.

41. Brandt, "Racism and Research," 333.

42. Eunice Rivers Laurie, interview, *The Black Women Oral History Project*, 229–230.

43. Eunice Rivers Laurie, interview, *The Black Women Oral History Project*, 232; see also 230–232; Jones, *Bad Blood*, 167.

44. Eunice Rivers Laurie, interview, *The Black Women Oral History Project*, 231.

45. Eunice Rivers Laurie, interview, *The Black Women Oral History Project*, 232.

46. Jones, *Bad Blood*, 164–165. Darlene Clark Hine found the explanations of James Jones

"compelling" but suggested the possibility that Rivers "viewed the study as a way of ensuring for at least some blacks an unparalleled amount of medical attention." Hine, *Black Women in White*, 156.

47. Stephen B. Thomas and Sandra Crouse Quinn, "The Tuskegee Syphilis Study, 1932 to 1972: Implications for HIV Education and AIDS Risk Education Programs in the Black Community," *American Journal of Public Health* 81 (November 1991): 1498–1505.

48. Jones, *Bad Blood*, 97, 188–189; Jay Katz, *The Silent World of Doctor and Patient* (New York: The Free Press, 1984), xvi, 1–4; David J. Rothman, *Strangers at the Bedside* (New York: Basic Books, 1991), 10, 47–48, 90, 247.

49. *Jet* [1973?], Eunice Rivers Laurie folder, Biographical Files.

RETHINKING THE TUSKEGEE SYPHILIS STUDY

Nurse Rivers, Silence, and the Meaning of Treatment

SUSAN M. REVERBY

More than twenty-five years after its widespread public exposure, the Tuskegee Syphilis Study continues to stand as the prime American example of medical arrogance, nursing powerlessness, abusive state power, bureaucratic inertia, unethical behavior, and racism in research. For historians of nursing and medicine, the so-called study's complexities still remain a site for continued reexamination as new primary research is explored and changing analytic frames are applied. The study was a forty-year (1932–72) "experiment" by the U.S. Public Health Service (PHS) to study "untreated syphilis in the male Negro"[1] The 399 men, who were positive for latent syphilis, thought they were being treated, not studied, for their "bad blood," a term used in the black community to encompass syphilis, gonorrhea, and anemia.

The study is often seen as a morality tale for many among the African American public and the nursing/medical research community, serving as our most horrific example of a racist "scandalous story . . . when government doctors played God and science went mad," as one publisher's publicity billed it.[2] This story has been told and taught in many different forms: in rumors, historical monographs, videos, documentaries, plays, poems, music, and an HBO Emmy–and Golden Globe award–winning movie, and at the ill-fated hearings on Dr. Henry Foster's nomination for the U.S. surgeon general's position in 1995.

For forty years the study went on as research reports were written and published in respected medical journals. The men were watched, examined, intentionally untreated, given spinal taps euphemistically referred to as "back shots," promised burial insurance, autopsied, misled, and lied to until 1972, when an Associated Press reporter broke the story nationwide. What followed was national outrage, a Senate hearing, a multimillion-dollar lawsuit filed by civil rights attorney Fred Gray, a federal investigation, and some financial pay-out to the survivors or their heirs that still continues. And in a White House ceremony on 16 May 1997, twenty-five years after the study ended, President Bill Clinton finally

Susan M. Reverby is professor of women's studies at Wellesley College.
Originally published in the Nursing History Review 7 (1999): 3–28. Reprinted by permission of the Nursing History Review.

tendered a formal federal government apology to all the men involved in front of a national television audience, a satellite hook-up to the Tuskegee community, and six of the remaining ailing and aging survivors and their families.[3]

With this moving formality, many may have considered the story of the study over. Yet in the glare of television lights, the pomp of the White House ceremony, the survivors' living memorial to racialized medicine, and the emphasis on emotionality in the media coverage, it is easy to elide what novelist Ralph Ellison differentiated between "shadow" and "act," to be uncertain what is "image" and what is "reality." Those categories, eloquently called forth by Ellison nearly fifty years ago to critique Hollywood's version of African American experiences, could not, however, be separated as simply as Ellison had hoped.[4] The "shadow" of the study, embedded in the "act" of the complex narratives of race, class, gender, medicine, and sexuality is, in the words of a Tuskegee colloquialism, "in the back, in the dark, in the corner, in the booth," even in the White House's East Room.[5]

The historian's task is to peer into those spaces, to explore why and how, and the consequences of the theatricality and narratives of race (embedded in class, sexuality and gender) as they are created in very specific historical circumstances.[6] With the Tuskegee study, historians have, for the most part, tried to understand judiciously the circumstances that shaped what is ultimately an experience of black victimization by racist means.[7] However, our understanding of the study can be deepened if we reconsider how we "listen" to the various stories and the analytic frames we self-consciously apply.

I will do this by listening attentively to the voice of one of key actors in this drama: public-health nurse Eunice Rivers Laurie. This will require a consideration of how race, gender, sexuality, and class are linked to create a politics of listening, representation, and experience that suggest what historian Evelynn M. Hammonds calls the differing "geometry" of the history of black women's representation/reality.[8]

My focus will thus be on the dilemmas for Nurse Rivers (as she was known throughout her professional life), who was the critical go-between, linking the African American men of the study to the PHS, Tuskegee Institute, and the state and local health department.[9] Nurse Rivers, who stayed with the study during its entire history, is often seen by many as its most disturbing figure, both functioning with invisibility and hypervisibility as the story is told.[10] Many have argued that she was duped, an African American Tuskegee-based public-health nurse kept ignorant of the real implications of the study and a nurse of her generation willing to do what the doctors ordered, especially when those orders came from the black physicians at Tuskegee, the white doctors of the PHS, and the local health department where she also worked. Others have seen her as the epitome of the race traitor, willing to use her class power within the black community to keep her job and sell out the rural men under her charge.[11] Any effort, however, to hear her explanations is very complicated; she spoke out very little after the story of the study broke and left few written documents.

Nurse Rivers' silences have seemed to make it possible for others to find the words for her, allowing her to be a cipher through which their own concerns and interpretations are written. She was, however, part of the tradition of black women who have spoken out—but whose choice of where to speak, what words to employ, and what silences to make use of require us to listen in ways our culture has taught many of us not to hear.[12] I will argue that by listening to how the concept of *treatment* is articulated, we can hear, not only as historian Evelyn Brooks Higginbotham notes how "these public servants encoded hegemonic articulation of race in the language of medical and scientific theory," but also a counternarrative produced by Nurse Rivers that reconfigures the race/medicine link through nursing and gender.[13]

To do this, we cannot just read Nurse Rivers' *testimony* (the little of it that does exist), as many historians and ethicists have done, nor merely imagine her thinking and rationales, as filmmakers, writers, and musical composers have done. Rather, we must attend to her *testifying*, what linguist Geneva Smitherman defines as "a ritualized form of communication in which the speaker gives verbal witness to the efficacy, truth, and power of some experience in which [the group has] shared."[14] If we listen to her testifying, I think we can obtain a deeper understanding of why an African American public-health nurse could become so enmeshed in this horrific study. And if we listen to this communal voice, we may begin to see how she used her experiences as a black woman and nurse to formulate an explanation of the study's dilemmas and to help the men caught in its web.[15]

To rethink the "study" and Nurse Rivers' role, the meaning of treatment itself must be reconsidered. In 1932, when the Tuskegee study first began, there were ongoing debates within the medical and nursing communities over the appropriate treatment for syphilis at its various stages, the accuracy of Wassermann tests, and the lack of randomization in the epidemiological evidence used to determine the prevalence of the disease.[16] The tensions between those who still thought that moral prophylaxis and rubber prophylactics (at best) were better than chemical treatments continued even after Ehrlich's discovery of Salvarsan. To be considered successful, these chemical treatments required sixty weekly visits (with anywhere from twenty to forty weeks considered necessary for any real impact) for often painful intramuscular injections.[17] Outside of major clinics and the particular practices of syphilologists, treatment was often uncertain at the hands of unskilled clinicians, follow-through was difficult, and the expense often a major deterrent to completion of the "cure." Medical uncertainty also existed over the treatment for latent syphilis cases, the supposed focus of the Tuskegee project.[18]

These debates took place within the economic realities of American medicine and the racial, class, and gender assumptions shaping medical understandings of the disease and the public-health strategies to combat it. In the face of overwhelming demand and increasingly limited funds, especially as the depression deepened, the reality of "treatment" for non-fee-for-service patients served by state and local health departments, came to mean no treatment at all, or minimal treatment "to render [patients] noninfectious to others, even though they had not themselves been cured."[19]

In Macon County, many of the local white physicians did not use intramuscular injections in their syphilis "treatment" and would not have provided care for indigent African Americans.[20] In many communities, physicians assumed that African Americans would not continue treatment (despite evidence that they would), although at the time "fully 80% of the entire American public could not afford syphilis therapy on a fee-for-service basis."[21] Beliefs that the disease was invasive in black communities because of supposedly inherent sexual promiscuity and medical assertions that blacks suffered from cardiovascular complications rather than neural ones, which they thought afflicted whites, suffused and shaped medical understandings of the disease and its so-called natural history.

When the actual Tuskegee study began, it was assumed at first that treatment in a medical sense would be provided, and even the PHS officials seemed to assure this. Both the local county health officer and the Tuskegee Institute officials who participated in significant ways discussed the extensive need for treatment in the community. Indeed, the men for the study were often "rounded up" (the term the officials used) at the very sites where others received their syphilis care.[22] The early exchange of letters among the PHS doctors, Tuskegee Institute officials, and the state and county health officials all show the kinds of treatment, however limited, that was being provided during the first year. It looked like a more or less typical PHS venereal disease control project.[23] But when it appeared that the money for treatment would run out, the PHS's Taliferrio Clark, the man who conceived the nontreatment study, wrote to a fellow physician at the Mayo Clinic in September 1932, bluntly declaring: "You will observe that our plan has nothing to do with treatment. It is purely a diagnostic procedure carried out to determine what has happened to the syphilitic Negro who has had no treatment."[24]

It was not just the PHS doctors, the local health department, and private physicians who agreed to the nontreatment. The Tuskegee Institute administrators, R. R. Moton, the institute's principal, and Dr. Eugene Dibble, the medical director of the institute's John A. Andrew Hospital, signed off on the "experiment." Their actions have to be seen in the context of the history of Tuskegee and its political culture.

Thus, this study did not just take place in some back corner of the rural South. Tuskegee as a place, both real and imagined, is central to the study's unfolding. It was and is a small southern city, serving as the urban center for Macon County,

Alabama, in an area of old plantations, sharecropping, sawmills, forests, and hard-scrabble living for the predominately black population.

As home to Tuskegee Institute, it has come to stand for both the incredible strength, endurance, and political savvy of African Americans and the site of one of the worst examples of American racism, co-optation, and exploitation. Its political culture was originally shaped by the old nineteenth-century "doctrine of reciprocity" between planter paternalism and seeming black submission that led to the founding of Tuskegee Institute (now Tuskegee University) under Booker T. Washington's iron-fisted leadership.[25] In the twentieth century, novelists Nella Larsen, Ralph Ellison, and Albert Murray powerfully captured the tensions that underlay the seeming calm of this culture, with its gradations of power between whites and blacks and within the black world (that were based on class, skin tone, education, urbanity, land ownership, gender, and a commitment to gentility).[26]

A generation of scholarship on the politics of Tuskegee has taught us that in everyday life and in hidden politics, such tensions gave way at times to compromises and at other times to grand eruptions of enormous political power.[27] It was in this layered world of surface cooperation with the Jim Crow system, coupled with the courting of white northern philanthropy and federal powers to subvert that system, that the Tuskegee Syphilis Study became a reality.[28]

In this political and cultural context, it may be that we can read both Moton's and Dibble's actions to mean that they hoped the study would actually show the lack of necessity for treatment in latent syphilis cases. They seemed to share the view of one of the PHS officials who told the federal investigating committee, "The study was conceived to try to determine if indeed the disease was worse than the treatment or vice versa."[29] Moton well may have thought it was a chance for the men to receive treatment when necessary, an opportunity for Tuskegee to participate in a study of international significance since there had been a retrospective study on whites in Oslo earlier in the century, possibly a way to show that other more cost-efficient forms of treatment might be found, or to screen out those who might not need extensive care. Moton himself (forever immortalized in part as President Bledsoe in Ellison's *Invisible Man*) was also well aware of class differences in the disease incidence in the black community, indeed proudly sharing with one of Tuskegee's white trustees that black secondary school students had an even lower rate of the disease than whites.[30]

Thus, both Moton and Dibble may have hoped that a different way to understand treatment, in the context of the reality of the southern black experience, might be possible. They may have also thought that this study would be one more nail in the coffin that would allow for the burial of the myth of black and white biological difference because of the comparison to whites in the Oslo study. As with the daily decisions that men like Moton and Dibble had to make at Tuskegee, and in following the traditions set up by Tuskegee's founder, Booker T. Washington, I suspect they merely transferred to another realm their daily efforts to find, what historian Martin Pernick called in another medical circumstance, an appropriate "calculus of suffering" that balanced financial exigencies with overwhelming need.[31] They may also have believed they were doing their best for the rural poor while trying to "uplift the race" through research.

As the study progressed, however, most of the men received neither a comprehensive course of the then-known medical treatments (nor penicillin when it became available in the late 1940s), nor did the autopsies show there was no need to treat even the latent cases, as evidence of the ravages of the disease was documented.[32] Indeed, the very language of the medical reports perpetuated the assumption that there was something "natural" about the failure to treat, with no acknowledgment of the role of the physician researchers in making sure this "natural" event happened.[33]

The men were never seen as individual patients because the lack of treatment was naturalized; it was the study's bedrock. As historian Susan Lederer has argued provocatively, the PHS researchers may have seen the men neither as patients nor as subjects, but as "cadavers, that had been identified while still alive," and the study as part of the longstanding use of indigent black men and women as "research animals."[34] As the PHS's Dr. Wenger put it bluntly: "As I see it, we have no further interest in these patients until they die."[35]

Despite the fact that the PHS officers thought they had a captured population that was supposed to be kept from treatment, some of the men both found ways to be treated and joined the great migration out of the rural South. Despite the PHS, for many of the men the study became one of *under*treated syphilis rather than purely untreated syphilis.

The exact numbers for whom there was undertreatment, rather than no treatment at all, shifted over time in the explanations given by the researchers. As the authors of the thirty-year report on the study somewhat reluctantly noted, "Approximately 96% of those examined had received some therapy other than an incidental antibiotic injection and perhaps as many as 33% had curative therapy."[36] Despite efforts made throughout the forty-year period to keep the men from treatment, some of the men (and we will never know how many) were able in various ways, often unknowingly, to slip out of the PHS's control to receive medicine for other ills that affected the course of their syphilis-related conditions as well.

For most of the men, their real experience with treatment revolved around the caregiving of public-health nurse Eunice Rivers Laurie. The PHS officials knew that any kind of research, just as in the real treatment programs for syphilis, would require the services of a public-health nurse who could be relied upon to reach out to the men and continue their interest.[37] "You belong to us," the men repeatedly told her as the study went on year after year.[38] Rivers did her work so well that even after the story of the study's deception broke, many of the men continued to call upon her and ask for her help. Twenty years later, survivors spoke movingly of her concern for them and her caregiving.[39] Others, of course, refused to have contact with her again.

Born in 1899 in Jakin, Georgia, Eunice Rivers was a Tuskegee Institute graduate with a good deal of public-health nursing experience by the time she was recommended for the "scientific assistant" position by Eugene Dibble, even though she told Dibble, " 'You know I don't know a thing about that.' "[40] She was thought to be one of the best nurses Tuskegee had produced. In her position with the PHS study (and with the support of Dr. Dibble and the institute's hospital), Eunice Rivers worked to find the subjects, drove them into Tuskegee for examinations, did the follow-up work, created the camaraderie that kept them in the study, helped in their assessment and in the provision of tonics and analgesics, assisted with the spinal taps, and encouraged the families to allow autopsies at the Tuskegee hospitals by promising and providing money for burial. She helped set up what was called "Miss Rivers' Lodge," an insurance scheme that guaranteed the men's families a decent burial in exchange for the men's participation in the examinations.[41] Although the doctors who were involved in the study changed regularly, Nurse Rivers was the constant.

When the story of the experiment broke in the press in 1972, Nurse Rivers retreated into a form of silence. She refused most interviews, did not give testimony before the Senate hearing, and only allowed herself to be interviewed once by the federal investigating team.[42] But two and a half years after the story came to light, she called her friends Helen Dibble (widow of the Tuskegee medical director) and Daniel Williams, Tuskegee's archivist, to her home one morning and began her "testifying." It is her testifying in 1975 to her friends, an interview with a former Tuskegee woman for the Schlesinger Library's Black Women's Oral History Project in 1977, her legal deposition, and her interview with historian James Jones that I will use to examine how she tells the treatment story.[43]

For Eunice Rivers, the men were patients, not subjects. Uncertain that she could really consider herself a "scientific assistant," she did feel comfortable as a nurse, even hanging the Nightingale Pledge on her living room wall.[44] Although she told Dibble she "didn't know much about that," she in fact learned.[45] She listened carefully to what the doctors told her. But she also wrote to the state health department's head nurse to ask for books on venereal disease.[46]

Describing the dangers of the 1930s treatment regimes, she claimed they were "really worse than the disease if it was not early syphilis," and again she said, "If syphilis was *not* active the treatment was worse than the disease."[47] Thus her narrative began with her view of treatment from a nursing perspective that sees the impact on the patient. She was aware of the pain and the suffering of the patient at the very moment of caregiving. In this way she differentiated early from late, latent syphilis, taking the uncertainty that existed in medical understandings of the disease to explain why it was appropriate to withhold treatment.

Nurse Rivers was doing the professional nursing work of caring. As an African American woman and member of the Tuskegee community, she was also healing, seeing that the men and their families got attention, bringing them baskets of food and clothing she could get from others. Although she maintained adamantly that as a nurse she never diagnosed, she argued equally that she cared.[48]

Reflecting on the data that suggests many of the men found various forms of treatment, she declared: "Now a lot of those patients that were in the study did get some treatment. There were very few who did not get any treatment."[49] She knew that "iron tonics, aspirin tablets and vitamin pills" are not treatments for syphilis. But she described these drugs as well as the physical exams as part of treatment. Within a very few minutes in one interview she emphasized the provision of these simple medications three different times. She said: "This was part of our medication that they got and sometimes they really took it and enjoyed it very much. And these vitamins did them a lot of good. They just loved those and they enjoyed that very very much." To emphasize her construction of these medications as "treatment," she pointed out others who tried to get into the study to get these "treatments." Her words suggest that she was choosing to emphasize the problems with the available drug regimens for the disease, the men's ability to be seen by a physician, and the provision of simple medications as a way to explain the kind of treating that was appropriate. Blinding herself from the idea that they were not directly treated for their syphilis, her sense of healing thus focused on her own caregiving role, the ways the men gained new knowledge about X rays and their own bodies, and the provision of "spring iron tonics" and aspirins they would not have gotten otherwise.[50]

Rivers' view of "treatment" was embedded in her conception of caring. For Eunice Rivers, above all, the work of the nurse was to care, especially for the African American community of which she was an integral part. In explaining her attraction to nursing, she declared: "I think if I had wanted to take medicine, I could have gone into medicine. . . . I never was interested in medicine as such. I was interested in the person, and it just never occurred to me that I wanted to be a doctor. I always felt that the nurse got closer to the patient than the doctor did, that was the way I felt about it."[51] Eunice Rivers found a way to solve what continued to be a dilemma for many public-health nurses: she saw herself as providing both preventive health nursing and "sick" nursing at the same time.[52] Well aware of the great needs of the impoverished community, she said directly, "These people were given good attention for their particular time."[53] And attention was what she gave: she listened to complaints, suggested ways to gain assistance, offered quiet comfort, provided simple medications. In a sense she was right. This was often more, and indeed a kind of treatment or healing, than many of the men she saw had ever had from health professionals. Indeed, if we think about the kinds of healing and therapeutics that were prevalent before the mid-twentieth century, we can even see Nurse Rivers' practice in a long line of caregivers.

We must consider, too, that her caring also brought power to Nurse Rivers.[54] She emphasized her role in bringing the men in, showing them around Tuskegee (which many of them had never seen), driving of a car. Laughingly, she reflected on how the men called their experience "Miss Rivers' study," but her chuckling suggests her sense that it was both not hers and hers in some real way.[55]

Nurse Rivers seems more troubled when she thinks about what penicillin meant for the treatment of syphilis (it became available by the late 1940s). When this topic comes up, her voice shifts and she speaks more slowly and directly about what the doctors have told her. She communicates in what sounds like a "just following orders" nursing voice.[56] She seems to be acknowledging that perhaps something may have been wrong; but then she immediately moves back into discussing the treatment of the early days. This suggests that when she is speaking about penicillin she is more directly troubled about the moral implications of withholding it.

Or, it can be surmised that she has lost the part of the nursing voice that gave her professional authority (the caring grounds) and shifted to the taking-orders position that, while morally protecting her in that time period, clearly troubles her years later.[57] Her shifting temporal sense suggests her moral qualms might have grown with the arrival of penicillin, but her views were so formed by the study's rationale and the earlier thinking that she almost cannot shift in her views, at least not in the 1940s.[58]

Rivers' language to explain her camaraderie with the men provides us with insight into her position, power, and the ways she negotiated her difficult middleground. In doing her work she spent hours in her car with the men, driving them into Tuskegee over rutted, muddy, and unpaved back country roads. For the men, the time with Nurse Rivers was also a break from the field work or day labor in the sawmills, small farms, and plantations that comprised their daily lives. In a short description of how the men joshed one another about "what they got" when they took their clothes off, she told historian James Jones about the following conversation in her car:

> I said, "Lord have Mercy." So what we did, we would all be men today, tomorrow, maybe we'll all be ladies. . . . Well, you see, when you've got one group together you can say anything. Tell 'em about anything. But if you got women and men, well you have to [be] careful about what you say, see. . . . You see. So when they want to talk and get in the ditch, they'd tell me, "Nurse Rivers, we're all men today!" . . . Oh we had a good time. We had a good time. Really and

truly. When we were working with those people, and when we first, and when we got started early that was the joy of my life."[59]

Thus when she described the talk in her car, she actually made a verbal gender shift and class switch that allowed her to join, or at least to hear, the men in their sexual bantering. Her position as a professional woman, representing what historian Darlene Clark Hine calls the "super-moral" black woman, would not normally make such a switch possible.[60] But Rivers, ever mindful of her position as a professional woman, caring for working-class men with a sexually transmitted disease, changed her verbal gender in order to shift, at least momentarily, her gendered class position. Although her place in the community and her representation is of a professional woman, in her car, while *she* was driving, literally moving liminally from rural country to the more urban Tuskegee, her gender, class, and sexualized hearing (if not her actually voicing) can invert in order for her to bond with the men.

Her description of her power also took on a shift of gendered racial power. It was within caring nursing work that Rivers saw her strengths. She entered nursing, at first, because of her father's suggestion. But, she said, "It was his decision but then it became a part of me. 'Cause really if it hadn't been, I never would have been a nurse. I had to make the decision within myself."[61] Although she worked within patriarchal authority and its influence, she did so with the belief that she shaped its limits and could indeed change her represented form when needed.

In order to understand how she saw her caring as a *form* of treatment, it is critical to see that she prided herself also on her ability to handle the white physicians. In these relationships, she is very much the "super-moral" black woman, responsible for representing the "race." She was the only one, she declared, who could control the temper of Dr. Wenger, one of the key PHS physicians in the study. She felt she could get the physicians to change their often insensitive and racist behavior toward the men. In her statements about the doctors and their relationships to the patients these themes of caring, power, and treatment come together. As she put it, she told the physicians: " 'Don't mistreat my patients. You don't mistreat them.' I said, 'Now, 'cause they don't have to come. And if you mistreat I will *not* let them up here to be mistreated.' "[62] Her use of the word *mistreat* three times in four sentences tells us that behavior in the provider-patient relationship is, for her, both caring and a form of treatment. The irony—that the major mistreatment in the study was the very absence or limited treatment in the clinical sense—is missing, however, from her words.

Rivers also told her Tuskegee students to maintain their dignity and their distance from the doctors. A public-health nurse she trained recalled that Rivers told her: "Never work with a physician who wants to use you. Don't let them pat you on the head because they'll think you want to drop your drawers. That way you can always stand up for what you believe."[63] Thus, while others have argued that she had to follow doctor's orders, this nurse's memories suggest that Rivers, like many nurses, knew there were ways to maintain one's dignity, limit the sexualizing of the nurse by the physician, and maintain respectability by setting careful limits on physicians' power.

Her respectability, dignity, and behavior are thus central to her sense of self in relationship to the doctors.[64] In dealing with the white doctors, she becomes not only hypervisible but also hypermoral, redefining black womanhood out of a sexual realm. In her car with the men, however, she shifted out of this gender position as a way to create a different sense of self and connection with the men, almost invisible and differently moral.

Rivers' form of code switching was thus between different gendered class positions. She was a devoted Tuskegee graduate, serving as president of Tuskegee's Nursing Alumnae Association and fighting to retain the school when it was threatened with closure.[65] As with other black professional women and in keeping with the Tuskegee spirit, she both separated herself from the "folk," given the caste lines that shaped the black experience in Tuskegee, and yet spoke their idiom (even if she had to change verbal gender to do so) and lived their lives in many ways. She demonstrated, when she had to, what historian Evelyn Brooks Higginbotham has called the "perceived centrality of female morality and female respectability to racial advancement."[66]

Rivers was a "race woman": someone whose whole life was devoted in her own terms to the betterment of African Americans as best she could. But our understanding of what this meant to her will have to be read in a complex and nuanced manner. Her tale of her upbringing emphasized her parents', and particularly her father's, efforts to make her see herself as different and important.[67] She described an attack upon her father by the Ku Klux Klan in Georgia for standing up to white oppression, his beating, and the shots that were fired into their home at night. Her father sent her off to a mission school but pulled her out before her last high school year. Rivers reports that he asked: " 'You all don't have anything there but white teachers?' " Linking these comments with his experiences with the Klan, Rivers narrates that her father then saw to it that she left the mission school to go to Tuskegee. Thus we can also read her belief in her ability to put the white doctors in their place and to shape how they treated the male "subjects" as her version of her father's commitment to the struggle against racism. As she stated in one interview, "Dr. Dibble knew that I really knew how to handle the white man."[68]

And it may also be that part of her story as a race woman and nurse is her silence. Evelynn M. Hammonds reminds us that "since silence about sexuality is being produced by black women and black feminist theorists, that silence itself suggests that black women do have some degree of agency."[69] Our understanding of Rivers' silence has to force us to hear both what she did and how she spoke about. Rivers' refusal to speak out and provide testimony may be because she had a different understanding of what had happened *and* because she was also felt she had to keep silent.

This is suggested in her struggle to explain her differences with one of the black physicians about whether she let patients get treatment. It is here that her testifying voice most clearly comes through. In his testimony before the federal investigating committee, Reginald James, who worked with Rivers on another venereal disease control out of the Macon County Health Department, claimed she would tell him not to treat patients who were in the study.[70] James's view is also corroborated by the repeated testimony of some of the surviving men who recalled that she kept them actively from getting treatment, even pulling one man out of the line at a penicillin treatment center in Birmingham in the late 1940s.[71] In her interview with her Tuskegee friends, Rivers declared:

> And Dr. James told folks up there in Washington I would not let him see the patients, that I would not let them get treatment. And when they told me that, I said I can't, I hate to dispute it. I said we're supposed to respect the medical profession but Dr. James is lying, saying, I, the only thing I would do, I would tell Dr. James this is one of the patients. Now it was up to him if he wanted to treat him. . . . So this is, ah ah, I don't know, but nobody knows what I went through here, you'd have thought I was a doctor mistreating the patients. [*her voice gets quieter*] And I, 'cause a lot of them, I don't know, I think that there was a lot of the jealousy with the medical profession and me, [*her voice gets stronger*] see, because they felt that I was not letting the patients get the treatment. I never told anybody that you couldn't get treatment. I told them, "So, go get . . . who's your doctor? If you want to go to the doctor, go and get your treatment." They didn't tell you you *couldn't* be treated. . . . They [the physicians] had to fall back on something, have an excuse, and maybe the medical profession was on them so they put it on me, that I wouldn't *let* the patients get the treatment.[72]

In a first reading this statement, it could be assumed that she was just forced to cover for the doctors and kept her silence. Her explanations resonate with the historic voice of many nurses who clearly understand the gender dynamics of the nurse/doctor relationship and who can articulate an anti-male or martyred nurse voice that serves as their form of resistance to oppression.[73] As in her other interviews, when she gets concerned about the study's moral morass, she retreats to "the nurse who just took orders and did not prescribe" voice.[74]

The use of interview sources and a rereading of archival materials suggests an alternative view of what her silences meant. Irene Beavers, a nurse who had been Rivers' student at Tuskegee and then her supervisor when she became director of nursing at the John A. Andrew Hospital at the Institute, provided a possible different interpretation. Mrs. Beavers described Rivers as a dignified "Harriet

Tubman" of nursing, an "underground railroad person who advised these people, not to be used." She recalled that Rivers told them during a lecture in her Tuskegee course on venereal disease control in the late 1940s (before the study was exposed):

> They [the men and their families] were not to tell that she had told them [that they were being used]. And there were several of them that . . . got treatment because she told the family to pick them up and bring them back. And take them to Birmingham . . . and they were treated for syphilis. . . . And she had to do it this way or she would have lost her job. . . . And the thing she was trying to get us to understand that as nurses you had a responsibility to yourself and to your counterparts and to your patients. . . . You had certain rights and there were some things you knew not to do. And you could make diagnoses too, although the physician felt he was the only person who could.[75]

Other public-health officials in Tuskegee said it would have been possible for her to have given the men penicillin from the local health department supplies, or to have gotten some of the other public-health nurses to provide it.[76]

One interview cannot, of course, serve as enough historical evidence for this way of understanding what Nurse Rivers might have done. Corroborative information would be necessary to at least suggest that she *might* have surreptitiously worked to get some men out of the study when she could. A hint of this comes briefly came from one of the federal investigating committee members, who, after interviewing her in 1972, wrote about her in a private letter to the committee's chairman. In the letter he stated that he both thought she followed doctors' orders and was "convinced . . . that she made treatment arrangements for any person in the untreated group upon his request."[77]

The third piece of evidence comes in a report from a PHS physician, Dr. Joseph Caldwell, who worked with her toward the end of the study. Writing to his superiors in 1970, he stated, "Once more, however, I began to doubt Nurse [Rivers] Laurie's conflicting loyalty to the project. Several times I have wondered whether she wears two hats—one of a Public Health Nurse, locally coordinating the Study and one of a local negro [sic] lady identifying with those local citizens—all of her race—who have been 'exploited' for research purposes."

Caldwell cited as his evidence a patient who had been lost to follow-up since 1944, but who somehow turned up in 1970 while Nurse Rivers was elsewhere. The man lived "four blocks from the old Macon County health department where all of [the] survey examinations were generally held." The man told Caldwell he and his wife were good friends of Nurse Rivers and her husband. Then the man told the PHS doctor, "He got penicillin shots, a full series, at the Macon County Health Department as soon as possible after 1944, when he first learned he had 'bad blood.' Perhaps I am being supersensitive," Caldwell concluded, "but this all seems to be a bit more than mere coincidence."[78]

Finally, when historian James Jones interviewed Rivers in 1977, he asked her directly about treatment. When they discussed the early forms of treatment (neo-arsphenamine and bismuth), she again emphasized her understanding of the nursing role, but she did so interestingly by answering him in the negative. "Nurses have so much responsibility today," she said. "But no, and I never told somebody *not* to take any medication." When Jones asked her the penicillin question by saying, "So how did you all go about keeping them from getting penicillin?" Rivers replied, "I don't know that we did." Jones then asked, "Did you try?" And Rivers answered: "No I did not try . . . to keep them, because I was never really told not to let them get penicillin. And we just had to trust that to those private physicians."[79]

All these differing sources suggest the possibility that while there was a "Miss Rivers' Lodge," to which the men paid with their lives and illnesses to gain a decent burial, there may also have been a "Miss Rivers' List" that got some of the men out of the study and into medical treatment.[80] We will never know how many men made it to the list. It could have been just this one man, perhaps, or it could have been many others, or none at all. In examining some of the patient records, I found that some of the men who left Macon County were treated elsewhere in the country; others actually got treatment at the Macon County Health Department. The PHS wanted total control over the men. But it was less complete in practice than we have been led to believe.

Rivers may also have been operating under a specific moral theory to make her decisions. First, following the arguments that ethicist and psychologist Carol Gilligan has made, we might agree that for Rivers "the moral problem arises from conflicting responsibilities rather than from competing rights and requires for its resolution contextual and inductive thinking rather than formal and abstract reasoning."[81] Second, historian Martin Pernick has argued that even before a rights' perspective developed around informed consent there was a sense of the importance of "truth-telling and consent-seeking" in medical practice in the nineteenth and early twentieth centuries.[82] While we could clearly argue there was little truth telling and no consent seeking on the part of the doctors, Rivers manifestly holds that she never lied and that she operated in a realm of mutuality. In this sense, she may have been operating from what other ethicists have called a " 'beneficence model' . . . where consent and disclosure comes primarily from an obligation to provide medical benefit rather than respect autonomy."[83]. While we could clearly argue that medical benefits were doubtful to nonexistent, Rivers clearly thought there was consent in the beneficence, but not in the rights, sense because the mutuality was one of nursing and caring.

Perhaps, after all, Rivers told only those she could trust. But choosing whom to trust was never easy for Nurse Rivers. In the context of the lawsuit that would bring compensation to the men and their heirs, she chose to testify as an martyred innocent, hinting at her moral agency, but primarily hiding by discussing "taking orders" or the dangers of some of the treatment for protection. In the face of the choice between naiveté and moral agency—but agency that would have implicated the black professionals in the conspiracy of knowledge and shown what a public-health nurse could do—she chose a careful line that erred on the side of duped innocence.

She avoided saying much about how her shifting gender position made possible her role in "treating" a sexually transmitted disease. The words to even explain this did not, of course, really even exist. As with many black women, as critic Mae Henderson has noted, Rivers had something to say but searched "for a way to say it" in a situation where "she had very little say."[84] She had to choose when to speak, with whom, and about what, a way of being that African American women have been practicing for generations.

In reality, we cannot really know about the extent of Rivers' own moral conflicts, especially after the study story broke. Those who were with her that fateful July day in 1972 when the media began to swarm said she retreated into a back room of the health department and wept.[85] The fragmentary evidence that does survive suggests that after 1972 she tried to reconsider her participation, to help the men as much as possible, and to rethink the meaning of treatment. Once Attorney Fred Gray began his legal proceedings, she retreated to almost complete silence. Mrs. Beavers stated Rivers was very savvy about legal issues in nursing and her silence and statements suggest just that.

In "testifying" about her position, she is giving "verbal witness to the efficacy, truth and power of some experience in which [the group has] shared."[86] In the context of Tuskegee in those years, with the lack of caring and health care available, she was truthfully providing treatment and care in a way that was understood by the Tuskegee doctors who had faith in her, by the men who truly loved what she did for them, and by the PHS physicians who were primarily grateful for her skills. She may have tried to find ways to work around class, race, and gender structures which shaped, but never totally controlled, her experience. As she told her students: "People may not like you for what you do, but if you are right they will respect you for what you do."[87]

I think we need to hear Nurse Rivers' words as representing the many voices that allowed her to accommodate and resist the pressures of race, class, profession, and gender at the very same moment in differing and subtle ways. The racism and sexism that provided the underpinnings for medical scientific arrogance has many differing faces, making possible many differing routes for resistance, and sometimes escape, for subjects and nurses. In the context of a Tuskegee culture that allowed for both racial accommodation and hidden resistance, perhaps Rivers really was finding the only position—a shifting one—she thought possible. That her changing position and multiple forms of speaking may also have created suffering and death alert us to the costs of expecting silence from a nurse and the dangers of an ethic of caring and beneficence without racial, gender, and class justice.

NOTES

Many people have contributed to this ongoing project during the last five years. Darlene Clark Hine first encouraged me to attempt this research and has kept me going. My gratitude for her faith in me is enormous. I also wish to thank Daniel Williams, Cynthia Wilson, James Jones, Evelynn M. Hammonds, Geeta Patel, Susan Bell, Barbara Rosenkrantz, Dixie Dysart, David Feldshuh, Jay Katz, and Allan Brandt for their ideas, suggestions, and insights. James Jones, in particular, has in this process been exceedingly generous with his materials, his time and his good counsel (even if I did not always take it). I am also grateful to the numerous colleagues, students, nurses, and physicians who have listened to me discuss this topic over the years and have provided continued information and correction.

Financial support for the research was provided by the Wellesley College Faculty Research Fund, the American Association of University Women Foundation, and the National Endowment for the Humanities. My year and a half at the Du Bois Institute for Afro-American Research at Harvard University was of particular and special support. I am grateful to Henry Louis Gates Jr., Dick Newman, and Patricia Sullivan at the Du Bois for the time they spent listening to me and for their special wisdom. Above all, I thank the people in Tuskegee who were willing to trust me with their stories. Any misreading of their understandings is my own failing.

1. The actual number of men in the study varies in the differing research publications. Most sources suggest there were approximately 399 men who had the disease and another 201 who were the "controls." However, some controls who developed syphilis were also switched into the study's other "arm." For an overview, the major monograph is James H. Jones, *Bad Blood: The Tuskegee Syphilis Experiment*, rev. ed. (New York: Free Press, 1993). See also Allan M. Brandt, "Racism and Research: The Case of the Tuskegee Syphilis Study," in *Sickness and Health in America*, 3d (rev.) ed., edited by Judith Walzer Leavitt and Ronald L. Numbers (Madison: University of Wisconsin Press, 1997), 392–404, and in this volume.

2. Jacket-copy language for Jones, *Bad Blood*. All subsequent citations to *Bad Blood* are from this first edition.

For perceptive analysis of the continuing importance of Tuskegee for African Americans and their health care, see Stephen B. Thomas and Sandra Crouse Quinn, "The Tuskegee Syphilis Study, 1932–1972: Implications for HIV Education and AIDS Risk Education Programs in the Black Community," *American Journal of Public Health* (hereafter cited as *AJPH*) 81 (November 1991): 1498–1505, and Vanessa Northington Gamble, "Under the Shadow of Tuskegee: African Americans and Health Care," *AJPH* 87 (November 1997): 1773–78, both in this volume.

3. For more details on the ceremony and how it was organized, see Susan M. Reverby, "History of an Apology: From Tuskegee to the White House," *Research Nurse* 3 (July/August 1997): 1–9.

4. Ralph Ellison, "The Shadow and the Act," in *The Collected Essays of Ralph Ellison*, edited by John F. Callahan (New York: Modern Library, 1995), 305. The essay originally appeared in *The Reporter*, 6 December 1949.

5. I am grateful to Cynthia Wilson of Tuskegee University for providing me with this colloquialism.

6. As Patricia Williams has argued, we will have to get beyond "voyeurism" and a tendency to "ritualize race as one-way theater," with whites only looking in. See her "World beyond Words," *Nation* 265 (22 September 1997): 10.

7. There have been numerous interpretations of the study, many of which are included in this collection of secondary and primary materials or listed in the bibliography.

8. Evelynn M. Hammonds, "Black (W)holes and the Geometry of Black Female Sexuality," *differences* 6, nos. 2–3 (1994): 126–45.

9. Nurse Rivers married when she was in her fifties. Although some of the community refer to her as Mrs. Laurie, for most of her life she was known as Nurse Rivers. Susan Reverby interview with Cynthia Wilson, Tuskegee, Alabama, 7 May 1997.

10. Hammonds, "Black (W)holes," uses these terms and is building on work by Audre Lorde on the invisibility/hypervisibility of black women. This analysis also reflects the importance of Evelyn Brooks Higginbotham's ground-breaking essay on the problem of the "metalanguage of race." See "African American Women's History and the Metalanguage of Race," *Signs* 17 (Winter 1992): 251–74. As Higginbotham puts it (p. 272): "Today, the metalanguage of race continues to bequeath its problematic legacy. While its discursive construction of reality into two opposing camps—blacks versus whites or Afrocentric versus Eurocentric standpoints—provides the basis for resistance against external forces of black subordination, it tends to forestall resolution of problems of gender, class and sexual orientation internal to black communities."

11. Jones, *Bad Blood*, devotes numerous pages and a chapter to Nurse Rivers. She is also the central figure in David Feldshuh's play, *Miss Evers' Boys* (Chicago: Chicago Theatre Group, 1991), and the subsequent HBO movie, *Miss Evers' Boys*, shown nationally for the first time on 22 February 1996. For interpretations of her role by three other historians, see Darlene Clark Hine, *Black Women in White* (Bloomington: Indiana University Press, 1989), 154–56; Susan L. Smith, "Neither Victim nor Villain: Nurse Eunice Rivers, the Tuskegee Syphilis Experiment, and Public Health Work," *Journal of Women's History* 8 (Spring 1996): 95–113); Evelynn M. Hammonds, "Your Silence Will Not Protect You: Nurse Eunice Rivers and the Tuskegee Syphilis Study," in *The Black Women's Health Book: Speaking for Ourselves*, 2d ed., edited by Evelyn C. White (Seattle: Seal Press, 1994), 323–31; also in this volume.

12. In thinking through Nurse Rivers' silence, I found helpful Nellie Y. McKay, "Remembering Anita Hill and Clarence Thomas: What Really Happened When One Black Woman Spoke Out," in *Race-ing Justice, En-gendering Power: Essays on Anita Hill, Clarence Thomas and the Construction of Social Reality*, edited by Toni Morrison (New York: Pantheon, 1992), 269–89, as well as all the essays in the Morrison collection; see also Hammonds, "Black (W)holes."

13. Higginbotham, "African American Women's History," 266.

14. Geneva Smitherman, *Talkin and Testifyin: The Language of Black America* (Boston: Houghton Mifflin, 1977), 58.

15. For use of Smitherman's terms, see Mae Gwendolyn Henderson, "Speaking in Tongues: Dialogics, Dialectics, and the Black Women Writer's Literary Tradition," in *Changing our Own Words: Essays on Criticism, Theory and Writing by Black Women*, edited by Cheryl A. Wall (New Brunswick: Rutgers University Press, 1989), 22.

16. See Allan M. Brandt, *No Magic Bullet* (New York: Oxford University Press, 1987); Elizabeth Fee, "Sin versus Science: Venereal Disease in Twentieth-Century Baltimore," in *AIDS the Burdens of History*, edited by Elizabeth Fee and Daniel M. Fox (Berkeley: University of California Press, 1988), 121–46; David McBride, *From TB to AIDS: Epidemics among Urban Blacks since 1900* (Albany: SUNY Press, 1991); and Jones, *Bad Blood*. In her review of Jones's book, Barbara Rosenkrantz raises the question of conflicting medical notions of treatment for syphilis but does not discuss Nurse Rivers; see her "Non-Random Events," *The Yale Review* 72 (1983): 284–96. For an example of how the debate on treatment could be used to justify the study, see R. H. Kampmeier, "The Tuskegee Study of Untreated Syphilis," *Southern Medical Journal* 65 (October 1972): 1247–51, both in this volume.

17. Fee, "Sin versus Science," 125.

18. It was assumed "that treatment in these cases could not reverse the injury of disease, although under favorable conditions arsphenamine and bismuth combined might abort progressive deterioration." William A. Hinton, *Syphilis and Its Treatment* (New York: Macmillan Company, 1936), 58, quoted in Rosenkrantz, "Non-Random Events," 292.

19. Fee, "Sin versus Science," 126.

20. Jones, *Bad Blood*, 147.

21. Michael M. Davis, "The Ability of Patients to Pay for Treatment of Syphilis," *Journal of Social Hygiene* 18 (October 1932): 380–88, quoted in Jones, *Bad Blood*, 259. Rosenkrantz, "Non-Random Events," 291, emphasizes the importance of Davis's finding and discusses the problem of asymptomatic but still contagious patients, while Jones puts it in a footnote. Rosenkrantz's review is the major discussion of the complexity of treatment in the study from a historical viewpoint.

22. "Deposition of Mrs. Eunice Rivers Laurie," for *Pollard et al. vs. United States of America* 20 September 1974, Tuskegee, Alabama, p. 113 (hereafter cited as Deposition-Laurie). The copy is missing from the courthouse records in Montgomery, Alabama. I am grateful to James Jones for providing me with a copy that was in his possession.

23. Jones discusses this in *Bad Blood* and the letters are in Records of the U.S. Public Health Service, Record Group 90, General Records of the Venereal Disease Division, 1918–36, Box 239, National Archives, Washington, D.C. (hereafter cited as PHS-NA).

24. Taliferrio Clark to Paul A. O'Leary, 27 September 1932, PHS-NA.

25. Robert J. Norrell, *Reaping the Whirlwind: The Civil Rights Movement in Tuskegee* (New York: Vintage, 1986), 14.

26. Ralph Ellison, *Invisible Man* (New York: Vintage, 1947, 1990); Nella Larsen, *Quicksand and Passing*, edited and introduction by Deborah McDowell (New Brunswick, N.J.: Rutgers University Press, 1986); Albert Murray, *South to a Very Old Place* (New York: McGraw Hill, 1971), and *Whistle Guitar Train* (New York: McGraw Hill, 1974).

27. Louis Harlan, "The Secret Life of Booker T. Washington," in *Booker T. Washington in Perspective: Essays of Louis R. Harlan*, edited by Raymond W. Smock (Jackson: University Press of Mississippi, 1988), 110–32.

28. But even when Tuskegee became central to both the legal and violent aspects of the civil rights movement in the 1950s and 1960s, the study continued unabated. See James Forman, *Sammy Younge, Jr.: The First Black College Student to Die in the Black Liberation Movement* (Washington, D.C.: Open Hand Publishing, 1986); and Norrell, *Reaping the Whirlwind*.

29. Testimony of Dr. Arnold Schroeter, U.S. Department of Health, Education and Welfare, Tuskegee Syphilis Study Investigating Committee Hearings, Washington, D.C., 1973, 1:25, Tuskegee University Archives (hereafter cited as HEW-TUA). See also Surgeon General H. S. Cumming to Dr. R. R. Moton, 20 September 1932, Moton Papers, General Correspondence, Box 180, Tuskegee University Archives, Tuskegee University, Tuskegee Alabama (hereafter cited as Moton-TUA). Jones, *Bad Blood*, 102, also cites this letter but does not emphasize the treatment question; Eugene H. Dibble, Jr. to R. R. Moton, 17 September 1932, Moton-TUA.

30. R. R. Moton to George Arthur, 17 February 1933, Moton-TUA.

31. I am borrowing here Pernick's book title for his work on the differential use of anesthesia, but it also fits the kind of process of political triage that was emblematic of the Tuskegee "machine"; see Martin S. Pernick, *A Calculus of Suffering* (New York: Columbia University Press, 1985). For an overview of Washington's mode of operation, see Louis R. Harlan, *Booker T. Washington: The Making of a Black Leader* (New York: Oxford University Press, 1972).

32. For a comprehensive listing of the medical reports on the study, see Jones, *Bad Blood*, 281–82. Ironically, perhaps, a reevaluation of the data from the original Oslo Study published in 1955 concluded: "It was estimated that between 60 and 70 out of every 100 of these patients went through life with a minimum of inconvenience despite no treatment for early syphilis. This gives no encouragement to withhold treatment because the final outcome in any individual cannot be predicted, and too, syphilis is still a transmissible disease when untreated and can cause serious difficulties among 30 to 40 out of each 100 who remain untreated." E. Gurney Clark et al., "The Oslo Study of the Natural History of Untreated Syphilis," *Journal of Chronic Diseases* 2 (September 1955): 343.

33. For a perceptive analysis of the rhetoric in the medical reports, see Martha Solomon [Watson], "The Rhetoric of Dehumanization: An Analysis of Medical Reports of the Tuskegee Syphilis Project," *Western Journal of Speech Communication* 49 (Fall 1985): 233–47, and in this volume. For the clearest example of use of this rhetoric to exonerate the PHS and to avoid any discussion of racism, see Kampmeier, "The Tuskegee Study of Untreated Syphilis."

34. Susan Lederer, "The Tuskegee Syphilis Study in the Context of American Medical Research," *Sigerist Circle Newsletter and Bibliography* 6 (Winter 1994): 2–4.

35. O. C. Wenger to Raymond Vonderlehr, 21 July 1933, PHS-NA.

36. Pasquale J. Pesare et al., "Untreated Syphilis in the Male Negro," *Journal of Venereal Disease Information* 27 (1946): 202; Stanley H. Schuman et al., "Untreated Syphilis in the Male Negro," *Journal of Chronic Diseases* 2 (1955): 551; Donald H. Rockwell et al., "The Tuskegee Study of Untreated Syphilis," *Archives of Internal Medicine* 114 (1961): 797.

37. For the clearest statement of her role before the story of the study broke, see Eunice Rivers et al.,"Twenty Years of Follow-Up Experience in a Long-Range Medical Study, *Public Health Reports* 68 (1953): 391–95, and in this volume. There are differing viewpoints on how much of this article Nurse Rivers actually wrote and no written evidence to evaluate the claims. (Personal communications with James Jones and Jay Katz.)

38. James Jones interview with Mrs. Eunice Rivers Laurie, Tuskegee, Ala., 3 May 1977, tape 2, p. 30 (hereafter cited as Jones-Laurie interview). I am grateful to James Jones for providing me with his transcription.

39. Herman Shaw interview with David Feldshuh, Notasulga, Ala., January 1992. I grateful to David Feldshuh for sharing this with me. Susan Reverby interview with Charles Pollard, Notasulga, Ala., 11 January 1994. See also Jones-Laurie interview.

40. Jones-Laurie interview, tape 1, p. 10. This assessment is based on my reading of her reports and my review of correspondence in the Tuskegee University archives and in the public health department records of the Alabama State Archives in Montgomery.

41. Eunice Rivers Laurie, "Oral History Interview" with Daniel Williams and Helen Dibble, 29 January 1975, Tuskegee, Ala., Tuskegee University Archives (hereafter cited as Tuskegee-Laurie Interview). I am grateful to David Feldshuh for informing me of this interview and to Daniel Williams for providing me with a copy of the tape. I made my own transcription with the able assistance of Carmen Bryant. (I believe this is the first transcription ever made of the tape, and I have left a copy in the Tuskegee University Archives. Feldshuh also had the tape transcribed.) Its first publication is in this volume.

42. In the fictional play and movie *Miss Evers' Boys*, Nurse Rivers is giving testimony before the U.S. senators investigating the scandal. This dramatic device allows her to reflect upon her experiences and to allow the drama to move back and forth in time. However, in the actual historical drama of the study, Nurse Rivers was never called to testify at the Senate hearing. See Susan Reverby interview with David Feldshuh, Ithaca, N.Y., 5 June 1992.

43. It is critical that we remember the Tuskegee-Laurie interview is an oral history, told to two people whom Nurse Rivers knew and trusted. She clearly wanted to leave another record of what she knew and thought. This interview gave her the chance (which she took) to leave her story in the institution she served and loved: Tuskegee University. I am aware that my transcription may have shifted some of the breaks in her narrative, although I have tried to stay as faithful as possible to her voice.

44. Eunice Rivers Laurie interview by A. Lillian Thompson, 10 October 1977, in *The Black Women Oral History Project*, edited by Ruth Edmonds Hill (New Providence, N.J.: K. G. Saur Verlag, 1992), 7:213–42, in the Schlesinger Library, Radcliffe College (hereafter cited as Schlesinger-Laurie Interview); Jones-Laurie Interview; Tuskegee-Laurie Interview.

45. Jones-Laurie Interview, tape 1, p. 10.

46. Eunice Rivers to Jessie Marriner, director of the Bureau of Child Hygiene and Public

Health Nursing, 9 September 1932, Alabama Department of Public Health, Administrative Files, 1928–35, Folder Macon County Miscellaneous 1930–33, Alabama State Archives, Montgomery, Ala.

47. Tuskegee-Laurie Interview, p. 12. In the Schlesinger-Laurie interview (p. 14), Rivers makes this position even clearer by saying: "And they never took anybody with early syphilis. And early syphilis was about three years or two years, that's considered early. After that, it was supposed to be late syphilis. What it as doing, it was doing it to you, you weren't transmitting it."

48. This theme of caring, not diagnosing, is a constant in all the interviews.

49. Tuskegee-Laurie Interview, pp. 5, 9, 12. All the quotes in this paragraph are from this interview, unless otherwise noted.

50. This view of what she was doing comes out most strongly in her deposition (Deposition-Laurie) and in her interview with historian James Jones (Jones-Laurie interview).

51. Schlesinger-Laurie Interview, p. 23.

52. On this dilemma, see Karen Buhler Wilkerson, *False Dawn: The Rise and Decline of Public Health Nursing, 1900–1930* (New York: Garland Publications, 1990).

53. Tuskegee-Laurie Interview, p. 16.

54. For a more theoretical discussion of some of these issues of power and empathy/caring (although primarily regarding medicine, not nursing), see Ellen Singer More and Maureen A. Milligan, eds., *The Empathic Practitioner: Empathy, Gender and Medicine* (New Brunswick: Rutgers University Press, 1994).

55. Tuskegee-Laurie Interview, p. 18.

56. This is, of course, my "reading" of her voice on the Tuskegee-Laurie Interview tape.

57. When I presented an earlier version of this paper to a nursing audience at Fitchburg State College, many of the older nurses in the audience responded with stories of their own "research" study experiences at major teaching hospitals. They voiced a clearly troubled sense that they often had no idea what they were giving the patients. One nurse made an insightful comment: "The only person who is blind in a double-blinded research study is the nurse."

In using these two voices, Rivers speaks in what Mae Henderson describes as "the internal dialogue with the plural aspects of self"; see Henderson, "Speaking in Tongues," 17.

58. This is the view most clearly articulated by Jones, *Bad Blood*: by the 1940s the study's rationale for nontreatment is so strong that even the presence of penicillin does not change the thinking of the study's supervisors.

59. Jones-Laurie Interview, tape 1, p. 31.

60. Darlene Clark Hine uses the term *super moral* to describe women like Nurse Rivers. See her "Rape and the Inner Lives of Black Women in the Middle West: Preliminary Thoughts on the Culture of Dissemblance," *Signs* 14 (Summer 1989): 915.

61. Schlesinger-Laurie Interview, p. 9.

62. Tuskegee-Laurie Interview, p. 19.

63. Mrs. Irene Beavers interview with Susan Reverby, Tuskegee, Ala., 10 January 1995 (hereafter cited as Beavers Interview). I am exceedingly grateful to Mrs. Beavers for her time and willingness to share her memories.

64. Hine, "Rape and the Inner Lives," 915.

65. Nursing School Records, Alumnae Association Folder, Box 2, Tuskegee University Archives.

66. Evelyn Brooks Higginbotham, "Beyond the Sound of Silence: Afro-American Women in History," *Gender and History* 1 (Spring 1989): 58–59. For further discussion of this differentiation within the black community, see Hazel Carby, *Reconstructing Womanhood* (New York: Oxford, 1987); Evelyn Brooks Higginbotham, *Righteous Discontent: The Women's Movement in the Black Baptist Church, 1880–1920* (Cambridge, Mass.: Harvard University Press, 1992); the essays in Darlene Clark Hine, ed., *Black Women's History: Theory and Practice*, 16 vols. (Brooklyn: Carlson Publishing, 1990); and, on health in particular, see Susan L. Smith, *"Sick and Tired of Being Sick*

and Tired": Black Women's Health Activism in America, 1890–1950 (Philadelphia: University of Pennsylvania Press, 1995).

67. Schlesinger-Laurie Interview, p. 20.

68. Ibid., p. 23.

69. Hammonds, "Black (W)holes," 137.

70. Testimony of Dr. Reginald G. James, HEW-TUA, pp. 59–60.

71. Rivers' sense of time here and her views are at odds with Jones's reading of Dr. Reginald G. James's comments from a *New York Times* interview published on 27 July 1972, the day after the Tuskegee story broke. Jones writes: "Between 1939 and 1941 he had been involved with public health work in Macon County—specifically with the diagnosis and treatment of syphilis." In his interviews James claims it was Rivers who kept him from treating some of the men in the study and that this left him " 'distraught and disturbed.' " He claims to have treated a man who never returned, presumably fearful of the loss of his benefits (Jones, *Bad Blood*, 6). I do not have the evidence to evaluate these differing claims. Several survivors have stated she *actively* kept them from treatment.

72. Tuskegee-Laurie Interview, p. 25 (italics mine).

73. For a fuller discussion, see Susan M. Reverby, *Ordered to Care: The Dilemma of American Nursing* (New York: Cambridge University Press, 1987).

74. See also Jones-Laurie Interview, p. 19.

75. Beavers Interview. See also Tuskegee-Laurie Interview, in this volume.

76. Amy and Walter Pack interview with Susan Reverby, Tuskegee, Ala., 11 January 1995. Both Walter and Amy Pack were working with Rivers when the story broke in 1972, and Walter Pack helped draft the public statement of the Macon County Health Department (hereafter cited as Pack Interview).

77. Seward Hiltner to Broadus Butler, 29 October 1972, U.S. Department of Health, Education and Welfare, Tuskegee Syphilis Study, Container 2, National Library of Medicine, History of Medicine Division, p. 5.

78. Joseph G. Caldwell to Dr. William J. Brown, 4 May 1970, Tuskegee Syphilis Study, Centers for Disease Control Papers, Box 8, Folder 1970, National Archives—Southeast Region, East Point, Ga.

79. Jones-Laurie Interview, p. 36.

80. I am grateful to Dick Newman of the DuBois Institute, Harvard University, for suggesting the parallel to Schindler. Unlike Schindler, Rivers was of the same racial/ethnic/cultural group as that of the victims. But she was of a different gender and class.

81. This view of Carol Gilligan's work comes from Mary Brabeck, "Moral Judgment: Theory and Research on Differences between Males and Females," in *An Ethic of Care*, edited by Mary Jeanne Larrabee (New York: Routledge, 1993), 34.

82. Martin S. Pernick, "The Patient's Role in Medical Decision-Making: A Social History of Informed Consent in Medical Therapy," in *Making Health Care Decisions: The Ethical and Legal Implications of Informed Consent in the Patient-Practitioner Relationship* (Washington, D.C.: GPO, 1982), 3:1–35.

83. Ruth R. Faden, Tom L. Beauchamp, and Nancy M. P. King, *A History and Theory of Informed Consent* (New York: Oxford University Press, 1986), 59.

84. I am paraphrasing critic Mae Henderson's analysis of the difficulties African American women have in explaining their lives in the face of explanations by others. Henderson writes: "In other words, it is not that black women, in the past, have had nothing to say, but rather that they have had no say" ("Speaking in Tongues," 24).

85. Pack Interview.

86. Smitherman, *Talkin and Testifyin*, 58.

87. Beavers Interview.

REFLECTIONS ON NURSE RIVERS

DARLENE CLARK HINE

In 1989, Darlene Clark Hine, John A. Hannah Professor of History at Michigan State University, published the path-breaking study of black nurses *Black Women in White: Racial Conflict and Cooperation in the Nursing Profession, 1890–1950* (Bloomington: Indiana University Press). The first of two selections that follow provides the beginning of Hine's consideration of Nurse Eunice Rivers. On 12 June 1993, Hine served as the chair and commentator on the papers of historians Susan Smith and Susan Reverby at the Berkshire Conference of Women Historians on a panel entitled "The Multiple Narratives of Nurse Rivers: The Tuskegee Syphilis 'Experiment' and the Problematics of African American Womanhood." The second selection reflects an editing of Hine's introduction and comments on this panel (revised versions of both Smith's and Reverby's papers appear in this volume).

Black Women in White

The racism, poverty, and myriad other forces that influenced black women's decisions to become nurses all receded once they were actually enrolled in the various training programs. Survival dictated that the student nurses imbibe a sense of the special nature and meaning of their calling. Black nurse supervisors and educators saw to it that their charges measured up to the highest ideals of nursing. If the young novices or probationers failed to be transformed, they were dismissed.

"To make a difference": this desire undergirded the thoughts and actions of most of the leaders and not a few of the practitioners in the black nursing profession. Perhaps Lillian Harvey, dean of the School of Nursing of Tuskegee Institute from 1944 to 1973, summed up best what it meant to be a nurse. As Harvey explained, one who can make a difference is

the nurse who can look at her patient, for example, and understand what is going on in that patient's body, anticipate some of the things and let the doctor,

Darlene Clark Hine is the John Hannah Professor of History at Michigan State University.
Sections originally published in Darlene Clark Hine, Black Women in White. *(Bloomington: Indiana University Press, 1989), 133, 134, 154–56, and given as commentary at the Berkshire Conference for the History of Women, 1994. Reprinted by permission of Indiana University Press and Darlene Clark Hine.*

the social workers and other persons know what is going on and what might possibly happen and then make herself the facilitator for getting the right people there to take care of whatever it is that is coming up. I feel that a nurse is really the patient's advocate. You are supposed to be there for the patient on the patient's side to look after the patient's best interests.[1]

. . . A powerful combination of parental prodding, head-on collisions with racial discrimination, and desire to reduce suffering encouraged not a few black women to consider a nursing career. Eunice Rivers Laurie, born in Early County, Georgia, on November 12, 1899, initially balked when her father suggested that she take up nursing at John A. Andrew Hospital at Tuskegee Institute. Rivers had pleaded, "But Papa, I don't want to be no nurse. I don't want folks dying on me." Undaunted, the father countered, "Well, Eunice, everybody's ain't gonna die on you. That's why should be a nurse. That's what is being a good nurse, so you could help save the people." Mollified, Rivers asserted to an interviewer, "Well I decided and he influenced me, but I made up my mind myself."[2]

. . . In many southern black communities, the black nurse, especially the public-health nurse, was the most prominent, if not the first professional, health-care giver to interact with the population. Thus it fell to her to establish the foundation and to define the nature of the professional-client relationship. As one writer put it, "The nurse, therefore, forms the hub around which much of a community's well-being revolves."[3] Black nurse Willa M. Maddux identified the requirements and characteristics black public-health nurses needed in order to work successfully with, as she phrased it, "the masses of untrained and indifferent people." Maddux contended, "It is imperative that the nurse be a person with broad sympathies, profound understanding and tact, and possess the requisite professional background." Writing in 1937, another black nurse from Florida observed similarly, "It is the job of the pioneer nurse to find an acceptable starting point to get the approval of the people that she hopes to serve."

Commencing in the late 1920s, black nurses began securing positions as public-health nurses with state, local, and federal health departments and agencies. Few of them possessed more than a nursing diploma, but this was more education than the majority of their clientele had received. On January 1, 1923, Eunice Rivers, having recently completed her training at Tuskegee Institute, reported for work, joining the three-member team of Alabama's Macon County Moveable School. The unit consisted of a teacher, carpenter, and nurse. Nurse Rivers had many wide-ranging responsibilities. She was expected to teach the rural tenant-farmer families the rudiments of home nursing, how to bathe a patient, how to take a temperature, how to give a massage. In summing up in an oral interview her decade of service with mothers and infants, she enumerated her accomplishments. In addition to teaching maternity care to new mothers, she trained the midwives how to deliver, how to wash their hands, cut their nails and . . . how to make the pads, how to prepare the bed for the delivery, because at that time most of the women had the babies on the floor. . . . We had an awful time trying to train the mothers to use the bed instead of the floor. We took paper— and there was no such thing as a draw sheet, a rubber sheet—so we carried old newspapers all the time, on the truck, and clean rags and this kind of thing, trying to teach the people how to do this. If we'd get in a home where we could find somebody who had an old ragged sheet, we'd show them how to make a pad, paper pad, to protect the bed. And also how to bathe the babies, feed them and prepare their meals, their bottles and this kind of thing.[4]

After nine years, Rivers left the Moveable School to become the nurse for the black men involved with the now-infamous government-run study of venereal disease, the Tuskegee Syphilis Experiment in Macon County, Alabama.

To achieve success as a public-health nurse required well-developed interpersonal-relations skills. None were more adept or possessed of more person-ality, tact, and determination than Eunice Rivers. Rivers overcame the fears and suspicions of Macon County rural blacks both during her years with the Moveable School and as the nurse with the Tuskegee Syphilis Experiment. Most of her clients evidenced a strong distrust of physicians, refusing to heed their advice or even to seek their services until it was often too late. Rivers lay part of the blame for this reluctance on the heads of the physicians, who quite often simply did not know how to talk to the people. She asserted that she won confidences by first acknowl-edging that "they're people as far as I'm concerned. I don't go there dogging them about keeping the house clean. I go there and visit a while until I know when to make some suggestions. When I go to the house, I accept the house as I find it. I bide my time." She continued, "Sometimes I don't do a thing but go there, sit down there and talk." This tactic proved especially effective and won for her the respect and admiration of not only the black people whom she served but also the black and white physicians with whom she worked.

The white doctors of the experiment marveled at Rivers' ability to get patients to obey instructions. On occasion, however, she even had to step out of the nurse's posture of professional subservience and deference to physicians' authority. In at least one instance she took to task a young white government doctor assigned to the syphilis study. She admonished him, "If anything happens that you can't get along, that you can't get it through their heads, just call me. We'll straighten it out. But don't holler at them. These are grown men; some of them are old men. Don't holler at them." The fact that she interceded and on occasion defended them won their trust. This perhaps explains why many of the black patients involved in the syphilis experiment continued to participate longer than they should have. Rivers was, of course, convinced that the experiment was a good and honorable effort.

Rivers admitted that as a nurse she was rewarded and sustained by the devotion and respect her patients showered upon her. "They depended on me . . . they would take whatever I said." Elaborating on her philosophy of the nurse-patient relationship, she added,

> After all, the doctor saw the patient and he was gone. And it was up to you to help that patient carry out his orders, do whatever the doctor suggested. The doctor said, you do so and so. . . . First thing, the patient doesn't know how to do it. He doesn't know what his reaction is going to be. He doesn't want to be stuck, this kind of thing. So the nurse plays an important part there. She's closer to the patient. Patients would get to the point where if they're not sure, they're going to ask you. They get you in the middle.[5]

Rivers was more than a good country nurse. Her forty-plus years' involvement in the Tuskegee Syphilis Experiment, in which treatment was deliberately withheld from patients, raises questions concerning relationships between the black nurses and the black community and between black nurses and white health-care professionals. Indeed, it is fair to say that without her the white "government doctors" would not have been so successful in engaging so many black males in such a detrimental and ethically bankrupt experiment. It was their unquestioning faith in Rivers as someone selflessly looking out for and protecting them that led the men to continue in the experiment for so many unrewarding years. Though they remained fundamentally suspicious of the motives of the "government doctors," they always tended to do what Rivers told them. According to historian James H. Jones, "More than any other person [Rivers] made them believe they were receiving medical care that was helping them."[6] They were not.

Rivers' motives for collaborating in this experiment and deliberately manipulating these black men are complex. It is possible that she viewed the study as a way of ensuring for at least some blacks an unparalleled amount of medical attention. Jones offers several compelling explanations for Rivers' complicity: As a nurse, she had been trained to follow orders, and probably it simply did not occur to her to question a—or, for that matter, any—doctor's judgment. Moreover, she was incapable of judging the scientific merits of the study. For Rivers, a female in a male-dominated world, deference to male authority figures reinforced her ethical passivity. Finally, and perhaps most significant, Rivers was black, and the physicians who controlled the experiment were white. Years of conditioning and living in the South made it virtually impossible for Rivers to have rebelled against a white, male government doctor, the ultimate authority figure in her world.[7] In this case the needs and interests of the black community of Tuskegee were not addressed and protected by the black nurse.

Nurse Eunice Rivers, Tuskegee Syphilis, and the Problematics of African American Womanhood

Few issues have aroused the black community's ire more forcefully than the Tuskegee Syphilis Study. The mere mention of the name sends angry tremors down the backs of even the most resolute black men and women. It has become the powerful symbol of black vulnerability in a white-dominated, capitalistic, patriarchal society. In its deepest sense, "Tuskegee Syphilis" is a potent metaphor for the multiple stratifications along the race, class, sex, and regional grids in twentieth-century America. . . .

We confront a challenge, however, when attempting to unravel the ironic dilemma of Rivers' pivotal role in the decades-long continuation of the black men's futile participation in the ethically bankrupt and useless Tuskegee Syphilis Study. We stand to learn a great deal about the intersections of race, gender, class, and regionality by coming to grips with Tuskegee Syphilis and Nurse Rivers.

The problem is, and I share Susan Smith and Susan Reverby's unspoken, but omniscient questions: Who was this woman, how representative was she of the African American women of her generation and similar class and professional status? The search for Nurse Rivers is an important quest, and the resolution may affect how black women in general are perceived and studied in the future.

Smith and Reverby take great pains to avoid simplistic dualisms as they seek the real identity of Nurse Rivers. Indeed, Reverby's cautious disclaimer that she doesn't "expect to find *a* truth about Nurse Rivers" is well placed. Moreover, both Smith and Reverby spare us the outmoded "two-ness" construction penned by the historian/activist W. E. B. Du Bois at the turn of the century. Further, Reverby uses to great effect Evelyn Higginbotham's analysis of the metalanguage of race.[8] Both scholars see clearly the ways in which our obsessive emphasis on race has tended to obscure issues of gender and class construction and their intersection.

To my knowledge this is the first panel ever developed by historians to focus attention on Nurse Rivers. This is not to say that others have neglected to remark on her role in Tuskegee Syphilis; it is only to underscore that who she was as a woman, an African American, a nurse, a professional black woman, a southerner, has not received nuanced examination. At the outset I must note the observation that I made in *Black Women in White: Racial Conflict and Cooperation in the Nursing Profession* that few African American women scholars have evidenced concern with Nurse Eunice Rivers Laurie. I am confident that the future will bring greater interest on their part.[9] There is a precedent. Until Nell Painter began working on Sojourner Truth, few African American women had studied one of "the most enigmatic women of the nineteenth century."[10] Painter argues that white feminists, on the other hand, embraced Truth with a passion. She embarked upon an intellectual journey to find out why. Yet, as Reverby effectively demonstrates,

Nurse Rivers has not wanted for attention, or suffered from invisibility. On the contrary, she has been the subject of a play and an Emmy award–winning HBO movie, the inspiration of a musical score, and the star of book chapters written by white male historians. She is featured in a traveling "Notable African American Women" exhibit, and was included in the black women's oral history project by the Schlesinger Library. So, what is the problem?

Could it be that, with few exceptions, black women scholars would like to ignore or dismiss Nurse Rivers for she may well reinforce negative stereotypes that prevail in our society, especially that of the ubiquitous Mammy, who, according to myth and wishful dreaming, was so willing to do the white man's bidding that she undermined her own community? Does Nurse Rivers hold up a mirror of self-hatred, the ultimate victim and villain combined into one horrible nightmare—a renegade black woman who does not serve her community, or sacrifice herself, who does not transcend her status and oppression, who is compliant and willingly assists in the exploitation of black men? No, better leave such women to the shadows, or to white feminist scholars!

But, then, what are white feminist scholars Susan Smith and Susan Reverby to do? In an essay in the *Journal of Women's History* I shared two laments.[11] I fretted that too little attention has been devoted to the real working-class status of black women and that the paucity of sustained analysis on the overwhelming poverty of the vast majority of black women has helped to foster erroneous impressions in the larger society of the mythical, heroic, transcendent black woman able to do the impossible, to make a way out of no way. But here is Nurse Rivers, who was neither heroic nor particularly transcendent of everyday racism and sexism. Yet as Smith and Reverby take pains to demonstrate, nor was she a villainous devil or mean-spirited witch. Dichotomous representations will always obscure black women and need to be avoided.

My second lament was an explicit call for more black women historians to write histories of white women, and an implicit challenge for white women historians to do likewise. My reasoning was that only through crossover history could we become more knowledgeable of each other and begin to break down intellectual and professional boundaries, to refine and to take even more seriously our methodologies of intersectional analysis.

Susan Smith and Susan Reverby have picked up the challenge, and they have wrought well. Reverby is very stand up about her quest: "Finding Eunice Rivers requires us to examine the use of race as a metalanguage to understand African American women and to analyze the narrow representations that have haunted their lives."

At the outset Susan Smith poses a series of critical questions. "What can this case study tell us about class difference among African Americans?" She uses her previous research on the black health movement in the early twentieth century to place Tuskegee Syphilis within the larger southern context of black disease and poverty, and racial exploitation. Her second critical question concerns Nurse Rivers and her role as a complex historical subject, not just as a victim or evil nurse. She asks, "What does it mean, then, to talk about the agency of Black women within racism and sexist social structures?" Again, Smith frames her investigation of this question by placing Rivers within the broader context of twentieth-century public-health work. She does a fine job of describing this work and the interpersonal relations skill that Rivers brought to it. She also captures well Rivers' desire to advance and to find secure regularized employment. Smith elaborates on how Rivers constructed a livelihood by knitting together several part-time jobs. Smith links Tuskegee Syphilis with white racism, and illuminates the differences between this study and the Oslo study that traced untreated syphilis in Norway. The difference needs underscoring. "The Oslo study was a *retrospective* study examining previous case records of white people whose syphilis went untreated, unlike the Tuskegee Study which was designed to deliberately withhold available treatment from Black people."

Smith makes two additional points that are important correctives to conventional misinformation: the study was not a government secret, kept hidden from health professionals, and a number of black health professionals engaged in the project for expedient reasons. The experiment on poor black men simply was not viewed as a problem by middle-class, professional black men. Class privilege blinded them to the study's immorality. I am curious as to whether the NAACP knew of the study, or other black protest groups. Was this study deemed less important because it concerned southern black men? Without such investigation we are left concluding that blacks were as culpable as were the whites who initiated the study. Obvious reliance on, and need of, government resources for other health projects led some black professionals to turn a blind eye to Tuskegee Syphilis. Is this a rationalization or explanation for their action?

I do question whether Rivers had the authority, as Smith suggests, to implement "the policy of the Public Health Service to prohibit the subjects of the study from receiving treatments for syphilis from anyone else, even after World War II when penicillin became available." There is a critical distinction between knowing about the experiment or study and failing to denounce it for purely expedient reasons, and actively directing or setting policy that in effect signed the death warrants of 100 men after a proven cure was available. In other words, I suspect there were limits to Rivers' agency. One reading of Smith's portrait evokes a Rivers who was knowledgeable, assertive, and hungry for employment and prestige, a woman who actually believed that the experiment served the best interest of the men fortunate enough to be involved. The problem is that if she is neither victim nor villain, as Smith has constructed her, are we now left to imagine that she was *in charge*? Here Smith goes out on a tenuous limb and seems in danger of minimizing how much race, sex, and class oppression operate and intersect to limit Rivers', and by extension any black woman's, agency. I would caution against taking Rivers' assertions of her innocence—"I know I didn't mislead anyone"—as the final word. Historians know that people deceive themselves all the time. Smith has given us much to think about in this intelligent presentation.

Reverby has written a multilayered essay that is distinguished by its use of "multiple narratives" of Nurse Rivers. Reverby's women's studies and historical approach begs examination of a much broader universe of sources and documents reflecting divergent perspectives on the significance of Rivers to the Tuskegee Syphilis Study. Accordingly, she provides an insightful analysis of the play by Dr. David Feldshuh, *Miss Evers' Boys*, which we saw together in Atlanta. She uncovered a new oral interview of Nurse Rivers, and has read all of the secondary historical works, and finally, she listened to original musical compositions. Thus she has an impressive command of what has been written and imagined about Nurse Rivers.

. . . Reverby's guarded reading of Rivers' own accounts *of* her story raised a number of questions. I applaud Reverby's delineation of the three substantial themes found in Rivers' own narrative. It is clear that she viewed herself as a competent caring professional whose work, including " 'treating' the syphilitic sharecroppers," helped to uplift the race. But try as she might, and she is to be commended for her intelligent effort, Reverby is doomed to remain frustrated in her quest to find the whole Rivers, I suspect, not only because of the black nurse's use of multiple voices and strategic silences, but also because Rivers dissembles with consummate skill.[12] While Rivers confuses caring with treatment, she cannot escape or explain away the fact that she denied penicillin to the men. This remains the ethical or moral horns of the dilemma upon which rests her significance as a historical figure. I suspect that she knew this.

And in one poignant passage, Reverby reveals that she is also knowing. "We are fascinated by her seeming innocence and her culpability. Despite our effort not to, I suspect we, and in this case me as a white woman and a nursing historian, still want her to have more power to serve as the talisman to absorb our moral uncertainties."

Reverby urges that we read Rivers' narrative as that of a "race woman" in order to understand her "gendered class attitudes." The works of two black women historians, Elsa Barkley Brown and Sharon Harley, may further illuminate this discussion.[13] Brown defines womanism as a consciousness that incorporates racial, cultural, sexual, national, economic, and political considerations into agency. To be a race woman, or a womanist, which entailed being both simultaneously, was a big order. It requires holding together many constituencies and multiple purposes all at once. The key question is this: Was Eunice Rivers a true race woman of the stripe of Maggie Lena Walker or Nannie Helen Burroughs?

Sharon Harley's essays on the black middle class help us to grasp more firmly the slippery concept of class. Harley distinguishes between the black upper-middle-class elite and the black middle class, whose "incomes were often too low, job security too elusive, and racial discrimination too widespread for most middle-class Black women to boast of being anything other than servants of their people."

Finally, I would like to reiterate one of Reverby's key points:

Her silences and inability to find the words, or the permission to utter them, to even explain her situation with James [a black physician involved in the study] suggest how powerful the pressures were to downplay the ways racism shaped the role of the black professional and Tuskegee Institute in the study. The overwhelming racism that motivated and perpetuated the study almost made it impossible to speak of the complexity of class and gender within the black community and made it almost impossible for her to find the words at all to explain what she thought had happened.

While Rivers may not have found her words to explain what happened, it is the task, or curse, of the historian to never stop trying. Whatever it takes, we must continue our pursuit of Nurse Rivers and her elusive truths.

NOTES

1. Interview with Lillian Harvey, 8 January 1976, conducted by Patricia Sloan. Original transcript is in the M. Elizabeth Carnegie Nursing History Archive, Hampton University School of Nursing, Hampton, Va. For a critique of the idealized images and unrealistic expectations of nurses, see Janet Muff, "Of Images and Ideals: A Look at Socialization and Sexism in Nursing," in *Images of Nurses: Perspectives from History, Art, and Literature*, edited by Anne Hudson Jones (Philadelphia: University of Pennsylvania Press, 1988), 197–200.

2. Interview with Eunice Rivers [Laurie], 10 October 1977, Schlesinger Library Black Women's Oral History Project, Radcliffe College, Cambridge, Mass.

3. Gerald A. Spencer, *Medical Symphony: A Study of the Contributions of the Negro to Medical Progress in New York* (New York: Arlain Printing Co., 1947), 107.

4. Interview with Eunice Rivers [Laurie].

5. Ibid.

6. Ibid.; James H. Jones, *Bad Blood: The Tuskegee Syphilis Experiment* (New York: Free Press, 1981), 160.

7. Jones, *Bad Blood*, 164–67.

8. Evelyn Brooks Higginbotham, "African American Women's History and the Metalanguage of Race," *Signs* 17 (Winter 1992): 251–74.

9. At the time this article was written, Evelynn M. Hammonds' article on Nurse Rivers was not yet available. However, it does appear in this volume.

10. Nell Irvin Painter, *Sojourner Truth: A Life, a Symbol* (New York: W. W. Norton, 1996).

11. Darlene Clark Hine, "Black Women's History, White Women's History: The Juncture of Race and Class," in *Journal of Women's History* 4 (Fall 1992): 125–33.

12. Darlene Clark Hine, "Rape and the Inner Lives of Southern Black Women: Thoughts on the Culture of Dissemblance," in *Southern Women: Histories and Identities*, edited by Virginia Bernhard et al. (Columbia: University of Missouri Press, 1992), 177–89. In the same volume, see

Cheryl Thurber, "The Development of the Mammy Image and Mythology," pp. 87–108. By "dissemblance," I mean the behavior and attitudes of black women that created the appearance of openness and disclosure but actually shielded the truth of their inner lives and selves from their oppressors.

13. Sharon Harley, "The Middle Class," in *Black Women in America: An Historical Encyclopedia*, edited by Darlene Clark Hine, Elsa Barkley Brown, and Rosalyn Terborg-Penn (New York: Carlson Publishing Co., 1993), 786–89; Elsa Barkley Brown, "Womanist Consciousness: Maggie Lena Walker and the Independent Order of Saint Luke," *Signs* 14 (Spring 1989): 610–33.

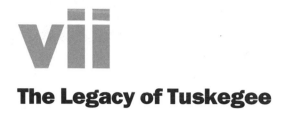

vii

The Legacy of Tuskegee

PROPER USES AND ABUSES OF THE HEALTH CARE DELIVERY SYSTEM FOR MINORITIES, WITH SPECIAL REFERENCE TO THE TUSKEGEE SYPHILIS STUDY

VERNAL G. CAVE

Since this 102nd Annual Meeting of the American Public Health Association is focused on minority health, you have heard and will continue to hear much about the proper uses and abuses of the health care delivery system in the United States as it pertains to the poor, the disadvantaged, the deprived minorities. The proper uses of what there is of a health care system should be the same for both the minorities and the majority of our society plus additional stakes for the minorities to address and correct the myriad factors that impact on good health. Despite pious platitudes, declarations of progress, assertions of recognition of the sacredness of human life and voiced concern for human dignity, abuses of the health care system for minorities abound. Among these is the abuse of minorities for human experimentation, sometimes for quite frivolous, poorly conceived and poorly monitored experiments, often without informed consent of the human subjects and indeed, not infrequently, without any consent of any kind.

Such abuse was perpetrated by the mighty government of the United States against its own black citizenry of Macon County, Alabama in the infamous Tuskegee syphilis tragedy. Mr. Peter J. Buxton, formerly a public health advisor for the United States Public Health Service and now an attorney in California, played a major part in bringing this story to the attention of the general public. In August, 1972, Jean Heller of the Associated Press broke the shameful story which was flashed around the world. Since then, the startling revelations and the awesome dimensions of this crime against humanity have become widely known but the surviving victims have not been treated well by their government and abuse continues.

Let us review some of the aspects of the Tuskegee tragedy which had its onset in 1933 A.D. Ironically, the events that lead to this tragedy were based on a commendable endeavor launched in 1929 by the Julius Rosenwald Fund, a Chicago based

Vernal G. Cave, M.D., was a noted public-health physician and a member of the Ad Hoc Tuskegee Syphilis Study Panel, Department of Health, Education and Welfare, in 1973. Originally published in the Journal of the National Medical Association 67 (1975): 82–84. Reprinted by permission of the National Medical Association.

philanthropic organization. The Fund set out to obtain health indices in Macon County and in five other rural counties of the South to provide the data to support the critical need for a program to upgrade the health and medical care of poor, rural blacks in the South. These counties, of which Macon County was perhaps the poorest and most depressed, had high incidences of diseases that resulted in large measure from the poor living conditions that prevailed in the area. There were high prevalences of syphilis, tuberculosis, pellagra, malnutrition, malaria and maternal and infant mortality. Macon County, of which Tuskegee is the county seat, had the third highest mortality rate among the 67 rural Alabama Counties in 1929.

According to the 1930 census the population of Macon County was 37,103 of which 82% were black. The county had only one black and nine white physicians engaged in private practice. This small number was located mostly in the central and northeastern portions of the county where most of the whites lived. The average income was one to two dollars a day. Even peripheral medical service was beyond the reach of most of the inhabitants. Roads and transportation were poor. Ignorance, superstition and dependence on folk remedies all contributed to the acceptance of excessive illness and short life spans as preordained. Many were only vaguely aware of the names, consequences and treatments of diseases that were common in the area. Convulsions or seizures due to various causes were dismissed as "fits" or "spells," miscarriages or stillbirths, possibly a consequence in some cases of congenital syphilis, were accepted without any procedures being performed to determine the cause; open sores were tolerated and only a vague knowledge of tuberculosis was evident in those who saw their children's bodies wracked by coughs and emaciated by "consumption." The attitudes of the inhabitants toward life, health, illness and death reflected a high degree of resignation and fatalism. This probably was a necessary psychological adjustment to the depressing reality of the futility of expecting anything approaching adequate medical care or any improvement in all of the various factors that can make for the good life. In 1932, Macon County with its socio-economic oppression was the perfect setting for the crime that was about to be perpetrated.

The Julius Rosenwald Fund program was the outgrowth of a genuine altruistic spirit. Armed with the knowledge that 35% of 3,684 individuals tested had reactive or positive tests for syphilis it undertook the commendable effort to examine and treat these cases. The United States Public Health Service cooperated in this project. In 1932, hardpressed for finance in the time of the Great Depression, the Fund had to relinquish its efforts at syphilis control and consequently transferred its program to the Public Health Service. Before withdrawing it had succeeded in demonstrating that relatively inexpensive mass treatment for syphilis was feasible. Indeed this demonstration has remained the cornerstone of all syphilis control efforts to this very day.

In October of 1932, the Public Health Service began to do its own thing on the black population of Macon County. In order to get a good response, schedules announcing the clinics set up for blood collecting were publicized using churches, schools, stores and other public gathering places. A total of 4,400 males and females over 18 years of age were tested. Twenty-two per cent were found to have positive blood tests. Out of this group, 412 who were known to have received no therapy and who were males of 25 years of age or older were chosen to be the original group for this study. To this day the Public Health Service has been unable to produce any semblance of a protocol showing the objectives of the study or how those objectives were to be achieved. Indeed there is some evidence that originally only some type of short-term study was contemplated. However, in 1933 another group of 200 black males of comparable ages to the first group but free of syphilis were chosen as controls. It is clear from what happened that from that point that the objective of the researchers was to follow the course of untreated syphilis through to the living end or more precisely, the dead end of the subjects.

Nowhere does the record show that the 412 syphilitic individuals were told in any meaningful way exactly what disease they had and the possible dangers of not being treated. All evidence points to the likelihood that they were never told and, therefore, were not in position to give knowledgeable or informed consent for their participation in this study. They certainly were not made aware of the disabling and fatal implications of untreated syphilitic infections.

To provide rapport and surveillance over the human subjects, a black nurse was employed to keep tabs on the human subjects. As members of "Miss River's Lodge," they thought of themselves as the chosen few. These unwitting victims were entitled to free medicine provided, of course, that it would not interfere with the relentless progression of their syphilitic states. This included "spring tonic," whatever in the world that might have been. The human subjects in this study were told that they would receive free examinations from the government yearly. On these days, they would be accorded free transportation in a "government car" and free hot meals on the days of examination. A magnanimous bonus was that they would be given opportunities to stop in town on the return trips to shop or visit with friends. At some point early in the study, the Milbank Memorial Foundation agreed to pay 50 dollars toward burial if the families made available the victims' bodies for autopsy. The final touch!

There was common medical knowledge in 1932 that untreated syphilitic infection produces increased disability and premature mortality. What did this study find? This study confirmed that untreated syphilitic infection produces premature mortality and increased disability.

The first report on this study entitled "Untreated Syphilis in the Male Negro, a Comparative Study of Treated and Untreated Cases" by R. A. Vonderlehr and others in 1936 contained, among others, the following observations: "Only 16% of the 399 syphilitic Negroes gave no evidence of morbidity as compared with 61% of the 201 presumably nonsyphilitic Negroes. The effect of syphilis in producing disability in the early years of adult life is to be noted by comparing the cases with no demonstrable morbidity under 40 years of age. This comparison shows that only one-fourth of the Negroes with untreated syphilis had no manifestations of disease whereas three-fourths of the uninfected persons were free of manifestations."

All subsequent reports represented monotonous reaffirmations that untreated syphilitic infection produces increased disability and premature mortality. It might be said that they proved a point, then proved a point, then proved a point. To quote Gertrude Stein, "A Rose is a rose, is a rose, is a rose."

In 1946, 14 years of non-treatment had elapsed. Penicillin, hailed as the miracle drug, was then available and utilized for the treatment of syphilis. At this time 25% of the syphilitic group and 14% of the controls of comparable ages had died. It was calculated by actuaries that at age 25 black male syphilitics allowed to remain untreated would have reduction in life expectancy of approximately 20%. Still the patients went untreated. The Public Health Service even continued to fail to treat for months after unanimous recommendation for immediate discontinuance of the study was made by the nine member Ad Hoc Tuskegee Syphilis Study Advisory Panel appointed on August 28, 1972 by Dr. Merlin K. Duval, Assistant Secretary for Health & Scientific Affairs of the Department of Health, Education and Welfare.

This in capsular form is an account of one of the flagrant abuses of the health delivery system. It is an exploitation in our nation's history whose immorality is so obvious that it can be quickly perceived by any but the hopelessly inconvertible bigots. All the survivors have now been located by the Public Health Service and have been offered the best medical care for the rest of their lives. But outrageously, the government is denying compensation to the victims. They have forced those who seek compensation into lengthy litigation. One would have thought that there would by now be federal legislative and executive agreement to compensate these aged victims rather than subjecting them to prolonged and agonizing trials. Yet this is the current status.

What should be done about this patient abuse? I offer a few suggestions:

A. PREVENTION. Prevention requires dealing with the root causes that make poor people susceptible to experimental human exploitation—poverty, ignorance, poor housing, unemployment, malnutrition, and now more recently inflation, to mention a few. It was stated in one of the reports by some of the researchers in this study that because of their lack of education, the human subjects could not be motivated by explaining to them that they would be contributing to humanity by taking part in this study. What irony! You can be sure that if the opposite condition existed; that is, if these human subjects were well educated, they likewise could not be persuaded to be sacrificial lambs for the rest of humanity.

B. LEGISLATION. Legislation is now pending to establish a National Commission for the Protection of Human Subjects of Biomedical and Behavioral Research. This legislation should be pushed and it should contain all or most of the recommendations of the Ad Hoc Tuskegee Syphilis Study Advisory Panel. This would include what can be called "ombudsmen" at the local levels to interpret for potential subjects of human experimentation just what they are getting themselves into.

C. COMPENSATION. Adequate compensation for the families and the surviving victims should be made and it should be done now. With all of the remaining victims in the late evenings of their lives, America has only a very short time left to make some type of material amends that can still be enjoyed by these victims. You and I can both cite examples of how speedily our government can act when it considers it important to do so. It would be extremely helpful if a resolution on this subject could come out of the deliberations of the Governing Council of the American Public Health Association at this session.

D. RECRUITMENT. Recruitment, training and retention of minority personnel in the health field is a must. For how else do you get physicians and other health workers in the Macon counties of our land? How else do you get a sufficient supply of health personnel to meet the needs of our indigent minorities in our urban ghettoes? And finally,

E. MINORITY PARTICIPATION. I would suggest that this is a signal example of the need for minority participation in every area of decision making in governmental involvement in health. It is difficult to conceive that our history would have been stained by the Tuskegee Tragedy if there had been minority representation when plans for this study were hatched in 1932. Our continual push for involvement is based not only on our desire to have a "piece of the action" at every level but more importantly on particular points of view that we can bring to any deliberations based on the milieu from which we come.

We can reduce the abuses and increase the proper uses of the health care delivery system for minorities. If we can move meaningfully on what is herein suggested, the victims of this American tragedy may become "Unknown Heroes for Change" who gave their lives so that others might live. May this be for all people everywhere.

THE TUSKEGEE SYPHILIS STUDY, 1932–1972

Implications for HIV Education and AIDS Risk Education Programs in the Black Community

STEPHEN B. THOMAS & SANDRA CROUSE QUINN

Background

AIDS among Black Americans

Since acquired immunodeficiency syndrome (AIDS) was first recognized and reported in 1981, more than 179,000 persons with AIDS have been reported to the Centers for Disease Control (CDC). Of these, more than 63% have died. Infection with the human immunodeficiency virus (HIV) has emerged as a leading cause of death among men and women under 45 years of age and children 1 to 5 years of age.[1]

By May 1991, there were 179,136 cases of AIDS reported in the United States. Of the reported cases, 97,329 (54%) were White and 51,190 (29%) were Black. Thus, although Whites still constitute a majority of the AIDS cases, Blacks are contracting AIDS in numbers far greater than their relative percentage in the population (Blacks constitute 12% of the US population). In addition, 52% of all children (under age 13 at time of diagnosis) and 52% of all women with AIDS are Black.[1] The best data available demonstrate that in the United States, HIV infection is spreading more rapidly among Blacks than among other population groups.

Because of the disproportionate impact of AIDS among Blacks, special emphasis must be placed on reaching this population with effective HIV education and AIDS risk reduction programs. To plan and evaluate these programs effectively, it is crucial to have an understanding of the behavioral risk factors and AIDS knowledge deficiencies in the Black community.

Public health professionals must recognize that the history of slavery and rac-

Stephen B. Thomas is associate professor of community health in the Department of Behavioral Sciences and Health Education, and director of the Institute for Minority Health Research at the Rollins School of Public Health at Emory University. Sandra Crouse Quinn is assistant professor of health behavior and health education at the School of Public Health, University of North Carolina, Chapel Hill.

Originally published in the American Journal of Public Health *81 (1991): 1498–1505. Reprinted by permission of the American Public Health Association.*

ism in the United States has contributed to the present social environment, in which those Blacks, whose behavior places them at greater risk for HIV infection, are also among the most disadvantaged members of our society. As we enter the last decade of the 20th century, the promises of opportunity and equality envisioned by the civil rights movement have failed to be realized for the vast majority of American Blacks. Blacks' consequent anger and despair in the fact of persistent inequality have contributed to the development of conspiracy theories about Whites (the government) against Blacks. These conspiracy theories range from the belief that the government promotes drug abuse in Black communities to the belief that HIV is a manmade weapon of racial warfare.

For example, The Nation of Islam has disseminated literature that describes AIDS as a form of genocide, an attempt by White society to eliminate the Negro race.[2] The mainstream Black media have also contributed to the discussion. "Tony Brown's Journal," a popular Public Broadcast System television show, aired a series of programs debating the issue of AIDS as a form of genocide. The *Los Angeles Sentinel*, the largest Black newspaper on the West Coast, ran a series of stories beginning March 9, 1989, suggesting that Blacks had been intentionally infected with HIV. *Essence* also ran a story titled "AIDS: Is It Genocide?"[3] In that article, Barbara J. Justice, MD, a New York City physician, asserted that "there is a possibility that the virus was produced to limit the number of African people and people of color in the world who are no longer needed" (p. 78). James Small, PhD, a Black studies instructor at City College of New York, was quoted as saying:

> Our whole relationship to Whites has been that of their practicing genocidal conspiratorial behavior on us from the whole slave encounter up to the Tuskegee Study. People make it sound nice by saying the Tuskegee "Study." But do you know how many thousands of thousands of our people died of syphilis because of that?[3]

The history of the Tuskegee Syphilis Study, with its failure to educate the participants and treat them adequately, helped to lay the foundation for Blacks' pervasive sense of distrust of public health authorities today. Fears about genocide have been reported by public health professionals and community-based-organization staff who work in Black communities. During his 1990 testimony before the National Commission on AIDS, Mark Smith, MD, from the School of Medicine at Johns Hopkins University in Baltimore, described the African American community as "already alienated from the health care system and the government and . . . somewhat cynical about the motives of those who arrive in their communities to help them" (p. 19).[4] Smith said that the Tuskegee Syphilis Study "provides validation for common suspicions about the ethical even-handedness in the medical research establishment and in the federal government, in particular, when it comes to Black people" (p. 20).[4]

Harlon Dalton, associate professor of law at Yale University and member of the National Commission on AIDS, eloquently describes the social basis for genocidal theories in his much quoted essay, "AIDS in Blackface."[5] Dalton believes that the Tuskegee Syphilis Study is a reflection of society's historical disregard for the lives of Black people. He accepts the commonly repeated distortion that "the government purposefully exposed Black men to syphilis so as to study the natural course of the disease."[5]

The continuing legacy of the Tuskegee Syphilis Study has contributed to Blacks' belief that genocide is possible and that public health authorities cannot be trusted. These fears and attitudes must be assessed in order to develop AIDS education programs for the Black community. For example, the Southern Christian Leadership Conference (SCLC), a leading civil rights organization founded by Dr. Martin Luther King, Jr., received funding from the CDC to provide HIV education through a national program titled RACE (Reducing AIDS through Community Education). In 1990, the SCLC conducted a survey to determine HIV education needs among 1056 Black church members in five cities (Atlanta, Ga; Charlotte, NC; Detroit, Mich; Kansas City, Mo; and Tuscaloosa, Ala). While 35% of the respondents believed that AIDS is a form of genocide, another 30% were unsure. Additionally, 44% believed that the government is not telling the truth about AIDS, while 35% were unsure. Furthermore, 34% believed that AIDS is a manmade virus, while 44% were unsure.[20]

The results of the SCLC survey strongly suggest that Blacks' belief in AIDS as a form of genocide and their mistrust of the government should be cause for serious concern among public health officials. Within this context, the health professionals responsible for HIV education must be made aware of the history of the Tuskegee Syphilis Study and its implications for HIV education and AIDS risk reduction programs in Black communities. Unfortunately, the details of the Tuskegee study are not well known. Therefore, we utilize the work of historian James Jones, who provides the most comprehensive description of the Tuskegee study in his book, *Bad Blood: The Tuskegee Syphilis Experiment—a Tragedy of Race and Medicine*.[6]

Factors Leading to the Tuskegee Syphilis Study

The Julius Rosenwald Fund, a philanthropic organization in Chicago, Ill, was dedicated to the promotion of the health, education, and welfare of Black Americans. In 1928, the fund's director of medical service approached the United States Public Health Service (PHS) in an effort to expand activities to improve the health status of Blacks in the rural South. At that time the PHS had successfully completed a study of the prevalence of syphilis in over 200 Blacks employed by the Delta Pine and Land Company in Mississippi. Twenty-five percent of the sample had tested positive for syphilis. The PHS collaborated with the Rosenwald Fund to provide treatment to these people. It was the success of this collaboration that led the PHS to submit a proposal to the Rosenwald Fund for expansion of syphilis control demonstration programs into five counties in the rural South. The Rosenwald Fund approved the proposal with the condition that a Black public health nurse be employed on the project.[6,7]

From 1929 to 1931, the Rosenwald Fund sponsored syphilis control demonstration projects in Albemarle County, Virginia; Glynn County, Georgia; Pitt County, North Carolina; Macon County, Alabama; and Tipton County, Tennessee. The primary goal was to demonstrate that rural Blacks could be tested and treated for syphilis. During the testing phase of the study, it was found that in Macon County, Alabama, 35% to 40% of all age groups tested were positive for syphilis.[6,7] Before the treatment phase of the project could begin, two things happened that led to the Tuskegee Syphilis Study.

First, there was much speculation in the scientific literature on racial differences in the natural history of syphilis. Although some theories suggested that syphilis affected the neurological functioning of whites, there was speculation that latent syphilis had an impact on the cardiovascular systems of Blacks. However, Dr. Bruusgaard in Oslo, Norway, conducted a retrospective study of white men with untreated syphilis which found that cardiovascular damage was common and neurological involvement was rare. This finding, published in 1929, was contrary to the prevailing scientific view in the United States.[6]

Second, the start of the Depression in 1929 devastated the Rosenwald Fund's financial resources, which were needed for the treatment component of the demonstration project. Without financial support from the Rosenwald Fund, the PHS simply did not have the resources to develop treatment programs in all five counties. It was thought that the best chance of salvaging anything of value from the project lay in the conduct of a scientific experiment.

Conflict between findings from the Oslo study and the prevailing scientific view in the U.S. on racial differences led Taliaferro Clark, M.D., of the PHS, to propose that a major improvement on previous syphilis research could be obtained by conducting a prospective study of living patients. Consequently, in 1932, Dr. Clark stated that "the Alabama community offered an unparalleled opportunity for the study of the effect of untreated syphilis" (p. 94).[6]

The original study population consisted of 399 Black men with syphilis and 201 controls. The study was intended to last for 6 to 9 months. However, as Jones demonstrates, the drive to satisfy scientific curiosity resulted in a 40-year experiment that followed these men to "end point" (autopsy). Jones eloquently describes the irony of the Tuskegee Syphilis Study:

[The] study would be an expression of concern for Negro health problems, keeping the PHS involved as a vital force in promoting medical attention to Blacks. The more damaging the disease was shown to be, the more pressure would build on Southern legislators to fund treatment programs. The study would also permit the PHS to maintain the momentum of public health work in Alabama by continuing the close working relationships with state and local health officials, not to mention Black leaders at Tuskegee Institute (p. 94).[6]

The Tuskegee Syphilis Study

Strategies Used to Recruit and Track Participants
The 40-year continuation of the Tuskegee Syphilis Study can be attributed to extensive collaboration among government agencies, along with an unprecedented community-based approach that demonstrated a degree of cultural sensitivity toward the poor Black target population in Macon County. The strategies used to recruit and retain participants in the study were quite similar to those being advocated for HIV education and AIDS risk reduction programs today. In addition to the PHS, which served as the lead agency, there was an impressive group of cooperating agencies from state and local levels:

- Macon County Medical Society
- Tuskegee Institute
- Alabama State and Macon County Boards of Health
- The Milbank Memorial Fund
- local Black churches and public schools
- local plantation owners

During the early phase of the project, the PHS decided to ask Tuskegee Institute to participate in the study. It was felt that because Tuskegee Institute had a history of service to Blacks in Macon County, its participation would not threaten white physicians in the county. Furthermore, the PHS felt that the use of Black physicians was necessary to facilitate the cooperation of subjects.[6] Tuskegee Institute benefited from this collaboration by receiving funds, training opportunities for interns, and employment for its nurses. Jones describes the complex political maneuvers involved in setting up the study:

[By persuading the Tuskegee Institute physicians to cooperate], the old syphilis control demonstration team of [PHS] clinicians would be reunited and the study would have the appearance of a revival of syphilis control work. The true purpose of the experiment would be totally obscured, leaving investigators free to trade upon the goodwill and trust that the Rosenwald Fund's syphilis control demonstration had generated among the Black people of the county and their white employers. Dr. Clark was not the least bit embarrassed by the deceit. (p. 100)[6]

The study included culturally sensitive grassroots approaches to ensure the involvement and continued participation of the men. The study employed Eunice Rivers, a Black public health nurse from Macon County, throughout the entire 40 years. As the primary contact person, she provided transportation, organized the men for examinations by the visiting PHS physicians, provided reassurance, and formed trusting relationships with the men and their families.[8]

The PHS was extremely successful in enlisting Black church leaders, elders in the community, and plantation owners to encourage participation. The plantation owners had an economic incentive to maintain the health of their employees. Often they would give permission for medical examinations while workers toiled in the fields.[7] In addition, physical examinations, including the taking of blood samples, were conducted in Black churches and schools. Jones describes the process through which subjects were recruited: "First the health officials won over local leaders. Then, they used schoolhouses and churches as makeshift clinics, with local schoolteachers and ministers serving as 'advance people' who spread the word about where and when the 'government doctors' would be in the area" (p. 69).[6]

In addition, the fact that Whites ruled Blacks in Macon County, coupled with the Black men's extreme poverty and almost total lack of access to health care, made the men willing subjects. As Dr. Frost, a Black physician from the Rosenwald Fund, stated, "as a group, they were susceptible to kindness."[6]

Lack of medical care in Macon County meant that many of the study participants had never been treated by a physician. The PHS physicians, believing that their patients would not understand clinical terms, did not even attempt to educate them about syphilis. Participants were not informed that they suffered from a specific, definable disease that was contagious and transmitted through sexual intercourse. Nor were they told that the disease could be transmitted from mother to fetus. The PHS clinicians translated medical terms into local language. Syphilis became "bad blood," a phrase that Black people of the rural South used to describe a variety of ailments.[9] Consequently, when the PHS physicians announced that they had come to test for "bad blood," people turned out in droves. The PHS also used incentives including free physical examinations, food, and transportation.[8] Burial stipends, provided by the Milbank Memorial Fund, were used to gain permission from family members for autopsies to be performed on study participants who reached "end point."[6]

From the historical and social perspective of the rural South in the early 1930s, the PHS strategies represented a high degree of understanding about the cultural milieu in which the study was being conducted. There is no doubt the approach was a sophisticated demonstration of cultural sensitivity coupled with political savvy and an impressive commitment by collaborating agencies. However, the tragedy was that a project originally intended to meet real health needs ended in a mere attempt to salvage scientific data.

How Did It Go On for So Long?

The Tuskegee study of untreated syphilis in the Negro male is the longest nontherapeutic experiment on human beings in medical history.[6] Numerous factors contributed to the continuation of this experiment over a period of 40 years. However, almost from the outset, its scientific merit was questionable.

The Alabama state health officer and the Macon County Board of Health extracted a promise from the PHS that all who were tested and found to be positive for syphilis, including those selected for the study, would receive treatment. It was understood by all, except the subjects, that the treatment given was less than the amount recommended by the PHS to cure syphilis. By the late 1930s some physicians began to raise concerns regarding the scientific merit of a study about untreated syphilis when it was clear that some subjects had received some form of treatment. In 1938, removal of these men from the experiment was briefly considered, but it was decided that in the interest of maintaining esprit de corps among the participants and in order to avoid suspicion, those men who had received minimal treatment would remain in the experimental group.[6]

The ultimate tragedy of the Tuskegee experiment was exemplified by the extraordinary measures taken to ensure that subjects in the experimental group did not receive effective treatment. During World War II, approximately 50 of the syphilitic cases received letters from the local draft board ordering them to take treatment. At the request of the PHS, the draft board agreed to exclude the men in the study from its list of draftees needing treatment.[6] According to Jones,

> [Preventing] the men from receiving treatment had always been a violation of Alabama's public health statutes requiring public reporting and prompt treatment of venereal diseases. . . . Under the auspices of the law health officials conducted the largest state-level testing and treatment program in the history of the nation [but] state and local health officials continued to cooperate with the study (p. 178).[6]

In 1943, the PHS began to administer penicillin to syphilitic patients in selected treatment clinics across the nation. The men of the Tuskegee Syphilis Study were excluded from this treatment for the same reason other drugs had been withheld since the beginning of the study in 1932—treatment would end the study. Once penicillin became the standard of treatment for syphilis in 1951, the PHS insisted that it was all the more urgent for the Tuskegee study to continue because "it made the experiment a never-again-to-be-repeated opportunity" (p. 179).[6]

In 1952, in an effort to reach subjects who had moved out of Macon County, the PHS utilized its entire national network of state and local health departments for the first time in its history in order to bring subjects in for examination. Over the next 20 years, state and local health departments cooperated in keeping the men in the study, yet denying treatment.

According to Jones, the ultimate reason why the Tuskegee Syphilis Study went on for 40 years was a minimal sense of personal responsibility and ethical concern among the small group of men within the PHS who controlled the study. This attitude was reflected in a 1976 interview conducted by Jones with Dr. John Heller, Director of Venereal Diseases at the PHS from 1943 to 1948, who stated, "The men's status did not warrant ethical debate. They were subjects, not patients; clinical material, not sick people" (p. 179).[6]

Jones details the following chronology of events leading to the end of the Tuskegee Syphilis Study:

- November 1966. Peter Buxtun, a venereal disease interviewer and investigator with the PHS in San Francisco, sent a letter to Dr. William Brown, Director of the Division of Venereal Diseases, to express his moral concerns about the experiment. He inquired whether any of the men had been treated properly and whether any had been told the nature of the study.
- November 1968. Buxtun wrote Dr. Brown a second letter, in which he described the current racial unrest prevalent in the nation. Buxtun made the point that "the racial composition of the study group [100% Negro] supported the thinking of Negro militants that Negroes have long been used for medical experiments and teaching cases in the emergency wards of county hospitals" (p. 193).[6] Dr. Brown showed this letter to the Director of the Centers for Disease Control. For the first time, health officials saw the experiment as a public relations problem that could have severe political repercussions.
- February 1969. The CDC convened a blue ribbon panel to discuss the Tuskegee study. The group reviewed all aspects of the experiment and decided against treating the men. This decision ended debate on the Tuskegee study's future: It would continue until "end point." The committee also recommended that a major thrust be made to upgrade the study scientifically.
- In the final analysis, it was Peter Buxtun who stopped the Tuskegee Syphilis Study by telling his story to a reporter with the Associated Press. On July 25, 1972, the *Washington Star* ran a front-page story about the experiment. It is important to note that the PHS was still conducting the experiment on the day when the story broke.

The story was picked up off the wire service and became front-page news and the subject of editorials in major newspapers across the nation. It did not take long for officials in the Department of Health, Education, and Welfare (HEW) and the

PHS to form a chorus of denunciation in concert with the public outcry condemning the study. Little effort was made directly to defend or justify the experiment. For example, Dr. Donald Printz, an official in the Venereal Disease Branch of the CDC, publicly stated that the experiment was "almost like genocide . . . a literal death sentence was passed on some of those people" (p. 207).[6]

Implications for HIV/AIDS Risk Reduction Programs in the Black Community

The historic 1972 disclosure of the Tuskegee study in the national press led to congressional subcommittee hearings held in February and March of 1973 by Senator Edward Kennedy. The result was a complete revamping of HEW regulations on protection of human subjects in experimentation. On July 23, 1973 a $1.8 billion class-action law suit was filed in the U.S. District Court for the Middle District of Alabama on behalf of the men in the study. In December 1974, the government agreed to pay $10 million in an out-of-court settlement. Jones provides a detailed description of the law suit consequences.[6]

There has been relatively little discussion of the Tuskegee Experiment within the public health professional literature since the historic 1972 disclosure of the study in the national press. For example, Cutler and Arnold's 1988 article titled "Venereal Disease Control by Health Departments in the Past: Lessons for the Present"[10] failed to make any mention of the Tuskegee study yet called upon readers of this journal to honor Surgeon General Parran who at one point directed the study. Silver described this omission as evidence of the continued inability to confront our racist past. Silver went on to state that

> the behavior of the PHS officers was no more than representative of the sentiments and prejudices of the times. But not to remember is to forget, and to forget is a disservice to those who suffered the indignities. . . . [In] calling upon us to honor [Paran], one of the participants, we should also mention the context in which the meritorious service was earned.[11]

Both Brandt[12] and Fee[13] emphasize the importance of history in the cultural meaning of disease. Therefore, as the pattern of HIV infection shifts and increasing numbers of Blacks are affected, it will be crucial to understand the historical context in which Black Americans will interpret the disease. The failure of public health professionals to comprehensively discuss the Tuskegee experiment contributes to its use as a source of misinformation and helps to maintain a barrier between the Black community and health care service providers. In presentations at public health professional meetings and interactions with Black community-based-organization staff members, the authors have consistently observed how the

Tuskegee Study is used to undermine trust and justify AIDS conspiracy theories. Although there is no evidence to support Dalton's assertion that the men were intentionally infected with syphilis,[5] this distortion continues to be disseminated through community discussions and the popular media. There is no need to misrepresent the facts of the study to recognize how it contributes to fears of genocide. Given that the conduct of the study demonstrated little regard for the lives of the men who participated, it is no surprise that Blacks today do not readily dismiss assertions that HIV is a manmade virus intentionally allowed to run rampant in their communities.

Now, almost 60 years after the experiment began, the Tuskegee Syphilis Study's legacy is a trail of distrust and suspicion that hampers HIV education efforts in Black communities. During testimony delivered before the National Commission on AIDS in December 1990, Alpha Thomas, a health educator with the Dallas Urban League, stated: "So many African American people that I work with do not trust hospitals or any of the other community health care service providers because of that Tuskegee Experiment. It is like . . . if they did it then they will do it again" (p. 43).[4]

Public health professionals must recognize that Blacks' belief in AIDS as a form of genocide is a legitimate attitudinal barrier rooted in the history of the Tuskegee Syphilis Study. Many public health authorities who work with Black communities are uncomfortable responding to the issue of genocide and the Tuskegee study. The common response is to ignore these issues. This approach may result in a loss of believability and further alienation. One culturally sensitive response would be for public health professionals to discuss the fear of genocide evoked by the AIDS epidemic. They must be willing to listen respectfully to community fears, share the facts of the Tuskegee study when it arises as a justification of those fears, and admit to the limitations of science when they do not have all the answers. This approach may help public health authorities to regain the credibility and the public trust they need to successfully implement HIV risk reduction strategies in the Black community.

The necessary public health science technology and experience exist for the development and implementation of effective community-based HIV education programs that are ethnically acceptable and culturally sensitive. Strategies such as (1) the use of program staff indigenous to the community, (2) the use of incentives, and (3) the delivery of health services within the target community were used to recruit participants in the Tuskegee Syphilis Study. These techniques are being implemented by AIDS risk reduction programs today. The value of these community-based strategies should not be diminished by their association with the Tuskegee study. The impact of HIV infection and AIDS in Black communities is exacerbated by the presence of other sources of poor health status and social inequities. Therefore, AIDS risk reduction programs must be built on solid assessments of community perceptions and needs, and must include ongoing involvement of community members in program planning and evaluation efforts.[14]

Successful HIV education and AIDS risk reduction will require a long-term commitment from and collaboration among federal agencies, state and local health departments, community-based organizations, private industry, philanthropies, and institutions of higher learning. Such collaboration must be based on trust between the agencies and the Black community. Given the legacy of Tuskegee, the credibility of public health service providers from outside the Black community is severely limited. Consequently, CDC's program to provide direct funding to Black community-based organizations (CBOS) to deliver HIV education represents a significant development in the effort to overcome distrust. However, while CBOS may have ready access to a community and may have established credibility with the target population, they often lack the infrastructure necessary for long-term success.[14] Consequently, CBOS will require consistent technical assistance and long-range funding from government and private agencies. To ensure that the specter of Tuskegee will not impede progress, it is crucial that decision-making power be distributed in such a manner that collaborating agencies allow CBOS to maintain control over program integrity.

Distrust of and resistance to involvement with public health programs have a legitimate basis in history; to overcome these feelings will require cultural sensitivity. In testimony before the National Commission on AIDS, Dr. Smith stated:

> [The Black] communities' perspective on medical research has a historical basis which sometimes outweighs the demonstrable integrity and commitment of individual investigators. . . . In light of the historical basis of the suspicion of being guinea pigs, it is particularly ironic to hear the cries for more access to experimental medicines. [This resistance] will only be overcome, frankly, with a more long-range effort to reassure African Americans that they will not be the victims of more Tuskegees.[4] (p. 31)

Public health professionals must support Blacks' increased access to clinical trials so that the AIDS knowledge base can be expanded and the benefits of potential treatments can be realized. The successful inclusion of Blacks in clinical trials will require researchers to conduct their investigations in convenient settings trusted by the Black community. In addition, investigators must recognize that simple compliance with protection of human subjects procedures is not sufficient. The researchers who conducted the Tuskegee study made a conscious decision to withhold information about syphilis from participants. Consequently, Blacks today may not believe that they are being told the whole truth about HIV. To overcome the distrust of community members, researchers must see that they are fully informed about research procedures, costs, and benefits, and that they have representation on research advisory committees. Investigators should conduct their work with an attitude of respect for the humanity of study participants, regardless of the social and cultural gulf that may exist between investigators and subjects. Ultimately, cultural sensitivity can best be manifested through the professional obligation to advocate AIDS policies that provide for the protection of civil rights and access to health care services.[15]

It must be acknowledged that public health research and practice operate in an environment influenced by societal values and political ideology. For example, needle distribution programs for intravenous drug users, along with HIV testing policies and counseling of HIV-infected women, are frequently the subject of political debate. Efforts to develop needle distribution programs have been stymied by political controversy, moral questions, and outraged claims that such programs have a genocidal impact on Black communities. In many communities where drug abuse is epidemic, needle distribution programs are perceived as contributing to the drug problem, particularly when such programs are promulgated in the absence of access to adequate drug treatment services. The image of Black intravenous drug users reaching out for treatment, only to receive clean needles from public health authorities, provides additional fuel for the genocide theory. The emphasis on HIV testing and counseling without adequate access to clinical trials and appropriate therapy for AIDS evokes memories of the deliberate withholding of treatment by the researchers in the Tuskegee study. Public health professionals must ensure that HIV testing and counseling are accompanied by specific informed consent, full discussion of treatment options, and appropriate referrals for primary care and clinical trials.

The reproductive rights of HIV-infected women cannot be separated from societal values, political ideology, moral issues, and concern over access to primary health care. In an effort to prevent perinatal transmission, the CDC and state health departments advocate HIV testing programs and counsel HIV-infected women to avoid pregnancy.[16] However, implementation of these public health policies in the Black community is potentially volatile and disastrous. The promotion of condoms as a means of preventing HIV infection is viewed with suspicion by Blacks. Levine and Dubler state that "many African Americans view any attempt to interfere with or discourage reproduction as part of a plan for genocide" (p. 333).[16] If health care providers demonstrate a lack of sensitivity to these views and continue to advocate HIV testing, contraception, and abortion, the fears of Blacks—who are already alienated from health care providers—will be reinforced.

AIDS in the Black community must be understood within the broader context of other leading causes of preventable death that may result in decreased population growth and decreased lifespan. The failure to close the gap in health status between White and Black Americans can be directly attributed to social inequities and Blacks' lack of access to health care. George Lundberg, editor of the *Journal of the American Medical Association*, attributes this lack of access to long-standing, institutionalized racial discrimination.[17] Although the PHS officials who conducted the Tuskegee study were clearly influenced by the racial prejudice of their time, it was their use of institutional power and resources that transformed prejudice into racism. We must guard against prejudicial assumptions about the race, class status, and lifestyle of people at risk for HIV infection. As Allan Brandt states, "the notion that science is a value free discipline must be rejected. The need for greater vigilance in assessing the specific ways in which social values and attitudes affect professional behavior is clearly indicated" (p. 27).[18] A failure to eliminate prejudice aggressively today could lead to repressive AIDS policies, cloaked as traditional public health practices designed to control the epidemic.

As the American public becomes increasingly aware of AIDS as a significant health problem in the Black community, there will be both opportunity and danger. The opportunity is to deal comprehensively rather than haphazardly with the problem as a whole: to see it as a social catastrophe brought on by years of economic deprivation and to meet it as other disasters are met, with adequate resources. The danger is that AIDS will be attributed to some innate weakness of Black people and used to justify further neglect and to rationalize continued deprivation. We must be mindful that the AIDS epidemic has uncovered the harsh reality of diminished economic resources, the limits of medical science, and confusion over how best to attribute responsibility for the prevention of HIV infection. It is within this context that public health must be used as a means for social justice.[19]

The AIDS epidemic has exposed the Tuskegee Syphilis Study as a historical marker for the legitimate discontent of Blacks with the public health system. In the absence of a cure for AIDS, education remains our best chance to stop the spread of HIV infection. We must discuss the feeling within the Black community that AIDS is a form of genocide, a feeling justified by the history of the Tuskegee study. This dialogue can contribute to a better understanding of how to develop and implement HIV education programs that are scientifically sound, culturally sensitive, and ethnically acceptable.

Acknowledgments

This study was supported in part by grant 14629 from the Robert Wood Johnson Foundation and a professional service contract from the Southern Christian Leadership Conference. Parts of this work were presented at the American Public Health Association Annual Meeting, New York City, October 1990; the Walter Reed Army Research Institute, Washington, DC, November 1990; and the Association for the Advancement of Health Education Annual Meeting, San Francisco, Calif, April 1991. The authors gratefully acknowledge the assistance of Patricia Mail and Peg Kopf, whose thoughtful criticism contributed significantly to this manuscript.

REFERENCES

1. Centers for Disease Control, *HIV/AIDS Surveillance Report*. June 1991. Atlanta, Ga.

2. Smith R. Muhammad warns Blacks to beware: social AIDS. *Eclipse: The Black Student News Magazine of the University of Maryland*. November 23, 1988;21:6.

3. Bates K. AIDS: is it genocide? *Essence*. September 1990;21:77–116.

4. National Commission on AIDS. Hearings on HIV Disease in African American Communities. 1990.

5. Dalton H. AIDS in blackface. *Daedalus: J Am Acad Arts and Sci*. 1989 (Summer);205–228.

6. Jones J. *Bad Blood: The Tuskegee Syphilis Experiment—A Tragedy of Race and Medicine*. New York, NY: The Free Press, 1981.

7. Parran T. *Shadow on the Land: Syphilis*. New York, NY: Reynal & Hitchcock; 1937.

8. Rivers E, Schuman S, Olansky S. Twenty years of followup experience in a long-range medical study. *Public Health Rep*. 1953;68:391–395.

9. Johnson C. *Shadow of the Plantation*. Chicago, Ill: University of Chicago Press; 1934.

10. Cutler J, Arnold R. Venereal disease control by health departments in the past: lessons for the present. *Am J Public Health*. 1988;78:372–376.

11. Silver G. AIDS: the infamous Tuskegee Study. *Am J Public Health*. 1988;78:1500.

12. Brandt A. AIDS: from social history to social policy. In: Fee E, Fox D, eds. *AIDS: The Burdens of History*. Berkeley, Calif: University of California Press;1988:147–171.

13. Fee E. Sin vs science: venereal disease in twentieth-century Baltimore. In: Fee E, Fox D, eds. *AIDS: The Burdens of History*. Berkeley, Calif: University of California Press;1988:121–146.

14. Thomas S, Morgan C. Evaluation of community based AIDS education and risk reduction projects in ethnic and racial minority communities: a survey of projects funded by the U.S. Public Health Service. *J Program Plan Eval*. 1991;14(4).

15. Quinn S. AIDS and HIV Testing: Implications for health education. *J Health Educ*. In press.

16. Levine C, Dubler N. Uncertain risks and bitter realities: the reproductive choices of HIV-infected women. *Milbank Q*. 1990;68:321–351.

17. Lundberg G. National health care reform: an aura of inevitability is upon us. *JAMA*. 1991;265:2566–2567.

18. Brandt A. Racism and research: the case of the Tuskegee Syphilis Study. *The Hastings Center Rep*. 1978;8:21–29.

19. Shannon I. Public health's promise for the future: 1989 presidential address. *Am J Public Health*. 1990;80:909–912.

WHEN EVIL INTRUDES

ARTHUR L. CAPLAN

Twenty years ago Peter Buxtun, a public health official working for the United States Public Health Service, complained to a reporter for the Associated Press that he was deeply concerned about the morality of an ongoing study being sponsored by the Public Health Service—a study compiling information about the course and effects of syphilis in human beings based upon medical examinations of poor black men in Macon County, Alabama. The men, or more accurately, those still living, had been coming in for annual examinations for forty years. They were not receiving standard therapy for syphilis. In late July of 1972 the *Washington Star* and the *New York Times* ran front-page stories based on Buxtun's concerns about what has been called the longest running "nontherapeutic experiment" on human beings in medical history and "the most notorious case of prolonged and knowing violation of subject's rights"—the Tuskegee study.[1]

Buxtun went public with his ethical concerns after years of complaining to officials from the Centers for Disease Control and the Public Health Service with no apparent effect. His decision to blow the whistle led to a series of sensational congressional hearings chaired by Senator Edward Kennedy in February and March of 1973. Legislators and federal officials expressed outrage over the immortality of a study in which poor, illiterate men had been deceived and given placebo treatment rather than standard therapy so that more could be learned about syphilis. Americans found it hard to believe that the Public Health Service had intentionally and systematically duped men with a disease as serious as syphilis—contagious, disabling, and life-threatening—for more than forty years.

The level of outrage about the Tuskegee study was enormous. One CDC official labeled the experiment akin to "genocide."[2] As a result of public anger over the immorality of the study, Congress created an ad hoc blue ribbon panel to review both the Tuskegee study and the adequacy of existing protections for subjects in all federally sponsored research. Even though the panel did not receive all the information about the study that the government had available,[3] they were still concerned enough about what had taken place to recommend the creation of a national board with the resources to reexamine all aspects of human experimenta-

Arthur L. Caplan is professor of bioethics at the University of Pennsylvania.
Originally published in the Hastings Center Report 22 (1992): 29–32. Reprinted by permission of the Hastings Center and Arthur L. Caplan.

tion in the United States. Congress, in 1974, created the National Commission for the Protection of Human Subjects of Biomedical and Behavioral Research which, in its seventeen reports and numerous appendix volumes, laid the foundation for the ethical requirements that govern the conduct of research on human subjects in the United States to this day.

Syphilis continues to challenge America's and the world's medical, public health, and moral resources. While there are a variety of antibiotics available to treat the disease, it has proven to be a stubborn and resilient foe. The Centers for Disease Control has found steady and alarming increases in the incidence of primary and secondary syphilis over the past decade. It is still a major public health problem in the United States today, especially among young black males.

The rise in the incidence of the disease has ensured that writings about the diagnosis, management, and treatment of syphilis are prominently featured in the professional literature of public health and biomedicine as well as in standard textbooks about venereal and infectious diseases. Ongoing concern about syphilis has led physicians and public health officials to draw upon as much information as they can about the course of the disease. One of the bitter if generally un-acknowledged ironies of the Tuskegee study is that, while it now occupies a special place of shame in the annals of human experimentation, its findings are still widely cited by the contemporary biomedical community.

In looking at instances of scientific misconduct and moral malfeasance with respect to research it is quite common to find the position advanced that good science is incompatible with bad ethics. When one wrestles with the horror of the medical abuse of vulnerable human beings it is somewhat comforting to believe that those who engage in such abuse could not produce anything of real value to medicine. Yet the continuing invocation of the findings of the Tuskegee study by those who diagnose, study, or treat syphilis shows that it is sometimes impossible to avoid a confrontation with the question of the ethics of relying on knowledge obtained in the course of immoral research.

The "bad ethics, therefore bad science" argument actually has two distinct components. One part of the argument holds that researchers engaged in obvious immoral conduct with their subjects could not generate useful or valid scientific findings. The second part holds that when the ethical conduct of research is egregiously immoral then any findings obtained ought not to be admitted into the body of scientific knowledge. While it may often be true that it is difficult to trust findings obtained using subjects who were abused or harmed (as was the case in Nazi concentration camp studies),[4] this part of the argument is not always true. Even a cursory glance through the literature of health care reveals that the Tuskegee study was and remains a key source of information about the diagnosis, signs, symptoms, and course of syphilis. No effort has been made to impugn its findings, and the biomedical community has relied upon them for decades.

James Jones, in his landmark book on the Tuskegee study, *Bad Blood*, notes that no researcher involved in the study ever published a single, comprehensive summary of its findings. The absence of such a review paper may have fostered the impression that no substantive findings of any real significance were obtained. But Jones also notes in the appendix to his book that Public Health Service scientists, physicians, and nurses associated with the study published a total of thirteen articles between 1936 and 1973 based solely upon its findings. These papers appeared in a wide variety of peer-reviewed journals, including *Public Health Reports*, *Milbank Fund Memorial Quarterly*, *Journal of Chronic Diseases*, and *Archives of Internal Medicine*.

It is a relatively simple matter to establish the importance assigned to the findings of the Tuskegee study by the contemporary biomedical community. The computerization on large data bases of the majority of the world's professional biomedical journals allows searches to be conducted to see which, if any, recent journal articles cite any of the thirteen papers presenting the findings of the Tuskegee study. An initial database search for the period January 1985 to February 1991 produced twenty such citations from a wide spectrum of journals, including American, British, and German publications. The twenty citations make reference to seven of the original thirteen papers.

A visit to any large medical library will also quickly reveal the importance assigned to the findings of the Tuskegee study in recent years. An informal random selection of twenty medical textbooks on sexually transmitted diseases, infectious disease, human sexuality, and public health published after 1984 turned up four books that made explicit reference to the study and cited at least one of the same thirteen articles. Three textbooks were published in the United States, one in England.

The range of journals in which contemporary articles on syphilis, venereal disease, and dementia directly cite the papers reporting the findings of the Tuskegee study is quite large. Direct citations of the Tuskegee study papers appear in articles in the *Journal of Family Practice* (1986), *The Lancet* (1986), *British Heart Journal* (1987), *New England Journal of Medicine* (1987), *Journal of the American Geriatrics Society* (1989), *The American Journal of Medicine* (1989), *American Journal of Public Health* (1989), and *Medical Clinics of North America* (1990), among others.

Nearly all the references in both the periodical literature and the medical textbooks use the Tuskegee study to describe the natural history of the disease. A recent review article on cardiovascular syphilis is typical of the way in which the Tuskegee study and its findings are cited:

In 1932, the United States Public Health Service initiated the Tuskegee Study to delineate further the natural history of untreated syphilis. A total of 412 men with untreated syphilis and 204 uninfected matched controls were followed prospectively. Vonderlehr (15), reviewing the autopsy material from the first years of the study, noted that only one-fourth of the untreated patients were without evidence of any form of tertiary syphilis after 15 years of infection. Moreover, cardiovascular involvement was the most frequently detected abnormality. Peters (16) analyzed the autopsy data from the first 20 years of the study. He found that 50% of patients who had been infected for 10 years had demonstrable cardiovascular involvement. Of the 40% of syphilitic patients who died during this period, the primary causes of death were cardiovascular or central nervous system syphilis (16). Of the 41% of survivors at 30 years of follow-up, 12% had clinical evidence of late, predominantly cardiovascular syphilis (17). Most of these patients had evidence of cardiovascular syphilis at the 15-year analysis (17). These data ... indicate that ... complications are usually evident 10 to 20 years after primary infection, and cardiovascular syphilis is the predominant cause of demise in those patients who die as a direct result of syphilis.[5]

The reference numbers 15, 16, and 17 in the excerpt are to three of the thirteen papers reporting the findings of the Tuskegee study.

Yet another representative example from the contemporary periodical literature of health care invoking the findings of the Tuskegee study appears in a review of neurosyphilis and dementia:

Neurosyphilis is rare as a manifestation of syphilis. Tertiary and late latent syphilis have been decreasing in incidence since the 1950s. There have been two studies of untreated syphilis: in the Oslo study neurosyphilis eventually developed in 7% of the patients, and in the Tuskegee study, syphilitic involvement of the cardiovascular system or the central nervous system was the primary cause of death in 30% of the infected patients, with cardiovascular involvement being much more common than neurosyphilis.[6]

Textbook references are quite similar to those that appear in the periodical literature. In giving an overview of the natural course of untreated syphilis one recent text states:

A prospective study involving 431 black men with seropositive latent syphilis of 3 or more years' duration was undertaken in 1932 (the Tuskegee study, 1932–1936) (16). This study showed that hypertension in syphilitic black men 25–50 years of age was 17 percent more common than in nonsyphilitics. Cardiovascular complications including hypertension were more common than neurologic complications were, and both were increased over control populations. Anatomic evidence of aortitis was found to be 25–35 percent more common in autopsied syphilitics, while evidence of central nervous system syphilis was found in 4 percent of the patients.[7]

Reference number 16 is to one of the thirteen papers in which the Tuskegee findings were presented.

These examples clearly illustrate the continuing importance assigned to the Tuskegee study by those concerned with understanding and treating syphilis. The case for the study's importance could be further bolstered by tracking down secondary and tertiary references to its findings. There can be no disputing the fact that contemporary medicine has accepted the findings as valid and continues to rely on them as a key source of knowledge about the natural history of the disease.

The acceptance of the Tuskegee study findings as valid refutes the argument that bad ethics is always incompatible with valid science, but the question still remains as to whether the data of the Tuskegee study should continue to be utilized. It may make sense in some situations to argue that data obtained by immoral means should not be used purely on ethical grounds. But even if it were wrong to cite data acquired by immoral means there is simply no way to purge the knowledge gained in the Tuskegee study from biomedicine. Too much of what is known about the natural history of syphilis is based upon the study, and that knowledge has become so deeply embedded that it could not be removed.

Still, the view that the study was immoral and therefore worthless has flourished. This is a cause for concern, because the belief that not much of value came from the Tuskegee study allows both medicine and bioethics to avoid examining such troubling questions as how immoral research could be conducted by reputable scientists under the sponsorship of the American government for forty years, how such research could be allowed to continue long after the promulgation of the Nuremberg and Helsinki Codes, and what the moral duties and responsibilities are of those in biomedicine who continue to cite the study's findings today.

While one of the textbooks that discusses the Tuskegee study does make reference to the ethical shadow hanging over the findings,[8] none of the others and none of the articles in the peer-reviewed periodical literature that directly cite the papers based on the study do so. Should the results of the Tuskegee study continue to be invoked in review articles and texts without some accompanying discussion of the manner in which the findings were obtained and the ethical impact that the study had on the subsequent responsibilities of researchers? Given that the study played a crucial role in causing Americans to rethink the ethics of human experimentation, it would seem morally incumbent upon those who discuss its findings in the context of textbooks and review articles to allot some space for a discussion of the ethical problems associated with it.

There are obvious limits to the extent to which anyone writing a scientific paper or book can review the circumstances and conditions under which scientific knowledge was obtained. The history of medicine is replete with examples of research, certainly considered immoral by contemporary standards, that generate findings still widely accepted and cited. Not every article in a scientific journal can be used as a vehicle for educating the reader about the morality of human experimentation.

But there are obvious forums in biomedicine, such as textbooks and review articles, where it makes sense for authors to include some discussion of the ethical circumstances surrounding morally dubious or blatantly immoral research. The obvious immorality of research methods should not blind us to the importance of noting and discussing them. If no place is made for discussions of the morality of studies such as Tuskegee, the research community may become complacent about the importance of its responsibilities toward human subjects at the same time as the public comes to believe that good science cannot emerge from immoral research.

REFERENCES

1. Stephen B. Thomas and Sandra C. Quinn, "The Tuskegee Syphilis Study, 1932 to 1972: Implications for HIV Education and AIDS Risk Education Programs in the Black Community," *American Journal of Public Health* 81, no. 11 (1991): 1498–1505, at 1501; Ruth Faden and Tom Beauchamp, *A History and Theory of Informed Consent* (New York: Oxford, 1986), p. 165.

2. James H. Jones, *Bad Blood: The Tuskegee Syphilis Experiment* (New York: Free Press, 1981), p. 207.

3. Jay Katz, personal communication, 1991.

4. See Arthur Caplan, ed., *When Medicine Went Mad* (New York: Humana, 1992).

5. J. D. Jackson and J. D. Radolf, "Cardiovascular Syphilis," *The American Journal of Medicine* 87 (October 1989): 428–29.

6. J. A. Rhymes, C. Woodson, R. Sparage-Sachs, and C. K. Cassel, "Nonmedical Complications of Diagnostic Workup for Dementia: University of Chicago Grand Rounds," *Journal of the American Geriatrics Society* 37, no. 12 (1989): 1157–64, at 1160.

7. G. L. Mandell, R. G. Douglas, Jr., and J. E. Bennett, eds., *Principles and Practice of Infectious Diseases*, 3rd ed. (New York: Churchill Livingstone, 1990), p. 1797.

8. K. K. Holmes, P. Mardh, P. F. Sparling, and P. J. Wiesner, *Sexually Transmitted Diseases*, 2nd ed. (New York: McGraw-Hill, 1990).

THE DANGERS OF DIFFERENCE

PATRICIA A. KING

It has been sixty years since the beginning of the Tuskegee syphilis experiment and twenty years since its existence was disclosed to the American public. The social and ethical issues that the experiment poses for medicine, particularly for medicine's relationship with African Americans, are still not broadly understood, appreciated, or even remembered.[1] Yet a significant aspect of the Tuskegee experiment's legacy is that in a racist society that incorporates beliefs about the inherent inferiority of African Americans in contrast with the superior status of whites, any attention to the question of differences that may exist is likely to be pursued in a manner that burdens rather than benefits African Americans.

The Tuskegee experiment, which involved approximately 400 males with late-stage, untreated syphilis and approximately 200 controls free of the disease, is by any measure one of the dark pages in the history of American medicine. In this study of the natural course of untreated syphilis, the participants did not give informed consent. Stunningly, when penicillin was subsequently developed as a treatment for syphilis, measures were taken to keep the diseased participants from receiving it.

Obviously, the experiment provides a basis for the exploration of many ethical and social issues in medicine, including professional ethics,[2] the limitations of informed consent as a means of protecting research subjects, and the motives and methods used to justify the exploitation of persons who live in conditions of severe economic and social disadvantage. At bottom, however, the Tuskegee experiment is different from other incidents of abuse in clinical research because all the participants were black males. The racism that played a central role in this tragedy continues to infect even our current well-intentioned efforts to reverse the decline in health status of African Americans.[3]

Others have written on the scientific attitudes about race and heredity that flourished at the time that the Tuskegee experiment was conceived.[4] There has always been widespread interest in racial differences between blacks and whites, especially differences that related to sexual matters. These perceived differences have often reinforced and justified differential treatment of blacks and whites, and

Patricia A. King is professor of law at Georgetown University.
Originally published in the Hastings Center Report 22 *(1992): 35–38. Reprinted by permission of the Hastings Center and Patricia A. King.*

have done so to the detriment of blacks. Not surprisingly, such assumptions about racial differences provided critical justification for the Tuskegee experiment itself.

Before the experiment began a Norwegian investigator had already undertaken a study of untreated syphilis in whites between 1890 and 1910. Although there had also been a follow-up study of these untreated patients from 1925 to 1927, the original study was abandoned when arsenic therapy became available. In light of the availability of therapy a substantial justification for replicating a study of untreated syphilis was required. The argument that provided critical support for the experiment was that the natural course of untreated syphilis in blacks and whites was not the same.[5] Moreover, it was thought that the differences between blacks and whites were not merely biological but that they extended to psychological and social responses to the disease as well. Syphilis, a sexually transmitted disease, was perceived to be rampant among blacks in part because blacks—unlike whites—were not inclined to seek or continue treatment for syphilis.

The Dilemma of Difference

In the context of widespread belief in the racial inferiority of blacks that surrounded the Tuskegee experiment, it should not come as a surprise that the experiment exploited its subjects. Recognizing and taking account of racial differences that have historically been utilized to burden and exploit African Americans poses a dilemma.[6] Even in circumstances where the goal of a scientific study is to benefit a stigmatized group or person, such well-intentioned efforts may nevertheless cause harm. If the racial difference is ignored and all groups or persons are treated similarly, unintended harm may result from the failure to recognize racially correlated factors. Conversely, if differences among groups or persons are recognized and attempts are made to respond to past injustices or special burdens, the effort is likely to reinforce existing negative stereotypes that contributed to the emphasis on racial differences in the first place.

This dilemma about difference is particularly worrisome in medicine. Because medicine is pragmatic, it will recognize racial differences if doing so will promote health goals. As a consequence, potential harms that might result from attention to racial differences tend to be overlooked, minimized, or viewed as problems beyond the purview of medicine.

The question of whether (and how) to take account of racial differences has recently been raised in the context of the current AIDS epidemic. The participation of African Americans in clinical AIDS trials has been disproportionately small in comparison to the numbers of African Americans who have been infected with the Human Immunodeficiency Virus. Because of the possibility that African Americans may respond differently to drugs being developed and tested to combat AIDS,[7] those concerned about the care and treatment of AIDS in the African American community have called for greater participation by African Americans in these trials. Ironically, efforts to address the problem of underrepresentation must cope with the enduring legacy of the Tuskegee experiment—the legacy of suspicion and skepticism toward medicine and its practitioners among African Americans.[8]

In view of the suspicion Tuskegee so justifiably engenders, calls for increased participation by African Americans in clinical trials are worrisome. The question of whether to tolerate racially differentiated AIDS research testing of new or innovative therapies, as well as the question of what norms should govern participation by African Americans in clinical research, needs careful and thoughtful attention. A generic examination of the treatment of racial differences in medicine is beyond the scope of this article. However, I will describe briefly what has occurred since disclosure of the Tuskegee experiment to point out the dangers I find lurking in our current policies.

Inclusion and Exclusion

In part because of public outrage concerning the Tuskegee experiment,[9] comprehensive regulations governing federal research using human subjects were revised and subsequently adopted by most federal agencies.[10] An institutional review board (IRB) must approve clinical research involving human subjects, and IRB approval is made contingent on review of protocols for adequate protection of human subjects in accordance with federal criteria. These criteria require among other things that an IRB ensure that subject selection is "equitable." The regulations further provide that:

> [i]n making this assessment the IRB should take into account the purposes of the research and the setting in which the research will be conducted and should be particularly cognizant of the special problems of research involving vulnerable populations, such as women, mentally disabled persons, or economically or educationally disadvantaged persons.[11]

The language of the regulation makes clear that the concern prompting its adoption was the protection of vulnerable groups from exploitation. The obverse problem—that too much protection might promote the exclusion or underrepresentation of vulnerable groups, including African Americans—was not at issue. However, underinclusion can raise as much of a problem of equity as exploitation.[12]

A 1990 General Accounting Office study first documented the extent to which minorities and women were underrepresented in federally funded research. In response, in December 1990 the National Institutes of Health, together with the

Alcohol, Drug Abuse and Mental Health Administration, directed that minorities and women be included in study populations,

> so that research findings can be of benefit to all persons at risk of the disease, disorder or condition under study; special emphasis should be placed on the need for inclusion of minorities and women in studies of diseases, disorders and conditions that disproportionately affect them.[13]

If minorities are not included, a clear and compelling rationale must be submitted.

The new policy clearly attempts to avoid the perils of overprotection, but it raises new concerns. The policy must be clarified and refined if it is to meet the intended goal of ensuring that research findings are of benefit to all. There are at least three reasons for favoring increased representation of African Americans in clinical trials. The first is that there may be biological differences between blacks and whites that might affect the applicability of experimental findings to blacks, but these differences will not be noticed if blacks are not included in sufficient numbers to allow the detection of statistically significant racial differences. The second reason is that race is a reliable index for social conditions such as poor health and nutrition, lack of adequate access to health care, and economic and social disadvantage that might adversely affect potential benefits of new interventions and procedures. If there is indeed a correlation between minority status and these factors, then African Americans and all others with these characteristics will benefit from new information generated by the research. The third reason is that the burdens and benefits of research should be spread across the population regardless of racial or ethnic status.[14] Each of these reasons for urging that representation of minorities be increased has merit. Each of these justifications also raises concern, however, about whether potential benefits will indeed be achieved.

The third justification carries with it the obvious danger that the special needs or problems generated as a result of economic or social conditions associated with minority status may be overlooked and that, as a result, African Americans and other minorities will be further disadvantaged. The other two justifications are problematic and deserve closer examination. They each assume that there are either biological, social, economic, or cultural differences between blacks and whites.

The Way Out of the Dilemma

Understanding how, or indeed whether, race correlates with disease is a very complicated problem. Race itself is a confusing concept with both biological and social connotations. Some doubt whether race has biological significance at all.[15] Even if race is a biological fiction, however, its social significance remains.[16] As Bob

Blauner points out, "Race is an essentially political construct, one that translates our tendency to see people in terms of their color or other physical attributes into structures that make it likely that people will act for or against them on such a basis."[17]

In the wake of Tuskegee and, in more recent times, the stigma and discrimination that resulted from screening for sickle cell trait (a genetic condition that occurs with greater frequency among African Americans), researchers have been reluctant to explore associations between race and disease. There is increasing recognition, however, of evidence of heightened resistance or vulnerability to disease along racial lines.[18] Indeed, sickle cell anemia itself substantiates the view that biological differences may exist. Nonetheless, separating myth from reality in determining the cause of disease and poor health status is not easy. Great caution should be exercised in attempting to validate biological differences in susceptibility to disease in light of this society's past experience with biological differences. Moreover, using race as an index for other conditions that might influence health and well-being is also dangerous. Such practices could emphasize social and economic differences that might also lead to stigma and discrimination.

If all the reasons for increasing minority participation in clinical research are flawed, how then can we promote improvement in the health status of African Americans and other minorities through participation in clinical research while simultaneously minimizing the harms that might flow from such participation? Is it possible to work our way out of this dilemma?

An appropriate strategy should have as its starting point the defeasible presumption that blacks and whites are biologically the same with respect to disease and treatment. Presumptions can be overturned of course, and the strategy should recognize the possibility that biological differences in some contexts are possible. But the presumption of equality acknowledges that historically the greatest harm has come from the willingness to impute biological differences rather than the willingness to overlook them. For some, allowing the presumption to be in any way defeasible is troubling. Yet I do not believe that fear should lead us to ignore the possibility of biologically differentiated responses to disease and treatment, especially when the goal is to achieve medical benefit.

It is well to note at this point the caution sounded by Hans Jonas. He wrote, "Of the new experimentation with man, medical is surely the most legitimate; psychological, the most dubious; biological (still to come), the most dangerous."[19] Clearly, priority should be given to exploring the possible social, cultural, and environmental determinants of disease before targeting the study of hypotheses that involve biological differences between blacks and whites. For example, rather than trying to determine whether blacks and whites respond differently to AZT, attention should first be directed to learning whether response to AZT is influenced by social, cultural, or environmental conditions. Only at the point where possible biological differences emerge should hypotheses that explore racial differences be considered.

A finding that blacks and whites are different in some critical aspect need not inevitably lead to increased discrimination or stigma for blacks. If there indeed had been a difference in the effects of untreated syphilis between blacks and whites such information might have been used to promote the health status of blacks. But the Tuskegee experiment stands as a reminder that such favorable outcomes rarely if ever occur. More often, either racist assumptions and stereotypes creep into the study's design, or findings broken down by race become convenient tools to support policies and behavior that further disadvantage those already vulnerable.

REFERENCES

1. For earlier examples of the use of African Americans as experimental subjects see Todd L. Savitt, "The Use of Blacks for Medical Experimentation and Demonstration in the Old South," *Journal of Southern History* 48, no. 3 (1982): 331–48.

2. David J. Rothman, "Were Tuskegee & Willowbrook 'Studies in Nature'?" *Hastings Center Report* 12, no. 2 (1982): 5–7.

3. For an in-depth examination of the health status of African Americans see Woodrow Jones, Jr., and Mitchell F. Rice, eds. *Health Care Issues in Black America: Policies, Problems, and Prospects* (New York: Greenwood Press, 1987).

4. See for example Allan M. Brandt, "Racism and Research: The Case of the Tuskegee Syphilis Study," *Hastings Center Report* 8, no. 6 (1978): 21–29; and James H. Jones, *Bad Blood: The Tuskegee Syphilis Experiment* (New York: Free Press, 1981).

5. Jones, *Bad Blood*, p. 106.

6. Martha Minow, *Making All the Difference: Inclusion, Exclusion, and American Law* (Ithaca, N.Y.: Cornell University Press, 1990).

7. Wafaa El-Sadr and Linnea Capps, "The Challenge of Minority Recruitment in Clinical Trials for AIDS," *JAMA* 267, no. 7 (1992): 954–57.

8. See for example Stephen B. Thomas and Sandra Crouse Quinn, "Public Health Then and Now," *American Journal of Public Health* 81, no. 11 (1991): 1498–1505; Henry C. Chinn, Jr., "Remember Tuskegee," *New York Times*, 29 May 1992.

9. Tuskegee Syphilis Study Ad Hoc Advisory Panel, *Final Report of the Tuskegee Syphilis Study Ad Hoc Advisory Panel* (Washington, D.C.: U.S. Department of Health, Education and Welfare, Public Health Service, 1973).

10. Federal Policy for the Protection of Human Subjects; Notices and Rules, *Federal Register* 56, no. 117 (1991): 28002.

11. 45 *Code of Federal Regulations* §46.111(a)(3).

12. This problem is discussed in the context of research in prisons in Stephen E. Toulmin, "The National Commission on Human Experimentation: Procedures and Outcomes," in *Scientific Controversies: Case Studies in the Resolution and Closure of Disputes in Science and Technology*, ed. H. Tristram Engelhardt, Jr. and Arthur L. Caplan (New York: Cambridge University Press, 1987), pp. 602–6.

13. National Institutes of Health and Alcohol, Drug Abuse and Mental Health Administration, "Special Instructions to Applicants Using Form PHS 398 Regarding Implementation of the NIH/ADAMHA Policy concerning Inclusion of Women and Minorities in Clinical Research Study Populations," December 1990.

14. Arthur L. Caplan, "Is There a Duty to Serve as a Subject in Biomedical Research?" *IRB: A Review of Human Subjects Research* 6, no. 5 (1984): 1–5.

15. See J. W. Green, *Cultural Awareness in the Human Services* (Englewood Cliffs, N.J.: Prentice-Hall, 1982), p. 59; Bob Blauner, "Talking Past Each Other: Black and White Languages of Race," *American Prospect* 61, no. 10 (1992): 55–64.

16. Patricia A. King, "The Past as Prologue: Race, Class, and Gene Discrimination," in *Using Ethics and Law as Guides*, ed. George J. Annas and Sherman Elias (New York: Oxford University Press, 1992), pp. 94–111.

17. Blauner, "Talking Past Each Other," p. 16.

18. See for example James E. Bowman and Robert F. Murray, Jr., *Genetic Variation and Disorders in People of African Origin* (Baltimore, Md.: Johns Hopkins University Press, 1981); Warren W. Leary, "Uneasy Doctors Add Race-Consciousness to Diagnostic Tools," *New York Times*, 15 September 1990.

19. Hans Jonas, "Philosophical Reflections on Experimenting with Human Subjects," in *Experimentation with Human Subjects*, ed. Paul A. Freund (New York: George Braziller, 1970), p. 1. Recent controversy in genetic research makes Jonas's warning particularly timely. See Daniel Goleman, "New Storm Brews on Whether Crime Has Roots in Genes," *New York Times*, 15 September 1992.

UNDER THE SHADOW OF TUSKEGEE

African Americans and Health Care

VANESSA NORTHINGTON GAMBLE

Introduction

On May 16, 1997, in a White House ceremony, President Bill Clinton apologized for the Tuskegee Syphilis Study, the 40-year government study (1932 to 1972) in which 399 Black men from Macon County, Alabama, were deliberately denied effective treatment for syphilis in order to document the natural history of the disease.[1] "The legacy of the study at Tuskegee," the president remarked, "has reached far and deep, in ways that hurt our progress and divide our nation. We cannot be one America when a whole segment of our nation has no trust in America."[2] The president's comments underscore that in the 25 years since its public disclosure, the study has moved from being a singular historical event to a powerful metaphor. It has come to symbolize racism in medicine, misconduct in human research, the arrogance of physicians, and government abuse of Black people.

The continuing shadow cast by the Tuskegee Syphilis Study on efforts to improve the health status of Black Americans provided an impetus for the campaign for a presidential apology.[3] Numerous articles, in both the professional and popular press, have pointed out that the study predisposed many African Americans to distrust medical and public health authorities and has led to critically low Black participation in clinical trials and organ donation.[4]

The specter of Tuskegee has also been raised with respect to HIV/AIDS prevention and treatment programs. Health education researchers Dr. Stephen B. Thomas and Dr. Sandra Crouse Quinn have written extensively on the impact of the Tuskegee Syphilis Study on these programs.[5] They argue that "the legacy of this experiment, with its failure to educate the study participants and treat them adequately, laid the foundation for today's pervasive sense of black distrust of public health authorities."[6] The syphilis study has also been used to explain why many African Americans oppose needle exchange programs. Needle exchange programs provoke the image of the syphilis study and Black fears about genocide. These

Dr. Vanessa Northington Gamble is associate professor of history of medicine and family medicine at the University of Wisconsin Medical School.
Originally published in the American Journal of Public Health 87 (1997): 1773–87. Reprinted by permission of the American Public Health Association.

programs are not viewed as mechanisms to stop the spread of HIV/AIDS but rather as fodder for the drug epidemic that has devastated so many Black neighborhoods.[7] Fears that they will be used as guinea pigs like the men in the syphilis study have also led some African Americans with AIDS to refuse treatment with protease inhibitors.[8]

The Tuskegee Syphilis Study is frequently described as the singular reason behind African-American distrust of the institutions of medicine and public health. Such an interpretation neglects a critical historical point: the mistrust predated public revelations about the Tuskegee study. Furthermore, the narrowness of such a representation places emphasis on a single historical event to explain deeply entrenched and complex attitudes within the Black community. An examination of the syphilis study within a broader historical and social context makes plain that several factors have influenced, and continue to influence, African Americans' attitudes toward the biomedical community.

Black Americans' fears about exploitation by the medical profession date back to the antebellum period and the use of slaves and free Black people as subjects for dissection and medical experimentation.[9] Although physicians also used poor Whites as subjects, they used Black people far more often. During an 1835 trip to the United States, French visitor Harriet Martineau found that Black people lacked the power even to protect the graves of their dead. "In Baltimore the bodies of coloured people exclusively are taken for dissection," she remarked, "because the Whites do not like it, and the coloured people cannot resist."[10] Four years later, abolitionist Theodore Dwight Weld echoed Martineau's sentiment. "Public opinion," he wrote, "would tolerate surgical experiments, operations, processes, performed upon them [slaves], which it would execrate if performed upon their master or other whites."[11] Slaves found themselves as subjects of medical experiments because physicians needed bodies and because the state considered them property and denied them the legal right to refuse to participate.

Two antebellum experiments, one carried out in Georgia and the other in Alabama, illustrate the abuse that some slaves encountered at the hands of physicians. In the first, Georgia physician Thomas Hamilton conducted a series of brutal experiments on a slave to test remedies for heatstroke. The subject of these investigations, Fed, had been loaned to Hamilton as repayment for a debt owed by his owner. Hamilton forced Fed to sit naked on a stool placed on a platform in a pit that had been heated to a high temperature. Only the man's head was above ground. Over a period of 2 to 3 weeks, Hamilton placed Fed in the pit five or six times and gave him various medications to determine which enabled him best to withstand the heat. Each ordeal ended when Fed fainted and had to be revived. But note that Fed was not the only victim in this experiment; its whole purpose was to make it possible for masters to force slaves to work still longer hours on the hottest of days.[12]

In the second experiment, Dr. J. Marion Sims, the so-called father of modern gynecology, used three Alabama slave women to develop an operation to repair vesicovaginal fistulas. Between 1845 and 1849, the three slave women on whom Sims operated each underwent up to 30 painful operations. The physician himself described the agony associated with some of the experiments:[13] "The first patient I operated on was Lucy. . . . That was before the days of anaesthetics, and the poor girl, on her knees, bore the operation with great heroism and bravery." This operation was not successful, and Sims later attempted to repair the defect by placing a sponge in the bladder. This experiment, too, ended in failure. He noted:

> The whole urethra and the neck of the bladder were in a high state of inflammation, which came from the foreign substance. It had to come away, and there was nothing to do but to pull it away by main force. Lucy's agony was extreme. She was much prostrated, and I thought that she was going to die; but by irrigating the parts of the bladder she recovered with great rapidity.

Sims finally did perfect his technique and ultimately repaired the fistulas. Only after his experimentation with the slave women proved successful did the physician attempt the procedure, with anesthesia, on White women volunteers.

Exploitation after the Civil War

It is not known to what extent African Americans continued to be used as unwilling subjects for experimentation and dissection in the years after emancipation. However, an examination of African-American folklore at the turn of the century makes it clear that Black people believed that such practices persisted. Folktales are replete with references to night doctors, also called student doctors and Ku Klux doctors. In her book, *Night Riders in Black Folk History*, anthropologist Gladys-Marie Fry writes, "The term 'night doctor' (derived from the fact that victims were sought only at night) applies both to students of medicine, who supposedly stole cadavers from which to learn about body processes, and [to] professional thieves, who sold stolen bodies—living and dead—to physicians for medical research."[14] According to folk belief, these sinister characters would kidnap Black people, usually at night and in urban areas, and take them to hospitals to be killed and used in experiments. An 1889 *Boston Herald* article vividly captured the fears that African Americans in South Carolina had of night doctors. The report read, in part:

> The negroes of Clarendon, Williamsburg, and Sumter counties have for several weeks past been in a state of fear and trembling. They claim that there is a white man, a doctor, who at will can make himself invisible, and who then ap-

proaches some unsuspecting darkey, and having rendered him or her insensible with chloroform, proceeds to fill up a bucket with the victim's blood, for the purpose of making medicine. After having drained the last drop of blood from the victim, the body is dumped into some secret place where it is impossible for any person to find it. The colored women are so worked up over this phantom that they will not venture out at night, or in the daytime in any sequestered place.[15]

Fry did not find any documented evidence of the existence of night riders. However, she demonstrated through extensive interviews that many African Americans expressed genuine fears that they would be kidnapped by night doctors and used for medical experimentation. Fry concludes that two factors explain this paradox. She argues that Whites, especially those in the rural South, deliberately spread rumors about night doctors in order to maintain psychological control over Blacks and to discourage their migration to the North so as to maintain a source of cheap labor. In addition, Fry asserts that the experiences of many African Americans as victims of medical experiments during slavery fostered their belief in the existence of night doctors.[16] It should also be added that, given the nation's racial and political climate, Black people recognized their inability to refuse to participate in medical experiments.

Reports about the medical exploitation of Black people in the name of medicine after the end of the Civil War were not restricted to the realm of folklore. Until it was exposed in 1882, a grave robbing ring operated in Philadelphia and provided bodies for the city's medical schools by plundering the graves at a Black cemetery. According to historian David C. Humphrey, southern grave robbers regularly sent bodies of southern Blacks to northern medical schools for use as anatomy cadavers.[17]

During the early 20th century, African-American medical leaders protested the abuse of Black people by the White-dominated medical profession and used their concerns about experimentation to press for the establishment of Black-controlled hospitals.[18] Dr. Daniel Hale Williams, the founder of Chicago's Provident Hospital (1891), the nation's first Black-controlled hospital, contended that White physicians, especially in the South, frequently used Black patients as guinea pigs.[19] Dr. Nathan Francis Mossell, the founder of Philadelphia's Frederick Douglass Memorial Hospital (1895), described the "fears and prejudices" of Black people, especially those from the South, as "almost proverbial."[20] He attributed such attitudes to southern medical practices in which Black people, "when forced to accept hospital attention, got only the poorest care, being placed in inferior wards set apart for them, suffering the brunt of all that is experimental in treatment, and all this is the sequence of their race variety and abject helplessness."[21] The founders of Black hospitals claimed that only Black physicians possessed the skills required to treat

Black patients optimally and that Black hospitals provided these patients with the best possible care.[22]

Fears about the exploitation of African Americans by White physicians played a role in the establishment of a Black veterans hospital in Tuskegee, Ala. In 1923, 9 years before the initiation of the Tuskegee Syphilis Study, racial tensions had erupted in the town over control of the hospital. The federal government had pledged that the facility, an institution designed exclusively for Black patients, would be run by a Black professional staff. But many Whites in the area, including members of the Ku Klux Klan, did not want a Black-operated federal facility in the heart of Dixie, even though it would serve only Black people.[23]

Black Americans sought control of the veterans hospital, in part because they believed that the ex-soldiers would receive the best possible care from Black physicians and nurses, who would be more caring and sympathetic to the veterans' needs. Some Black newspapers even warned that White southerners wanted command of the hospital as part of a racist plot to kill and sterilize African-American men and to establish an "experiment station" for mediocre White physicians.[24] Black physicians did eventually gain the right to operate the hospital, yet this did not stop the hospital from becoming an experiment station for Black men. The veterans hospital was one of the facilities used by the United States Public Health Service in the syphilis study.

During the 1920s and 1930s, Black physicians pushed for additional measures that would battle medical racism and advance their professional needs. Dr. Charles Garvin, a prominent Cleveland physician and a member of the editorial board of the Black medical publication *The Journal of the National Medical Association*, urged his colleagues to engage in research in order to protect Black patients. He called for more research on diseases such as tuberculosis and pellagra that allegedly affected African Americans disproportionately or idiosyncratically. Garvin insisted that Black physicians investigate these racial diseases because "heretofore in literature, as in medicine, the Negro has been written about, exploited and experimented upon sometimes not to his physical betterment or to the advancement of science, but the advancement of the Nordic investigator." Moreover, he charged that "in the past, men of other races have for the large part interpreted our diseases, often tinctured with inborn prejudices."[25]

Fears of Genocide

These historical examples clearly demonstrate that African Americans' distrust of the medical profession has a longer history than the public revelations of the Tuskegee Syphilis Study. There is a collective memory among African Americans about their exploitation by the medical establishment. The Tuskegee Syphilis

Study has emerged as the most prominent example of medical racism because it confirms, if not authenticates, long-held and deeply entrenched beliefs within the Black community. To be sure, the Tuskegee Syphilis Study does cast a long shadow. After the study had been exposed, charges surfaced that the experiment was part of a governmental plot to exterminate Black people.[26] Many Black people agreed with the charge that the study represented "nothing less than an official, premeditated policy of genocide."[27] Furthermore, this was not the first or last time that allegations of genocide have been launched against the government and the medical profession. The sickle cell anemia screening programs of the 1970s and birth control programs have also provoked such allegations.[28]

In recent years, links have been made between Tuskegee, AIDS, and genocide. In September 1990, the article "AIDS: Is It Genocide?" appeared in *Essence*, a Black woman's magazine. The author noted: "As an increasing number of African-Americans continue to sicken and die and as no cure for AIDS has been found some of us are beginning to think the unthinkable: Could AIDS be a virus that was manufactured to erase large numbers of us? Are they trying to kill us with this disease?"[29] In other words, some members of the Black community see AIDS as part of a conspiracy to exterminate African Americans.

Beliefs about the connection between AIDS and the purposeful destruction of African Americans should not be cavalierly dismissed as bizarre and paranoid. They are held by a significant number of Black people. For example, a 1990 survey conducted by the Southern Christian Leadership Conference found that 35% of the 1056 Black church members who responded believed that AIDS was a form of genocide.[30] A *New York Times*/WCBS TV News poll conducted the same year found that 10% of Black Americans thought that the AIDS virus had been created in a laboratory in order to infect Black people. Another 20% believed that it could be true.[31]

African Americans frequently point to the Tuskegee Syphilis Study as evidence to support their views about genocide, perhaps, in part, because many believe that the men in the study were actually injected with syphilis. Harlon Dalton, a Yale Law School professor and a former member of the National Commission on AIDS, wrote, in a 1989 article titled, "AIDS in Black Face," that "the government [had] purposefully exposed Black men to syphilis."[32] Six years later, Dr. Eleanor Walker, a Detroit radiation oncologist, offered an explanation as to why few African Americans become bone marrow donors. "The biggest fear, she claimed, is that they will become victims of some misfeasance, like the Tuskegee incident where Black men were infected with syphilis and left untreated to die from the disease."[33] The January 25, 1996, episode of *New York Undercover*, a Fox Network police drama that is one of the top shows in Black households, also reinforced the rumor that the US Public Health Service physicians injected the men with syphilis.[34] The myth about deliberate infection is not limited to the Black community. On April 8, 1997, news anchor Tom Brokaw, on "NBC Nightly News," announced that the men had been infected by the government.[35]

Folklorist Patricia A. Turner, in her book *I Heard It through the Grapevine: Rumor and Resistance in African-American Culture*, underscores why it is important not to ridicule but to pay attention to these strongly held theories about genocide.[36] She argues that these rumors reveal much about what African Americans believe to be the state of their lives in this country. She contends that such views reflect Black beliefs that White Americans have historically been, and continue to be, ambivalent and perhaps hostile to the existence of Black people. Consequently, African-American attitudes toward biomedical research are not influenced solely by the Tuskegee Syphilis Study. African Americans' opinions about the value White society has attached to their lives should not be discounted. As Reverend Floyd Tompkins of Stanford University Memorial Church has said, "There is a sense in our community, and I think it shall be proved out, that if you are poor or you're a person of color, you were the guinea pig, and you continue to be the guinea pigs, and there is the fundamental belief that Black life is not valued like White life or like any other life in America."[37]

Not Just Paranoia

Lorene Cary, in a cogent essay in *Newsweek*, expands on Reverend Tompkins' point. In an essay titled "Why It's Not Just Paranoia," she writes:

> We Americans continue to value the lives and humanity of some groups more than the lives and humanity of others. That is not paranoia. It is our historical legacy and a present fact; it influences domestic and foreign policy and the daily interaction of millions of Americans. It influences the way we spend our public money and explains how we can read the staggering statistics on Black Americans' infant mortality, youth mortality, mortality in middle and old age, and not be moved to action.[38]

African Americans' beliefs that their lives are devalued by White society also influence their relationships with the medical profession. They perceive, at times correctly, that they are treated differently in the health care system solely because of their race, and such perceptions fuel mistrust of the medical profession. For example, a national telephone survey conducted in 1986 revealed that African Americans were more likely than Whites to report that their physicians did not inquire sufficiently about their pain, did not tell them how long it would take for prescribed medicine to work, did not explain the seriousness of their illness or injury, and did not discuss test and examination findings.[39] A 1994 study published in the *American Journal of Public Health* found that physicians were less likely to give pregnant Black women information about the hazards of smoking and drinking during pregnancy.[40]

The powerful legacy of the Tuskegee Syphilis Study endures, in part, because the racism and disrespect for Black lives that it entailed mirror Black people's contemporary experiences with the medical profession. The anger and frustration that many African Americans feel when they encounter the health care system can be heard in the words of Alicia Georges, a professor of nursing at Lehman College and a former president of the National Black Nurses Association, as she recalled an emergency room experience. "Back a few years ago, I was having excruciating abdominal pain, and I wound up at a hospital in my area," she recalled. "The first thing that they began to ask me was how many sexual partners I'd had. I was married and owned my own house. But immediately, in looking at me, they said, 'Oh, she just has pelvic inflammatory disease.' "[41] Perhaps because of her nursing background, Georges recognized the implications of the questioning. She had come face to face with the stereotype of Black women as sexually promiscuous. Similarly, the following story from the *Los Angeles Times* shows how racism can affect the practice of medicine:

> When Althea Alexander broke her arm, the attending resident at Los Angeles County-usc Medical Center told her to "hold your arm like you usually hold your can of beer on Saturday night." Alexander who is Black, exploded. "What are you talking about? Do you think I'm a welfare mother?" The White resident shrugged: "Well aren't you?" Turned out she was an administrator at usc medical school.

This example graphically illustrates that health care providers are not immune to the beliefs and misconceptions of the wider community. They carry with them stereotypes about various groups of people.[42]

Beyond Tuskegee

There is also a growing body of medical research that vividly illustrates why discussions of the relationship of African Americans and the medical profession must go beyond the Tuskegee Syphilis Study. These studies demonstrate racial inequities in access to particular technologies and raise critical questions about the role of racism in medical decision making. For example, in 1989 *The Journal of the American Medical Association* published a report that demonstrated racial inequities in the treatment of heart disease. In this study, White and Black patients had similar rates of hospitalization for chest pain, but the White patients were one third more likely to undergo coronary angiography and more than twice as likely to be treated with bypass surgery or angioplasty. The racial disparities persisted even after adjustments were made for differences in income.[43] Three years later, another study appearing in that journal reinforced these findings. It revealed that older Black patients on Medicare received coronary artery bypass grafts only about a fourth as often as comparable White patients. Disparities were greatest in the rural South, where White patients had the surgery seven times as often as Black patients. Medical factors did not fully explain the differences. This study suggests that an already-existing national health insurance program does not solve the access problems of African Americans.[44] Additional studies have confirmed the persistence of such inequities.[45]

Why the racial disparities? Possible explanations include health problems that precluded the use of procedures, patient unwillingness to accept medical advice or to undergo surgery, and differences in severity of illness. However, the role of racial bias cannot be discounted, as the American Medical Association's Council on Ethical and Judicial Affairs has recognized. In a 1990 report on Black-White disparities in health care, the council asserted:

> Because racial disparities may be occurring despite the lack of any intent or purposeful efforts to treat patients differently on the basis of race, physicians should examine their own practices to ensure that inappropriate considerations do not affect their clinical judgment. In addition, the profession should help increase the awareness of its members of racial disparities in medical treatment decisions by engaging in open and broad discussions about the issue. Such discussions should take place as part of the medical school curriculum, in medical journals, at professional conferences, and as part of professional peer review activities.[46]

The council's recommendation is a strong acknowledgment that racism can influence the practice of medicine.

After the public disclosures of the Tuskegee Syphilis Study, Congress passed the National Research Act of 1974. This act, established to protect subjects in human experimentation, mandates institutional review board approval of all federally funded research with human subjects. However, recent revelations about a measles vaccine study financed by the Centers for Disease Control and Prevention (CDC) demonstrate the inadequacies of these safeguards and illustrate why African Americans' historically based fears of medical research persist. In 1989, in the midst of a measles epidemic in Los Angeles, the CDC, in collaboration with Kaiser Permanente and the Los Angeles County Health Department, began a study to test whether the experimental Edmonston-Zagreb vaccine could be used to immunize children too young for the standard Moraten vaccine. By 1991, approximately 900 infants, mostly Black and Latino, had received the vaccine without difficulties. (Apparently, 1 infant died for reasons not related to the inoculations.) But the infants' parents had not been informed that the vaccine was not licensed in the

United States or that it had been associated with an increase in death rates in Africa. The 1996 disclosure of the study prompted charges of medical racism and of the continued exploitation of minority communities by medical professionals.[47]

The Tuskegee Syphilis Study continues to cast its shadow over the lives of African Americans. For many Black people, it has come to represent the racism that pervades American institutions and the disdain in which Black lives are often held. But despite its significance, it cannot be the only prism we use to examine the relationship of African Americans with the medical and public health communities. The problem we must face is not just the shadow of Tuskegee but the shadow of racism that so profoundly affects the lives and beliefs of all people in this country.

NOTES

1. The most comprehensive history of the study is James H. Jones, *Bad Blood*, new and expanded edition (New York: Free Press, 1993).

2. "Remarks by the President in Apology for Study Done in Tuskegee," Press Release, the White House, Office of the Press Secretary, 16 May 1997.

3. "Final Report of the Tuskegee Syphilis Study Legacy Committee," Vanessa Northington Gamble, chair, and John C. Fletcher, co-chair, 20 May 1996.

4. Vanessa Northington Gamble, "A Legacy of Distrust: African Americans and Medical Research," *American Journal of Preventive Medicine* 9 (1993): 35–38; Shari Roan, "A Medical Imbalance," *Los Angeles Times*, 1 November 1994; Carol Stevens, "Research: Distrust Runs Deep; Medical Community Seeks Solution," *The Detroit News*, 10 December 1995; Lini S. Kadaba, "Minorities in Research," *Chicago Tribune*, 13 September 1993; Robert Steinbrook, "AIDS Trials Short-change Minorities and Drug Users," *Los Angeles Times*, 25 September 1989; Mark D. Smith, "Zidovudine: Does It Work for Everyone?" *Journal of the American Medical Association* 266 (1991): 2750–2751; Charlise Lyles, "Blacks Hesitant to Donate; Cultural Beliefs, Misinformation, Mistrust Make It a Difficult Decision," *The Virginian-Pilot*, 15 August 1994; Jeanni Wong, "Mistrust Leaves Some Blacks Reluctant to Donate Organs," *Sacramento Bee*, 17 February 1993; "Nightline," ABC News, 6 April 1994; Patrice Gaines, "Armed with the Truth in a Fight for Lives," *Washington Post*, 10 April 1994; Fran Henry, "Encouraging Organ Donation from Blacks," *Cleveland Plain Dealer*, 23 April 1994; G. Marie Swanson and Amy J. Ward, "Recruiting Minorities into Clinical Trials: Toward a Participant-Friendly System," *Journal of the National Cancer Institute* 87 (1995): 1747–1759; Dewayne Wickham, "Why Blacks Are Wary of White MDs," *The Tennessean*, 21 May 1997, 13A.

5. For example, see Stephen B. Thomas and Sandra Crouse Quinn, "The Tuskegee Syphilis Study, 1932 to 1972: Implications for HIV Education and AIDS Risk Education Programs in the Black Community," *American Journal of Public Health* 81 (1991): 1498–1505; Stephen B. Thomas and Sandra Crouse Quinn, "Understanding the Attitudes of Black Americans," in *Dimensions of HIV Prevention. Needle Exchange*, ed. Jeff Stryker and Mark D. Smith (Menlo Park, Calif.: Henry J. Kaiser Family Foundation, 1993), 99–128; and Stephen B. Thomas and Sandra Crouse Quinn, "The AIDS Epidemic and the African-American Community: Toward an Ethical Framework for Service Delivery," in *"It Just Ain't Fair": The Ethics of Health Care for African Americans*, ed. Annette Dula and Sara Goering (Westport, Conn.: Praeger, 1994), 75–88.

6. Thomas and Quinn, "The AIDS Epidemic and the African-American Community," 83.

7. Thomas and Quinn, "Understanding the Attitudes of Black Americans," 108–109; David L. Kirp and Ronald Bayer, "Needles and Races," *Atlantic*, July 1993, 38–42.

8. Lynda Richardson, "An Old Experiment's Legacy: Distrust of AIDS Treatment," *New York Times*, 21 April 1997, A1, A7.

9. Todd L. Savitt, "The Use of Blacks for Medical Experimentation and Demonstration in the Old South," *Journal of Southern History* 48 (1982): 331–348; David C. Humphrey, "Dissection and Discrimination: The Social Origins of Cadavers in America, 1760–1915," *Bulletin of the New York Academy of Medicine* 49 (1973): 819–827.

10. Harriet Martineau, *Retrospect of Western Travel*, vol. 1 (London: Saunders & Ottley; New York: Harpers and Brothers; 1838), 140, quoted in Humphrey, "Dissection and Discrimination," 19.

11. Theodore Dwight Weld, *American Slavery As It Is: Testimony of a Thousand Witnesses* (New York: American Anti-Slavery Society, 1839), 170, quoted in Savitt, "The Use of Blacks," 341.

12. F. N. Boney, "Doctor Thomas Hamilton: Two Views of a Gentleman of the Old South," *Phylon* 28 (1967): 288–292.

13. J. Marion Sims, *The Story of My Life* (New York: Appleton, 1889), 236–237.

14. Gladys-Marie Fry, *Night Riders in Black Folk History* (Knoxville: University of Tennessee Press, 1984), 171.

15. "Concerning Negro Sorcery in the United States," *Journal of American Folk-Lore* 3 (1890): 285.

16. Ibid., 210.

17. Humphrey, "Dissection and Discrimination," 822–823.

18. A detailed examination of the campaign to establish Black hospitals can be found in Vanessa Northington Gamble, *Making a Place for Ourselves: The Black Hospital Movement, 1920–1945* (New York: Oxford University Press, 1995).

19. Eugene P. Link, "The Civil Rights Activities of Three Great Negro Physicians (1840–1940)," *Journal of Negro History* 52 (July 1969): 177.

20. Mossell graduated, with honors, from Penn in 1882 and founded the hospital in 1895.

21. "Seventh Annual Report of the Frederick Douglass Memorial Hospital and Training School" (Philadelphia, Pa.: 1902), 17.

22. H. M. Green, *A More or Less Critical Review of the Hospital Situation among Negroes in the United States* (n.d., circa 1930), 4–5.

23. For more in-depth discussions of the history of the Tuskegee Veterans Hospital, see Gamble, *Making a Place for Ourselves*, 70–104; Pete Daniel, "Black Power in the 1920's: The Case of Tuskegee Veterans Hospital," *Journal of Southern History* 36 (1970): 368–388; and Raymond Wolters, *The New Negro on Campus: Black College Rebellions of the 1920s* (Princeton, NJ: Princeton University Press, 1975), 137–191.

24. "Klan Halts March on Tuskegee," *Chicago Defender*, 4 August 1923.

25. Charles H. Garvin, "The 'New Negro' Physician," unpublished manuscript, n.d., box 1, Charles H. Garvin Papers, Western Reserve Historical Society Library, Cleveland, Ohio.

26. Ronald A. Taylor, "Conspiracy Theories Widely Accepted in U.S. Black Circles," *Washington Times*, 10 December 1991, A1; Frances Cress Welsing, *The Isis Papers: The Keys to the Colors* (Chicago: Third World Press, 1991), 298–299. Although she is not very well known outside of the African-American community, Welsing, a physician, is a popular figure within it. *The Isis Papers* headed for several weeks the best-seller list maintained by Black bookstores.

27. Jones, *Bad Blood*, 12.

28. For discussions of allegations of genocide in the implementation of these programs, see Robert G. Weisbord, "Birth Control and the Black American: A Matter of Genocide?" *Demography* 10 (1973): 571–590; Alex S. Jones, "Editorial Linking Blacks, Contraceptives Stirs Debate at Philadelphia Paper," *Arizona Daily Star*, 23 December 1990, F4; Doris Y. Wilkinson, "For Whose Benefit? Politics and Sickle Cell," *The Black Scholar* 5 (1974): 26–31.

29. Karen Grisby Bates, "Is It Genocide?" *Essence*, September 1990, 76.

30. Thomas and Quinn, "The Tuskegee Syphilis Study," 1499.

31. "The AIDS 'Plot' against Blacks," *New York Times*, 12 May 1992, A22.

32. Harlon L. Dalton, "AIDS in Blackface," *Daedalus* 118 (Summer 1989): 220–221.

33. Rhonda Bates-Rudd, "State Campaign Encourages African Americans to Offer Others Gift of Bone Marrow," *Detroit News,* 7 December 1995.

34. From September 1995 to December 1995, *New York Undercover* was the top-ranked show in Black households. It ranked 122nd in White households. David Zurawik, "Poll: TV's Race Gap Growing," *Capital Times* (Madison, Wis.), 14 May 1996, 5D.

35. Transcript, "NBC Nightly News," 8 April 1997.

36. Patricia A. Turner, *I Heard It through the Grapevine: Rumor in African-American Culture* (Berkeley: University of California Press, 1993).

37. "Fear Creates Lack of Donor Organs among Blacks," *Weekend Edition,* National Public Radio, 13 March 1994.

38. Lorene Cary, "Why It's Not Just Paranoia: An American History of 'Plans' for Blacks," *Newsweek,* 6 April 1992, 23.

39. Robert J. Blendon, "Access to Medical Care for Black and White Americans: A Matter of Continuing Concern," *Journal of the American Medical Association* 261 (1989): 278–281.

40. M. D. Rogan et al., "Racial Disparities in Reported Prenatal Care Advice from Health Care Providers," *American Journal of Public Health* 84 (1994): 82–88.

41. Julie Johnson et al., "Why Do Blacks Die Young?" *Time,* 16 September 1991, 52.

42. Sonia Nazario, "Treating Doctors for Prejudice: Medical Schools Are Trying to Sensitize Students to 'Bedside Bias.' " *Los Angeles Times,* 20 December 1990.

43. Mark B. Wenneker and Arnold M. Epstein, "Racial Inequities in the Use of Procedures for Patients with Ischemic Heart Disease in Massachusetts," *Journal of the American Medical Association* 261 (1989): 253–257.

44. Kenneth C. Goldbert et al., "Racial and Community Factors Influencing Coronary Artery Bypass Graft Surgery Rates for All 1986 Medicare Patients," *Journal of the American Medical Association* 267 (1992): 1473–1477.

45. John D. Ayanian, "Heart Disease in Black and White," *New England Journal of Medicine* 329 (1993): 656–658; J. Whittle et al., "Racial Differences in the Use of Invasive Cardiovascular Procedures in the Department of Veterans Affairs Medical System," *New England Journal of Medicine* 329 (1993): 621–627; Eric D. Peterson et al., "Racial Variation in Cardiac Procedure Use and Survival following Acute Myocardial Infarction in the Department of Veterans Affairs," *Journal of the American Medical Association* 271 (1994): 1175–1180; Ronnie D. Horner et al., "Theories Explaining Racial Differences in the Utilization of Diagnostic and Therapeutic Procedures for Cerebrovascular Disease," *Milbank Quarterly* 73 (1995): 443–462; Richard D. Moore et al., "Racial Differences in the Use of Drug Therapy for HIV Disease in an Urban Community," *New England Journal of Medicine* 350 (1994): 763–768.

46. Council on Ethical and Judicial Affairs, "Black-White Disparities in Health Care," *Journal of the American Medical Association* 263 (1990): 2346.

47. Marlene Cimons, "CDC Says It Erred in Measles Study," *Los Angeles Times,* 17 June 1996, A 11; Beth Glenn, "Bad Blood Once Again," *St. Petersburg Times,* 21 July 1996, 5D.

SELECTIONS FROM THE UNITED STATES SENATE COMMITTEE HEARINGS FOR THE NOMINATION OF DR. HENRY FOSTER FOR SURGEON GENERAL OF THE UNITED STATES, MAY 1995

Pages 21–23:

[SENATOR] KENNEDY: . . . Dr. Foster, I'd like, if you would, to outline a bit about your service in [Tuskegee]. After you finished your medical profession, you decided to go to [Tuskegee], and I'd be interested in hearing from you about how you decided it, why you decided it, sort of what you found. I think we will have an opportunity to go into the details of your professional record. I'm enormously impressed with it, personally. I think part of these hearings, as well, is that American people want to get a sense about the individual—what kind of person you are. And I'd be interested, if you could tell us. It's a number of years ago. Why did you decide to go there, what did you find, what was life like? Could you share that with the committee?

[DR.] FOSTER: Yes, sir, Senator Kennedy, I shall. A significant part of my residency training at Meharry was conducted at [Tuskegee]. That was a part. It had inputs from Emory University. We had faculty that alternated faculty from Meharry. And [Tuskegee] had a very busy OB/GYN service. So, as a consequence, I went there. And the most striking thing was—so many patients—I almost never saw anyone that had prenatal care. They would come, either when they were terribly ill, convulsing with toxemia, or in labor, which they thought was okay to do, but there was no real concept of prenatal care.

I was very influenced, the most, by Dr. John Daniel Thompson, who was then the professor and chairman of the Department of OB/GYN at Emory University. Dr. Thompson was a southerner, a white man from Columbus, Georgia, who drove 300 miles round-trip twice a month, alternating with other faculty at Emory, to help us address that situation. And in good conscience with the high-quality

Dr. Henry Foster is professor of obstetrics and gynecology at Meharry Medical College. In 1995, he was President Bill Clinton's unsuccessful nominee for surgeon general.

U.S. Senate Hearings for the Nomination of Dr. Henry Foster for Surgeon General of the United States, May 1995, pp. 21–23, 35–36, 39–41, 79–83, 98–99, 130–134.

training I felt—it would have been the worst turning my back that I could do—those women were poor, destitute.

I said, "They need something." I was glad that Dr. Eugene Dibble, who was then, who kept that hospital going, hired me. He said, "Foster, this is where you have to be." And I agreed. So we went there [in 1965].

Pages 35–36:

SENATOR JEFFORDS: . . . Let me go on to another area that I have a question. That is the Tuskegee Syphilis Study. I have listened to the FBI and I am confident that you were not there that evening, but I'm also come from a rural community, and it would amaze me that being in a small group of doctors that if something was that controversial, that there would not have been some discussion about it or something that you would have been aware of the nature of that study. And, I'd just like your own statements on that, because, as I say, if it was that controversial, and that exciting, or maybe it wasn't at the time, and by the nature of things, that controversial. But, I'd like to know, it's hard for me, and I'd like to hear from you that you didn't really learn anything about [it] until I guess '72.

FOSTER: Senator, I can make it very simple. The reason there was no controversy, because there was no subject, there was no topic. Nothing has offended me more than this. That study became known to everyone in Tuskegee, in 1972. It was I who had become president of the Macon County Medical Society. The writings show that it was I who called the meeting to help the CDC identify these men, so they could be treated. I was outraged quite frankly. I didn't believe it was happening in America, a quarter of a century after the Nuremberg. I didn't believe it, and if anyone in Tuskegee had known about it, Senator, I think the place would have gone ballistic. Tuskegee is a place where there's a depository of all racial lynchings that have ever occurred in this country, kept as we sit here. No one knew about that study until 1972. I was outraged then, if I had found out in '71, or '70, or '69, I would have been equally outraged. It was awful.

Pages 39–40:

[SENATOR] COATS: . . . In at least three areas, the words of Doctor Foster and the public record are disturbingly at odds. On the issue of abortion, on the issue of involuntary sterilization, and on the issue of the Tuskegee syphilis experiments. Each case raises serious questions of candor, credibility, and ethical judgment of the nominee, and I believe deserve thorough examination. Throughout this entire nominating process we have been given conflicting and confusing statements. Both by Dr. Foster and by this administration.

. . . And there are serious questions of whether he [Dr. Foster] knew of the Tuskegee experiments before he made any public criticism. The administration claims that Dr. Foster was in the mainstream of these issues. That is highly questionable. But it also begs an important question. The issue is not simply what is permissible, but what is principled. The calling of the surgeon general [is that he] must not only understand what is legally permissible, he should [also] represent the highest ideals of his profession.

Page 41:

. . . Dr. Foster claims that he did not know any details of the infamous Tuskegee Syphilis Study prior to 1972. He asserts that he was first informed by the media of that study in July of that year. However, I'm disturbed that the numerous official government documents and statements by witnesses that the committee's investigation has uncovered, which raise questions about Dr. Foster's assertions. These documents suggest that two institutions of which Dr. Foster was a member knew of this Tuskegee experiments.

Dr. Foster was chief of obstetrics at the Tuskegee Institute while the Public Health Service was urging cooperation from the hospital. Official documents suggest that the institute and its physicians were well aware of the syphilis study. In February of this year, Dr. Foster denied that he was an officer of his county's medical society. Documents, however, show that he was the vice president of the small, ten-member, medical society in 1969, and became its president in 1970.

Official Public Health Service documents, and at least one witness, indicate that the Public Health Service met with the society membership and gave each member of the society detailed information about the study, including a list of surviving participants of the study. Dr. Foster has insisted that he did not attend the meeting and that he had never heard of the study before 1972. It is a fact, in 1970, that Dr. Foster became president of the Macon County Medical Society. A state health official has given a deposition claiming, at that point, that he informed Dr. Foster of the Tuskegee experiments. And I quote, "I had discussed this matter with him on a subsequent time in connection with a comprehensive health-planning meeting, as I recall now."

And he says, referring to Dr. Foster, "Well, we think we ought to treat them." That was the proper sentiment, I would suggest, from Dr. Foster. But it was a sentiment allegedly expressed well before Dr. Foster claims to have [had] any knowledge of the matter. In fact, it was over a year before Dr. Foster made any public criticism of the Tuskegee scandal. This nomination has turned into something difficult and disturbing. . . .

Pages 79–83:

[SENATOR] KASSEBAUM: . . . I'd like to go to another area where, again, asking what your responsibility was at a given time. Was briefly, the Tuskegee study was briefly mentioned yesterday, Dr. Foster. And I would just like to ask a few follow-up questions on that issue. You told the committee yesterday that you knew nothing about this study until it became a public controversy in 1972. And that actually nobody in the community knew or they, there would have been outrage.

And, at that point, there was a great outcry, in 1972, over the study which denied medical treatment to 400 black men suffering from syphilis for a period almost [forty] years. I certainly can understand why you, in the earlier period of time, might not have known. There are depositions from some who did know after 1970, because they were involved in it and they lived there. But, not to get into all of the problems, because you were not [the] one directing the program—it was under the direction of the Center[s] of Disease Control. But, I think, it is important to know, what, after you knew about it, was done.

You said you did not attend the May '69 meeting in which top officials of the Center[s] for Disease Control briefed the Macon County Medical Society on the study and no one ever raised this issue with you before it became a public issue. Were all of these records that were part of CDC's interpretation of what they wished or didn't wish to do, have not been [????]* is controlled initiative at this time. But in 1974, the state health officer for Alabama, Dr. Ira Myers, said in a court deposition, that he discussed this issue with you in 1970, before it became public. In his statement, I just would like to ask you—is that correct? Do you recall a conversation with Dr. Myers in 1970?

FOSTER: No, I recall no such conversation. What—maybe this would be helpful, when I first became aware of the Tuskegee study, it was in 1972, and I was in a meeting with Dr. Ira Myers, when we learned, together, at least I learned, we were at a state planning meeting in Montgomery. And a note was put under us that there were camera crews that wanted to talk to us. And we went out, and I'm sure Dr. Myers, and I discussed the case then, but that was in 1972. We were together when the story broke.

KASSEBAUM: Well, regardless then of what one knew when, and it's hard for me to believe that nobody knew about this in Macon County at that time, but regardless of that, once it became public in 1972, I believe you were president of the Medical Society in 1972 in Macon County, is that correct?

FOSTER: Yes, ma'am.

KASSEBAUM: What did you do then, at that point, when you knew, in 1972, in July of 1972, that this was a problem?

*Unclear in the hearing transcript

FOSTER: I called a meeting, I called a meeting of the physicians in the society, and I told them that we had learned that the CDC had agreed and would treat these men. And that we should devise a mechanism to help them identify them.

KASSEBAUM: And, did you demand that treatment be given at that point? It was about, it's my understanding there was about eight months' period of time, from the time you identified the men until treatment was started.

FOSTER: I don't know the time interval, Senator. But I do know, at the time the CDC had said they would treat the men.

KASSEBAUM: And I could understand that's the CDC's responsibility. On the other hand, you were the president of the Macon County Medical Society at the time, there was general outrage about what was happening, and I guess I would like to know if you assumed responsibility to say you, too, were outraged and make that clear to the Centers for Disease Control, that they indeed had to start that treatment immediately.

FOSTER: I, I did, I thought, the very best thing, and that was to help identify the men. Some of the men were patients of the doctors in the medical society. I did not, I'm an obstetrician/gynecologist, and the [????] once that was done, Senator, quite honestly, I had no reason to feel that the CDC would not follow through on its word. After all, that study had started even before I was born, and I think the atmosphere—and I went back to working forty hours a day and trying to run my OB service. And of course, you do know that a few months thereafter that I left Tuskegee.

KASSEBAUM: That's right. Thank you, Dr. Foster, my time is up. Senator Kennedy?

KENNEDY: Thank you very [much], Dr. Foster, and welcome again. An interesting point as even in the meeting of 1969, and we'll come back to where you were at the time. None of the doctors that were there, that were interviewed, had any information, understanding, awareness, that treatment was being denied. They've all told that. To [investigators]. They never, they said that they had no understanding that treatment was being denied. So they had never understood that it was being denied of the first notification. It was only at the time that you were briefed, as I understand, [Dr.] Myers. And that is true with [Dr. Luther McCrae], who is one that says that you were there.

The man, the one person that says you were there, the other doctors don't even remember being there, the one person that says you were there has stated that he does not ever remember being told by the CDC that treatment was denied. If you don't know, I'm so interested, if you don't know, how you're supposed to be exercised about this. I thought, when you did know, you took the steps in terms of demanding there's going to be treatment. I mean that's, at least my understanding of the record. Is that your understanding as well?

FOSTER: Yes, sir, Senator Kennedy. And I have always wondered why this [????] continues. None of the doctors who remember the meeting said anything was ever said about treatment being withheld. So I don't see what there was to cover up. But I can tell you, when I learned it was in 1972. It's also interesting, as you know, Senator, that this precipitated a class-action suit, and during the discovery process this medical society was found completely nonculpable in this, and I think that's very important.

KENNEDY: Now, let me come to the question about the May 19 meeting, when, allegedly you were at that meeting. In May 19, 1969, and it took a long time to finally get the record, I don't know how many of us could say where we were in May of 1969 at a particular time when you're out there delivering all those babies all over the county. But, finally, it has come out, and I put in the record last night, the affidavit about where you were on the May 19 meeting. We have an affidavit, which I put in the record yesterday, stating that you delivered a baby that night, and that is where you were on May 19. I have a statement, which I'll include in the record, from Minnie Jam[e]ison, who was the mother of that baby . . .

FOSTER: . . . [laughter] . . .

Pages 98–99:

[SENATOR] FRIST: Let me briefly turn to the Tuskegee study. Its credibility, you know its credibility, that we got people on both sides saying different things. Let me just add for the record if I could, Madam Chair, an article from the *Nashville Banner* by Bill Snyder who independently interviewed a number of people. We've had access to certain records in terms of testimony that's been given about people who are present or not present in 1969 at a meeting you denied being present at.

Let me just briefly read from this particular article. It says that you make the statement that you knew nothing about this until 1972, which you've reiterated today.

FOSTER: Absolutely correct.

FRIST: Let me read the article.

FRIST: "However, a former colleague, Dr. Luther Mc[C]ra[e], says Foster learned about the study during a 1969 meeting at the Macon County, Alabama, Medical Society and voiced no objections to it. One man's word against another. Not quite. Two doctors who remember attending the 1969 meeting with officials of the U.S. Public Health Service say that government officials did not discuss the most troubling aspects of the research, which began in 1932." Quotation begins: " 'They never mentioned anything about denying these people treatment,' says Dr. John Hue, a Tuskegee orthopedic surgeon. 'They only said they were checking on them since they hadn't been treated.'" New quotation: "This view is supported by the two surviving public health service officials who attended the meeting. 'I don't recall any elaborate or extensive discussion concerning this study,' recalls Dr. Alfonso [????], a former official of the Communicable Disease Center[s] in Atlanta, [a] new part of the public health service."

I'd like to make that entire article part of the record, if I could. Is that accurate?

FOSTER: Not before 1972.

Pages 126–29:

COATS: . . . Let me get to a question that really is nagging at me, Dr. Foster, and I want to tell you why it's nagging me, at me, because of an editorial in the *Washington Post*, not an unsympathetic newspaper to your nomination. This editorial, dated March 1, 1995, it says the following: "Dr. Foster, recently, Dr. Foster's name has become linked to the infamous forty year Tuskegee experiment in which hundreds of black men with [syphilis] were deliberately left untreated in the name of medical research. At issue, is what [in then] Dr. Foster knew about the study before it was publicly exposed, in 1972. We heard the answer is that Dr. Foster and the White House maintained that he was not informed about the study until the story broke. To have known earlier and not insisted on proper treatment for the innocent patients would disqualify any candidate for the surgeon general's post. The Tuskegee [syphilis] study conducted by the U.S. Public Health Service in Macon County, Alabama, was a terrible case of cruelty in science. It is crucial to pin down when Dr. Foster learned about the study. The question of his fitness for the job hangs on it."

[????]: Madam Chairman, I ask consent that this editorial from the *Post* be published in the record.

COATS: That—

KASSEBAUM: Consented.

COATS: That is what prompts my questions here, because it's not just this, Senator, but it is a respected newspaper and I think it reflects the opinions of many Americans that it is crucial that, that, we pin this down. Now, Dr. Foster, you testified that you had no knowledge to this prior to 1972. In fact, yesterday you stated that if anyone, uh, in Tuskegee had known about the study, the place would have gone ballistic, that's the quote from your testimony yesterday. What troubles me, and what nags at me, uh, is that that statement is, uh, appears to be in contradiction of a number of official government documents, that you'd leave there and think a reasonable person to conclude that either you did know about this or, if you didn't, um, um, you weren't at all attuned to what was going on in the county at the time and in the medical society at the time. For instance, an official Public Health Service summary of the meeting that took place on February 6, 1969, indicates that Dr. Myers of the state health department said "the society," said "the medical society," the society is the Macon County Medical Society, "had been very reasonable to work with. Some of the fears of real troublemaking have not come to pass. The Macon County Health Department and the Tuskegee Institute have been fully cognizant of the study." Dr. Kaiser, who is a senior member of the task, of the technical staff, for the [Milbank] Foundation. They are the ones, apparently, who paid for the autopsies of the, of the [syphilitic] patients that died.

Uh, Dr. Kaiser said, um, um, asked the question about what the Tuskegee Institute thought of the study, Dr. [Olansky], who's a professor at Emory University, explained that the Tuskegee Institute knew of the study. You were the head of the institute at that time, I believe, and, uh . . .

FOSTER: No, I've never been head of the Tuskegee Institute.

COATS: Alright, he asked what the Tuskegee, what is your connection with the Tuskegee Institute?

FOSTER: I was chief of O/G services at John Andrew Hospital.

COATS: Okay, I, I, I, I stand corrected on that. You were vice president of the county medical society at the time.

FOSTER: That's correct.

COATS: Uh, Dr. [Olansky] explained that the Tuskegee Institute knew of the study. The patients had been taken to the institute's hospital. Apparently, that's the hospital you were working at. Physicians at the institute, says, physicians at the institute knew of the study. Then, another official Public Health Service document, a letter from a Dr. Brown of the Public Health Service, to Dr. Robertson of the [Milbank] foundation, dated November 19, 1969, indicates that the county medical society, and I quote here, "assured Public Health Service officials of their cooperation in continuing the study." In addition, the letter states that Public Health Service furnished each of the Macon, each of the Macon County Medical Society's members with a list of surviving participants in the Tuskegee study. In a deposition taken on September 1974, in connection with a lawsuit filed against the federal government, Dr. [Sencer], who was then director of the Center[s] for Disease Control, is quoted as saying, "For the first time in a good number of years, and after the meeting of 1969, we did meet with the physicians who would be treating the bulk of these individuals." Another document dated April 15, 1969, from Dr. [Sencer] to Dr. [McCrae], then-president of the medical society when you were vice president, states, "Dr. Ira Myers has discussed with you the study that has been conducted in Macon County for the past thirty years." You had indicated in your testimony [no one] in Macon County was aware of the study. These documents would suggest otherwise. Another official document, dated March 13, 1969, a letter from Dr. Myers to Dr. William Brown, states that the Alabama State Board of Health notified the Public Health Service that it was "referring this matter to the Macon County Medical Society for its decision regarding continuity." The letter identifies Dr. [McCrae], Dr. Settler, as officers of the society, and of course you were an officer then, too. The official government summary of the meeting on February 6, 1969, is Macon Medical, Macon County Medical Society, states that the Public Health Service, "should increase its contact with both the Macon County Health Department and the Macon County Medical Society to help them, to assist more fully, in the continuance of the study." Dr. Myers had indicated in another official document that he thought it was a good idea to keep the local medical society informed as to what we're doing, "and what we wish to achieve, to work closely with them, and keep them informed of, everything that, everything that we do."

Dr. [Sencer] is quoted in another document. He said, "If we establish good liaison with the local medical society, there will be no need to answer criticisms."

COATS: . . . Dr. Smith suggested the doctor go to the county medical society meeting, bring up these points, pro and con, "they might think the same way," he says, "if the local physicians agree there is no need for treating these patients, that would be good public relations." Another document says, "uh, Dr. [Sencer] said he gathered the group, uh, gathered that the group felt better rapport should be established as soon as possible with the local medical society as well as the Health Department to enlist their cooperation in furthering study." Now, I've got five more pages, of official documents, and Madam Chairman, I would ask unanimous consent that all of these documents be placed in the record. My question, Dr. Foster, is, what would you do if you were me, and you agreed with the editors of the *Washington Post*, that this was a critical question, and your staff presented you with ALL this testimony, ALL these documents of respected individuals, director of disease control, state public-health service doctors, a professor from Emory University, a doctor from the foundation that was paying for some of the study, uh, president of the Macon County Medical Society, all these individuals indicating that this study was discussed, that a plan was put in place to inform ALL the doctors of the society. That meetings were held. People were sent to the community to discuss it. That, uh, uh, lists were given out of the patients in the study. Um, it, it, it just presents, such a, such a contrast to your statement that you didn't know anything about it. That nobody knew anything about it, and that if someone had known the place would have gone ballistic, but nobody knew, and it just presents, uh, eh, a great problem to me. You have provided honorable service to the most needy of our society, and you have a career that is exemplary in many, many ways, but this is an extraordinarily troubling question that I have and I just can't overlook it and I wish one more time you would address this question for the record.

FOSTER: Senator Coats, of all the things that have transpired over the past three months, I find nothing more offensive than what you deliberately just put forth. This was clearly a dastardly experiment conducted under the auspices of the U.S. government, and someone would have the audacity to try to put that on the black people in Tuskegee beggars description. I know that that study, in 1972, implicated Dr. Ira Myers, and I took the action that I thought was appropriate. Do you want to know how to answer it quote to quote? Look at the facts! I, I, I never heard anything mentioned about the fact that those people who do remember the meeting stated exclusively nothing was ever said about any treatment being withheld. Even the Dr. ???? said there was nothing said about treatment being withheld. That is the story! If that's the story, I worked with those doctors. I knew their commitment. That, that is the most unbelievable thing that ever happened. What happens [????] the legal [????] of a class-action suit that would [????] $7 million. There was, the suit says there was no implication, whatsoever, of the medical society with doctors. I was outraged in 1972! I would have been equally outraged in 1971, '70, '69, '68, '67. It was the American government, and that was an outrage, and they cleared it up. Nobody else at Tuskegee knew about it, and the doctors that I worked with—plus the fact, as I said the other day, Tuskegee is the center, that the repository for all racial lynch[ings] that have occurred in the, this country reside right now—nobody, that study started before I was born and the government covered it up, and that's what the study showed. They covered it up. They hoodwinked somebody else for twenty years. Why couldn't they have hoodwinked me, hoodwinked me, for two years? It seems logical!

COATS: So, it, it, it's your testimony then that the documents that we have, the statements that we have, the, that, that, the statements from the various doctors that I quoted and others is incorrect.

FOSTER: Under oath, incorrect, wrong, wrong, wrong, sir.

Pages 130–34:

COATS: Can you see why it's troubling to me, and why the question needs to be pursued? I mean, that's why I'm here. It, it, and I don't, we're not talking about the Center[s], the director of Center[s] for Disease Control, the president of the medical society, the head of the state public-health service, um—

FOSTER: Well, Senator, in all due respect, why is it, you, nothing is mentioned about the fact that nothing was ever said at these so-called meetings about any therapy? Isn't that central? I'm not a legal mind, but to me that's the story. If there was nothing said, what is there to cover up? I don't understand.

COATS: Well, Dr. [McCrae] had indicated, specifically, that he had talked to you about it.

FOSTER: He hadn't. He had not, Senator. If I did, Senator, he didn't have anything to talk about, because there was nothing about a cover-up.

[COATS]: OK, I'm just saying, he said that he talked to [you], you said that he didn't, and we'll have to rest, let it rest at that. We have one individual, actually a group of individuals, testifying one way, and you testifying another way. I'm trying to clarify the record to find out what the answer is.

SIMON: Madam Chairman, I, I think part of the clarification of the record is the article that Senator Frist put in the, put in the record earlier from the *Nashville [Banner]*, where all the other physicians who were there said they do not recall this being, uh, uh, this being said.

COATS: I, uh, I misspoke. I said, "Dr. [McCrae]." I meant Dr. Myers testified that he had spoken to you.

FOSTER: Do you think I'm a scapegoat?

KASSEBAUM: All right, I, I think—

FOSTER: I mean, really, we do!

KASSEBAUM: Uh, we have all of the documents, of course. I think that's the complication that Senator Coats has, that there's all the documents that have been available to the press and to the committee, and to anybody who wishes to see them, and we did extensive work in compiling all of the documents together. We did not do a compilation. Senator Kennedy, it's your time for questions.

KENNEDY: I welcome the fact that, uh, those documents are going to [be] made available right away, and out there because in the preliminary review, there is virtually no reference to Dr. Foster mentioned in there. There is no reference to Dr. Foster having any knowledge that treatment was denied. I'll ask the senator, is there any reference in any of those documents that would indicate that Dr. Foster knew that treatment was being denied?

COATS: Well, Senator—

KENNEDY: Is there, or isn't there? That is, basically, the question and the challenge to which you put. When you recount those document[s] you said, "How do you react to these documents?" and I am saying right now, and those documents will be made available to the press, whether there is any evidence in those, in ANY of those documents, that Dr. Foster knew that treatment was being denied?

COATS: Well, I'm happy to respond to Senator Kennedy. I said I was troubled by the fact that a member of respected individuals, including the director for the Center[s] for Disease Control, indicated that everyone in the medical society was provided a list of patients, that the medical society had been informed on numerous occasions that, uh, Dr. Foster as vice president and then president of the medical society, it just, it seems, unusual to me in the extreme that somewhere along the line, in between 1969 and 1972, that all of these contacts, all of these would lead to the medical society, that Dr. [McCrae] would not have been aware, it was based on his statement, that he said if anyone in Tuskegee had known about the study the place would have gone ballistic. It is clear there were many people in Tuskegee that knew about the study. We have that as an official record. It is true. It is true, Senator Kennedy. There is no specific mention that, other than, other than Dr. Myers. Dr. Myers said that he did inform Dr. Foster of this, and Dr. Foster, uh, indicated that was not the case.

KENNEDY: Now wait, now wait, Madam, uh, Chair. Facts are there is no reference in any of the documents that have just been held up that are so troublesome to the senator that he made them public that there is any information. Most of them are self-serving documents and Public Health Service documents. There is not a reference in any of those documents that Dr. Foster understood that, uh, that treatment was being withheld, number one. Two, I would just refer back to, uh, so that people understand, that testimony and the inclusions that, uh, uh, Senator Frist put into the record, which have been sustained by the record of these hearings, and that is that the doctors who attended the 1969 meeting, and they have been inquired of, were told of the study, and NONE OF THEM WERE TOLD that treatment was being denied. So, this is nothing new, and the final point is, in the statement of Mr. [McCrae], Ira Myers and Foster were both at the state planning, in 1972, is completely consistent with the, what Dr. Foster says, that he was notified at the planning meeting, and the senator cannot tell this committee or the members of the United States Senate that that particular meeting was prior to the time in 1972, because Mr. Myers doesn't remember, and that's the testimony. So, uh, I have felt, Madam Chair, that the statement, that, and response that Dr. Foster has given, uh, was more than adequate in terms of responding to these questions, but it does seem to me that, uh, when members hold up documents and saying how are we going to react and respond to these documents, and they are self-serving documents, none of which, none of which challenges the position and the statement of Dr. Foster of the other information which has been provided in terms of the series of events which have been proceeded as to uh, uh, as to be worthy of, uh, pointing out, and I think it's, uh, if the Senator has a difference with that characterization and that series of, of, representation, then I'd welcome, in whatever time is, uh, is here for him, to, to make it.

COATS: Well, Senator Kennedy, I think I stated very clearly what my question to Dr. Foster was. The question was whether there was knowledge of such a study. Dr. Foster said he had no knowledge, that no none in Tuskegee had knowledge, or the place would have gone ballistic.

KENNEDY: The treatment was withheld.

COATS: My statement—

KENNEDY: "The treatment was withheld" is the, is the key operative word. There's no one who's questioning that there was a study. The other members knew that the study, the question was when did he know that they weren't providing treatment?

COATS: Were you aware that there was a study, Dr. Foster?

FOSTER: After, I know now . . .

COATS: Well, that's my question of, uh, Senator Kennedy.

FOSTER: I didn't, I'm not going—

COATS: It wasn't a question of whether treatment was withheld. It was a question of whether, Dr. Foster, my question is, was he aware that there was a study?

FOSTER: I became aware, Senator Coats, in 1972, the first time I ever heard of the Tuskegee study in any kind of shape, form, or fashion, . . .

COATS: Yes, sir.

FOSTER: . . . and I was outraged.

COATS: I understand that.

FOSTER: I couldn't imagine it!

COATS: I am trying to reconcile your understanding of whether or not there was a study with a significant volume of documents and indications that there was knowledge of a study among the medical society among the doctors in Tuskegee, uh, from '69 to '72. That is my question.

KASSEBAUM: Do you have any further comment, Senator Kennedy?

KENNEDY: Just, uh, the, uh, not at this time, Madam Chairman. I would like to make just a brief, uh, after the senator's conclusion, make a brief closing comment.

JEFFORDS: Yes, I'd like to make a few comments, uh, first of all, I want to commend the chairman for how she has handled these hearings, uh, we have listened to. I think now that, uh, the final issue that, uh, um, has been very well put forth with all the possible vigor by Senator Coats on the issue of the Tuskegee Study. . . . I am convinced, uh, with respect to the Tuskegee situation, that uh, you were not aware and the key question, as I remember from that *Washington Post* editorial, was the question I had, too, as others, and I can't disagree with the, um, *Washington Post* editorial which said if you were aware, and you did nothing, you shouldn't be approved, and you don't disagree with that, and I don't disagree that, and yet, as Dr. Frist pointed out, um, and from our review of the documents, there is absolutely no evidence up 'til '72, that you were aware of the, that the truth was being withheld, so, I uh, I find, that, that I agree with the chairwoman that we, uh, that was a key issue, and I think that that, in my line, was what satisfied. . . . You know if this question to us today was whether the White House had put forth the information in a way that would give me confidence in approving your nomination, I would say they have failed miserably, but that's not the issue before us. The issue before us is Dr. Foster, and his ability to pursue the job of surgeon general, and the questions do I have confidence in that, and, uh, you've been very forthcoming during these hearings. You have corrected previously inaccurately forwarded information or misstatements, and, uh, your answers have addressed the questions and concerns to my mind. And, I, uh, know you have a lot of support from the medical community [????], a record of achievement in addressing problems. So, I would just like to say at this time, uh, I am positive in my own mind that, that you ought to be approved by this committee, and I hope that you do go before the full Senate and let them examine the facts that we all have here. Thank you.

FAMILIES EMERGE AS SILENT VICTIMS OF TUSKEGEE SYPHILIS EXPERIMENTS

CAROL KAESUK YOON

Tuskegee, Ala., May 9, [1997]—It has been 25 years since the nation learned that more than 400 black men infected with syphilis went untreated for decades in a federally financed experiment in this rural southern town laced with sandy roads and pine forests.

These men, who are expected to receive a Presidential apology on Friday in Washington, have been the subject of countless academic studies, news articles and books, as well as a play and a made-for-television movie.

Yet their families—the wives and children they may have unwittingly exposed to the disease—have remained largely unseen and unheard, bearing in silence a legacy of anger and shame as well as possible damage to their health. In an acknowledgment of the harm that may have been done, the Federal Government, since 1975, has been quietly running a small program that provides medical benefits to family members infected with syphilis.

"You get treated like lepers," said Albert Julkes Jr., 55, whose father was a participant in the project the Government called the Tuskegee Study of Untreated Syphilis in the Male Negro. "People think it's the scourge of the earth to have it in your family."

Mr. Julkes, a retired customer service agent for a gas and electric utility, recounted his father's ordeal as he sat in the kitchen of his home just across the border in Columbus, Ga. "It was one of the worst atrocities ever reaped on people by the Government," he said. "You don't treat dogs that way."

In 1974 the Federal Government began making well-publicized reparations to the men who participated in the experiment, in which they were led to believe they were receiving free medical care, when its actual purpose was to study the long-term effects of untreated syphilis on black men. But since 1975, the Government has also been making amends to some of the families, providing lifetime medical benefits to the 22 wives, 17 children and 2 grandchildren with syphilis they may have contracted as a direct result of the lack of treatment accorded the men in the study.

Carol Kaesuk Yoon is a reporter at the New York Times.
Originally published in the New York Times, *12 May 1997, pp. A1, A12. Copyright © 1997* New York Times. *Reprinted by permission.*

"What they deserve is the best medical care we can provide," said Dr. Bill Jenkins, who in 1969, while a statistician with the National Center for Health Statistics in Washington, was among several people who unsuccessfully tried to end the experiment.

Dr. Jenkins, who said he was appalled by the experiment and haunted by his unsuccessful effort to halt it, is now an epidemiologist and devotes himself to running the Government's program to provide medical benefits to the men and eligible family members. "I try to give them the care that I would want to give to my mother," Dr. Jenkins said.

In addition to providing care to the family members, the program, at the Federal Centers for Disease Control and Prevention, called the Participants Health Benefits Program, also serves the eight surviving men. The program, formally known as the Tuskegee Health Benefits Program, cost the Federal Government $2.1 million last year, Dr. Jenkins said.

But while the program treats physical ills, the family members' emotional wounds have gone largely unrecognized, some relatives say. The pain of Tuskegee is still very real even among grandchildren of the study participants, some of whom had not even been born when the study was officially ended after its existence was widely reported in the press in 1972.

"I'm angry about it, very, very angry about it," said Carmen Head, whose grandfather, Freddie Lee Tyson, participated in the study. Miss Head, who is 22 years old and lives in Fairfax, Va., said family members had told her very little about her grandfather's participation. The subject is taboo, particularly with her grandmother, she said, adding, "It's a painful issue in my family."

Miss Head's mother, Lillie Head of Waterbury, Conn., is one of many family members no longer living in the South. Mrs. Head said she had never learned whether her father was one of the more than 400 participants with syphilis or if he was one of some 200 men without syphilis who were in a control group.

"It was something to be ashamed of, so it wasn't talked about," said Mrs. Head, 52, a high school physical education teacher. "We were really very disturbed after we found out my father was a part of it."

Martha Jernigan, 49, a home health aid in Tuskegee, said she has two cousins who are descendants of men in the experiment and knows many other relatives of participants who are living in the same area. "They thought we were animals, stupid, that we didn't know better," she said. "Times haven't changed when it comes to blacks."

Herman Shaw, 94, a survivor of the study still living on his family farm in Tuskegee, sat on his front porch on Thursday sifting through photographs of his late wife, Fannie Mae. Mr. Shaw was able to offer one of the few memories of a wife's reaction to learning the truth about the study. "She was somewhat shocked, may I say," he said, "because it was a disease. It wasn't anything that we'd heard about and nobody seemed to know about."

Dr. Vanessa Northington Gamble, a medical historian and physician who directs the Center for the Study of Race and Ethnicity in Medicine at the University of Wisconsin medical school, said such reactions are common among family members.

"There is a lot of pain that people still express and feel about what the Government has done to them and their family members, their community," said Dr. Gamble, who has studied the experiment for years and is chairwoman of the Tuskegee Legacy Committee, a group of experts formed last year to press for an official apology.

"I talked to a woman in Wisconsin who knew that I'd been studying this," she recalled. "All of a sudden she started crying, saying her uncle was also in the study."

The lingering shame and a distrust of the Government may be one reason that the number of family members in the Participants Health Benefits Program has never been high. Originally, 106 men who were in the experiment began receiving benefits in 1974, Dr. Jenkins said, but the number of wives appears never to have been very large. He said that in 1975, at what was probably the peak of participation by wives, only 50 had been tested. Of those, 27 were found to be positive for syphilis and eligible for the program.

In the study, which began in 1932, more than 600 men were recruited by the Government health workers, who led them to believe they were receiving free medical treatment. Throughout the 40-year study, the men were never told of the experiment and those with syphilis were never told they were infected. They never received any treatment for the disease, even when the use of penicillin became routine in the 1940's. When participants died, researchers offered their families free burial in exchange for the rights to do autopsies so they could gather their final data for the study, which researchers say was scientifically flawed from the start.

Dr. Jenkins said that when the true nature of the study became known, some family members became so distrustful of the Government that they refused to be tested for syphilis. No effort was ever made to track down sexual partners of the men, other than their wives.

When the study was under way, some wives tried to enroll, believing the project was a reliable source of medical care. When they were turned away, many were upset, according to Dr. Jim Jones, a historian at the University of Houston and the author of "Bad Blood" (Free Press, 1993), which historians regard as the definitive account of the experiment.

Dr. Jenkins said another reason the number of wives in the program might be low is that the men chosen for the study were supposedly in a latent, noninfectious stage of syphilis, unable to transmit the disease to their wives. That point, however, is still being debated.

"It's unclear what stage of the disease the men were at," Dr. Gamble said. "So that brings the issues around to the women and children."

Nowadays, the Tuskegee experiment is so notorious that scientists resist doing anything that could be construed as continuing the so-called research. "No one has ever studied the health consequences to the families, not to my knowledge," Dr. Jenkins said. "We will not compile the data in any way to make an assessment of them as a group. It would seem too much like another study." If such an effort is organized, he added, "I don't want to have anything to do with it."

But Jenkins said even if researchers knew how many family members were infected with syphilis, there is no way to be certain whether the syphilis was contracted from the men in the study. The test for syphilis is a blood test for antibodies to the disease. A positive result indicates only that a person had syphilis at some point in their lives, with no indication of when or from where the infection arose.

Fred David Gray, a lawyer who has represented the participants in the study since 1972, winning them an out-of-court settlement totaling $10 million, said that in 1974, as part of that agreement, the Government was ordered to provide lifetime health care for participants as well as some family members.

"I hope to see and I think what the men would like to see is some final closure," Mr. Gray said in an interview on Thursday in his Tuskegee office. He said in the last 23 years, he has given out settlement payments to some 6,000 heirs and participants. Despite the fact that the apology is expected Friday, and Mr. Gray as well as four of the elderly survivors are planning to attend, Mr. Gray said he is continuing to press for the President to change the site of his apology to Tuskegee.

It was soon after Mr. Gray and some of the survivors of the experiment held a news conference here in April to request the Government apology that the White House said one would be forthcoming. Dr. Gamble said the study legacy committee she heads had been pressing for months for an official apology.

But Dr. Jenkins said any form of apology should be seen as not an end but a beginning.

"There's a tendency to believe that African-Americans are reluctant to participate in research because of this one study and I think that belittles the concerns of the African-Americans," Dr. Jenkins said. "They are concerned about public health research because they're alienated from American society in any number of ways and this study is the bellwether. It's much bigger than just this study and we're going to have to do a lot more work than just apologize for this."

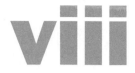

viii

Key Actors Rethink the Study

SUMMARY OF AD HOC COMMITTEE TO CONSIDER THE TUSKEGEE STUDY, PUBLIC HEALTH SERVICE, CENTERS FOR DISEASE CONTROL, U.S. DEPARTMENT OF HEALTH, EDUCATION AND WELFARE, FEBRUARY 6, 1969

Memorandum

Department of Health, Education, and Welfare, Public Health Service, Health Services and Mental Health Administration
TO: For the Record
FROM: Director, CDC
SUBJECT: Summary of Ad Hoc Committee to Consider the Tuskegee Study, February 6, 1969

An ad hoc committee meeting was convened Thursday, February 6, 1969, at 1:00 p.m., in Conference Room 207, National Communicable Disease Center, to examine data from the Tuskegee Study and offer advice on continuance of this Study. Participants included:

Committee Members:
Dr. Gene Stollerman
    Chairman, Dept. of Medicine
    University of Tennessee, Memphis
Dr. Johannes Ipsen, Jr.
    Professor
    Dept. of Community Medicine
    University of Pennsylvania, Philadelphia
Dr. Ira Myers
    State Health Officer
    Montgomery

This committee was convened by the Centers for Disease Control in 1969 to discuss the study's data and consider its future.
Summary of Ad Hoc Committee to Consider the Tuskegee Study, 6 February 1969, Centers for Disease Control Papers, Tuskegee Syphilis Study, Box 6, Folder 1969, National Archives–Southeast Region, East Point, Ga.

Dr. J. Lawton Smith
  Associate Professor of Ophthalmology
  University of Miami
Dr. Clyde Kaiser
  Senior Member Technical Staff
  Milbank Memorial Fund
  New York City

Resource Persons:
Dr. Bobby C. Brown, VDRL, NCDC
Mrs. Eleanor V. Price, VD Branch, NCDC
Dr. Joseph Caldwell, VD Branch, NCDC
Dr. Paul Cohen, VDRL, NCDC
Dr. Sidney Olansky
  Professor of Medicine
  Dept. of Internal Medicine
  Emory University Clinic, Atlanta

Recorders:
Dr. Leslie C. Norins
  Chief, VDRL, NCDC
Mrs. Doris J. Smith
  Secretary to Dr. Norins, VDRL, NCDC

Attending:
Dr. David J. Sencer
  Director, NCDC
Dr. William J. Brown
  Chief, VD Branch, NCDC
Dr. U. S. G. Kuhn, III, VDRL, NCDC
Miss Genevieve W. Stout, VDRL, NCDC
Dr. H. Bruce Dull
  Assistant Director, NCDC

The purpose of the meeting was to determine if the Tuskegee Study should be terminated or continued.
  Considerations were:

1. Current welfare of study participants
2. Adequacy of follow up of study participants
3. Original purposes and design of study in 1932

At the time of this meeting there were only seven patients whose primary cause of death was ascribed to syphilis.

The potential benefits to be achieved from continuing the study at this time were:

1. Clarification of the relationship of serology to morbidity from syphilis.
2. Clarification of the relationship of syphilis to pathological findings.
3. Clarification of a variety of risk factors associated with morbidity and mortality from late syphilis.

Full treatment of the survivors originally in the syphilitic group was considered. The dangers to patients suffering from cardiovascular or neurological conditions from late Herxheimer's reactions were emphasized.

The meeting was terminated with several salient points:

1. Treatment for these patients was not indicated unless they had signs of active syphilitic disease.
2. Medical follow up of all survivors should be intensified.
3. Knowledge of medical value could be gained by continuing to record information gained either through medical follow up or from pathological examinations in the study group.
4. The Macon County Health Department and the Tuskegee Institute have been fully cognizant of the study. The Public Health Service should increase its contact with both the Macon County Health Department and the Macon County Medical Society to help them to assist more fully in the continuance of the study.
5. This type of study would never be repeated.

David J. Sencer, M.D.
Assistant Surgeon General

Recorders:
Dr. Leslie C. Norins
    Chief, VDRL, NCDC
Mrs. Doris J. Smith
    Secretary to Dr. Norins, VDRL, NCDC

Attending:
Dr. David J. Sencer
    Director, NCDC
Dr. William J. Brown
    Chief, VD Branch, NCDC
Dr. U. S. G. Kuhn III, VDRL, NCDC
Miss Genevieve W. Stout, VDRL, NCDC
Dr. H. Bruce Dull
    Assistant Director, NCDC

Dr. Sencer opened the meeting by asking each person to introduce himself. He then gave a brief summary of the Tuskegee Study. This Study was begun in 1932, in Macon County, Alabama, a rural area with a static population, and with a high rate of untreated syphilis, to evaluate the effect of untreated lues, and it was conducted by the Venereal Disease Division of the United States Public Health Service.

Dr. Sencer then said the question has come up: Should we terminate the Study or should we continue it? It becomes a political problem. At the time the Study was begun there was no concern about racial problems, discrimination, etc. At that time there was no problem about not treating the disease. "We want your advice in making a decision. We are here to discuss this problem."

The meeting was then turned over to Dr. Bobby Brown.

Dr. Brown said we were here to take three looks:

1. The study as it was set up in 1932
2. What has happened to the individuals
3. Focus on the survivors

He then explained that he had spent the past 4–5 days going over clinical records of patients, and had prepared charts to inform the participants on the present status of the Study. He then showed a number of slides.

The original study group was composed of 412 male Negroes who had received no therapy, and who gave historical and laboratory evidence of syphilis; 204 men comparable in age and environment were selected for the control group.

The first findings were published in 1936 by Vonderlehr *et al.*; complete re-evaluations in 1938 and 1939 showed many of the patients had received treatment. The last evaluation (35th year) of this group occurred in 1968. At that time there were 36 controls and 53 syphilitics—a total of 89 still living; 373 in all groups are known dead to date, out of a total of 625 patients. Eighty-three showed some evidence of syphilis at time of death. Dr. Brown believes that syphilis was a primary cause of death in only seven as shown at autopsy. Many had lesions, several showed aortic insufficiency; some died of strokes. Many died from other causes: TB, renal failure, accidents (mostly auto accidents), knifings, etc.

There was much discussion concerning correctness of diagnosis, pathology reports, survival rates, etc. Dr. Olansky explained about the 1952 evaluation, how difficult it was to communicate with the patients; could not reach them by mail, some were picking cotton and could not find them. He told about Nurse Rivers and the active part she has played in the Study.

The participants then discussed the ages of the patients. The youngest is now 59 years old; the age range goes up to 85 years; one patient claims to be 102. Dr. Kaiser told of a study being conducted on the East Coast with a group of executives to learn the incidence of heart disease mortality. He said the executives get the best of medical attention; most die of heart disease. He was amazed at the survival rate in the Tuskegee Study.

The group then discussed autopsy findings. Dr. B. Brown explained about situations at times of death—many patients had lain in state 4 or 5 days, many had been embalmed; it was difficult to gain access to the bodies. This could contribute to lack of findings of autopsies, inaccuracies, cursory examinations, etc.

Dr. Stollerman was concerned about medical findings, and patients deserving of treatment. Dr. Smith then said we are here to decide three proposals, important at the moment. What information can we derive from this study? He summarized as follows:

1. Stress pathology
2. Silver stains
3. Animal inoculations

Dr. Smith said serological and epidemiological workups were good. The weak link in the chain is *pathology*. He suggested tremendous emphasis be put on this Study. In the next few years the patients were going to be gone. He thought it would be worthwhile to have a competent pathology flown in upon notification of death; do stains on organisms. He said there was no reported information on whether organisms are present in tissues. He then said when he participated in the 1967 evaluation he found one "control" patient with Argyll-Robinson pupils. He thought the Armed Forces Institute of Pathology would become interested in this Study. He urged that animal inoculations be done. "You may find seronegative patients in this group. But I don't think it will make any difference whether you treat them or not. First, stress pathology; get away from serology. You will never have another study like this; take advantage of it."

Dr. B. Brown said he had been in communication with the National Institutes of Health. Slides and blocks are available from them; this laboratory has frozen tissues. Dr. Smith then said he thought it would be worthwhile to do eye examinations, stating he had fundus pictures, neurological examinations of the patients from the 1967 evaluation. "20 years from now, when these patients are gone, we can show these pictures." Dr. Smith said he would be willing to go back to Tuskegee, go to their homes, explain to them what we were doing, do eye examinations on those who agree, take rabbits, get fluids from patients and inject into rabbits "on the spot." "I would stress:

"A. Pathology
"B. Eye studies, silver stains
"C. No treatment (I doubt if you could cure them)."

"This is a golden moment. Turn this Study into pathology studies." Dr. Stollerman thought there was a moral obligation here to treat patients for neurosyphilis.

The participants then discussed the dangers of treatment—Herxheimer reactions, fibrillations, etc. Dr. Stollerman thought we were obliged to set criteria for treatment. Dr. Olansky said if we insisted on spinal taps we would not have any patients.

Dr. Stollerman asked about the incidence of hypertension. He was told it was very high "but they are living with it." Blood pressures are virtually all high; all showed evidence of cardiac abnormalities.

The group then discussed remuneration to patients. When the Study started, payments were $50.00; "the undertaker got that." Most of the patients now have burial insurance. Dr. Myers said they pay 50 cents a week until they die.

Dr. Sencer asked about the Macon County Health Department situation. Dr. Myers said the Macon County Medical Society is composed mostly of Negro physicians. "There has been a complete social change. The county health officer is serving two or three counties; she is a former medical missionary to Nigeria, very competent." Dr. Myers said the County Health Department is understaffed.

Dr. Smith suggested giving the patients more money—"$200.00—explain that the study is being upgraded; ask them for permission to do examinations, give them shots of penicillin at the same time. I think an investment of $18,000.00 would be good to get the examinations." Dr. Sencer thought this suggestion ghoulish. Dr. Myers mentioned that this group did not like handouts.

Dr. Stollerman thought the patients should have a complete hospital checkup. It was explained that they had complete checkups at the VA Hospital in 1952 and 1958. They still receive treatment when indicated.

Dr. Sencer outlined on blackboard the possible courses of action:

ACTION	STUDIES
I. None	1. Survival Tp with treatment
II. Discriminate	After Negative without treatment
III. Total	2. Accurate incidence of pathology lesions
	3. Relation Syphilis Longevity

Dr. Stollerman then said he thought the data that had been presented was wonderful, but pathology would be open to criticism.

Dr. Myers was asked if he thought we could get permission to treat the patients. He said, "No, I haven't seen this group, but I don't think they would submit to treatment." Dr. Olansky said he would question the wisdom of treatment at this point, mentioning catastrophic consequences.

Dr. Myers said regardless of what your decision will be, if you raise a question at this time, the whole program will fold. Dr. Sencer then asked Dr. Myers what were the limitations of the County Medical Society. He said they had been very reasonable to work with; some of the fears of real troublemaking have not come to pass.

Dr. Smith said he had a good rapport with the younger Negro physician at

Tuskegee. Dr. Myers thought it a good idea to keep the local medical society informed as to what we were doing and what we wished to achieve; "work very closely with them and keep them informed of everything that we do."

Dr. Ipsen said there were only 10 physicians in Macon County at the beginning of the Study. Dr. Myers said there is now a new group in the Society—it is composed of 5–7 Negro physicians, and one white physician.

Dr. Dull then asked how you could answer criticisms for not treating these patients. Dr. Sencer said if we established good liaison with the local medical society there would be no need to answer criticisms.

Dr. Myers said at this stage he thought we should only take better care of the patients. Dr. Smith recalled when he was there in 1967 he found two cases of glaucoma and brought them to treatment. If he had not, they would have gone blind. "I think the patients appreciate this."

Dr. Olansky reiterated that the original policy of the Study was that when medical treatment was indicated, they were pulled out of the Study and were given treatment.

Dr. Myers stated that Macon County is now being promoted as a Negro center of culture. "I don't know where you will be able to study this kind of group. No populations are that stable these days. These patients are over 70; they do not move anymore."

Dr. Kaiser asked what Tuskegee Institute thought of this Study. Dr. Olansky explained they knew of the Study; the patients had been taken to the Institute's hospital. Dr. Myers replied that the Institute is now coming into a new era. Dr. Dibble, former medical director of the Institute, who died last year, was depended upon to keep the State Health Department informed. But now they are more progressive; he explained Nurse River's good relations with the Institute; her husband had been in on the first of the Study; she has now retired, due to age, infirmities, etc. But physicians at the Institute knew of the Study. He said the school has been active in Civil Rights Movement—"they have brought themselves up by their own bootstraps and are trying to do what we have failed to do."

Dr. Olansky replied that as weak as the Study is, it is still a good study.

Dr. Sencer remarked that our mechanism has broken down; Nurse Rivers is getting old, gets lost when she goes to visit patients. "We do not have the mechanism at this time." He then asked Dr. Myers about the state's appropriations to counties. Dr. Myers said appropriations run $10 or $11 thousand per county, requiring each county to put up 50–50 matching funds; the State Health Department does have supervision over the county health departments.

Dr. Sencer then asked what if we subsidized a person in the Health Department. Dr. Myers said, "Very good. We want to see the job done. That would be very good."

Dr. Sencer then asked, "Do you think that treatment of this Study group is indicated? Dr. Stollerman thinks there may be criticisms for not treating." . . . "In other words, you think cardiovascular disease is an indication for treatment?"

Dr. Stollerman replied that he thought it was. "I am not questioning your data, but I think they should be treated."

Dr. B. Brown then stated that we had no criteria for treatment. Dr. Sencer asked Dr. Caldwell if the man who has aortic regurgitation is getting good treatment. Dr. Caldwell said, "no. We told him he had to get to a doctor to get better care. That's all we could do."

Dr. Sencer said he thought additional resources would have to be put into the Study. "And take into consideration Dr. Stollerman's theory. If this Study is to be continued, CDC has to establish a relationship with the medical men in the area; find a way to increase the resources of the Health Department. We are going to have to establish better rapport; better follow-up on patients. The man who needs digitalis could be taken where he could get it. I think we ought to outline what we are going to do in the future."

Dr. Smith suggested a doctor go to the County Medical Society meetings, bring up these points, pro and con. "They might think the same way." —— "If the local physicians agree there is no need for treating these patients, this would be good public relations."

Dr. Stollerman said he thought when a patient has aortic regurgitation or indications of cardiovascular disease, you had to make an exception due to the medical nature of the group. "I think you should treat each individual case as such, not treat as a group."

Dr. Myers remarked that so far as he knew there had not been a physician in the area for all of the length of the Study. "I think we should establish rapport with the County Medical Society; talk to one physician in the Society before you talk to them as a group."

Dr. Sencer then asked, "What about the medical officer?"

Dr. Myers said she may lean toward treatment. "Dr. Barrett is a good pediatrician; —— very interested in research."

Dr. Sencer then asked how she was accepted by the local medical group. Dr. Myers said she had very good relations with them. "She loves the people in the area. She's very good to them."

Dr. Sencer then asked if this would be a good place to start—with her. Dr. Myers answered by saying she was serving several counties, but he would find out.

Dr. Kaiser then said he was quite impressed with the reprints that had been given to him—then reviewed them, mentioning that the last report in 1964, which summarized previous reports, emphasized the deleterious effects of syphilis. He recalled that about 2 years ago Dr. Robinson (head of Milbank Fund) wrote to Dr. W. J. Brown and made a proposition: "give a lump sum and terminate all obligations." Dr. Brown rejected this offer, and suggested taking lump-sum increments over periods of 5, 10, 15 years. Dr. Robinson then wrote back, suggesting that the Milbank Fund "go along on the old basis."

Dr. Sencer remarked he was not thinking of financial aid. He then asked what Dr. Kaiser's thoughts were on the political, racial overtones, etc.

Dr. Kaiser replied, "This is not a Study that would be repeated now. The public conscience would not accept it. —— If you could combine treatment with the present Study. —— I am impressed with the plan —— but I don't know whether the Fund would up the ante."

Dr. Sencer: "What has been the expense: $50.00 is not enough? Is it the sophistication of the place?" [Handwritten over the last word is "people?"]

Dr. B. Brown then mentioned the number of autopsies being performed today; compared DeKalb and Fulton Counties; "DeKalb has a higher rate of autopsies—perform more than they do at Grady."

MEDICARE was then mentioned. This plan now takes care of the older patients.

Dr. Myers summarized by saying, "You have seen the older doctors die out, Nurse Rivers is getting old and is inactive, the problems are increasing. Unless you pour new life blood into this Study, it will die out." He then went on to explain the coroner system in Alabama. They have a poor system—an MD signs death certificates, the coroner signs (in desperation), or a health officer could sign, but not likely. All death certificates are on file in Montgomery, not in the counties.

Dr. Sencer then said he gathered that the group felt there was:

1. merit in continuing the Study;
2. treatment is not indicated, but if patients have indications of active syphilitic disease, they should be treated;
3. better rapport should be established as soon as possible with the local Medical Society, as well as with the Health Department, to enlist their cooperation in furthering the Study.

Sencer: "It would be my feeling we are going to have to resubsidize a new person in the Health Department (work with Health Department) but also have the responsibility to help us improve and speed up pathological examinations. I would be personally opposed, from a psychological standpoint, in trying to raise the contribution. You have a good point, but the man who died yesterday got $50.00, and the man who dies today gets $200.00." Dr. Sencer then suggested getting another nurse "to give preferential treatment."

Dr. Myers suggested giving the money to the doctor who performs the autopsy. Dr. Olansky asked if it would not be a good idea to get one of the doctors in the County Medical Society to perform the autopsies.

Dr. Sencer reiterated that we would have to get a public health nurse; "Whether we do it through Dr. Myers—this is one of the details we will have to work out."

Dr. Sencer continued, "First and foremost, we have to establish rapport with the County Medical Society and the Health Department."

Dr. B. Brown asked how we answer criticisms. Dr. Sencer replied that people outside Atlanta do read medical journals, and this could be blown up out of all proportions, but if we established rapport with the local health officials, he did not think we would have a problem.

Dr. Kaiser asked if the medical records were kept 'at the medical center.' Dr. B. Brown explained they were kept here in Atlanta (at the Venereal Disease Branch): "In very good shape—I have seen poorer-kept records in hospitals in Atlanta." Mrs. Price explained that clinical data are kept on McBee cards.

Dr. Sencer then said that this should be a joint effort with the Health Department, Dr. Brown, and himself. Dr. Myers said he would be happy to work with us.

Dr. Stollerman then asked what the group thought of the possibility of isolating treponemes.

Dr. W. J. Brown explained about the seminar held last week on spiral organisms, stating that Dr. Smith has shown that penicillin treatment has had no effect on spiral organisms, even after massive doses.

Dr. Stollerman asked Dr. Smith if he had ever found organisms in humans who have never had treatment. Dr. Smith said he did not want to say; he then mentioned the study of Dr. Yobs on the persistence of treponemes in late syphilis. Dr. Smith said he liked Dr. Norins' summarization: "After treatment of syphilis the outward lesions go away, but are all organisms eradicated throughout the body?" Dr. Smith said he thought we were going to come out of this Study with "some tremendous information"; he recalled that we have better techniques now; 42% of patients going through eye clinics, with inflammatory eye diseases, suffer from eye problems caused by spiral organisms. "I think we may come up with some treatment for them."

Dr. W. J. Brown said we have learned a great deal from Dr. Smith's work and it should urge all of us to try to find and treat everyone in a primary and secondary stage. Then he thanked each one who came to help us. "The advice you have given has been invaluable."

Dr. Sencer then said he thought everyone understood the sense of what we wanted to accomplish, "and we are going to do it. We will lean heavily on Ira." (Dr. Myers).

Meeting adjourned at 4:10 p.m.

THE LAWSUIT

FRED GRAY

I have been involved with the Tuskegee Syphilis Study since July 27, 1972, when Mr. Charlie Pollard came into my office and asked me if I read the newspaper about the men who were involved in the syphilis tests for "bad blood." He said he was one of the men. He related that a few days before, he was at a stockyard in Montgomery and a newspaper woman found him and questioned him about the Tuskegee testing program, and asked him if he knew Nurse Eunice Rivers. The reporter engaged him in a conversation about his involvement in a health program since back in the thirties. During our conference, Mr. Pollard related in detail his involvement in the experiment. As a result of our discussion, I agreed to represent Mr. Pollard in a lawsuit against the government and others who were legally responsible for operating and maintaining the experiment.

Mr. Pollard's statement confirmed the story I had read while flying from Washington, D.C., to Montgomery a few days earlier. As we saw in the previous chapter, that wire service article by Jean Heller was the first public exposure of the Tuskegee Syphilis Study, although as it developed there was considerable documentation of the Study in the medical literature and there were many doctors, health personnel, undertakers, white employers, college administrators, and draft board members in the Macon County area who had knowledge if not complete understanding of the Study.

When Mr. Pollard came into my office on July 27, 1972, my life was already quite busy. I had many civil rights cases pending in addition to my general practice of law; I was minister of a church; Bernice and I had four small children; I was trying to be a good husband; and I was in the middle of a legislative term, in which I served as one of the first two African Americans elected since Reconstruction to the Alabama House of Representatives.

My legislative service was complicated by the fact that voting rights litigation, which I had been involved in myself, led to a judicial decree that Alabama's unfair state electoral districts would be replaced by single-member districts based on an

Fred D. Gray Sr. is a distinguished civil rights attorney in practice in Tuskegee and Montgomery, Alabama. He has served as the lawyer for the study's survivors and heirs in their lawsuit since 1972. Originally published in Fred D. Gray, The Tuskegee Syphilis Study: The Real Story and Beyond *(Montgomery: Blackbelt Press, 1998), 80–99. Reprinted by permission of the Blackbelt Press.*

473

equal apportionment of the population. Under the old system, which had been in force since the 1901 Alabama Constitution effectively disfranchised African Americans, legislators were elected to the House of Representatives from multi-member districts and the representation was not proportional to the population. This allowed the big planters from the small predominantly African American rural counties to dominate the political process since they had as much power as the representatives from the large urban counties but were accountable mainly to themselves and their cronies. In 1965, African Americans obtained the right to vote, and we had a majority in the district encompassing Macon, Bullock, and Barbour counties. In 1970 I was elected, along with Thomas Reed, the other African American serving in the State Legislature.

I could tell many stories about this period and I did in my first book, *Bus Ride to Justice*. These were very interesting years in Alabama, to put it mildly. In any event, in 1974 there would no longer be two House seats from the district of Macon, Barbour, and Bullock counties. This meant a vigorous campaign against Thomas Reed in the spring of 1974. My wife, Bernice, had some real strong feelings about my running for re-election. She knew I was more qualified than Thomas Reed, but she believed that he was a better politician. She felt that he would probably win the election and that in reality he was more suited for the political shenanigans that went on in the Legislature. She felt that by the time my term ended, I would have proved to the white community and to all that I was an effective legislator, and that African Americans could serve in the Legislature with distinction. I would have made my contribution, and then I could return and do my work in the church and the law office.

The Tuskegee Syphilis Experiment was just one pending case at Gray, Seay and Langford, the law firm that I had built, with my partners Solomon Seay and Charles Langford, into the largest African American law firm in Alabama at that time. We had offices in Montgomery and Tuskegee and we had many civil, criminal, and civil rights cases. However, I recognized that the Tuskegee Syphilis Study was one of the largest cases I had. Bernice recognized that, too, and she thought, rather than for me to be involved in politics or trying to do so much in the Legislature, I needed to be devoting my time and effort towards this big and very important case. Bernice kept me focused on this case. She would not let me forget it, not put it on the back burner. She was determined that I devoted the time and effort to this case, because it could be my biggest case. She was right.

Of course, I thought I should stay in the Legislature. So I made up my mind to run for re-election and, as Bernice predicted, I lost the election to Thomas Reed. This turned out to be one of those cases where pride goeth before a fall, but in this case, at least, the fall was for the best because it allowed me to devote my full attention to the lawsuit that was beginning to gather steam.

Conclusions, 1972–1973

As a result of our initial investigation into the case, we reached the following conclusions:

1. The United States government violated the constitutional rights of the participants in the manner in which the study was conducted.
2. The government knew the participants had syphilis and failed to treat them—even after penicillin became available.
3. The Public Health Service failed to fully disclose to the participants that they had syphilis, that they were participating in a study, and that treatment was available for syphilis.
4. The Public Health Service led the participants to believe that they were being properly treated for whatever diseases they had, when in fact, they were not being meaningfully treated.
5. The Public Health Service failed to obtain the participants' written consents to be a part of the study.
6. The Study was racially motivated and discriminated against African Americans in that no whites were selected to participate in the Study; only those who were poor, uneducated, rural and African-American were recruited.
7. There were no rules and regulations governing the Study.

We believed those were the key issues to be resolved in a lawsuit. Of course, once the lawsuit was filed, we must prove our allegations, and in a case involving as many plaintiffs and defendants and stretching over as long a time span as this one, we knew that would be a Goliath-sized task for our David-sized law firm.

Search for Assistance

The work involved in developing this case was tremendous. I was reminded of advice given me by my law school adviser, Professor Samuel Sonnenfield. He encouraged me to seek assistance of other more experienced lawyers, and be willing to share a fee with them, particularly during the early years of my practice. As I had done with civil rights cases throughout my career, I tried to find someone to assist me in this case.

Finding and obtaining assistance was more difficult than I ever imagined. For almost a year, I telephoned and traveled all over the country, looking for someone to help me with this potentially historic case. I needed help in conducting legal research, drafting pleadings, filing briefs, and financing the case.

With previous civil rights cases, I was usually able to obtain such assistance from the NAACP or the NAACP Legal Defense Fund. But both organizations are non-profit corporations, whose policies did not permit them to assist in fee-generating cases.

It was going to take a substantial amount of money to develop this case. I could not find anyone who was willing to give me assistance in my two areas of need.

With a recommendation from Jack Greenberg, director counsel of the NAACP Legal Defense Fund, I sought out Michael I. Sovern, then dean of Columbia Law School, and one of his professors, Harold Edgar. They agreed to assist me with legal research.

I still had the responsibility of financing the case. I went to my local banker, James Allan Parker, president of Tuskegee's Alabama Exchange Bank, discussed my problem, and he indicated a willingness to make a loan. It was not a loan on a contingent fee basis. No banker would have done that. I would have to pay the bank regardless of the result of the lawsuit. However, he was willing to wait until there was a resolution of the case before the loan would become due. With these two components in hand, I was now ready to file the lawsuit.

Plaintiffs and Defendants

On July 24, 1973, the lawsuit was filed. Jurisdiction was invoked under (1) the Fourth, Fifth, Eighth, Ninth, Thirteenth and Fourteenth Amendments to the U.S. Constitution; (2) the civil rights laws 42 USC Section 1981, Section 1985(3) and Section 2000(D); (3) the Federal Torts Claims Act, 28 USC 2671; (4) the federal common law, and (5) the Constitution, statutes, and common law of Alabama.

This lawsuit was to redress grievances by damages and injunctive relief in order to secure for the plaintiffs themselves, and the class they represented, protection against continued or future deprivation of their rights by the defendants. The goal was to get the government's full attention. Originally, $1.8 billion in damages was sought for the surviving participants and the heirs of those who had died.

In the complaint as finally amended (on August 1, 1974) we had four categories of plaintiffs:

1. Living syphilitics
2. Living controls
3. Personal representatives of the estates of deceased syphilitics
4. Personal representatives of the estates of deceased controls.

The named plaintiffs included Charlie Pollard, Carter Howard, Herman Shaw, Price Johnson, and others. My law partner, Solomon Seay, Jr., assisted with the case. Cleveland Thornton, a young white lawyer from Barbour County and a member of our firm at the time, also assisted me in this case.

The defendants were the United States of America, Casper Weinberger as Secretary of the Department of Health, Education, and Welfare, Dr. Ira L. Myers, State Health Officer; Dr. John R. Heller, individually; Dr. Sidney Olansky, individually; and others. The defendants were represented by William J. Baxley, then Attorney General of Alabama, James T. Pons, Kenneth Vines, Calvin Pryor, Lawrence Klinger, Herman H. Hamilton, Jr., Champ Lyons, W. Michael Atchinson, and Oakley Melton, Jr.

Over the years, I have been asked why I did not include Nurse Eunice Rivers Laurie and Tuskegee Institute as defendants in this case? Isn't it a fact that each of them played a part and should bear some of the blame in connection with the Tuskegee Syphilis Experiment? Did I fail to add them as defendants because they were black and all of the other defendants were white? Did I fail to add them because all of the plaintiffs were African Americans? Isn't it a fact that if I had named them as defendants it would have adversely affected the allegations that the Tuskegee Syphilis Experiment was racist?

All of these questions are related and are fair questions to be considered.

Nurse Rivers was a lone African American female working on a health program financed by the federal government. She was working directly with white doctors from Washington, D.C. Neither the racial climate nor society's attitudes toward government encouraged her questioning the activities of white government officials. She did not question the fact that the government was financing and supporting the program.

She believed she could help, and at the same time she would be helping the federal government. Miss Rivers was powerless to have either begun, continued, or stopped the program. She worked in an environment where all of her superiors were white, while she worked directly with African American men. Even after penicillin became available, Nurse Rivers had no voice as to whether or not these men would be given penicillin. In 1969, a committee was formed to consider whether or not the program she had worked on for more than three decades—and had been the most constant aspect of for more than three decades—should continue. Nurse Rivers was not invited to participate in that discussion or to be a policy-maker in that decision. She was not even consulted. The white doctors from Washington concluded that the experiment should continue and that the participants still should not be treated for syphilis. The Alabama Department of Public Health, for which she also worked, again under the direction of white male doctors, went along with this program from the beginning to the end.

So you have one lone African American female, who from 1932–1972 was supervised by white doctors from Washington and by the white health officer from Macon County, in a program sponsored by the federal government. It would have been unrealistic for Nurse Rivers to express any views opposing the State of Alabama, the Macon County Health Department, white doctors from Washington, D.C., and the

United States government. I felt Nurse Rivers was misled, betrayed, and was also a victim of the Tuskegee Syphilis Study. In preparing the lawsuit, after reviewing the facts and circumstances, I was not going to subject her to being a defendant in the case. She was not the moving force in organizing, maintaining, or perpetuating the experiment. She was nothing more than one of many lower-level government employees who were involved in the Study but not named as defendants.

I did not include Tuskegee Institute as a defendant. In the 1930s, during the Great Depression, Tuskegee Institute was an African American educational institution struggling for its very existence. The federal government came to the institution and requested that some facilities of the college hospital be used for the purpose of examining the participants in a health care program. Tuskegee Institute was being asked to cooperate with the federal government in providing health care for the participants. The cooperation was being sought in a study that began as an outgrowth of the Rosenwald Fund survey in Macon County, which was a project of one of Tuskegee Institute's significant benefactors. As with Nurse Rivers, I felt that it would have been unrealistic to expect Tuskegee Institute to refuse to cooperate with the government. Tuskegee Institute administrators were asked to provide facilities and services; they were never invited to review or set policy. I felt the same about Tuskegee Institute as I did about Nurse Rivers—that the Institute and its officials were misled, betrayed, and taken advantage of as she had been.

Interestingly, President Bill Clinton took this same position twenty-five years later when he said:

> Medical people are supposed to help when we need care, but even once a cure was discovered, they were denied help, and they were lied to by their government. Our government is supposed to protect the rights of its citizens; their rights were trampled upon. Forty years ago, hundreds of men were betrayed, along with their wives and children, along with the community in Macon County, Alabama, the City of Tuskegee, the fine university there, and the larger African American community.

So the President, in his apology to surviving Study participants on May 16, 1997, recognized that Tuskegee Institute, along with these participants, and the whole community were lied to and betrayed by the federal government.

The Allegations

In our complaint, we alleged the following basic facts:

1. The participants were poor, Southern, rural, African Americans, of limited education, who knew nothing of their roles as experimental subjects.

2. The Tuskegee Syphilis Study began in 1932 and was announced by employees of the U.S. Public Health Service as a new health care program beginning in Macon County, Alabama. The notices were circulated throughout the county by mail, at African American schools, and African American churches. Only African Americans were given the notices, and only African American males were subsequently selected to participate in the program. None of the participants in the Study were meaningfully treated for syphilis.

3. The participants were never told that they were being solicited to be used in an experiment.

4. The employees of the government purposely did not inform the participants when they were found to have syphilis, and intentionally withheld this information from them.

5. The government represented to the participants, or gave the impression by words and actions that they were receiving adequate medical treatment for all of their ailments. Such representations or impressions were false and were known to be false by the government. However, each of the participants reasonably believed such representations and participated in the experiment for over forty years.

6. The participants were never advised that any of them had syphilis, and they were never treated for syphilis.

7. The participants never gave their informed consent to be subjects in any such experiment.

8. No white persons were solicited or used in the Study.

9. Those selected were used in a program of controlled genocide solely because of their race and color in violation of their rights, secured by the Constitution and laws of the State of Alabama.

10. The government exploited the participants in violation of rights guaranteed under the Fifth, Ninth, Thirteenth, and Fourteenth Amendments to the Constitution of the United States, and Article 1, Section VI of the Alabama Constitution of 1901. Plaintiffs further alleged that they were injured physically and mentally. They were afflicted with distress, pain, discomfort, and suffering. Some died as a result of participating in the Study.

Theory of the Case

The theory of the case was that the government had breached its duty to the participants in failing to obtain informed consent, inform them of the nature and purposes of the experiment, and inform them of the possible hazards and effects upon the health of the participants which might result from their participation.

The government had a duty to the plaintiffs once penicillin became available to treat those who had syphilis, which it failed to do. The government violated the civil rights of the plaintiffs in that it and state officials acted under color of State law by denying them their constitutional rights of equal protection, of due process, and of privacy. The government was negligent in conducting the Tuskegee Syphilis Experiment without any established protocol for conducting the experiment, thus subjecting the participants to unnecessary risks.

Defendant Dr. R. L. Myers, State Health Office, filed an answer on September 29, 1973, substantially denying the basic allegations and raising, as a second defense, that there was insufficient information to determine whether or not all of the subjects were African American, poor, and uneducated.

On May 14, 1974, the defendant United States answered the complaint, and alleged as defenses:

1. The action was barred by the statute of limitations.
2. The injuries and damages alleged by the complaint were caused without the fault, carelessness, or negligence on the part of the defendant or any of its agents, servants, or employees acting within the line and scope of their employment.
3. It denied that the injuries and damages to the participants, as alleged in the complaint, were caused by acts of negligence, or carelessness on the part of the government.

The government substantially denied all of the material allegations of the complaint. The United States admitted, however, that the Experiment began in 1932, that the participants were African American and were in the Study; that the Study was conducted by the federal government, and that some participants had died since 1932. It denied that the causes of death were related to the Study. That was the position of the United States of America when the suit was filed in 1973.

Discovery

One major problem in preparing the case for trial was the matter of obtaining discovery. According to the federal rules of civil procedure, after a lawsuit is filed, and prior to trial, a party may obtain any and all information which the other party has that may be relevant to the lawsuit. This is called discovery. We utilized several forms of discovery including depositions, interrogatories, requests for admissions, and requests for production. Interrogatories are written questions which must be answered in writing and sworn to under oath the same as if the answers were given orally in court. Interrogatories were propounded to the known living doctors involved in the Study and proper officials of the Public Health Service and to the government, but many of the answers were inconclusive. The response to the motion to produce documents during the early part of the study was met with a "no records available so far as the government knew."

The plaintiffs then undertook to try and find those records. As a result of our independent efforts, I met Jim Jones, a medical researcher, who had located the early records of the study, from 1931–1939, scattered through some 410 boxes in the National Archives. He literally searched through each individual box and picked out the information that was applicable to the Tuskegee Syphilis Study. Jim Jones's work was significant and made my task less difficult. He later wrote an excellent book about the study entitled *Bad Blood* and is now a professor of history at the University of Houston.

Opening Estates for Deceased Participants

During the course of our litigation, we were confronted with many legal problems. As indicated early during the discovery period, the government did not know and could not locate the early documents that would give us the facts concerning the origin of the Study. There were questions as to whether or not this was an appropriate class action suit. There were serious questions concerning the suit being barred by the statute of limitations. There were major problems of standing—who had the legal right to bring the action on behalf of the deceased participants in the Study.

The original complaint was filed on behalf of the widows and heirs of deceased participants. The defendants raised the issue of standing, saying that under Alabama law, the only person who could sue for a deceased person is the personal representative of the individual estate. That meant, in the cases of participants who had died without wills, it would be necessary to file a petition in the Probate Court of Macon County in each case and have someone appointed personal representative of that person's estate. Under Alabama law, in addition to filing an application for Letters of Administration, a bond must be filed in an amount twice the value of the estate prior to the Court granting Letters of Administration. The person who petitioned for the Letters of Administration must be a resident of the State of Alabama. Many of the deceased participants had died outside of Alabama.

This was a serious problem. The Court entered an order stating that the personal representative was the proper party to file a suit on behalf of the deceased participants, and gave us a short period of time in which to have them appointed. This was a difficult task. We needed to have appointed personal representatives for each of the deceased participants. There were 463 deceased participants. Under most circumstances this would have been an impossible task. First, we had to find individuals who were familiar with the deceased participants, for example, wives, children, close relatives, or friends. In instances where we could find none, we asked people we knew if they would serve as personal representatives of the estates of deceased participants. This required tremendous cooperation between people in the community. These men lived in all parts of Macon County. We began to talk with persons throughout the county and lined up persons who signed individual petitions, and had individuals to sign bonds so the administration could be completed.

In addition to the community involvement and finding persons to serve as administrators, we also had to locate persons who would sign bonds on behalf of these petitioners. The Judge of Probate of Macon County, in the final analysis, had to sign the order approving the bonds and appointing a personal representative on each of these estates. How could our Probate Office with its limited resources be able to accomplish such a task? I discussed this entire matter with the Honorable Preston Hornsby, Judge of Probate of Macon County. He knew the families of many of these men. In addition, he was the best politician in the county. Prior to the time he was elected Probate Judge, he was Sheriff of Macon County. In the first major campaign where blacks were able to vote, he openly solicited African-American votes and was elected Sheriff of Macon County. After successfully serving in that capacity, he ran for and became Judge of Probate.

After I discussed this matter with Judge Hornsby, he understood, was sympathetic, and gave whole-hearted support to our efforts. We literally moved a part of the Probate Office out of the Courthouse and into our office where we were able to prepare all of these documents. Within the time frame appointed by the Court and with the assistance of Judge Hornsby, we were able to have personal representatives appointed on the estates of each of the deceased participants. When the complaint was amended and filed on August 1, 1974, we had personal representatives of the estates of deceased syphilitics and personal representatives of deceased controls as plaintiffs in the suit.

What Our Research Proved

The mountain of documents eventually unearthed showed that, unquestionably, government doctors knew from the inception of the Study that the participants believed they were in a treatment program. Along with letters from the project nurse indicating this, they received letters from participants' friends asking to be included in the government treatment program.

What was done to participants in order to secure information about untreated syphilitics? Among the overreaching steps by the United States in the early years were:

1. The United States' doctors wrote and visited every local doctor in the area, gave them a list of patients in the study, syphilitics and controls, and secured their cooperation in the study. This cooperation included not treating anyone for syphilis because it would spoil the data.

2. United States' doctors sent these participant lists to "prominent lay people" (almost certainly white employers) to facilitate follow-up.

3. The doctors sent annual letters to participants telling them the federal doctors were coming again to treat their bad blood, and to find out whether past treatment had improved their condition.

4. Public Health Service personnel stopped participants from receiving treatment from the traveling State public health clinics and at other opportunities for treatment.

5. The Public Health Service wrote, through the Alabama Board of Health, to the local draft boards in 1941 to make sure that these men were not called for wartime physicals which would disclose syphilis and make treatment mandatory. Initially, the persons thus deprived included not only the original syphilitics, but also controls who had developed syphilis in the intervening years and had received no treatment for it. No effort was made to assure that these persons' wives and children had been treated.

6. The doctors and nurse handed out substantial quantities of painkillers such as aspirin and tonics, as well as some codeine, as an inducement to stay in the program, knowing the participants thought it was curative treatment for their ills.

7. The doctors did all this while their own medical records and reports they published were demonstrating unequivocally that the syphilitics were dying faster, and experiencing higher rates of heart morbidity than were the controls. That point was clear to the doctors from the very beginning, and it was duly monitored by articles that plotted participants' "death curves." Notwithstanding their own knowledge of the heightened death curve of the non-treated syphilitics, the deliberate and affirmative program of nontreatment was continued. Moreover, an intentional decision was made not to monitor the patients for a variety of other ailments, including, most tragically, neurosyphilis.

In summary, from 1933 on, the Study strayed far from its original short-term goals. Unlike the initial one-shot survey, the long-term research design was not evaluated carefully, and the rights of the humans involved were completely submerged to the researchers' desires to get just a little more return on their invested capital. This was the progression: the 1932 survey data, coming from syphilitics only, showed that untreated syphilitics had severe health problems, and much more complex ones than had been expected. That finding raised this question:

How much damage was syphilitic in origin, and how much was the product of adverse environment? Further, the 1932–33 findings of massive heart abnormalities could be undercut if heart specialists challenged the diagnostic techniques used. To preclude challenge to the Study's conclusions on either ground, the solution was to select a group of controls from the surveyed non-positive-Wassermann Negroes, and follow both groups for a while in order to "bring the material to autopsy." The doctors would confirm the initial 1932 diagnoses, reject the environmental hypothesis, and additionally measure interim syphilitic damage.

This was the long-term study plan and its effectuation, as unconscionable then as now. The Tuskegee experiment was not done with therapeutic hopes. There is not the slightest question but that the doctors who established and ran this program believed, based upon the careful Rosenwald records, that the then current medications posed trivial risks compared to the consequences of untreated syphilis. CDC's effort in 1972 to portray this study in its early years as potentially beneficial given the perceived dangers of mercury and arsenicals is inaccurate. Exactly the opposite is true. The doctors were so sure that untreated syphilis was a deadly serious problem, and that treatment was efficacious, that they wanted to prove it beyond question by control group comparisons and autopsies that would rule out any other possible explanation of data. Based on the documents, this process permitting these participants to suffer and die, seems never to have concerned the doctors in the least. The program doctors simply failed to think of the patients, their wives, or their children as human beings. This program of non-treatment then lasted forty years.

As far as later doctors were concerned, in relation to this group, penicillin's discovery was a regrettable event, worrisome lest it pollute the sample. In their 1955 article, "Untreated Syphilis in the Male Negro," Schuman, et al., analyzed participants' treatment status. The authors note that eight of the men had received adequate penicillin treatment by 1951 (with seroreversal in three cases), and mention no ensuing complications. They further note that the surviving syphilitic group is now 70 percent untreated, 22.5 percent inadequately treated, and 7.5 percent adequately treated. But they argue that those patients who have had some treatment should be followed still:

> [In] 1952 they are veterans of an aggregate of 5494.5 man-years of untreated disease, in comparison to only 28.5 man-years of adequately treated disease.
>
> Since the man-years of adequately treated disease represents such a small part of the total years of observation, and in most patients the treatment was administered many years after the date of the initial infection, it is felt that the antibiotic era has not defeated the purpose of the study.

The authors' perception of the significance of penicillin in terms of whether it spoiled the research ought to be juxtaposed against their other findings:

[T]he single most striking feature distinguishing the syphilitic group from the nonsyphilitic is that the death rate is higher among the syphilitic group. Exactly how and why more of the syphilitic group has died is not clearly discernible, but the penalty which the syphilitic patients have paid in terms of life expectancy is well-documented.

How could this disregard of human safety and life capacity have been allowed to continue? By the 1950s, a patient discovered to have latent syphilis would have been treated with antibiotics by almost every doctor in the United States, using bismuth if necessary to control adverse reactions, reactions that can occur only if the treponemes are alive and potentially dangerous.

So far as can be ascertained from the documents, no course of treatment was formally or informally considered for these African Americans until a young Public Health Service worker began complaining in 1966. Literally, not one single piece of paper out of the thousands of pages discussing every aspect of the study discusses whether treatment ought to be given. The documents reveal that the doctors believed in 1952 that a twenty-year investment should not go to waste, that this was the last opportunity to study untreated syphilis, and incredibly, that having shortened the lives of so many, they should press on with the work even though it might mean further premature deaths and disability. Even in 1969, treatment was rejected by a committee for reasons which patently included the desire to continue the Study and obtain just a little more information from the group. Compelling evidence that the 1969 determination was not made on the basis of the patients' medical needs is that each and every one of these very same participants was uniformly urged to get treated in 1972 after the Study was exposed.

The new doctors, in the 1960s, worked and acted in an era where the requirement of informed consent for experiments was formal and unambiguous. They knew perfectly well they did not have consent, and that these men were "at risk," albeit the risk may have been lower for the participants whose syphilis was still latent after thirty years of non-treatment. Moreover, statistics hide individual cases. One terribly potent indictment is that the subjects, ever since 1932, would have nothing to do with spinal taps. Those first taps, Vonderlehr's Golden Needle treatment, performed without anesthetics, were exceptionally painful. The Study's internal documents often treat the fearful reactions to this pain as proof of some rural superstitions of the participants.

Our investigation, however, led us to believe, that Dr. Vonderlehr did the taps poorly, a view shared by Nurse Rivers. Dr. Vonderlehr was tired, overworked, and very anxious because he had to get all the taps done before word of what was happening spread among the participants. After the initial taps, most of the participants made it very clear they would never submit to such a procedure again, so the PHS officials early abandoned any hope of making spinal taps a routine part of the annual checkup and the five-year surveys, fearing the Study would collapse. The doctors acknowledged they could not use the only effective diagnostic procedure available to test the presence of one of the more serious complications of syphilis. Yet the doctors knew the threat of neurosyphilitic was real: 23 percent of the participants had it in 1932 when the first survey was done. Of the first participants examined once the Study ended, 16 percent had neurosyphilis.

Finally, doctors who knew penicillin was a remedy for syphilis permitted the Study to proceed because of apparent statistical safety based on the controls' death rates. The use of the controls' life-expectancy as the test of safety was questionable. It assumed the comparability of the two groups except for syphilis, an assumption later doctors expressly made. However, the survey techniques utilized by Vonderlehr to get his initial sample were weighted to pick up syphilitic persons of greater than average hardiness, in that they had survived syphilis thus far and were out doing heavy work. Field hands and manual workers were sought out by Vonderlehr so that he would not have to waste his Wassermann tests on women.

The later doctors assumed comparability because they had never read the file on how the syphilitics were selected. They made the mistake of relying on their predecessors' writings, including its reports of the participants volunteering in droves at churches and schools. But the doctors stopped working at churches in January 1933, because for every man presenting himself, three women would seek testing. If the doctors refused to treat women, the men refused to cooperate because they thought the doctors were from the Army. So the doctors went to the saw mills, the Public Works employment centers, and into the fields with Keidel tubes. The Wassermann positive rates with Keidel tubes were well below those at the churches, indicating that those syphilitics capable of doing heavy work were more than usually sturdy. It should have been no surprise, given the relative hardiness required to get into the two sample populations, that syphilitics in later years might even be doing better than controls.

Nothing the doctors might have learned about untreated syphilis could possibly justify this calculated mistreatment of a group of United States citizens. An added dimension of this tragedy is that the study was poorly done in scientific terms. Nearly all these patients were given some treatment with arsenicals or mercury, and often with both, in the course of the initial 1932–33 survey. The amount was believed too small to have much effect on the disease, but it ruined the study as one of untreated syphilis. The doctors botched the sample doing the short-term study, securing it by going through the motions of treatment, before a long-term study was even contemplated. Rather than call it quits, the doctors falsified the sample selection procedure in their initial papers by arbitrarily defining the little treatment as no treatment at all. Although it baffled later doctors how so many patients had gotten some, albeit obviously inadequate, treatment, no one had read the files. The files were found in the National Archives, meaning that an on-going medical experiment was conducted with no one involved even knowing where the papers pertinent to its initial design and early years were kept.

The Settlement

The government did not begin to discuss the possibility of settlement until after we obtained much of the information detailed in the earlier chapters of this book and made it known by appropriate court pleadings and briefs.

Ultimately, we were successful in getting financial compensation for each of the living participants and the heirs of deceased participants in the Tuskegee Syphilis Study. In addition, the government was ordered to continue its health care program for the living participants and widows and children of any participants who tested positively for syphilis.

While the final $10 million settlement was not what I had hoped to receive for my clients, considering all of the facts and circumstances, it was in my opinion fair and reasonable. This study started in 1932. There were a multiplicity of legal problems that would have to be resolved if there had been a trial. If this case were discovered today under the same facts and circumstances, the value of the case would be substantially higher. When the proceeds from the settlement were paid into court, the funds were placed in an interest-bearing account. It took a number of years to locate all the participants, and after the recipients had received the principal amount there was accumulated interest to disburse. Thus, we had to verify again whether the participants were living or dead, and if dead, whether there were living heirs, and in all cases we had to find current addresses. This case is still pending.

The settlement was divided into four categories:

1. Living syphilitics received $37,500.
2. Heirs of deceased syphilitics received $15,000.
3. Living controls received $16,000.
4. Heirs of deceased controls received $5,000.

The persons who suffered most and whose lives were at risk were the syphilitics. Though many received some incidental or even accidental treatment over the years, they were never treated for syphilis during the experiment, not even after penicillin became available. The controls did not have syphilis. Neither they nor their wives and children were at risk. That is why there was a difference in the amounts for the syphilitics and the controls.

When the proceeds from the settlement were paid into court, the funds were placed into an interest-bearing account. The next task was to locate the living participants and the heirs of the deceased participants. This was a major task and it took years to accomplish. Originally, we did not know who the heirs of the deceased participants were, so we had to find them. When we began to find heirs and people realized there was money involved, it became necessary to have hearings to determine who were the legitimate heirs. The principal amount of funds were finally completely distributed in 1992, except for interest payments. Then, the process started all over again to distribute the interest payments. Many who were paid principal amounts had died and we had to locate their heirs. However, more than six thousand persons have received compensation. We are still looking for some heirs to distribute interest money.

When it became generally known that money was available, some men and women claimed falsely to have been in the Experiment. In instances where participants were deceased, some falsely claimed to be heirs. As a result, during the time when claims were being litigated, the court held hearings on conflicting claims dealing with heirs.

In addition to the financial settlements, the government was ordered to continue providing other benefits including free health care for living participants and to the families of syphilitic participants, as well as free burial expenses for participants based on the cost of living index at the time of their deaths.

OUTSIDE THE COMMUNITY

HAROLD EDGAR

Twenty years ago, when the *Washington Star* told the public that the United States Public Health Service had, since 1932, maintained a study of untreated syphilis in the Negro male that was *still* going on, my reaction was, How could people have done this? I later worked on the participants' lawsuit, and I learned of the study's many complexities. In the end, though, the best explanation of "how" it could have happened is the obvious one: the researchers did not see the participants as part of "their" community or, indeed, as people whose lives could or would be much affected by what the researchers did.

Looking back on those events after two decades, there are a number of observations I'd like to make.

Tuskegee under the Law

First, I should like to describe some aspects of the legal landscape of the Tuskegee litigation. The injustices done to the participants did not fit easily into the framework of an adjudicable lawsuit. The issues that faced Fred Gray, an Alabama civil rights lawyer, and me could have filled a book. Among them: the United States cannot be sued in tort without its consent. However, in 1946 by act of Congress the government became responsible in damages, like any employer, if an employee exercising a nondiscretionary authority causes an injury cognizable under *state* law. Did the act permit recovery for harm done between 1932 to 1945 to people (many of whom were dead by 1946), on the theory that there had been an ongoing project whose success depended upon keeping the facts secret from the participants? Second, could unwitting (and unwilling) service in an experiment give rise to a contract claim against the government, or even a claim that government had taken property and owed compensation? Third, what relevancy, if any, did Nuremberg have? There, the United States had conducted in its own name criminal proceedings against German doctors on the theory that their criminal

Harold Edgar is professor of law and director of the Julius Silver Program in Law, Science and Technology at the Columbia University School of Law.
Originally published in the Hastings Center Report 22 *(1992): 32–35. Reprinted by permission of the Hastings Center and Harold Edgar.*

homicides and assaults could not be justified by their desire to gain useful information by experiments. Fundamental principles of medical ethics recognized everywhere, the prosecutors claimed, permitted experiments only with informed consent. Had our government's conduct, therefore, violated the fundamental principles of liberty and justice embodied in the American conception of due process? If so, can the United States be held responsible for its employees' "constitutional torts" under the 1946 act on a theory that "state" law includes federal law?

How could we prove damages, particularly when people had died from causes not obviously related to syphilis? Could we use in evidence against the government the chief finding of the study—that syphilis seems to cause pervasive medical problems previously not thought to have been caused by syphilis? If so, could we shift the burden of proof to the government and require it to *disprove* the relationship between syphilis and any individual's medical condition? If not, could we use aggregate data about the men as a group (so much extra heart disease, for example), and then value the excess and award it proportionally to individuals?

The complexity of sustaining such a suit through a verdict and appeals was matched by its futility, if the ambition was to put money into the hands of those who had personally suffered injustice. Even if ultimately successful, litigation would take years, and fewer people would actually have the advantage of monetary payment. And yet was it fair to settle the action on a class basis without regard to individualized damages? We believed there were major barriers to any recovery, and it was futile to attempt to ascertain the medical damages each person sustained. The victims' class representatives themselves made the decision to settle, and I had no doubt then nor do I now that this was a wise thing to do. As further proof that law marches to the slowest of beats, it is just this past year that the last payments to a few persons pursuant to the settlement agreements have been made.

As a result of the settlement, however, the Tuskegee litigation made no new law. The extremely interesting issue of how government misbehavior in conducting medical experiments should be analyzed for purposes of constitutional law went unanswered and remains unanswered to this day. The problem has been raised in litigations involving CIA experiments, and military experiments exposing servicemen to radiation, among others, but the Supreme Court passed over its chance to comment on the problem. In *United States v. Stanley*, the Supreme Court held that the courts were closed to a serviceman injured by surreptitious administration of LSD.

The Tuskegee study was, however, surely a major force in the development of American bioethics. Among other things, it was a direct cause of the National Research Act in 1974, which required the establishment of institutional review boards at institutions receiving federal grants. These IRBs have been transformed from peer group meetings in which controversial research might be discussed into legally mandated, professionally diverse, and bureaucratically independent centers that have the power to shape and regulate research within an institution. Increasingly, conventional product regulation, such as the FDA's regulation for commencing testing of insignificant risk devices, builds on the presence and protective capacities of IRBs. And yet who gets on IRBs, the extent to which they are subject to institutional controls, how successfully they carry out their mission, and at what costs, remains, I submit, largely a mystery. Nonetheless, the core IRB concept—an institutionally based, multidisciplinary ethics committee—has been adopted as the paradigmatic American response to bioethics dilemmas.

Science by Deception

Apart from its violation of human rights, the Tuskegee study was a serious incident of what is now called "science misconduct." The story is told brilliantly by Jim Jones in his book *Bad Blood*. Jones found and organized the physicians' and the study's early papers in the National Archives. These materials showed not only that the study was ethically wrong measured by the ethical standards of the 1970s, but that it had been, from the start, a program built upon deception. In 1932 the researchers told participants they were getting free medical treatment. Without that promise, the researchers could not get participants' cooperation in giving blood and undergoing spinal taps. The subsequent program built on that lie, although it was a complicated lie.

The central fact about the forty-year study was that its scientific rationale made no sense. The fact that the government was running a long-term study when no person in charge had any idea of what the original protocols were, or where they were, is itself shocking. On reading the protocols, moreover, it is apparent that the forty-year study was an afterthought.

The initial plan was simply to go to Alabama for a one-shot visit to take a snapshot of secondary syphilis in a population. The snapshot would show, for example, whether people who had had syphilis for ten years were much worse off than those who had had syphilis for five years. (Some readers may not realize that the government did not infect the participants; they had the disease already. The men ranged in age from their twenties to their sixties when the study started.) The initial plan rested on a highly dubious premise, namely, that the participants were capable of giving adequate information about how long they had been infected. When they got the data, however, the physicians could not read their snapshot. Although they had generated a lot of data, no one knew whether the X-ray pictures that seemed to reveal massive amounts of heart damage were either accurate or, if they were, indicated syphilis rather than other causes. Only after doubts came up about the interpretability of data was a decision made to go back to Alabama to create a control group of age-matched nonsyphilitics, and "bring the material to autopsy." The goal was to learn by autopsy whether the heart problems were indeed caused by syphilis.

The forty-year study then proceeded upon a false claim that the men had not been treated. They were treated in 1932, although completely inadequately, by then-current standards. They were treated with as much mercury and arsenicals as the government doctors doing the first work in 1932 could get—the only limit on treatment was the availability of drugs. The participants' cooperation was obtained by providing such treatments. The researchers then administered a spinal tap with no anesthetic, called it treatment, and left town. How did it happen that the long-term study explained itself as a study of "untreated" syphilis?

Despite their having administered drugs, and thus destroyed the sample, the researchers pressed on. Moreover, they did what people still do today: they assumed their error had no biasing impact. Interesting also, for it too has its modern analogy, was their reasoning, which was shaped by their capacity to measure. Since modest amounts of arsenicals and mercury did not cause seroconversion of the blood (the Wassermann tests still were positive), they assumed that treatment had no possible effect upon syphilis. Whether it did or not is impossible to tell, because among other things, in later years, they had no way to control for who was getting what antibiotics in private medical visits. The aggregate data suggest, however, that the younger men did not do as badly when measured against the control group as did the older ones. Sampling biases, however, could readily account for the difference, inasmuch as one would predict that sicker people, among those who were in their forties and fifties in 1932, would find more attractive the promise of free treatment and thus show up in greater numbers.

This was bad science. It was also unethical medicine. It was during the first fifteen years of follow-up that the most outrageous incidents occurred, including switching newly infected control subjects into the participant group while making no effort to protect them or their families, and keeping participants from becoming aware of their disease or of treatment available for it when new public health efforts were launched again after the Depression.

Yet, one of the worst faults of the project in later years had nothing to do with whether administering penicillin was a good idea: that point was complicated initially by the question of whether the massive doses required were safe, and by the belief that the disease was probably benign in people who had had it so long. The harm came from the failure aggressively to follow up on diagnosed medical problems having nothing to do with syphilis, while simultaneously handing out placebos that many men understood to be medical care. By the end of the study, a number of participants had private doctors, but many others did not, and the failure to follow up adversely affected controls as well as syphilitics.

For reasons I do not understand, front page news coverage results today when science fraud occurs. Why there should be surprise that misdeeds, let alone dumb mistakes, happen in a billion-dollar business I do not know. And yet if one looks to standards in the recent past, one realizes that contemporary scientists are vastly more alert to these problems than were people who were highly regarded in their own day. It is, therefore, not the case that things are always getting worse.

The Racial Difference

One irony about Tuskegee is that the study was racist to the core, in that no such program could possibly have continued so long but for the central fact that participants were African Americans. (Indeed, I believe race injected itself in the decision whether to shut the program down in the 1960s. Sadly—for the government should have legal authority to keep its promises—there was no easy way to secure payments of death benefits to the participants unless there was an ongoing study. The men rightly counted on them as burial insurance, and if they stopped, the story might become public. So I believe the research kept going in part to keep the story private.) Despite the centrality of race, however, the researchers were not personally vicious racists. They sought and secured research help in the African-American community, and they were personally committed to vastly expanded public health services for African Americans.

I disagree with one of Jones's conclusions, however. He suggests the physicians believed that blacks and whites were different in terms of how syphilis affected them, and that the study was intended to shed light on this difference. The former proposition is true, but my recollection is that the latter had nothing to do with the enterprise. What drove the physicians was an attempt to undermine the conclusion of the best prior study of untreated syphilis, a study done in Oslo, Norway. It may well be that, as Jones recounts, the Oslo data suggested neurosyphilitic complications were less common among whites than supposed. That was not, however, the conclusion that attracted American attention. The Oslo study suggested that if the individual infected does nothing about syphilis, in two out of three cases *nothing* adverse happens to him. The Oslo data were subject to all sorts of sampling biases, and the American doctors didn't believe them. If true, however, the proposition had implications for how one spent the limited funds available for public health during a depression.

On the issue of racial impact of the disease, the physicians involved unquestionably believed both before the study and as a result of the study's data that syphilis does affect different groups differently. They believed neurosyphilis is a less common outcome among blacks than whites, and that crippling heart disease is more common among blacks than whites. Indeed (and I thought it was cause for grievance), they used that belief to justify continuing the study even though they could not monitor for neurosyphilis because the participants would never again accept a spinal tap. I do not know whether their beliefs about the relative impact of the two complications among blacks and whites are true. The physicians did not think that their belief in this regard was particularly interesting or surprising, however. Nor was this specific belief a prop for a broader, more systemic set of beliefs about blacks.

There has been a sea-change in attitude about such matters today. At present, any assertion of group difference is always a potentially explosive issue. The horrors of the Holocaust and the pervasive racism that still afflicts American life make it impossible for many people even to contemplate that different groups may be different in lots of ways. Acknowledging that fact may permit others to urge social policies that are frightening, and so the intellectual leadership suppresses the observations in order to keep control of the inappropriate inferences that others might draw. Yet what the Tuskegee doctors could contemplate—group differences—will be forced upon the medical world in the effort to understand problems ranging from why some people get lung cancer while others do not, to how come the French eat so much fat and do not get our rates of heart disease. Indeed, the fact that groups may be different (why does a vaccine work in Finland and not in Alaska?) may have major implications for how we appraise "research" as opposed to "experimental therapies," for we draw lines between these categories more sharply than the reality makes desirable.

Finally, the Human Genome Project will bring to the forefront of human consciousness awareness of the range of variability not only among individuals, but among groups. To acknowledge those differences, while insisting on their irrelevance to respect for individual dignity and equality of right, is a challenge we shall have to face.

VENEREAL DISEASE CONTROL BY HEALTH DEPARTMENTS IN THE PAST

Lessons for the Present

JOHN C. CUTLER & R. C. ARNOLD

Introduction

As one reviews the history of public and professional responses to epidemic diseases before and after and discovery of effective methods of control, one realizes that the acquired immunodeficiency syndrome (AIDS) problem, while obviously new, has many parallels in the past. Throughout history civilization has been confronted with pandemics such as influenza, smallpox, plague, cholera, syphilis, and others, but only within the past century have there been specifics to deal with them. Even in recent history, we have experienced problems similar to AIDS, notably the spread of venereal disease (VD) during World Wars I and II. Thus patterns of programs for VD control developed during the past have relevance now.

Whatever approach may be taken in dealing with the AIDS problem, it must be, as learned from past experiences, both non-judgmental and non-moralistic if it is to be effective. There may be a classic parallel in our World War I and WWII handling of the problems associated with the explosive spread of venereal diseases in both the military and civilian populations and the resultant obstructions to the war effort. Because of the wartime needs in both the military and civilian populations, it was obvious and accepted that the problem had to be approached from a medical point of view rather than avoided because of value judgments. At that time, diagnostic and treatment procedures for syphilis and gonorrhea were complex, time-consuming, expensive, heavily dependent upon individual initiatives, and "primitive" according to today's advances. However, the "public health" approach to control, utilizing existing knowledge and resources, proved to be highly effective in lowering incidence and prevalence rates.

It should be noted with respect to AIDS that pathogenic agents evolve or mutate,

Dr. John C. Cutler is emeritus professor of international health at the University of Pittsburgh School of Public Health. He was one of the Public Health Service physicians involved in the study. Dr. R. C. Arnold is a retired assistant surgeon general in the Public Health Service who worked on research on treatment of syphilis with penicillin.
Originally published in the American Journal of Public Health 78 (1988): 372–76.
Reprinted by permission of the American Public Health Association.

and that resultant new challenges to the health community constantly appear. This may be illustrated by the pandemic of influenza of World War I, by frequent emergence of new strains of viruses and bacteriae, the development of chemotherapeutic and antibiotic resistance, as with the gonococcus. Such recurrent events calls for control efforts based upon earlier experience, existing knowledge about the agents, and evolution of new or modified control measures. In addition, there are continuing changes in the risk of disease transmission within various geographic, social, and age groups because of the changing patterns of transportation, food movement, travel and, in particular, changes in social behavior such as age at onset and patterns of sexual activity, patterns of marriage and break-up, public reaction to sexual behavior, etc. Over the decades, the public health sector has been able to respond to the impact of these various factors. Within the United States, continuing and/or evolving patterns of disease and disability, life expectancy, etc., reflect the successes and failures, as well as the constantly changing challenges to the health of the community.

A review of the response of all levels of government to the problem of syphilis might be useful in charting a course for control of AIDS today. There are remarkable parallels between the two diseases, including a long latency period before the disabling or fatal clinical symptoms become manifest. The challenges posed by syphilis to the medical/public health professions in developing patterns of cooperation in educational and research programs and in methods for securing and implementing effective public and professional involvement in the VD control effort, clearly have relevance to the problems posed today by AIDS.

The Impact of World War I

At the outset of World War I, when VD was a leading cause of incapacitation or rejection for active duty, public concern was sufficient to override the previous moralistic judgmental inhibitions against VD control efforts. In retrospect, these earlier attitudes seem once again to complicate a rational approach to the problems of the present AIDS epidemic. Because of the overriding concerns with the war effort it was possible under the leadership of the United States Public Health Service (USPHS) in 1917 to initiate a cooperative control program among state and local health departments and the private sector, including medical practitioners, the hospital system, and voluntary agencies. It was viewed by the public as necessary, in support of the war effort, to keep the military fit for duty rather than restricted or incapacitated by syphilis and gonorrhea and the scheduling requirements of existing treatment regimens. The essential elements of the WWI VD control effort included case reporting, widespread availability of testing (using the relatively costly and varied procedures then available), the provision of arsphenamine (for treatment of syphilis) at public expense, promotion of prophylaxis—both chemical and use of condoms by the military, in particular—establishment of treatment facilities, and a public education program, all basically centered in the state health departments.

Within a year, the seriousness of the problem was sufficiently appreciated to result in enactment of the Chamberlain-Kahn Act in 1918 which established a formal basis for cooperative efforts within the federal government—specifically between the USPHS and the Army and Navy. In addition, the legislation provided for a VD Division within the Public Health Service, authorized grants to states for VD control programs, and provided specifically for VD research. The law was written so as to promote the establishment and implementation of minimum standards of program efficiency by the grantees. Because of the perceived significance of such a cooperative and interdependent control program in promoting the war effort, the program enjoyed wide public acceptance as long as the wartime conditions prevailed. This has been documented in fascinating detail by Brandt.[1]

With the winning of the war, the attitudes toward VD control changed. In light of the present public attitudes, a quotation from Vonderlehr and Heller[2] is most relevant for it mirrors the importance of public and professional attitudes and the resultant government programs:

A change in the attitude of the people was observed with the return of the troops after World War I. This change was reflected in Congress. Once the Versailles Treaty was signed the people of the United States assumed that the Germans had been beaten for all time. When the U.S. Army was demobilized a similar assumption was made regarding the defeat of the spirochete and the gonococcus, and the VD problem was forgotten. In the third year of existence of the new Division of Venereal Diseases, the grant-in-aid program dwindled to $100,000 and thereafter was discontinued altogether. The activities of the Public Health Service in venereal disease control were reduced to research investigations. Venereal disease control was in the doldrums and remained there for about fifteen years.

An incident which portrays the prudish attitude once taken by the public and even by the medical profession toward the venereal diseases, occurred during the early experiences of one of our preeminent specialists. Thirty years ago, Dr. P. S. Pelouze read his first scientific paper on gonorrhea before a meeting of physicians. One of them rushed up to Dr. Pelouze and said: "Pelouze, you are making a grave mistake in letting yourself become known as one interested in gonorrhea; it will ruin you."

Dr. Pelouze replied, "Do you mean that a doctor who shows an interest in a disease that afflicts millions of human beings and has been so badly neglected by our profession that our lack of knowledge upon it is our greatest medical blot, will be ruined?"

The physician replied, "Most assuredly."

"Don't you think, then," said Dr. Pelouze, "that it is time a few of us were ruined?"

Most physicians felt as Dr. Pelouze's colleague, and they reflected the attitude of the public generally. Most people would rather not have their family doctor, or a doctor related to them, associated with venereal disease.[2]

Renewed Interest in VD Control

By the mid-1930s the seriousness of the VD problem was beginning to come back in to the medical and public consciousness, primarily because of the leadership of Dr. Thomas Parran who became Surgeon General of the USPHS in 1936, a year in which the USPHS budget for VD control was $58,000. By then the serious problems of disability, death rates, and costs of long-term effects of syphilis alone were again evident nationwide. A gradual, well-planned move to reestablish a full-fledged national VD control program began. It is relevant to remind ourselves that the problems Dr. Parran faced then are sharply mirrored in the current public and professional attitudes about AIDS. For instance, because of the planned use of the word "syphilis" in a radio program to be broadcast nationally, the Surgeon General of the USPHS was denied permission to air a program. However, shortly after this episode, the *Reader's Digest* was concerned and farsighted enough to publish an article entitled "Why Don't We Stamp Out Syphilis?" which focused national attention on the extent of the problem. There was a highly supportive public response, matched by strong support from the medical and public health communities which were aware of the problem but had been unable to move effectively because of the lack of adequate financial and political support. It should be noted also, as is evident today, that in the period before the resurgence of public interest and availability of governmental funds for research and program implementation, the medical and public health schools and the voluntary agencies had been carrying out basic and clinical research on syphilis and gonorrhea as well as public health control studies. Support for such work came primarily from voluntary agencies, such as the Milbank Memorial Fund, the Rockefeller Foundation, the Rosenwald Foundation, the Reynolds Foundation, and others, showing their recognition of the significance of the problem and the need for action. As is often the case, this private sector interest paved the way for later governmental action. Much had been learned from these pioneering projects, but nationwide, applications of the knowledge that had been acquired could come only when there was widespread and active public support to provide the funding required.

As a result of the growing public concern and interest, a national conference was called by Surgeon General Parran in December 1936, which put forward plans for a revitalized national VDL control program. The VD control program was restarted the same fiscal year when funds became available through Title VI of the Social Security Act. This is best summarized by a quote from the History of the USPHS.[3]

The Social Security Act of 1935 marked the beginning of an important public health era in the United States. Included in the Act was Title VI which authorized general health grants to States by the Public Health Service. . . .

Under Title VI of the Social Security Act the Public Health Service was authorized to allot $8,000,000 annually in grants-in-aid to State health departments. The appropriation of $2,000,000 annually for scientific research was also authorized. The law further provided that the distribution of funds to the States should be based proportionately upon population, financial need, and the existence of special health problems. These funds were not given without what may legally be termed a consideration, as the States were required to match dollar for dollar the sums appropriated for general health services and special health problems. A part of the grant-in-aid appropriation was reserved for the training of State and local health personnel. Funds allotted for training, however, did not have to be matched. Regulations for the administration of grants-in-aid funds under Title VI of the Social Security Act were promulgated by the Public Health Service after conference with the State and Territorial health authorities. Funds authorized by the Social Security Act first became available on February 1, 1936, when Congress appropriated $3,333,000 for the remaining five months of that fiscal year.

Thus, for the first time in the history of the United States, the Federal government entered into a partnership with the States and Territories for the protection and promotion of the health of the people. For the first time the Public Health Service was under legal authority cast in the role which it had so long wished to play, that of partner, adviser, and practical assistant to the State health departments, and through them to municipal and local health services to be accomplished with Federal aid, and to leave the administration of these activities to the States. Consultant and technical services have been provided for the States in the planning of both general and specific programs. Personnel of the Public Health Service frequently have been assigned to the States upon request to administer health programs.

In 1938 the Lafayette-Bulwinkle Act, approved May 24, implemented the attack upon syphilis and gonorrhea through grants-in-aid to the States and expansion of research specifically upon these diseases by the Public Health Service. In 1939 amendments to the Social Security act raised the ceiling of grants-in-aid to the States under Title VI to $11,000,000, with provision that the increases should be utilized in the States for special health problems. The National Health Conference in 1938, in which the Public Health Service participated, proposed not only an expansion of public health services but also the construction of hospitals and studies of methods, needs, and resources of public medical care for the indigent.[3]

The program, inaugurated by Dr. Parran, was based upon the nine basic principles of public health control of syphilis which he had formulated:

- A trained public-health staff;
- Case finding and case holding;
- Premarital and prenatal serodiagnostic testing;
- Diagnostic services available;
- Treatment facilities available;
- Distribution of drugs for treatment;
- Routine serodiagnostic testing;
- A scientific information program;
- Public education.

It should be noted that concurrent with the public health concerns about syphilis and the resultant political and public health program responses there had been a highly active and productive research program carried out both nationally through cooperative efforts within the university community and the USPHS and, internationally, through the Health Organization of the League of Nations. Through these efforts, new arsenical preparations were developed and treatment programs worked out which cut treatment time from the previous 18–24 months to as few as five days. All of these new treatment procedures had a high rate of toxic reactions, and rare fatalities, but they were accepted realistically then in light of the long-term effects of the untreated disease and the accompanying social and economic costs.

In spite of treatment modalities that were complex and toxic by today's standards, the well-planned and coordinated national program made real headway. Through cooperative programs made possible by increased funding from both federal, state, and local government, a massive national VD control program was mounted thanks to the Social Security Act of 1935 and the leadership of the national public health community.

World War II and After

With the beginning of World War II, the need for large scale application of the shortened, intensive arsenical-based treatments requiring up to 10 weeks in hospitals was recognized: the increased patient mobility in civilian as well as military populations due to wartime needs caused problems in completing therapy. Starting in 1942, so-called Rapid Treatment Centers (RTCS) were begun and by 1946 had been established in 35 states and the District of Columbia, most of them under state health department management but with federal financial support and strong professional cooperation. By 1946 the USPHS had been given congressional responsibility for national administration of the program; $5 million was appropriated to subsidize the centers and to pay the local general hospitals which were also important resources for treatment—usually local-government administered. A total of 59 projects in 37 states—50 state or locally operated and nine projects USPHS operated—were in existence. In 1945, of the 183,000 cases of syphilis reported nation-wide, 52,000 (29 per cent) were treated in the RTCS.

The entry of the US into WWII had served as a catalyst to the national program, again because of the high rates of rejection of draftees due to syphilis and because of the high rates of absence from duty of military manpower resulting from syphilis and gonorrhea. As in WWI, cooperative agreements were set up between the USPHS and the military. In the same fashion, working through the Conference of State and Territorial Health Officers, plans were made for the nationwide program to protect the national well-being and health. In so doing, the classic approach was taken: case finding through screening of hospital admissions, etc. The system of contact interviewing and tracing was developed, utilizing well-trained personnel, designated as VD investigators or epidemiologists. This represented a break with past tradition that had held that only a professional such as a physician, nurse, or social worker could interview and do contact tracing. In addition, the significance of the voluntary organization in the total public health program was fully recognized, and the American Social Hygiene Association (ASHA), now called American Social Health Association, played a very important role in community program operations, education, and building community support.

The importance of the federal-state cooperative effort was fully recognized and further implemented through the assignment of USPHS personnel to state and local health departments so as to assure the availability of necessary professional staff. The significance of and need for research was also recognized and resulted in increased federal support of a number of highly productive academic centers as well as several existing USPHS centers. One of the latter, the Venereal Disease Research Laboratory (VDRL) at the Marine Hospital at Staten Island, NY had the clinical resources of the large population of merchant seamen. Here, Mahoney, Arnold, and Harris had made the discovery of penicillin therapy for syphilis and developed the VDRL test for syphilis.[4]

It was understood that research was of no value unless its findings could be put to use, so that with federal VD funds a number of university programs were supported which not only conducted basic and applied research but also provided training for the physicians, nurses, laboratory personnel, and administrators needed at the various levels of control programs. At the same time, within the USPHS, there was a highly productive ongoing program that assigned commissioned officers to universities for advanced training in VD control, research, etc.

World War II brought about national recognition of the adverse effects of VD, particularly syphilis, and permitted the plans that leaders such as Parran and others had developed to be realized. Public antipathy to the VD patient and to control programs was dissipated to a large extent and the health professional, financial, and administrative resources needed to establish an effective national program were made available. This is best summarized by a quote from the Military History of World War II which epitomizes the complexity and the interdependence of the public health program for the control of a disease.[5]

> The relationship between the US Public Health Service and the Army from 1940 to 1945 was highly satisfactory and mutually advantageous. To a varying extent, every activity of the Venereal Disease Control Division of the Public Health Service during World War II affected the Army's program. Only the history of that division's activities (in the files of the US Public Service) can tell the complete story of that collaboration and assistance. The success of the Army venereal disease control program in the Zone of Interior was due in no small measure to the active support and cooperation provided by the Public Health Service. The program of the Public Health Service constituted one of the most valuable contributions to venereal disease control during World War II. Important phases of this program were liaison activities at service command headquarters; cooperation in the contact and separation programs; support of State and local control programs by allocation of funds and assignments of personnel; distribution of educational literature, films, and posters; analysis of statistical data; support of legislation; establishment of rapid treatment centers; organization of public meetings; and extensive research activities.[5]

Paradoxically, the aftermath of the successes of WWII and the advances in penicillin therapy which permitted a single-injection cure of syphilis as well as of gonorrhea was the loss of both public concern about and medical and political interest in VD. The feeling in Congress was that since there existed a "single-shot" cure for syphilis there was no longer any need for the support of the full-scale public health approach which had been so successful. Appropriations for VD control were cut sharply (Table 1).[6]

The authors have a very personal reaction to these budgetary cuts. For we well remember that during the 1955 budget hearings the Director of the USPHS VD Division, who was requesting funding so as to make further advances, was asked,

TABLE 1. *Federal Appropriations for Venereal Disease Control, 1945–64, and VD Appropriations as a Percent of Total Public Health Service Appropriations*

Fiscal Year	Total V.D. Appropriation	Total Public Health Service Appropriation	% V.D. of Total
1945	$12,339,000	$ 127,725,073	9.66
1946	11,949,000	142,305,380	8.40
1947	16,909,000	103,797,686	16.29
1948	17,324,500	191,283,100	9.06
1949	17,370,000	237,053,500	7.33
1950	16,000,000	320,528,803	4.99
1951	12,863,500	225,069,280	5.72
1952	11,653,360	231,343,508	5.04
1953	9,800,000	221,607,250	4.42
1954	5,000,000	210,619,500	2.37
1955	3,000,000	251,310,000	1.19
1956	3,626,000	391,440,500	.93
1957	4,195,000	534,141,000	.79
1958	4,415,000	565,757,797	.78
1959	5,400,000	758,177,208	.71
1960	5,400,000	840,314,152	.64
1961	5,814,500	1,039,052,837	.56
1962	6,000,000	1,369,656,118	.44
1963	8,000,000	1,581,540,000	.51
1964	9,588,000	1,608,723,000	.59

Sources: V.D. Appropriations obtained from the Venereal Disease Branch, Communicable Disease Center, U.S. Public Health Service. Public Health Service Appropriations obtained from U.S. Public Health Service. Background material concerning the Mission and Organization of the Public Health Service, prepared for the Interstate and Foreign Commerce Committee, House of Representatives, April, 1963. Washington, D.C. Government Printing Office, 1963.

"Doctor, why do you need all this money; haven't you heard that it is now possible to cure syphilis with a single shot of penicillin?" This comment was the result of a report from the Venereal Disease Research Laboratory of the USPHS widely quoted in the press just before the hearings which showed the effectiveness of a single injection with long-acting penicillin. In spite of the subsequent explanations and discussions, Congress took the approach that the total control program was no longer needed. Starting in 1958, the budget cuts were reflected in the rise in rates of reported syphilis resulting from the fact that at state and local levels the VD control programs were forced to curtail the comprehensive approach (Tables 1 and 2).[6]

TABLE 2. *Civilian Case Rates per 100,000 Population for Primary and Secondary Syphilis by Race, United States Summary (known military cases excluded), Fiscal Years 1941–63*

Fiscal Year	Total	White	Non-White
1941	51.7	24.7	287.9
1942	57.0	26.0	325.3
1943	63.8	27.5	373.6
1944	61.6	27.7	348.5
1945	60.5	27.0	340.3
1946	70.9	34.7	376.9
1947	75.6	36.9	404.9
1948	55.9	25.8	308.5
1949	37.1	16.4	211.2
1950	21.6	9.4	123.4
1951	12.1	5.0	70.9
1952	7.9	3.3	45.5
1953	6.2	2.7	35.6
1954	4.9	2.1	28.0
1955	4.1	1.8	22.5
1956	4.1	1.6	25.0
1957	3.8	1.6	21.8
1958	3.9	1.6	22.6
1959	4.7	2.0	26.6
1960	7.1	3.1	38.7
1961	10.4	4.0	60.6
1962	11.0	3.8	66.7
1963	11.9	3.8	73.7

Source: U.S. Public Health Service. V.D. Statistical Letter Supplement: Trends in Morbidity and Epidemiological Activity, December 1963. Table 1b.

Conclusion

The levels of public and professional interest in and support of the VD control activities at all levels of government are mirrored in federal, state, and local budgets, university training and research activities, public attitudes toward VD education and control programs promoting prophylaxis and condom usage. Thus the present public and health-community reaction to AIDS reproduces a pattern which has been well demonstrated in the past: increased federal funding in support of research and treatment, promotion of self-protective sexual behavior and practices such as condom usage and discrimination in patterns of sexual behavior, and the attempt by public health professionals to approach the problem as one of health and related economic costs, rather than to assume a judgmental, moralistic attitude. In light of past experience with syphilis and successes even before the advent of simple penicillin therapy, this approach to AIDS management, if implemented, may be expected to slow the spread of the disease. Eventually, as such an approach is strengthened and modified, as more is learned about cause and therapy, it can be expected to begin to bring the disease under control. We use the word "control" guardedly. For it is to be noted that even with simple curative therapy for syphilis and gonorrhea, the rates have fluctuated greatly, reflecting public attitudes and resultant control program changes. In the light of past experience, "control" not eradication, is the most that can be expected. The public health approach must be modified to integrate new discoveries in diagnosis, treatment, and prophylaxis as they are made, but must once again be developed to deal with the current judgmental and even panic-like reactions of the public and some health professionals to the patient needing care or the individual at risk of infection. In so doing, it must be recognized that involvement of all levels of government, the community at large, and the medical, educational, industrial, and social work sectors is essential for success.

In conclusion, we feel that a quotation from the presentation made by Dr. Raymond A. Vonderlehr, Chief of the VD Division of the USPHS, during a critically important period of progress is highly relevant with respect to AIDS, just as it was with respect to syphilis. At the World Forum of Syphilis and Other Treponamatisos in 1962 he made the following statement:

And, finally, as a senior citizen and one who has spent the great majority of his professional career in this struggle against syphilis, I feel it appropriate that I sound a word of warning. It is a well understood precept in a free society that the price of liberty is eternal vigilance. And, if we in our time are to free this nation of syphilis infection, we must remain ever steadfast in our will and determination to see this current struggle through to a successful conclusion. If we have learned anything from the past, it is the fact that syphilis will not just go away because we would wish it so. We should now be aware and ever remain aware that this highly contagious disease will require our eternal vigilance and vigorous effort when the trend line of syphilis incidence inevitably approaches the end point of eradication. For it will be in this critical period that pressures will develop from many quarters to cease and desist the great impetus that is now being built up. Unless there is raw courage, rare determination, and a united will, the forces of reaction and complacency will gain the upper hand and history will again be repeated. This must not happen in a civilized society. I am firmly convinced that you assembled here, your associates at home and the people everywhere will stand up and be counted to the very end—no matter what the cost nor how great the effort must be—so that this generation can say with justifiable pride, "Syphilis we have no more. . . .

The philosophy expressed by Dr. Vonderlehr is one which can serve as a guide to the public health professions as they move forward to deal with AIDS as well as with the many other sexually transmitted diseases.

REFERENCES

1. Brandt AM: No Magic Bullet: A Social History of VD in the US since 1880. New York: Oxford University Press, 1985.

2. Vonderlehr RA, Heller JR Jr: The Control of Venereal Disease. New York: Reynal & Hitchcock, 1946; 5–8.

3. Williams RC: The United States Public Health Services 1798–1950: Commissioned Officers Association of the USPHS. Bethesda, MD USPHS, 1951; 154–156.

4. Mahoney JF, Arnold RC, Harris A: Penicillin treatment of early syphilis: A preliminary report. Vener Dis Inform 1943; 24:355–357.

5. US Army Medical Dept: Preventive Medicine in World War II, Communicable Diseases. Washington, DC: Office of the Surgeon General, Dept of the Army, 1960; 158.

6. Anderson OW: Syphilis and Society—Problems of Control in the United States 1912–1964. Chicago, IL: Center for Health Administration Studies, Health Information Foundation, Research Series 22, 1965.

THE INFAMOUS TUSKEGEE SYPHILIS STUDY

GEORGE A. SILVER

I read the April 1988 issue of the Journal with interest, finding it informative and useful.

Perhaps a bit discouraging to many of your readers, however, was a bit of evidence of our continued inability to confront our racist past. I have reference to the article by Cutler and Arnold,[1] in which no mention is made of the infamous "Tuskegee Study." That was the "scientifically controlled experiment," from 1932 to 1972, in which hundreds of Black patients from Macon County, Alabama, with syphilis, were carefully observed, but untreated. The object of the experiment was to determine the effect of untreated syphilis on human subjects. The Public Health Service officers as well as the local and state health officials who participated in this noxious "experiment," whose subjects neither knew nor consented to their experimental role, suffered no pangs of conscience. One of the overseers of the project when asked about it said, "There was nothing in the experiment that was unethical or unscientific."[2] However, when the information did appear a few years ago, the topic became a cause célèbre and a book about the matter[2] had wide circulation.

I call attention to the topic at this time without rancor. After all, the behavior of the PHS officers was no more than representative of the sentiments and prejudices of the time. But not to remember is to forget, and to forget is a disservice to those who suffered the indignities. It seems to me, therefore, that in calling upon us to honor one of the participants, we should also mention the context in which the meritorious service was earned.

REFERENCES

1. Cutler JH, Arnold RC: Venereal disease control by health departments in the past: Lessons for the present. Am J. Public Health 1988; 78:372–376.

2. Jones JH: Bad Blood. New York: The Free Press, 1981: 8.

George A. Silver is an emeritus professor of public health, Institution for Social and Policy Studies, at Yale University.

Originally published in the American Journal of Public Health 78 (1988): 1500. Reprinted by permission of the American Public Health Association.

DR. CUTLER'S RESPONSE

JOHN C. CUTLER

I understand and accept Dr. Silver's feelings about the Tuskegee Study. However, there seemed to be no reason to mention this or any other study in our article; all of the studies contributed to the program developments which led to the successes of the national VD control program.

I hope we can apply the knowledge gained from our past errors as well as our past successes. We need to deal with AIDS in the same non-judgmental public health manner that made our past accomplishments in the control of gonorrhea and syphilis possible.

Originally published in the American Journal of Public Health *78 (1988): 1500. Reprinted by permission of the American Public Health Association.*

DEADLY MEDICINE

TOM JUNOD

The infection, if it doesn't destroy you, becomes part of you. The spirals of rot, the tiny worms of decay—if they live inside you long enough, burrow deep enough under your skin, your body accepts them and somehow learns to live with them. That is why, says the Old Doctor, treatment is sometimes worse than the disease. That is why, says the Old Doctor, with his eager, desperate grin, you don't give medicine to men who have endured infection their entire life. They have survived; their disease is dormant. Why would you want to treat them *now*, when they have grown old with the sickness inside them? Why would you want to kill the infection *now* and risk poisoning them with its debris? They have come this far, gone so long—why can't you just leave them alone?

Oh, they are all old or dead now, the doctors and the men they called their patients, whom others called their victims. It's been sixty-one years since they were first joined, in unnatural collaboration, sixty-one years since the United States Public Health Service—the government and its best physicians—commenced what was to become known as the Tuskegee Syphilis Study, or, in popular parlance, the Tuskegee Experiment. The "natural history" of syphilis is what the government doctors sought to chart, the "natural course of the disease," "the eventual outcome of untreated syphilis in the male Negro"—and to that end, they found hundreds of black syphilitics in and around Tuskegee, Alabama, did what they could to prevent them from getting treatment and then watched them die. . . . Watched them die for ten, for twenty, for thirty, for forty years, until 1972, when a reporter finally wrote about the Study and the outcry forced the government to shut it down.

Yes, they are old now, most of the doctors and the men who survive, old enough for their pasts to ring across time and reverberate, in the present, as history. The men? There were 622 of them—431 with syphilis and 191 who served as a basis for comparison—and of these, but 20 still draw breath, octogenarians, nonagenarians, living ghosts, haunted witnesses. The doctors? They are harder to count, because, unlike the men, they were never numbered, never identified in scientific papers as No. 194 or No. 329 or No. 495. Public servants, soldiers in the war on disease, the

Tom Junod is a freelance writer whose articles have appeared in numerous journals and magazines. Originally published in Gentlemen's Quarterly *(1993): 164–71, 231–34. Copyright © 1993 Tom Junod. Reprinted by permission.*

doctors filed in and out of the Tuskegee Study in military procession, following their orders, fulfilling their obligations, executing what someone else had started, always able to move on, move out and deny responsibility for what they left behind: men whose hearts blew up and brains broke down, a residue of distrust and an experiment that would somehow never properly die.

It wasn't *supposed* to die. It was meant to go on, to outlast the doctors who worked on it, to generate data until it calculated some elusive final sum. It wasn't supposed to die, in fact, until the last of the men did. This is how the Tuskegee Study worked: In life the men would be observed, and in death they would be harvested—brought in for autopsy and made to disclose their ultimate secrets. Time was its engine, death its point: hell, it would still be going on, now, today, had it not been forcibly interrupted, and even now, today, one of the doctors laments its end, says that the tragedy of the Tuskegee Study was its premature cessation, because the doctors were *learning* things from it, interesting things, important things. . . .

Continuance, then, was Tuskegee's curse. It wasn't supposed to die, and it has not died in the places where racial memory matters. The transaction between doctor and patient has always depended on trust, and Tuskegee is trust's toxin. There are black children who go unvaccinated because of Tuskegee. There are black men and women who believe that AIDS is the government's genocidal instrument because of Tuskegee. There are black men and women with AIDS who won't take AZT because of Tuskegee. People are *dying* because of Tuskegee. Penicillin killed the old scourge, killed syphilis. It cannot kill the new scourge, however. It cannot kill AIDS, and it cannot kill Tuskegee.

Nothing can. Even the Old Doctor knows that now. He has tried to grin it away, explain it away, push it away with silence and forgetting, yet Tuskegee is always there, waiting for him. Why him? The others have gotten away with it. The other doctors in the procession—they are everywhere, in private practice, academia and business, in Kentucky, Maryland, Massachusetts, New Jersey, Ohio, Pennsylvania, Rhode Island, South Carolina and Texas—they, by and large, have been spared history's judgment. It is a comforting thing for an old man to believe: that what's past is past, that time can settle what human beings cannot. Why did history wait so long to rob Dr. Sidney Olansky of that notion? Such a nice man. Why did he have to learn at 79 years of age that history is not the past—that it is the present and that the present is what kills you in the end?

The Old Doctor is terminal. He will tell you this grimly, unabashedly, without humor or irony, this jaunty little man with the dented nose and the big ears and the white brush-cut hair and the fifty-year-old penchant for bow ties; this peppery fellow whom his nurses pinch on the cheek and call Dr. Sid. "This thing is going to be the death of me," he says. "When I die, my death certificate will say 'KILLED BY

TUSKEGEE STUDY.'" It gnaws at him, he says. It keeps him awake at night. It gives him diarrhea. It is the claw scraping at his stomach, and he does not go five minutes without thinking about it. "It's a hell of a thing," he says.

How do you involve yourself in the thing that will be the death of you? It has to be the life of you first, and for a long time the study of syphilis and the Public Health Service were the life of Sid Olansky. See, his life had been so *good*, so full of struggle and triumph, so full of travel and adventure, so full of love and family, so full of work and—why not say it?—service. It's what he was, it's how he saw himself: as a servant, dispensing his knowledge to the people who needed it. He could have been anything, this son of Russian-Jewish immigrants, who grew up poor in the Roxbury section of Boston. He could have been a baseball player (he was a catcher who hit home runs, and the Red Sox offered him a minor-league contract); for God's sake, he could have been Somerset Maugham's consort, had he been so inclined (Maugham, Olansky says, tried to pick him up when he was a young med student in Europe)—but no, he wanted to be a doctor. There was a war on, and he wanted to serve.

The war against the Nazis was on its way, of course, but this war—this was the war against disease. You had to have come up back then, Dr. Sid says, to know what it was like, the potential, the *promise*, that America and its doctors could beat the ancient plagues, the killers and the cripplers, the age-old pestilences. Even syphilis! The Great Pox. Used to be you couldn't even whisper the word in polite company, but in 1937 Thomas Parran, then the U.S. surgeon general, wrote a book about it, *Shadow on the Land: Syphilis*, which demystified it, broke the silence, made stamping out the epidemic every American's patriotic chore. Why, in a chapter titled "White Man's Burden," Parran even wrote about the damage syphilis was inflicting on "the Negro" in Macon County, Alabama, home of the fabled Tuskegee Institute, where public-health officers found about one syphilitic for every three blacks tested. Fortunately, Parran wrote, there was treatment available, and "the Negro instinctively trusts the white man. . . . He trusts the Government, because . . . he has believed that the Government is a friend of his and tries to help him. 'The government health doctor' therefore has an entrée. . . ."

The government health doctor—that's what Sid Olansky would be. He had been denied a scholarship to Columbia University because he was a Jew; he had gone to medical school in Scotland because he was broke; now he would be one of America's elite. He joined the Public Health Service during World War II, when the PHS was made a part of the military. He was stationed in Panama, treating soldiers, when he received the call to run the Washington, D.C., rapid-treatment clinic for syphilis, because the clientele, he says, was "mostly black, and they had a boy from Mississippi running it, and they were afraid he wouldn't get along too well."

Dr. Sid got along just fine. He made a name for himself in Washington and was asked, in 1950, to run the Venereal Disease Research Lab (VDRL) of the U.S. Public

Health Service. He was 37 years old, with an international reputation in syphilology, and he was working for the country that had developed the A-bomb to beat the Axis and penicillin to beat the Pox. He was a busy man, an important man, and he did not ask whether what the government had bestowed on him was a blessing or a curse.

No, Sidney Olansky loved his new job: the travel, the research, the camaraderie among PHS officers—all of it. He didn't even mind directing a study he inherited—the Tuskegee Syphilis Study. Was he enthusiastic about the study? No, he says now, never—"but to be honest, I wasn't unenthusiastic, either." He had heard of the Tuskegee Study, of course—who hadn't? It had been running for eighteen years and was already, as Olansky was to write later, "one of the longest continued medical surveys ever conducted." It wasn't as if the Study was a secret. Parran had blessed it, and the doctors who worked on it wrote about their findings, such as they were, in journals published by the American Medical Association. The Milbank Memorial Fund, in New York City, knew all about it, too, because in order to keep the subjects in the Study, the PHS had offered them "burial insurance"—$35 for the family, $15 for the undertaker—and the foundation put up the cash every time one of them died. Hell, the doctor who performed the autopsies was from the all-black Tuskegee Institute, and Eunice Rivers, Miss Rivers, the nurse who cared for the men, who tracked them down on the dirt roads of Macon County and rounded them up for examinations, was black herself—how bad could the Study be? Besides, the damned thing was already up and running, and all Sidney Olansky had to do was . . . continue it.

Of course, that's all anybody associated with the Tuskegee Study had to do. That's what it was *about*, almost from the start. Initiated by Drs. Taliaferro Clark and Raymond Vonderlehr of the Public Health Service's Venereal Disease Branch in 1932, the Study was supposed to last six months. It was supposed to demonstrate that syphilis was killing black people and move legislatures to fund testing and treatment. True, it began with a lie—the doctors told the men, who were mostly unschooled sharecroppers, that they would be receiving treatment for "bad blood" and then gave them aspirin and vitamin tonics—but at least the Study had a reason for being. Nearly twenty years later, its only reason for being was the preservation of its own existence.

A study of untreated syphilis? By the mid-1940s, there was a treatment for syphilis. There was a *cure* for syphilis. In the old days, in the Thirties and early Forties, physicians treated syphilis with a kind of chemotherapy, injecting patients with derivatives of arsenic; while the treatment killed the bacteria, it required a year's worth of shots and exacted a hell of a toll on the body. During the war, though, doctors at the VDRL found that two weeks of penicillin essentially cured syphilis, in all its forms. By the time Olansky became the director of the lab, doctors were prescribing penicillin for everything from pneumonia to strep throat, and even Macon County's board of health was sending busloads of syphilitics to Birmingham for the drug. A study of untreated syphilis? The nation was mounting a drive to treat syphilis and eradicate it once and for all. It was becoming increasingly difficult to *find* people with untreated syphilis. The men in the study— they were oddities, throwbacks. Their numbers were dwindling, and their like would never come again. The PHS officers knew this and, beginning as early as 1950, acknowledged in their speeches and correspondence that the Tuskegee Study of Untreated Syphilis in the Male Negro "can never be duplicated since penicillin and other antibiotics are being so widely used." Yes, the Study was one of a kind; a once-in-a-lifetime opportunity, and the PHS had a responsibility, "a high moral obligation," one officer wrote, to "those who served," a responsibility to keep the Study alive even as the men died.

Did Dr. Sid ever question the wisdom, or morality, of withholding penicillin from the men? No. Nobody did. "It was a study of *un*treated syphilis," says Dr. John Cutler, who helped run the Study from the PHS's Washington headquarters in the 1950s. That was the answer; there was no need to ask questions. It was a study of untreated syphilis, and it was, says Olansky, "part of my job, so I did it." Most of the men, 70 percent or 80 percent, would do all right without penicillin . . . and the ones who wouldn't—well, they wouldn't, that's all, and you can never know if penicillin would have helped them anyway, because they had *late* syphilis, and, in Olansky's words, "the damage had been done." The Study had other problems— scientific problems, administrative problems—and *those* Dr. Sid was prepared, was qualified, to solve. He bumped up the burial insurance to $100; he tried to figure a way to make the men sit for spinal taps, as they had when the Study first started. Twice—and only twice, he will say, he will insist—he visited Tuskegee to help draw blood from the men, to participate in what he calls "the bloodlettings." He remembers the "picnic-like atmosphere," the men singing songs, the lack of hostility, the kindness. He remembers the weather, the beautiful clear skies. He remembers the poverty. He does not remember much else.

Olansky left the PHS in 1955 and promptly forgot about Tuskegee. Oh, sure, once, right after he'd quit the lab, he mentioned the Study in a speech at the University of Virginia, and a young doctor named Count Gibson wrote to him, saying the Study "cannot be justified on the basis of any accepted moral standard: pagan . . . religious . . . or professional." Olansky wrote him back, immediately, that when he first became involved in the Tuskegee Study, "all the things that bothered you bothered me at that time. After seeing these people, knowing them & studying them & the record, I honestly feel that we have done them no real harm & probably have helped them in many ways." And that was the last Dr. Sid had to think about it—for years. He went from the PHS to Duke University, and from Duke to Emory University, in Atlanta, where he settled. In 1969, the Centers for Disease Control, which by that time was running the Study, convened what it called a "blue-ribbon committee" to decide whether the Study should continue. Seemed there was a problem: a field-worker in the San Francisco office, a young bearded chap, comparing the Study to something cooked up by the Nazis. Well, the CDC needed to hear an authoritative voice on the subject, so it turned to Dr. Sid. The committee met on February 6, and of the seventeen people in the room, only one doctor recommended that the men receive treatment. It was not Dr. Sid. Dr. Sid was, as ever, stalwart; even with all its flaws, Tuskegee was, he said, "a good study." Dr. Sid insisted that there were no medical grounds for treating the men, that for the most part their syphilis was inactive and that giving them penicillin could incur "catastrophic consequences." The Study, of course, would go on.

Three more years. The young bearded chap from San Francisco, Peter Buxtun, finally found a way to make himself heard: In 1972, he talked to an Associated Press reporter about Tuskegee, and the reporter launched the Study into history. One year later, Fred Gray, an attorney from Tuskegee, sued on behalf of the men and their heirs. Calling the Study "a program of controlled genocide," Gray sued the United States of America and the Milbank Memorial Fund and Caspar Weinberger (then secretary of the Department of Health, Education and Welfare) and a host of other officials and—as one of the only two Tuskegee Study doctors mentioned by name—Sidney Olansky. "A million and a half bucks I didn't have"—that's what Olansky was being sued for, all because his name appeared on more research papers than any other name did, and because he happened to be alive. He was lucky, though: He "escaped." The government settled, disbursing a total of $9 million to a class of several hundred claimants—and not only did Olansky not have to pay a dime, he didn't have to think about Tuskegee anymore.

Farrakhan—he's the one who brought it all back, in Dr. Sid's opinion. The Honorable Louis Farrakhan of the Nation of Islam. Nearly twenty years after the damned thing had died, eighteen years after Olansky had put it out of his mind, Farrakhan was on TV, rabble-rousing, linking Tuskegee to AIDS, citing Tuskegee as proof of the white man's genocidal intentions. Some black activists were even saying that Olansky and his cohorts *gave* the men syphilis. . . . Well, such a charge, it was irresponsible. "We didn't give them anything," Dr. Sid would say. "They earned it, I assure you." In fact, when the producers of ABC's *PrimeTime Live* asked him to appear on their show, he was pleased because he thought he would have a chance to "set the record straight" and silence the ghosts of Tuskegee once and for all. His four children—and especially his sons, David and Alan, with whom he shares a dermatology practice—*begged* him not to get in front of the camera, but Dr. Sid has always, in the words of his son Alan, relied on his greatest gift, the "gift of instantaneous rapport." People respond to him and the smile that flares constantly across his face. He would smile on TV. He couldn't help it—smiling is what Dr. Sid calls his "nervous mannerism." But, according to David, "he honestly thought that if he could sit down with people, he could convince them that he would never hurt anyone."

On February 6, 1992, Sidney Olansky got his chance. On February 6, 1992—twenty-three years to the day after he sat down with the CDC's blue-ribbon committee—Dr. Sid got a chance to sit down with 10 million people across the United States of America.

Alicia Newton played the tape and heard a woman gasping in the crowd. The man on the screen—the Old Doctor, with the white hair and the white lab coat and the bow tie—was *smiling*, and from the audience there came this sound of alarm, this exhalation of horror. This wasn't the first time Alicia had played the tape of *PrimeTime Live*. She had, in fact, made it her mission to play the tape for as many black audiences as she could, to talk about it on the radio, to bring it before the students at Atlanta's Morehouse University. God, she could remember the first time she'd seen it and realized that the Old Doctor lived and worked in Atlanta. Alicia was "in shock," watching this "animal," this "Mengele," *grinning* as he defended the Tuskegee Study, as he said "Syphilis was not such a bad disease," as he called the men "a pack of sheep." But her shock was nothing compared with that of the woman who ran up to her on this night at the end of the tape, "*shaking*, she was so devastated," and said "Sidney Olansky is my dermatologist!"

Why didn't she know? That's what the woman, Anisa—she doesn't want her last name used—couldn't understand. She had gone to Princeton, she subscribed to eighteen magazines, she'd read about Tuskegee years ago. . . . How could she not have known about Dr. Sid? Why did Anisa have to hear about her dermatologist's past from Alicia Newton at Africa House, a place for Afrocentric education? Why hadn't she heard about Dr. Sid from her endocrinologist, the man who'd recommended the Olanskys in the first place? He knew about Sidney Olansky, she thought, he *had* to have known.

It was a betrayal. What else could she call it? Anisa is a woman of color. Anisa—along with Alicia Newton—counts herself among the 35 percent of the African-American population that, according to Dr. Stephen Thomas, believes that AIDS is the result of a genocidal conspiracy and, to a lesser extent, that Tuskegee was the conspiracy's trial horse, its statement of purpose. Thomas, a professor at the University of Maryland, has traveled from city to city, church to church, housing project to housing project, to educate black people about AIDS. He has polled 6,000 black Americans and has found that the conspiracy theory "has taken on a life of its own as a disaster myth that helps people cope with a calamity that has befallen them." Not everyone he polls knows about Tuskegee, at least not by name; "they just know something terrible happened way back when."

Oh, but Anisa knew Tuskegee by name, and she believed that it was a "template" for what is happening now with AIDS, for the dissemination of an engineered virus—a man-made, gene-spliced technological marvel—into populations that threaten the perpetuation of the white race: homosexuals and people of color. Of course she knew about Tuskegee! As a black woman, she has made herself vigilant about medical issues because that's what black women have to be, to protect themselves and their families—vigilant and knowledgeable when they deal with white doctors. Her vigilance is what got her involved with the Olanskys. She needed a good pediatrician, and her endocrinologist recommended Marion Olansky, who turned out to be "one of the best physicians I ever had," says Anisa. Such a nice woman, such a *good* woman and "such a caring physician." When Anisa had a skin problem, she didn't hesitate to visit Marion's husband, and when Dr. Sid was busy, she didn't hesitate to visit his son David. She felt she could *trust* them. That's why, when she found out that Dr. Sid had been involved in the Tuskegee Experiment, she was "stunned, absolutely stunned." The Olanskys were good people, she says—how could the family countenance a "Josef Mengele" in their midst? And how could she trust another doctor when the best she'd ever had was married to the man who spoke of Tuskegee with a smile?

Josef Mengele? A Nazi? Sid Olansky was a Jew. How could he be a Nazi? Nazis pulled people out of their home and burned them to ash. All Dr. Sid did was his job. An animal? A criminal? No, Dr. Sid would say, here's what he was: a chump, a fall guy. His family told him not to go on TV; he didn't listen. He thought he could make people understand. Schmuck! Here he was, 78 years old, working in the same office with his sons, relaxed and happy—all he had to do was keep his mouth shut and he would have been free to grow old and die with his past still his prisoner. Instead, he received bomb threats, death threats. Instead, he had to change the route he drove to work so he could avoid black neighborhoods. Instead, Alicia Newton distributed fliers in the lobby of his office building, urging people to "Stop Olansky." Well, he didn't care about her, and he didn't care about Farrakhan anymore, either. He didn't care about anyone but his family. Everyone else—they were using him, for politics, for propaganda. Even the dermatology department at Emory University, the department *he'd* started, the department *he'd* built from nothing, wanted to take his name off the Sidney Olansky Dermatology Library.

They met last November, at Olansky's request—Dr. Sid, his sons and the faculty and residents of the dermatology department. Twenty years at Emory, and suddenly they wanted to wipe his name off the walls, erase the syllables by which he hoped to be remembered, as they would some scrawled obscenity, unless he could recant on the matter of Tuskegee, like a heretic before the fire. But he had staked his life in defense of Tuskegee, and it was this, his life, that he offered up for inspection by the bright young men and women of the department. His life, his career: How could they judge him by something that had occupied so little of his time so long ago?

They could. They had to. They had done their homework, the bright young men and women. They had examined the documents, read the books, summoned an ethicist and a theologian to help guide their inquiry. All they wanted now was for him to acknowledge, to understand, that the Tuskegee Study was unethical. But no. Dr. Sid acknowledged no such thing, and indeed, in the words of department chairman Dr. Thomas Lawley, he seemed to have trouble "grasping certain issues." A nice man and a hell of a physician: The faculty and residents had to grant that to Sid Olansky. But when the meeting was over, they were still stumped by the question they had asked the ethicist and the theologian to help them answer: If a man is involved in a historical evil, is he then, by necessity, an evil man?

"Don't forget, they listen to their granddaddies," Thomas Parran wrote in *Shadow on the Land* as advice to those who would seek to test and treat blacks for syphilis. He was right, of course. The way Sandra McDonald grew up, what her grandfather and grandmother told her was important. It settled deep in her memory, as a connection to what she calls the "collective memory" of her race. What her grandfather and grandmother told her was this: Don't ever let a doctor do an experiment on you.

Sandra often recalls those words, for she now stands at the center of an epidemic, where access to medical experiments is often necessary for survival. She runs Outreach, Inc., an organization that—mouth to mouth, door to door—is dedicated to telling Atlanta's black population one thing about AIDS: that it is killing them. She is a stocky woman with preternatural energy, and when people challenge her with their suspicion that AIDS is a genocidal conspiracy, she likes to respond "When your house is on fire, what are you gonna do? You gonna sit in that house and say 'Oh, white people don't like me, they set my house on fire'? Or are you gonna get out of that house and save yourself? Well, baby, our house is on *fire*."

Sandra can talk, all right. She knows, however, that her voice all alone cannot allay the suspicions of the people who come to Outreach, because there is another voice guiding them, the voice of *their* parents and grandparents and great-grandparents. Hell, the voices of millions of parents and grandparents and great-grandparents, the span of generations, the sum of their wisdom and pain, are all distilled into the one bitter counsel Sandra calls her "soul voice": the intuition that you get as a black person, the gooseflesh that rises on your arms when you know something's *not right*. See, the center of the epidemic is not the center of America; the center of the epidemic is the margin of America. The center—and the future—of the epidemic has wound up at places like Outreach, and the soul voice has lifted itself up in full alarm.

You want to see the margin of America? Come to the HIV-positive support group at Outreach's bleak storefront on the south side of Atlanta, off a road very few white people have cause to travel. There are twenty-eight people in the room, sitting on steel folding chairs around tables with torn contact-paper tops. There are steel racks filled with pamphlets, and inspirational messages on the walls. The walls are beige, and the carpet has been trod into a color beyond naming. Twenty-seven of the twenty-eight are black. There are flamboyant queens, burly trans-vestites, ex-cons, ex-junkies, ex-athletes, fathers holding down jobs, mothers hold-ing children, HIV-positive mothers with HIV-positive babies. The ones who have developed AIDS from their infection have whittled faces and eyes hungry for hope. The whole group applauds any hint of good news or even any expression of resolve. They are determined to live, doomed to die.

On this day, they are talking about research studies and experimental drugs. Sandra steps in front of them and asks "How many of you know about something called the Tuskegee Experiment? Raise your hands if you know."

About a third of the group raises their hand.

"Isn't that when they gave syphilis to those men?" someone asks.

"I won't even drive *through* Tuskegee," a man named Jimmy says.

"Okay," Sandra says, "how many of you think that AIDS is genocide? Raise your hands."

There issues from the group a low buzz, along with a reflex-quick assemblage of hands raised straight and tall. In all, about two thirds of the group believes that AIDS is genocide.

"Okay, now, how many of you grew up with your grandparents or parents or your aunt or somebody telling you not to let anybody experiment on you?"

Twenty-seven hands reach for the ceiling.

"See?" Sandra says. "You might not know Tuskegee, but in the back of your mind, that's that soul voice talking to you."

It is the soul voice that speaks in the margin of America, the center of the epidemic. In Atlanta, 80 percent of the black women who should have been taking AZT and other anti-retroviral drugs weren't doing it, according to a survey con-ducted by the AIDS Research Consortium of Atlanta in 1990, and as a result, they were dying. "It wasn't a matter of them not being offered the drug," says Terri Creagh of ARCA. "It was a matter of them refusing it" because they thought it was "poison" or because they distrusted the medical Establishment or because they were estranged from the very idea of seeking care for themselves.

In Baltimore, doctors at Johns Hopkins University Hospital have told Creagh that people in the surrounding neighborhoods "believe that the doctors will come and snatch their children and experiment on them."

In Washington, D.C., and the black communities of Maryland, where Stephen Thomas does a great deal of his work, "if an AIDS vaccine came out tomorrow," Thomas says, "a significant number of blacks would not [take] it."

In New York City, Dr. Lawrence Brown, an attending physician at Harlem Hospital, a professor at Columbia and the head of medical services at a large drug-treatment program headquartered in Brooklyn, says that Tuskegee "comes up 25 percent to 33 percent of the time when you ask a patient why [he] won't participate in research."

And in Atlanta, Anisa, the patient of Marion Olansky, will not allow her children to be vaccinated. Not for measles. Not for mumps, not for the flu or meningitis. Not even for tetanus.

The soul voice.

"If I'm gonna die of HIV, I'm gonna die of HIV," says a young woman, the mother of HIV-positive twins, at the Outreach meeting. "I'm not gonna let anyone practice on me."

God knows, the soul voice has heard of more than Tuskegee. God knows, the soul voice has heard of doctors who practiced their craft on the poor . . . doctors not from the Tuskegee Study but from the Tuskegee generation. In 1972, when the Tuskegee Study came to its end, it was a defining moment in the history of medicine; the world was cleaved, and the past fell away from the present. It was not until Tuskegee died that modern standards of informed consent came to live; it was not until Tuskegee died that an *apparatus*, fixed and permanent, was established to protect the rights of patients involved in human experimentation.

The doctors of the Tuskegee generation did not have to contend with that apparatus, and consequently the doctors of the Tuskegee Study did not have to write their protocol on paper or subject it to civilian scrutiny. There was no such thing as civilian scrutiny; physicians regulated themselves, answering only to one another. They heeded the call of the many by sacrificing the few, and the charity ward, the prison and the military became the proving grounds of modern medicine.

"Poor people, and especially poor black people, are the basis upon which our present-day clinical medicine is built," says Count Gibson, the physician from the University of Virginia who challenged the morality of Tuskegee in his 1955 letter. Gibson is a professor emeritus at Stanford University now; he is of the Tuskegee generation, and he remembers his days as a resident, when poor patients sometimes checked into the hospital and, if they were "interesting" cases, checked out only after doctors had researched whatever had caught their interest. "It salves the conscience of the medical Establishment to dump on Sidney Olansky," Gibson says. "But he was part of the mood and ethos of the land. Those that were being sacrificed . . . let's say that none of them were members of the Century Club. There was a feeling that people in ward services in a general hospital owed something back to medicine and to society to balance, quote-unquote, what we were doing for them."

Yes, that's what the men of the Tuskegee Study were: frontline fodder in society's war against disease, "volunteers with social incentives." That's how they were characterized in the research papers of the Olansky era, and that's how Dr. John

Cutler, professor emeritus at the University of Pittsburgh, characterizes them today: "They served their race very well," he says. Cutler is a tall, tweedy, genteel man, with pinkish skin and white hair and unkempt white eyebrows that shift like clouds over his pale-blue eyes. He regrets both what he regards as the premature close of the Tuskegee Study and the restrictions on human experimentation that it engendered. Yes, he has done research on prisoners, in an influential study of syphilis conducted at Sing-Sing in the 1950s: "It gave them a sense of value for once, that they were contributing something to society." Yes, he has compared the men in the Tuskegee Study to soldiers: "If I may make an analogy," he once told a newspaper reporter, "it's like sending men off to war and knowing some will die. It's in the interest of the total society." And no, he does not regret his involvement in the Study, not at all: "You had to make those value judgments, you had to pick your patients when you were carrying out a study. . . . We had the responsibility, the job had to be done, and we did it. . . . [The men] were given tender loving care by Nurse Rivers. And when they died, they were given a dignified burial."

Don't ever let a doctor do an experiment on you.
Out of the past and into the future, the soul voice has been speaking all night long. It speaks, among the twenty-eight at Outreach, when a young woman says that when she goes to the local public hospital, where the doctors are often medical students, she doesn't know whether she's being helped or studied. It speaks again when a man in a red hat and red sweats and red sneakers stands up and testifies about why he, in contrast, volunteers for research studies: "I didn't get into the studies for me. I got into the studies for the person behind me. I'm alive 'cause somebody did it for *me*—a real good brother who didn't even know me. And I'm gonna let them experiment with *me* because *he* thought enough of someone he hadn't seen to let them experiment with *him*. 'Cause we're in a battle, y'all. I know for a fact that I'm living on the prayers of someone else. I'm living off the experiments of long ago."
There's one thing the soul voice doesn't know, however, and when the meeting ends and the hands reach for chips and cups of coffee, a man in women's clothes and another in an *X* hat and warm-ups approach a white man who came that night to Outreach. The experience that they spoke of tonight—hasn't that been his experience, too? His parents and grandparents—didn't they tell him not to let anyone experiment on him? They ask these questions, and their eyes, hungry for hope, appear surprised and hurt when he replies that no, that has not been his experience at all.

It's because they were doctors. They took his name off the library, and that shook up Sid Olansky, because he respected them. If they had been civilians, he could have spat in contempt and said they were all just ignorant, and if they were reporters, he could have said, as he still said of the *PrimeTime Live* people a year after their Tuskegee broadcast, that "they were out to deliberately destroy me."

But they were doctors, and because of that Sid Olansky had to listen to them, had to wonder if maybe he were not missing something after all, and one night he sat and watched "Deadly Deception," an investigation of Tuskegee on PBS's *Nova*.

Oh, it was biased, to a degree—they all are. How could it not be, with a title like that? But, well, he had never actually bothered to learn much about Tuskegee. He had never read *Bad Blood*, James Jones's meticulously documented book on the subject, and he had never given much credence to the newspaper and magazine articles that often drew from Jones's research. It was all propaganda, he said, and everyone told him not to trouble himself. So he was shocked, he says, shocked and embarrassed, when he watched *Nova* and heard one of the men from Tuskegee, Herman Shaw, reading from something even Dr. Sid had to admit was hard proof that the old black man had been deceived.

What Herman Shaw read was a letter he had received in 1932, on stationery that bore the name of the Macon County Health Department and the inscription "ALABAMA STATE BOARD OF HEALTH AND U.S. PUBLIC HEALTH SERVICE COOPERATING WITH TUSKEGEE INSTITUTE":

> *Dear Sir:*
> *Some time ago you were given a thorough examination and since that time you have gotten a great deal of treatment for bad blood. You will now be given your last chance to get a second examination. This examination is a very special one and after it is finished you will be given a special treatment if it is believed you are in a condition to stand it.*

The "special treatment" was a spinal tap, an often-excruciating diagnostic procedure with no therapeutic application. The letter ended "REMEMBER THIS IS YOUR LAST CHANCE FOR SPECIAL FREE TREATMENT."

So they had been deceived—duped. Not just Herman Shaw but Dr. Sid, too! "Volunteers with social incentives": That's what he had called the men. Well, he was wrong, and he had to live with his error. Twenty years of his life defending a lie. Twenty years of his life defending something his son Alan now conceded was a historical evil. "Tuskegee's not as bad as the Nazis," Alan said after watching *Nova*. "It's almost as bad. It goes against every tenet of medicine."

What could Dr. Sid say? Nothing. For three days he was nearly silent around the office, speaking only to his patients. And after the three days were up, Emory's Thomas Lawley received a letter. The letter stated that the Olansky's "finally realized that the patients in the study were deliberately and systematically deceived and that the study was designed, promoted and initially run by a racist." That this "all was a revelation to Sid." That Sid now "admits that he made a mistake in not believing that the patients should have been given penicillin," a "feeling based on the belief that the penicillin would not help them physically." That "we all feel horrible about this and wish it could be undone."

The letter was signed by Alan Olansky, M.D.

The old man was a giant. He was tall and quiet and gentle, and he worked all day in the sun under a big hat and his garden was always green. The children who passed his house on their way to school looked upon him with awe and wonder, as they would upon some blessed hermit, for they knew that God had lavished gifts upon him. How else could Mr. Shaw's collards always grow so big and pretty if he didn't have the help of God? How else could such an old man stand so straight and work so long if God were not lifting him up? How else could he cheat the sun and conjure the rain if he were not one of the chosen few? "I swear, you'd be coming down the road in the summertime, and it would be all hot and dry, and all of a sudden the road would be wet, like it had just rained or something, and then it would be dry again, and you'd be, like, 'Whoa, that was Mr. *Shaw's* house,' " says Greg Potts, one of those awestruck children, now a security guard at the V.A. hospital in Tuskegee. "Like—I don't know—it only rained on *his* house or something."

The children could not know that Mr. Shaw had been chosen for something else, by men in distant cities, men whose ultimate purpose would remain as elusive as any design of the Deity. Mr. Shaw and the others, they did not know about the Study, of course; they did not know about syphilis. It was, in rural Alabama, a sign of sin, a word swallowed by silence. Even today, even after all that has happened, silence is what blooms in Tuskegee, blooms and covers and abides. The doctors came here long ago, with silence as their method; they didn't tell the men about their syphilis, and the men, very often, went to their grave without knowing, without telling their children. It is hard to meet a person in Tuskegee who did not have some acquaintance, by friendship or lineage or simple proximity, with one of the men involved in the Study.

"You know your ancestors were slaves," says Cecilia White, whose great-great-grandfather and great-uncle went in the Study. "You know this. You know that black women nursed white babies. You know *that*. But it hurts to know that my great-great-grandfather was experimented on like a dog, like an animal, like a guinea pig, like some *thing* at the vet school. It's . . . degrading."

In 1972, when news of the Study broke, Greg Potts heard that Herman Shaw had been one of the men. "I was, like, 'Mr. Shaw? Our Mr. Shaw? They did that, to *that* man?' Then no one is safe; they can do it to anyone. Then you say to yourself, Wait a second, *that's* why it rained on his garden and no one else's. He has been called to do this. It was like God said to those doctors 'You can do what you want, he's my chosen one and you can't hurt him. He's going to outlive you all, and he will be my witness, and that's why his garden grows so green.' "

The way syphilis kills you, it destroys in silence. In its primary stage, it appears as a sore, a chancre; in its secondary stage, when it is spreading to the rest of your body, it usually appears as a rash; in its latent stage, it disappears from sight, and if you are lucky, if you are in the majority, if your body develops an immunity to the bacteria, it never returns. If you are unlucky, however, the bacteria hide in your bones or your skin or your heart or your brain and eat you alive. You cannot do much about it by the time syphilis shows itself to you for the third time, for by then it already may have ruined your joints, ulcerated your skin, blinded your eyes, pitted your heart or softened your brain. By then, as Sidney Olansky has often said, "the damage has been done."

How much damage has been done by the Tuskegee Study? The CDC's official verdict was that between 28 and 100 of the 431 syphilitic men died as a result of their untreated disease. The life expectancy of all 431 of the men was reduced by 20 percent, and they were subject to a host of other ills—what the doctors called "increased morbidity." Most of those who died suffered from cardiovascular syphilis; the infection scarred and weakened the aorta, which would sometimes leak and deplete the men slowly, or else develop aneurysms and blow out in an instant. Some men wound up in insane asylums. Although it is not clear that penicillin was developed in time to save them, as late as 1968 some were showing signs of neurosyphilis, and such complications probably could have been averted had someone in the late Forties or early Fifties given them penicillin. In all, the majority of the men were essentially unscathed by their syphilis and died the way most people die: cancer, car accidents, clogged arteries, old age. Such a result is no credit to the Tuskegee Study, of course; the men were simply fortunate that the disease was more merciful than the doctors.

And the doctors? Dr. Sid? How much has the Study damaged him? Like syphilis, like sin, history can bide its time before it presents you with its complications, can trap you with peace before it forces you into penance. Has the damage been done, in the heart of Dr. Sid, or has the germ of his past expressed itself in time for treatment? Tuskegee's most prominent defender for twenty years, he is, at this late date, the only one of the doctors to have offered any sort of public recantation. "I'm sorry I was involved in it," he says, "even though I didn't start it and I didn't finish it. I'm terribly sorry. I wish it had never started. It didn't accomplish any of the things I wanted it to or thought it might. Sure I'm sorry. It has cost me a great deal."

He wants to put it behind him now; he has apologized, and he has explained his participation in the Study by saying that he did not know the men had been deceived. It is a plausible explanation, his son Alan says, reasonable . . . and yet there is evidence that he *had* to have known of the deception, just had to, in a 1952 letter that informed Dr. Olansky that it would be hard to persuade the men to sit for spinal taps, because they remembered the "special gold needle treatment with considerable awe and dread" from the first time. Does Dr. Sid remember those words? "Well, I realized they used some kind of deception, but I was not aware of the fact they lied to them—that's my point. . . ."

Spare him. Spare the Old Doctor the dissembling, the feeble excuses. He has made it clear that he was just doing his job, and if history has made *anything* clear, it's that others would have done the same. Indeed, in the matter of Tuskegee, others did do the same, and worse. The curse of Tuskegee was not that it was hard to do or required of its participants some sort of extraordinary conviction; the curse of Tuskegee was that it was easy. Because all the men had to do was die. And all the doctors had to do was let them.

ix

Imagining the Tuskegee Syphilis Study

SELECTIONS FROM *MISS EVERS' BOYS*

DAVID FELDSHUH

ACT ONE

Scene 4

1932. Outside the Possom Hollow Schoolhouse. Six months later. Celebration. The men are massaging each other's backs with mercury. Evers guides them. The Victrola is playing. Douglas watches.

DOUGLAS. What's going on?

EVERS. Treatment. Mercury treatment. "Miss Evers' Style." *(To the men.)* Rub hard now. The Macon County Victrola Gillie Competition champions got to work. Squeeze that mercury into those muscles 'til they yell—

MEN. *(All together, enjoying themselves, a shout.)* "Please!"

EVERS. *(Miss Evers passes out more salve.)* Here you are now. Willie, go crank up that champion Victrola.

WILLIE. Yes, ma'am. I just love the feeling of being able to hear music just by moving a needle. *(He turns the handle on the Victrola.)* And thanks for the new record, Dr. Douglas.

DOUGLAS. How'd you break the Charleston Rag record?

WILLIE. We didn't break it. *(Enjoying himself.)* We wore it out. *(Music starts; Willie looks at Douglas.)*

DOUGLAS. *(Guessing, to Willie.)* The Red Onion Jazz Babies?

WILLIE. Yes, sir. That's it. This man is right on the money.

HODMAN. *(Interrupting, to Ben.)* Why do I always get stuck with you? I got obligations, you know. Rub harder. Ouch.

BEN. That hard enough?

HODMAN. Hey, don't shred me.

EVERS. *(Enjoying herself.)* Lord, oh lord. You men are feeling frisky.

HODMAN. Hot blood. *(The others agree.)*

BEN. *(Delighted.)* That's it.

Dr. David Feldshuh is an emergency-room physician, playwright, and director of the Cornell Theatre Arts Program, Cornell University.

Originally published as David Feldshuh, Miss Evers' Boys *(New York: Dramatist's Play, 1995), Act 1, Scenes 5, 6; Act 2, Scenes 1, 2, 7; Epilogue; pp. 39–54, 63–71, 87–89, 93–98. Reprinted by permission of David Feldshuh.*

EVERS. *(Enjoying herself; the men respond with ad libs to her observations.)* And you look good. Just like you should. Every one of you. You look healthy. *(Sharp silence and freeze. Tableau. Music out. Light up on Evers. Downlight on the men. Evers looks at them for a moment and then speaks to the audience, as testimony.)* Those first six months . . . those men were winning every which way. Until the government pulled the string and the bottom fell out. *(Set change. The men exit. Dr. Brodus enters. Douglas crosses to Brodus' office as the set changes around him and the dialogue continues. Evers follows him.)*

Scene 5
1932. Memorial Hospital. The office of Dr. Eugene Brodus. Evers waits, listening. Two weeks later.

DOUGLAS. *(As if continuing an argument.)* There's no more money. It's as simple as that.

BRODUS. And if it were Manhattan and not Macon.

DOUGLAS. Dr. Brodus, I'm just telling you what I've been told to tell you. Washington tells me. I tell you. I'm as disappointed and frustrated as you are. I've given six months to this treatment program.

BRODUS. Yes, you have. *(Polite but cool.)* Thank you.

DOUGLAS. *(Stung.)* I'm just reminding you whose side I'm on.

BRODUS. *(Even more polite.)* Thank you, then. For reminding me.

DOUGLAS. Thousands of patients. Each patient requiring forty injections over two years. . . . *(Calming himself.)* Dr. Brodus, it's simply too much disease for the budget.

BRODUS. Those patients need that treatment.

DOUGLAS. Yes, sir, they do. Of course, they do. . . . And no one is going to get it for them, if we don't.

BRODUS. We.

DOUGLAS. Yes, sir. We. You and I and Nurse Evers and every person working on this project, and all those patients, all of us; we're all hanging onto Washington's attention by a single thread.

BRODUS. And that thread is. . . ?

DOUGLAS. A suggestion. Just a suggestion. A temporary solution. A way to keep Washington's attention. A way to salvage this situation until Washington appropriates more funds.

BRODUS. To continue treatment?

DOUGLAS. Yes, sir. To continue treatment for those men. *(Sincere, dedicated.)* I believe that what we have here, in Macon County, is an extraordinary opportunity to catalogue the effects of untreated syphilis in the Negro.

BRODUS. Untreated syphilis?

DOUGLAS. We have a perfect laboratory here: a fixed population, virtually untreated disease. A study could be created and carried out with minimal expense. And it would be the most important study of its kind ever conducted. More important than the Oslo research because we'd be dealing with living patients not paper records.

EVERS. Oslo?

DOUGLAS. Nurse Evers, in Oslo, Norway, they studied the autopsy records of three hundred Caucasian patients who had died from untreated syphilis. To see what the disease had done to them. They studied the Caucasian. I believe the Negro should have a chance to be studied too. . . . That's my suggestion.

EVERS. Those patients need medicine.

DOUGLAS. And we are the only people who can get it for them. But we've got only one thing on our side, Nurse Evers: the disease itself. We follow these patients for six months. We catalogue what this disease untreated does to them. And then we let the facts speak for themselves. The Public Health Service could use those facts to educate, to motivate, to create new priorities. New money. For treatment. Not just for our patients but for every syphilitic in the country. A revolution in health care. *(Dedicated.)* And, Dr. Brodus, our research could prove conclusively if the disease differentiates along racial lines.

BRODUS. What if it proves that Negro and Caucasian are equal? That the disease affects both races in exactly the same way? How would Washington feel about that suggestion?

DOUGLAS. *(Matching him.)* Dr. Brodus, it doesn't matter how they'd feel, does it? If that data came from the best damned study ever done.

BRODUS. *(Considering as he works on a tabulation.)* The high and mighty Dame Syphilis: the Italians called it the "French disease," the French called it the "Neapolitan disease," the Russians called it the "Polish disease." Do you know what they're all calling it now, up there in Washington?

DOUGLAS. No, sir.

BRODUS. Come now, Dr. Douglas, what are they all calling it now?

DOUGLAS. *(Trapped.)* "The Negro disease."

BRODUS. That's right. That's what they're calling it. But that's not what I call it. I call it, "God's disease." God has given it to man. To all men. Equal . . .

DOUGLAS. Yes, sir, I agree. Yes, sir. Yes. And we could prove that. Once and for all we could prove that what the disease does, it does to all of us, colored and white.

BRODUS. You know what else they say up there, in Washington?

DOUGLAS. No, sir.

BRODUS. *(A hint and a challenge.)* "Money," Dr. Douglas, "money."

DOUGLAS. *(Facing the challenge.)* "Don't throw white money—

BRODUS. *(Finishing it for him.)* —after a colored man's disease."

DOUGLAS. *(An admission and a challenge.)* That's right. That's what else they're saying. . . . Now are we going to let that kind of talk stand, Dr. Brodus, or are we going to fight it?

BRODUS. *(After a moment.)* What would your role be, Dr. Douglas?

DOUGLAS. I'd coordinate all the data and come down periodically for examinations. Liaison between Washington and Macon.

BRODUS. Physician and scientist.

DOUGLAS. Yes.

BRODUS. That can be a uneasy combination.

DOUGLAS. Isn't that how you see yourself?

BRODUS. I'm a skeptic, Dr. Douglas. I'm the Voltaire of pelvic literature.

DOUGLAS. You have some doubts?

BRODUS. Yes, I do. Always. . . . Would Washington match Oslo?

DOUGLAS. I've already spoken with them. . . . Washington needs your help, Dr. Brodus.

BRODUS. I see. . . .*(A change.)* The Negro man must be studied in exactly the same way they study the white. Periodic examinations—

DOUGLAS. Yes, sir.

BRODUS. X-rays?

DOUGLAS. Of course, yes. And blood work.

BRODUS. And spinal taps. Just like Oslo?

DOUGLAS. *(Dealing.)* Just like Oslo. Dr. Brodus, every patient in our study would have a spinal tap to test for neurologic syphilis. Equal.

BRODUS. *(Considering.)* Six months?

DOUGLAS. A year. Two years at the most. Just until we can force more money to continue treatment.

BRODUS. *(Not a question.)* Two years at the most.

DOUGLAS. Just until we get that money for treatment.

BRODUS. *(Considering.)* What was the title of the article reporting the Oslo research?

DOUGLAS. *(Rapidly.)* "*Uber das Schicksal der nicht spezifisch behandelten Luetiker.*"

BRODUS. "The Fate of Syphilitics Who Are Not Given Specific Treatment." That's an unwieldy title.

DOUGLAS. *(Having thought about it previously.)* "A Study of Untreated Syphilis in the Negro Male." That title's clear, uncluttered and to the point.

BRODUS. "The Tuskegee Study of Untreated Syphilis in the Negro Male"? I want "Tuskegee" in there.

DOUGLAS. *(A guarantee.)* That's what it will be called. The Tuskegee Study. . . . We'll need new blood work—

EVERS. *(Interrupting, unable to remain silent; quietly trying to separate Brodus from Douglas.*) Dr. Brodus, I promised the men treatment. Now we just going to let 'em go? Just leave 'em with nothing?

BRODUS. *(To quiet her.)* It's not nothing.

EVERS. *(Half to herself.)* It sounds like nothing to me.

DOUGLAS. *(Continuing.)* Nurse Evers, we'll need baseline blood work first. Then the spinal taps.

EVERS. The patients don't know what a spinal tap is, Dr. Douglas. And when they find out it's not treatment, they won't come.

DOUGLAS. Then they can't find out.

EVERS. You explain it to them. That it's for their own best good. Maybe then they'll come.

DOUGLAS. *(Gently.)* Better call the spinal taps something else. This is for the good of the men. You understand that, Nurse Evers? We have nothing else. You understand that, don't you?

EVERS. Dr. Brodus, if we—

BRODUS. The patients must believe that nothing has changed.

EVERS. *(Disbelieving.)* What about contagion?

DOUGLAS. We will only keep patients in the study who have non-contagious syphilis. Any patient found contagious is taken out of the study.

EVERS. *(To brodus.)* And the arsenic injections? The mercury rubs?

DOUGLAS. *(Gently.)* Use heat liniment.

EVERS. *(Caught in the middle.)* Heat liniment?

BRODUS. *(Gently.)* Nurse Evers . . . please.

EVERS. Yes, sir.

DOUGLAS. Nurse Evers, those men need help. Don't they?

EVERS. Of course, they do.

DOUGLAS. Would fifty dollars be of help to those men?

EVERS. Fifty dollars is a lot of money in Macon County, Dr. Douglas.

DOUGLAS. Would fifty dollars life insurance convince those men to stay with this study?

BRODUS. A decent burial would mean a lot to those men. They're buried in feed sacks by the city dump.

DOUGLAS. As long as this research continues, any study patient that dies for whatever reason receives fifty dollars, for burial. I could fight and get that much money, Nurse Evers, if it would convince those men to stay in the study.

BRODUS. *(Quietly.)* You'll be able to keep nursing those patients and their families and take those men to the hospital free of charge if they get sick and know that they're all signed up, right up front, first in line, when the treatment money comes through. . . . There's a lot of detours on this road, Nurse Evers. But as long as we're going in the general, forward, direction, we got to keep on traveling, don't you think? *(Privately.)* We have one thread tugging at

Washington's money. If that thread breaks, then we have nothing. Really nothing.

EVERS. I'm afraid for those men, Dr. Brodus.

BRODUS. Push past that fear, Nurse Evers.

EVERS. I can't.

BRODUS. We don't have a choice here.

EVERS. Seems not. . . . First in line?

BRODUS. First in line.

EVERS. *(After a moment.)* All right.

BRODUS. Good.

DOUGLAS. *(A sudden solution.)* "Backshots," Nurse Evers. We don't want to frighten the men. Better call those spinal taps, "backshots." *(Brodus and Douglas purposefully exit, leaving Evers alone. She comes forward to a testimony area.)*

EVERS. You've got to go back, Senator. You've got to appreciate Macon County, Alabama, in 1932, to understand what "caring" meant in those times. You've got to think like we thought then. . . . You're talking about civil rights. I'm talking about people just trying to stay alive. And some other people trying their best to help them. If you want to walk where I walked, you got to be walking that messy middle ground. *(Lights crossfade to Scene 6. Posters appear advertising for treatment. Evers crosses to Caleb.)*

Scene 6

1932. Outside the Possom Hollow Schoolhouse; morning, two weeks have passed. An examining table and a dressing screen have been set up. Evers, in a white gown, is cleaning and sterilizing instruments and getting records ready for the spinal taps. Caleb, the first patient on the first day of this procedure, stands by the screen in mock defiance.

EVERS. *(Busy, not at all threatened; enjoying the interaction.)* And I said take off your shirt.

CALEB. And I said no.

EVERS. Caleb Humphries, take, off, your, shirt. *(Caleb mimics her.)* This is a serious medical procedure, this backshot, Caleb. Now you got to stop this playing around just 'cause we're in this schoolhouse, and you start acting like this here's a hospital and when I ask you to take your shirt off, I'm asking in a medical not a personal way.

CALEB. *(Matching her gravity.)* Then I'll take it off in a medical way, not a personal way.

EVERS. Caleb Humphries, I'm sorry I'm without a piece of shale from Orange Creek at this moment . . . so I could throw it upside your head . . . in a medical way. Now get undressed; we got four more patients after you this morning. *(He goes behind the screen and starts taking things off; enjoying himself.)*

CALEB. Everything off?

EVERS. Everything.

CALEB. You goin' to stay around?

EVERS. Usually do.

CALEB. What for?

EVERS. Take notes.

CALEB. Can't Dr. Douglas remember on his own.

EVERS. It goes faster if I'm helping . . . *(Clothes are hanging over the screen.)* Pants now.

CALEB. What you gonna give me in trade?

EVERS. *(Still busy working, she takes a gown to him.)* Put this gown on.

CALEB. Gown? *(Pause.)* This don't got no buttons up front.

EVERS. That's not the front. You've got it on backwards; turn it around.

CALEB. Good. *(Pause.)* Now what kind of thing is this; my back's open.

EVERS. Hold it closed with your hand, Caleb.

CALEB. Now the front's riding up over my . . . riding up too high.

EVERS. Then just leave it, Caleb. I've been a nurse for eight years. I don't think nothing will be surprising me none. *(Caleb enters; he makes his way to the table. Deliberately not paying him much attention.)* Looks good. Now come on out here and sit on the table with your legs hanging over the side while I'm readying things.

CALEB. *(Getting on the table.)* What's this gonna be?

EVERS. I suppose you'd call this, well, a "backshot," Caleb. It's like a shot with a needle *(Touching his lower back.)* down here, at this part of your back, so we can check your spine fluid.

CALEB. It gonna hurt?

EVERS. Probably.

CALEB. You don't do much pretending do you, Nurse Evers?

EVERS. I want my patients to believe what I'm saying, Caleb. They wouldn't be doing that if I told them it wasn't gonna hurt and then it hurt.

CALEB. I believe you.

EVERS. You do?

CALEB. Of course.

EVERS. Good. . . . Come on now, let's get you ready for Dr. Douglas.

CALEB. I don't like that man much. He talks to me like I'm stupid. He says, "Be there on time." I say, "All right." Then he says, again, "Now you be there on time." And I say, "I said, all right." Then before I can get out, he says again, "Now you be sure to be there. . . . On time." They always talking to us like that.

EVERS. Macon's like a foreign country to him, Caleb. He's learning as fast as he can. (*Caleb remains unconvinced.*) Now just sit there, with your hands on your lap and don't be touching back here once I start sterilizing it. (*She puts on a face mask and starts painting rubbing antiseptic solution in a circular motion on his lower back.*)

CALEB. That's cold.

EVERS. Has alcohol and iodine in it.

CALEB. Go easy now.

EVERS. I ain't doing nothing.

CALEB. (*Frightened, seeing the mask for the first time.*) What's that mask about?

EVERS. It's about not breathing on your back when I clean it. Keep your head in that direction. Come on. Stop turning.

CALEB. I want to get a look at you. I figure a look at you is good medicine.

EVERS. Didn't know you were into honey talking, Caleb.

CALEB. Why, Nurse Evers, Mama was always complaining to me: "Boy, you got a diploma in smartness at the mouth."

EVERS. That right?

CALEB. Yes, ma'am. . . . Too bad she's gone. And my wife. And my child.

EVERS. That's what makes you so angry?

CALEB. I look around this place and all I see is everything and everybody broken down; no one ever getting ahead. Folks around here, they just get scraped and scratched every which way 'til they're all worn down. I'm angry 'cause I want to be using my brain and my mouth instead of my hands and my back.

EVERS. You want to get ahead, you gotta first ask yourself what you do well and then go out and try to use it. You're a "talkin' man" so you have to go out and find a way to use that gift for talking, like a salesman or something.

CALEB. You know I was raised Baptist and I'm thinking that when you're raised Baptist you got a better chance of being a "talkin' man" 'cause if you got a good preacher preaching at you each week, you get a feeling for it.

EVERS. That's what you had?

CALEB. Yes, ma'am. Every week. Reverend Banks he was a fine preacher. As far back as I can remember, I can remember his preaching. When I was six years old a big lightning storm touched down by the church. The church members said that the lightning was just plain jealous of the voice of Reverend Banks. Well, an old oak tree was cut down by that lightening and fell on the outhouse behind the church. The next Sunday I climbed up on that oak tree and started taking off on the Reverend to the other children. "Raise out of hell"; "keep you eyes on the Lord"; then I warmed up, didn't care what I was saying anymore: "this here tree has brushed this here outhouse 'cause it smelled; smelled; smelled so bad" . . . I'm goin' on like that in the biggest, deepest voice a six year old can put on and the Reverend hear me and my mother hear me and the whole choir that's practicing just inside the church while we kids is playing outside, they hear me too. And I was lashed for the wages of sin. This backshot can't hurt worse than that day. After that, every time we were alone, all those children would be yelling at me "Caleb, Caleb, do the Reverend. Do the Reverend." Now I "do the Reverend" for the fun of it.

EVERS. You are a talking man.

CALEB. Think so?

EVERS. Yes. Yes, I do. *(Douglas enters rapidly, wearing a gown, mask and gloves.)*

DOUGLAS. Sorry to keep you waiting, Nurse Evers. Good morning, Caleb. Nice to see you. *(Caleb stands. Evers helps Douglas adjust his mask. Douglas is efficient but anxious. He wants things to go well.)* So you're our first patient our first day?

EVERS. Yes, sir. . . . Is that good?

DOUGLAS. *(Reassuring.)* Absolutely. We're fresh, we're rested, we're ready to work. Yes, it's good. Of course it is. Now here's how we do this: You just keep sitting the way you are, Caleb. I'm going to locate that spot between the vertebrae in your lower back and make a small needle puncture. Not much to it really.

CALEB. Good.

DOUGLAS. First I'm going to ask you to bend your head over. Good. Now. Just a little further. Good. Very good. Now. Here's the most important part: you're going to have to sit very still. Nurse Evers will help you. Especially once the needle is inside your spinal canal; don't move then or that needle might injure the nerves to your legs.

CALEB. To my legs?

DOUGLAS. That's right. You understand?

CALEB. Of course, I understand.

DOUGLAS. That's why we don't want you to move.

CALEB. Don't worry, I'm not movin'.

DOUGLAS. All right; now, here we go. *(To Evers.)* All set?

CALEB. Yes, sir.

DOUGLAS. Caleb?

CALEB. Yes, sir.

DOUGLAS. Good. Now, I'll just take that needle Nurse Evers.

CALEB. Let me see it—it's big . . .

DOUGLAS. Not to worry, Caleb. Only a little part will go in. Just this first little part here at the front. . . . So. *(Douglas starts to position the needle.)*

CALEB. What's it made out of?

DOUGLAS. Gold. It's made out of gold.

CALEB. Well, that's good.

DOUGLAS. Yes, it is. . . . So. Here we go. *(Douglas is standing behind the table focused on Caleb's lower back; each time the needle goes in or comes out, it is searingly painful.)*

CALEB. *(Controlling the pain.)* Aah. You goin' too far.

DOUGLAS. I have to try to find the spinal canal. *(Calmly, repositioning the needle.)* I'll be as gentle as I can. Please, just sit still. All right, here we go now. *(Douglas focuses intently; he doesn't want to miss again.)*

CALEB. *(He resists moving and, trying to ignore the intermittent bursts of pain which occur only when the needle is pushed in, automatically falls into his preaching voice; his anger is stronger than the pain and it is this anger that makes his words clear and resonant, despite the procedure.)* Ahhh. . . . That needle is the work of the devil . . . it's sharp and burning and greedy gold in color . . . ahh . . . *(A catechism.)* What color was Job? Black. What color was Jeremiah? Black. Who was Moses' wife? An Ethiopian. David said he became like a bottle in the smoke. What's natural? It's as natural to be black as the leopard to be spotted. . . . Ahhhh . . .

DOUGLAS. *(Silence; all stop for a moment.)* What in the world are you saying, Caleb?

CALEB. *(Afraid but not in pain.)* Catechism of the Church of the Living God founded by William Christian in Wrightsville, Alabama, in 1889.

DOUGLAS. Does it help?

CALEB. It keeps my mind from violence, Dr. Douglas.

DOUGLAS. Then just keep saying it. . . . One more time now. Hold it. *(Needle in suddenly; the next four lines come at once.)*

EVERS. Dr. Douglas—

DOUGLAS. *(Quieting her.)* Please, Nurse Evers.

CALEB. Ahh; no more, I'm getting off this here table now.

DOUGLAS. *(Alarmed.)* No.

EVERS. *(Taking charge.)* Caleb Humphries don't you move, you hear me; you sit there and don't move; you gotta be a walkin' man, not a cripple man; now you sit there and don't move. Stop moving.

CALEB. Ahhhh.

EVERS. Dr. Douglas—

DOUGLAS. *(Over her, triumphant, relieved.)* Got it. There we go. We're all set. *(Carefully.)* Now I'll just collect some fluid if you will be so kind as to give me the test tube, Nurse Evers.

EVERS. Don't move.

DOUGLAS. *(Douglas puts tube under the needle and collects a small amount of fluid.)* There we are. *(He pulls out the needle. The removal of the needle stings.)*

CALEB. What you doing?

DOUGLAS. Just removing the needle. Well. Now if you don't want a bad headache, Caleb, take my advice and sit here for a while. Just sit right here.

CALEB. Why'd you do that to me?

DOUGLAS. I didn't do anything to you, Caleb. It's not uncommon that the exact entrance to the spinal canal can't be found the first time. Unfortunately, that can cause some pain.

CALEB. Dr. Douglas?

DOUGLAS. Yes, Caleb?

CALEB. Practice.

DOUGLAS. I beg your pardon.

CALEB. I said practice, sir, 'cause you're not gonna have a next patient if you go stickin' them the way you stuck me. How many patients you think'll come here when they find out what you're doin' feel like getting a hot screwdriver twisted in your back?

DOUGLAS. There was nothing wrong with the way I performed that spinal tap . . . (*Correcting himself.*) backshot. And if you warn the other patients away from this, you'll be depriving those men of government care.

CALEB. I don't have to warn 'em about nothing, sir. They can hear. They hear it once, they start wonderin'. They hear it twice, and you and Nurse Evers are gonna be out of patients as fast as those men can stampede back home and tell their neighbors about them "spinal taps." That ain't no tap, let me tell you. Not what you're doing.

DOUGLAS. I'll just check this fluid, Nurse Evers.

EVERS. Yes, doctor.

DOUGLAS. Thank you for the advice, Caleb. I'm sorry that hurt so much.

CALEB. Well, maybe you didn't mean it to hurt.

DOUGLAS. No, I didn't. Of course I didn't. I'm just trying to help. (*Douglas exits with the fluid.*)

EVERS. Will you tell the others?

CALEB. Hurts like hell.

EVERS. Dr. Douglas will get better.

CALEB. How? By practicing?

EVERS. That's how you get better.

CALEB. Well, next time you should put me at the end of the line. . . . You think I should?

EVERS. What?

CALEB. Tell the others.

EVERS. You're looking for something that I can't answer for you, Caleb.

CALEB. Why not?

EVERS. I'm a nurse. I'm here to help Dr. Douglas get done what needs to be done. That's my job.

CALEB. We need to be healthy. That's what needs to be done. Right?

EVERS. Yes.

CALEB. I'm just asking you, if this is making me healthy? (*Evers is preparing for the next patient. Caleb watches her for a few moments.*) See, Nurse Evers, I don't trust the white. You gotta watch them. So they don't be sneaking up on you. No white folks with money come around when my wife took ill or my baby was born sick.

EVERS. Hanging onto that anger won't help you win, Caleb.

CALEB. *(Evers is cleaning the wound. It stings.)* Nurse Evers, I gotta keep angry to work my place, to save my money . . . sometimes just to get up in the morning.

EVERS. I can understand that.

CALEB. You can? You don't seem like a get-up-in-the-mornin'-angry to me.

EVERS. I'm not. I'm more the go-to-sleep-angry kind.

CALEB. I can't seem to do that. Can't get to sleep when I'm angry.

EVERS. You must be up a lot of nights.

CALEB. I am. Yes, I am.

EVERS. Got to trust somebody, Caleb.

CALEB. Maybe.

EVERS. Sometime. How else you going to live? No one can make it just on their own.

CALEB. *(Pause.)* You been a good friend to people around here.

EVERS. They're my family.

CALEB. You never been married?

EVERS. Too busy.

CALEB. Getting an education. Getting trained as a nurse so you can polish silver.

EVERS. Now there's some anger that I went to sleep with a few nights. But I was patient. Now here I am doing what I was trained to do. . . . And I got a job offer. A nursing job. In New York City.

CALEB. You taking it?

EVERS. Thinking about it. I've started thinking seriously about it.

CALEB. I'd take it if I was you.

EVERS. You would?

CALEB. In a minute. And take me with you.

EVERS. What about the gilleein'?

CALEB. Take them too. We'll hire a bus. Dance up in Harlem. . . . You got a first name?

EVERS. Yes.

CALEB. You gonna tell me what it is?

EVERS. Why you want to know?

CALEB. When I talk about this saintly woman with God's gift of beauty and compassion, it's gonna lose something if I can't make a direct connection by using your first name.

EVERS. When you going to be doing that kind of talking?

CALEB. To myself. When I need the company of a woman I respect.

EVERS. It's unusual.

CALEB. Lorraine?

EVERS. No.

CALEB. Madelaine?

EVERS. No.

CALEB. Sally Ann?

EVERS. Eunice.

CALEB. That's a fine name. Sounds like it got "nice" in it, don't it?

EVERS. You can God-talk and sweet-talk, can't you, Caleb?

CALEB. I don't have to be pepper all the time. And you don't have to be alone all the time neither.

EVERS. I got the work.

CALEB. That ain't a person.

EVERS. No. But it's my life. The work with you all is my life. (*They look at each other for a moment.*)

CALEB. No time for specials . . . Eunice?

EVERS. (*Struggling.*) No, Caleb. No time. I got to treat all my patients the same.

CALEB. (*Direct.*) I'll be putting my trust in you. If you don't mind.

EVERS. (*Troubled.*) Caleb . . .

CALEB. If you don't mind . . .

EVERS. (*Recovering.*) Well. Sure. I don't mind. Of course, I don't. (*Trying to end the conversation with a smile.*) I've never seen no patient, ever, preach gospel through it all.

CALEB. I told you. It just comes on out. Natural like.

EVERS. Well, you take off that gown, "talkin' man."

CALEB. You meanin' that in a medical way or a personal way?

EVERS. And then get dressed . . . behind the screen. (*She continues preparing for the next patient. As Caleb crosses behind the screen, he looks over his shoulder and starts singing "Children, Don't Be Afraid" to Evers, a modest, simple serenade. After a while, Evers crosses to Dr. Brodus' office with the spinal tap data as the lights fade.*)

ACT TWO

Scene 1

1946. Simultaneously, three separate playing areas appear. On one part of the Stage, Willie in a pool of dim downlight is quietly testing his legs by practicing his dance turns again and again to perfection. Caleb, Hodman, and Ben holding their instruments stand in the shadows, watching Willie. The play of light and shadow is not realistic.

On another part of the stage Brodus and Douglas are dimly revealed surveying slides using two microscopes in Brodus' office. By turns they enter plot points on a large graph they have created on a blackboard. The work is quiet and methodical. This setting and activity will continue throughout the treatment center scene until interrupted by Willie's arrival in Brodus' office.

Evers stands between these two settings downstage center.

WILLIE. *(A private whisper, as he practices.)* Da, da, da . . . da, da.

EVERS. *(As testimony.)* When you're up close for fourteen years, you don't notice the changes. . . . Unless they catch you by surprise. But even then, after a while, those surprises get familiar and it almost seems like nothing has changed. . . . Those men looked healthy. No pain or nothing like that. And they felt good. You wouldn't believe anything was wrong with them. That's the kind of disease it was, see. Hidden. Some people in this room might have syphilis at this very moment and you wouldn't know it. No offense meant, Senator.

I'm not saying there weren't consequences. I'm just saying it wasn't that simple. The disease was not predictable. And there was no money. And the treatment was dangerous. Convulsions. And teeth would fall out. It was ridiculous. I came to believe that if a person looked good, you best just leave them be.

But 1946 changed all that. Something new arrived, something that changed everything. The "silver bullet," they called it: penicillin. Meningitis, cured. Pneumonia, cured. Finally. And now, syphilis, cured. A national treatment program. And my patients were going to be first in line.

(Day 1.)

BRODUS. *(Lights up; looking up from his work.)* That's not possible. *(Evers turns to Douglas and Brodus.)*

EVERS. First in line. That's what we said. That's what you told me. That was the promise.

DOUGLAS. *(Reasonable.)* First we must stop the disease from spreading. Contagious patients first. *(Brodus and Douglas continue to plot graph numbers on a large blackboard.)*

(Day 2.)

(Lights up; Willie suddenly stops dancing and grabs his legs.)

WILLIE. Help. Help. *(Lights change. Evers moves to him, alarmed. Evers is fearful that it is syphilis that is starting to cripple Willie but she is uncertain as to diagnosis and desperately seeks hope in that uncertainty. The men and Evers gather around Willie.)* I'm sorry I yelled like that. I couldn't see what I was doing my eyes were watering so bad. . . . Like a baby. Yelling.

EVERS. *(Cradling Willie.)* You were in pain. It's OK to yell, Willie. *(She rolls up his pants legs.)* I'm losing it. I'm spooked.

CALEB. Don't say that.

HODMAN. You the star attraction, Willie.

BEN. You lose it. We lose it too.

EVERS. Rest, Willie. Let me look after that leg for you. *(She begins to massage his legs.)*

WILLIE. Bad. Real bad. I'm losing it all.

EVERS. *(Determined.)* No, you're not. You'll be all right, Willie. You're not going to lose it all. You can't be thinking like that. Come on now. Let's work on this leg. *(The men quietly attend to Willie. Evers speaks to Brodus and Douglas, determined. The men do not hear her. She continues to work on Willie until the argument pulls her to Brodus and Douglas.)*

(Day 3.)

EVERS. *(To Brodus and Douglas.)* Willie's beginning to drag his leg.

BRODUS. Who?

EVERS. Willie Johnson. I don't know what's wrong with him . . .

BRODUS. And?

EVERS. I want to know what's wrong with him. I want to bring him here. To be examined. By both you gentlemen.

BRODUS. Why?

EVERS. Dr. Brodus, he's one of the study patients.

BRODUS. I see. . . . Bring him.

EVERS. I will. I sure will.

(Day 4.)

(Evers is suddenly pulled into the men's scene by Willie's cry and Caleb's command.)

WILLIE. *(In pain.)* Ahhhh.

CALEB. *(Angry.)* You need some doctorin', boy.

EVERS. *(Stung.)* He got some.

CALEB. Well, it ain't doing him no good.

BEN. What you mad at her for?

HODMAN. Caleb—

CALEB. These legs are walking out of here for all of us. Without Willie, we're nothing.

EVERS. I'll speak to Dr. Douglas.

CALEB. I'm not talking about more back rubs. I'm talking about something different. Something new. For his leg.

EVERS. I said I'll speak to Dr. Douglas when he comes down next week. And I've already spoken to Dr. Brodus. I'll get them both to examine you, Willie. Personally. To see what's bothering you. For right now you need some of those pink aspirin pills, that's for sure. But you got to know exactly what's bothering you before you can treat it permanent, see? You got to give it a name: like arthritis, or rheumatism, or gout, or just plain too much hard work. You got to name it before you can fix it, see? Now you're under my care, Willie. I've watched after you all these years. Haven't I? And your wife, Hodman? And your niece, Caleb? Ben? You all have been doing all right, haven't you?

CALEB. *(Sharply.)* We gotta get these feet moving right, Nurse Evers. Now.

EVERS. I know, Caleb. I know.

BEN. What you fussin' at her for? What's wrong with you?

CALEB. Don't nobody do nothing for you. You gotta do it for yourself. Willie, you gotta get some new doctorin'.

EVERS. No, Caleb.

WILLIE. Can't afford it.

CALEB. You gotta afford it. Ain't nothing more important to you than your legs. Sell that heifer you got.

WILLIE. *(Willie works on his legs.)* I'm waiting. Waiting for the Lord to put his hands on my shoulders.

CALEB. *(Sharply.)* No, Willie. You don't have no waiting time left. None of us do. Now stop thinking and start movin'. You're not rich enough to feel sorry for yourself. Come on. Get moving. "Gotta work." Come on.

HODMAN. Willie, drink you a quart of May tea at the beginning of the month.

CALEB. What are you selling him?

HODMAN. I seen it work. You see what I'm saying to you, Willie?

WILLIE. All I see is grandpa laying in the dirt.

CALEB. You got dying on the brain, Willie Johnson.

WILLIE. It preys on my mind, Caleb.

BEN. It don't have to. We got our own burial society. That's right, ain't it, Nurse Evers?

EVERS. Yes, Ben. That's right.

CALEB. If you're dead it don't matter what they do to you.

EVERS. Got your Aspiration, don't you, Willie?

WILLIE. That Aspiration ain't won nothing in seven months.

CALEB. Come on. You got to work that pain out of those legs.

EVERS. That's it, Willie. That's what you got to do. *(Willie begins to stand up. Evers is now caught between the two scenes.)*

(Day 5.)

EVERS. Dr. Brodus, my patients have waited the longest. They need penicillin the most. It would help them.

BRODUS. Penicillin can't undo the damage that has already been done.

EVERS. It might stop them from getting worse.

BRODUS. Perhaps. Or it might kill them.

EVERS. *(Stands.)* Penicillin?

BRODUS. The Herxheimer reaction.

EVERS. *(Crossing to Douglas and Brodus.)* Herxheimer?

BRODUS. An allergic reaction that could kill a chronic syphilitic with a single injection of penicillin.

EVERS. Like the arsenic?

BRODUS. Worse.

DOUGLAS. Washington is researching the question now. To determine the degree of risk.

(Day 6.)

(Willie is standing, holding his legs.)

CALEB. Gotta work.

EVERS. *(To Willie.)* Come on, Willie. You got your Aspiration, don't you?

WILLIE. Yes, ma'am. Nothing's going to beat me out of my ticket to the Cotton Club. *(Willie tentatively tests his legs.)*

EVERS. *(To Brodus and Douglas.)* And if there's no risk, then he'll get the penicillin. Right?

CALEB. Do that one again, Willie.

EVERS. Don't look down, Willie. Look straight out and dance through the pain. . . . *(To Brodus and Douglas.)* How long until Washington decides the risk?

DOUGLAS. You can't hurry this kind of investigation. It's too dangerous. You make mistakes.

CALEB. "Gotta work."

EVERS. Come on, Willie. *(Hoping.)* There's nothing wrong with that leg.

HODMAN. Willie, do like you always do.

EVERS. Dance that pain down, Willie.

HODMAN. Come on, Willie. Gotta work.

CALEB. Gotta work.

EVERS. *(To Brodus and Douglas.)* How long? Exactly how long are they going to have to wait?

BRODUS. As soon as there's a decision to do so, we'll move to treat every patient in the study.

MEN. Gotta work . . . gotta work. *(Quietly but insistently the men use their instruments and the phrase "gotta work" to create a rhythm to push Willie to dance. The words become embedded in a combination of vocal sounds and driving hand and foot percussion. There is desperation in this crusade. The sounds are sharp and tinged with anger. Willie forces himself to dance through the pain. The pain is always there but the determination to ignore it grows during the following lines. This combination of word and sound underscores the following dialogue.)*

EVERS. Got to fight it, Willie. Got to fight it hard . . .

WILLIE. *(Determined.)* Gotta work, gotta work . . .

EVERS. *(To Brodus and Douglas.)* These men need all the help they can get. Right now.

DOUGLAS. Right now, you better look after those men. If the spirochete is embedded in the heart muscle and penicillin kills the germ, holes could be left in that muscle and the heart might disintegrate—

EVERS. What?

WILLIE. *(Willie dances past the pain and shouts, triumphant.)* You hear me, Grandpa. I'm gonna win 'cause I'm going to do that double fly step, the one you taught me, you hear.

EVERS. What? *(A cry.)* Dr. Brodus?

BRODUS. The heart might explode. *(Light change.)*

EVERS. *(Turning into the new scene; a frightened shout.)* There's two men in this treatment center who have no place being here. *(Lights crossfade to Scene 2 as Evers moves to the rapid treatment center and Brodus and Douglas continue working. Hodman and Ben exit. Willie and Caleb move into the next scene.)*

Scene 2

1946. A Birmingham rapid treatment center. One month later. The setting is defined by two benches. Caleb and Willie are waiting in line behind one bench. Evers is standing on another bench. In the background, Douglas and Brodus continue smoothly plotting points on the graph.

EVERS. *(Continuing as the setting changes around her.)* Is there a patient here named, Willie Johnson? Is there a patient in this treatment center named Caleb Humphries?

WILLIE. *(Willie stands on the bench and yells to Evers across the room.)* Yes. I'm here. Over here. Behind you, Nurse Evers. *(She turns to him.)* You're wearing a new hat.

EVERS. *(Yelling.)* What you doin' here, Willie Johnson?

CALEB. *(Caleb stands on the bench next to Willie.)* We're here to get a hip shot of that penicillin, Nurse Evers.

EVERS. No, sir. No sir, you're not. You're government patients. You're not supposed to be here. Now come on over here so we're not disturbing all these people. *(The men and Evers come together.)*

WILLIE. The doctor sent us to come.

EVERS. What doctor? That doctor didn't know you were a United States Government patient. If that doctor knew that, he wouldn't have sent you. Now you get on that bus and go on back to Tuskegee. Penicillin ain't for you. And what are you doing here, Caleb?

CALEB. Sam Heart's brother's here. He's getting a shot. Tom Daniel's cousin's here. He's getting it. I talked to those men. You know what they got?

EVERS. What?

CALEB. Bad blood. That's what I got, ain't it? They're getting a hip shot of that penicillin. That's what I'm getting. And Willie.

EVERS. No. You're not.

CALEB. Yes. I am.

EVERS. Caleb. That shot could kill you.

CALEB. They're all still standing. Over there in the other room.

EVERS. They're different from both of you.

CALEB. They got bad blood. Just like us.

EVERS. No. It's different. They just got it. You all had it for years. They're not in danger from this penicillin. You all are. It could make holes in you heart. Make it explode. And there's nothing bothering you, Caleb.

CALEB. Nothing. Now.

EVERS. That's right. Nothing. And, Willie, this is not the kind of chance you want to take.

CALEB. We don't see it like that.

EVERS. Well, I do. *(To Willie.)* You know what penicillin is?

WILLIE. Some kind of medicine.

EVERS. It's a mold.

WILLIE. A mold?

EVERS. Like you find under a tree. . . . It's a mold.

WILLIE. And it can kill you, you say?

EVERS. We don't know. That's why we have to wait. Until we're certain it's safe. Please. We got to wait.

CALEB. I'm not waiting.

EVERS. You're a government patient.

CALEB. I don't want to be no government patient no more.

EVERS. And you won't be if you get that shot. If you live.

WILLIE. Mold ain't goin' to be doin' me much good, I don't guess.

EVERS. We ain't givin' you no mold in Macon County. Come on. *(Willie moves to leave with Evers.)*

CALEB. You stay right here, Willie.

WILLIE. What's wrong with you? You heard what she said.

CALEB. I don't trust the government.

WILLIE. I'm not talking to the government, Caleb. I'm talking to Nurse Evers. *(Evers and Willie start to leave.)* Come on, Caleb. Let's go. That stuff no good for us.

EVERS. I'll tell them not to give you that shot.

CALEB. You do that. I'll get it somewhere else.

EVERS. I'm worried for you, Caleb. Please.

CALEB. No. That may be the only word I have left to me, Nurse Evers. But I can still use it. . . . No. *(He sits.)*

EVERS. Come on, Willie.

CALEB. *(Desperate, calling after him.)* Willie . . . Willie . . . *(Evers escorts Willie to Dr. Brodus' office as lights crossfade and Caleb exits.)*

Scene 7

1946. Dr. Brodus' office. Two months later. Throughout the scene, Willie is quietly practicing and counting as he moves; at intervals he stops only to start again with renewed determination; he is not part of the scene in the office. During the first part of the scene, Evers hears Brodus and Douglas but continues to stare at Ben.

WILLIE. Over the top.

DOUGLAS. Penicillin won't help them. It's too late. The damage is done.

BRODUS. It would stop them from getting worse. . . . We're giving penicillin to every other syphilitic in the country regardless of how many years they've had the disease.

DOUGLAS. They're different.

BRODUS. How?

DOUGLAS. They're not in the study.

EVERS. *(As testimony.)* Mr. Benjamin Washington died at seventy-four years of age. *(Ben exits.)* A long life. But not a good one . . . I got Mr. Washington that coffin. He looked serene and peaceful.

WILLIE. Over the top. *(Evers notices Willie and is then pulled back into the scene by Douglas' line.)*

DOUGLAS. *(Coming over the end of Willie's line.)* We cannot invalidate fourteen years work and the sacrifice of all those patients with a single injection that might be useless or lethal.

BRODUS. We have fourteen years of data.

DOUGLAS. *(Sharply.)* Fourteen years is not end point. It's scientifically incomplete if not taken to end point.

EVERS. End point?

DOUGLAS. If we're going to match the Oslo study we have no choice. . . . It's no longer our decision. It's Washington's decision. This study must go to end point.

EVERS. And how far is that?

DOUGLAS. Autopsy. The facts in this study must be validated by autopsy.

EVERS. My patients shouldn't have to make that sacrifice.

DOUGLAS. *(Losing his patience.)* They already have. Each year we get closer to unraveling the secrets of this disease because those few men have sacrificed for something greater than they'll ever understand. We owe it to those men to make this the best study possible.

EVERS. I promised before God not to harm my patients. I promised before God to devote myself to the welfare of my patients.

DOUGLAS. Nurse Evers . . . I'd appreciate a follow-up call to every physician in the Tuskegee area. Make sure they understand that they're not to treat those men with penicillin. By mistake. *(Douglas exits.)*

WILLIE. Gotta work, gotta work.

EVERS. I've lied to those men because you told me to. I've misled them because I thought I could trust you with their welfare. Those men need penicillin. No one will help them if we don't. No one will help them if we don't.

BRODUS. I understand your passion, Nurse Evers.

EVERS. I'm not going up over that next hill, Dr. Brodus.

BRODUS. *(Cutting her off, an explosion.)* You think you're the only person who feels? *(To Evers.)* You got your burden and I got mine. You serve the race in your way. I serve it in mine. I can't rock the boat while I'm trying to keep a people from drowning. There are trade-offs you can't even imagine. Don't you see that? *(In the background, Willie's practicing becomes more desperate.)* You spend your time around the colored. Good. Well, I spend mine tiptoeing around the white. But I ain't there to shine no shoes. And I ain't no Uncle Tom. And I ain't no shufflin' nigger. *(After regaining control, he looks at Evers.)* Is that colored enough for you, Nurse Evers? *(Brodus looks at Evers for a moment, turns and leaves. Willie is seen and heard simultaneous with Brodus' exit.)*

WILLIE. *(Reaching past the pain.)* Da, da, da, da, da.

EVERS. *(Lights change as Evers cries out through her own pain to both the exiting Brodus and to Hodman as he enters.)* We've got a choice right now.

Epilogue
1972. *Outside the Possom Hollow Schoolhouse. A crisp American flag and a printed sign are tacked to the decaying wood. The sign reads: "United States Senate Testimony Site; Location: (written in by hand.) Possom Hollow School; Date: (written in by hand.) April 24, 1972." Brodus and Douglas are sitting waiting to testify.*

EVERS. *(As testimony.)* Those that got out were safe. Mr. Willie Johnson left Macon county for Tipton County, Tennessee, in 1956. He got that hip shot of penicillin in Tipton and that's why he can use a cane now instead of crutches. Mr. Caleb Humphries got out too. He became a preaching man, with a traveling circuit. I lost track of them after they left Macon. . . . We used to tell the men that this disease had three parts: you get it, you forget it and then you regret it twenty or thirty years later when it comes back to haunt you. That's how it's been with me too. I tried to stop thinking about it after 1946. The men were set apart from the thousands that were treated with penicillin and the study continued. "The Tuskegee Study of Untreated Syphilis in the Negro Male" had acquired a life of its own. It had become . . . familiar. Each spring I prepared a report on the number of patients remaining: four hundred and twelve in 1946; three hundred and sixty ten years later; one hundred and twenty-seven this year, 1972. *(Evers sits. Caleb enters from the schoolhouse on his way to get Willie. Caleb sees Douglas and stops.)*

CALEB. You into pork, Dr. Douglas?

DOUGLAS. That statement was taken out of context.

CALEB. And a very down-home way of puttin' it: "A great hog has been made out of a very small pig."

DOUGLAS. I was commenting on a statement by the mayor of Tuskegee; the original statement was not mine.

CALEB. But very down-home it was, nonetheless. And you agreed with it. From listening to your testimony inside, I mean. And as soon as I heard what you said I knew I had to ask you one question.

DOUGLAS. All right, what question?

CALEB. You got any more pigs cookin'? 'Cause if you do I hope you learned the difference between treatin' and watchin'.

DOUGLAS. Mr. Humphries—

CALEB. Reverend Humphries.

DOUGLAS. Reverend Humphries, those were not racial decisions: those were research options that were appropriate at the time.

CALEB. *(Stopping him.)* Don't get me wrong, Dr. Douglas. I don't think it was forty years of "garbage science" or whatever the newspapers are calling it. Because I got something useful out of all this.

DOUGLAS. You did?

CALEB. Fourteen dollars. And that certificate of participation for being a good patient for fourteen years. *(He takes out the certificate.)*

DOUGLAS. That seems pretty useless to me.

CALEB. Well, that's what I thought. But I searched for that certificate for two days when all this blew up. I said to myself, Dr. Douglas, I said; "I gotta find that certificate. I gotta find it and give it to my lawyer." *(Caleb exits. Evers, Brodus, and Douglas sit in silence.)*

EVERS. *(To Dr. Brodus.)* What will they do to you?

BRODUS. Nothing. At my age I've got nothing to lose. *(Ironic.)* Except my good name. *(They wait.)*

DOUGLAS. That data has been used and will be used again and every time it is used that researcher is saying I believe in that study. *(Pause; no one speaks.)* Dr.

Brodus, that data proved that black and white are affected in exactly the same way. That's what you wanted to prove, wasn't it? Those statistics helped you stand up against racial bias.

BRODUS. *(Eye to eye.)* Those men could have been given a choice.

DOUGLAS. Those men were serving their race. *(Silence. Douglas, Evers and Brodus sit and wait. Caleb enters with Willie who is using a cane. Caleb is carrying the Victrola and walking with Willie toward the schoolhouse where Willie will testify. Willie's walk must not be exaggerated. It consists of a slight limp and weakness in one leg. He uses his cane to compensate for this disability. He walks slowly but with dignity. Evers hears the following dialogue.)*

CALEB. *(To Willie.)* That's what that newspaper article was saying, Willie. That's what "guinea pig" means. They were all just watching us to see what the bad blood would do.

WILLIE. Nurse Evers?

CALEB. She took you out of that Birmingham line, didn't she? That penicillin could have saved Ben and Hodman and made you a dancin' man.

WILLIE. *(He is still uncertain.)* Nurse Evers?

CALEB. Nurse Evers, and that man there and that man. And all those doctors from Washington. Watchin' and waitin'. Waitin' for us to die. *(Guiding him toward the schoolhouse.)* Come on.

WILLIE. *(Pause; refusing to accept completely what Caleb is saying, he looks at Evers and moves toward her. To Evers.)* Nurse Evers. . . . You was a friend to me.

EVERS. I am a friend to you, Willie.

WILLIE. What kind of friend could do what you did?

EVERS. Understand, Willie. You have to try to understand.

WILLIE. You try to understand me. That penicillin would have made it so I could walk without pain and maybe even Jackspring. And they didn't give that to me in Birmingham because you pulled me out of that line so I could be a part of Miss Evers' Boys and Burial Society. So you all could do your watching while I wake up past midnight not feeling my legs or else feeling pain, burning pain like a hot iron pressin' on my skin, 'til I shout, "Take this pain away, Lord, please, take this pain away." My body was my freedom. You hear me? MY BODY WAS MY FREEDOM. *(He takes the Victrola from Caleb and puts it down.)* You all wanna watch. Watch now. Watch and think what I used to do with my feet and what I could have done; how my feet sounded faster than this here music could have pushed them. You all want to watch? Watch. *(With difficulty Willie starts the music. Caleb remembers the music. The two men enjoy the remembrance for a moment.)* "Drop over, double step; drop over, double step; drop over step, step, strut." Lord, you remember that, Caleb? *(They laugh; but as Willie listens to the music, and as he remembers the way he used to be able to dance, his rage increases. This memory becomes more vivid as he turns to Evers and recites the patter he used to say.)* "Drop over, double step"? *(Standing still, sharply, to the others.)* You watching'? "Gillee strut, down, drop; gillee strut down, drop, drop." Watch. You watch this now. *(Spurred by his own anger, he forces himself to tap his cane and slightly shuffle one foot, a broken suggestion of his former skill. He can do no more and refuses to humiliate himself by trying. He stands with dignity and recites.)* "Gillee, drop, drop, drop, drop, down, drop, down, drop, down . . ." Watch. *(Willie stops tapping his cane and foot. Keeping an eye on them, he uses the patter to make them watch his stillness.)* "Drop, down, drop, drop, drop, down; *(A shout of anguish; he doesn't move.)* WATCH, and remember: drop, down, down, down, down . . ." *(Willie gives up the memory and hits the Victrola with his cane, stopping it. Silence. Willie stands perfectly still. Evers moves to comfort Willie.)* NO. NO HELP. *(Willie moves away; to Evers, tapping his cane.)* . . . I can walk pretty good on this stick. *(Willie exits into the schoolhouse. Caleb follows him. Douglas exits. Brodus exits. After Willie is gone, Caleb returns to retrieve the Victrola. Evers sits and avoids his glance. Caleb begins to exit toward the schoolhouse.)*

EVERS. *(Suddenly.)* I LOVED YOU MEN. I looked after you as if you were my own. I got you free care and doctorin' that no one could afford back then.

CALEB. And you got us buried.

EVERS. Yes, that too. You're too far away now to recall what a decent burial meant in those days. You're just one step, too far away.

CALEB. And if I hadn't taken that step, I'd never have gotten penicillin.

EVERS. Those men had some peace and some suffering. Who's to say they wouldn't have had the suffering without the peace if I hadn't come along.

CALEB. *(Trying to understand.)* What made you do it? . . . What made you do it?

EVERS. NURSING WAS MY LIFE, Caleb. You know that. Those ideals have guided my life.

CALEB. What ideals?

EVERS. Treat every patient the same. Follow what the doctors say.

CALEB. *(Looking at her.)* Eunice Evers . . . Eunice Evers, you did those ideals proud. *(He exits; Evers waits; we hear Caleb's car start and drive away. Evers comes forward; all lights dim except for a spotlight on Evers.)*

EVERS. In the testimony today, there was a man gracious enough to wonder what effect the scandal, as he put it, might have on the public health nurse who had worked with the participants and who lived in Tuskegee. "She has been known throughout the program as a selfless woman," he said, "who devoted her entire career to this project." And then he was kind enough to hope that it would "not be necessary for her to share any of the blame."

Well, now there's big blame and then there's little blame. The big blame— that seems to be going to the government and those doctors.

Some people in Macon are even saying the government gave those men that disease in the first place. I can't let myself be thinking about that. I got enough thinking to do just handling the little blames.

Those are the blames that got nothing to do with talk about right and wrong and black and white and guinea pigs and money. Those little blames are when you go back to where you live, lived for your whole life, and catch your friends looking at you for no seeming reason, and people walk by you and don't say "good morning" and they don't use your name when they're giving you change as if using it would dirty their mouths up some. Newspapers don't publish stories about these little blames but they mount up and they're strong and they push you to live a new way of life. *(Strong, not apologetic or self-pitying.)* I loved those men. Those men were susceptible to kindness. *(A snare drum is heard. In the shadows Ben and Hodman and Caleb appear in white tux and tails dressed as they might have appeared if they had ever made it to the Cotton Club. Miss Evers' Boys are a silent, antique still photograph. Willie re-enters to the fragile rustling of the snare drum. Willie, also dressed for the Cotton Club, dances smoothly between the shadows of the other characters, a dry leaf scattering brilliant turns and twists into the wind. Evers looks then turns away facing the audience. The drum fades to silence. Willie's graceful, haunting dance continues.)*

WILLIE. *(Whispered.)* Da, da, da, da, daaaaaaa. *(Lights fade.)*

END OF PLAY

TUSKEGEE EXPERIMENT

SADIQ

1. while Sydney Bechet was
   pullin' pistols in Paris,
   Nurse Rivers, who even
   had a car to shuffle her
   syphilitic children across
   Macon County, her "bad
   blood" cotton pickers,
   the "joy" of her life,
   was clearly chosen.
   an appointment befitting
   this darkest century.

2. a Dr. Clark conviction
   a Dr. Wenger coversion
   a Dr. Vonderlehr conception
   a Dr. Peters spinal puncture
   A Dr. Dibble hanging from
   his ankles in the town square,
   the Surgeon General's *schwartzegeist* rising,
   while Tuskegee falls asleep.

3. bring them to autopsy
   with ulcerated limbs,
   with howling wives,
   bring them in, one coon corpse at a time.
   (says Dr. Dibble,)
   "a dollar a year for forty years
   to watch these shadows rot."

Sadiq Bey is a New York–based poet.
Originally published and performed on Don Byron's compact disc Tuskegee Experiments
(Nonesuch Records), 1991.
Reprinted by permission of Sadiq Bey.

"they didn't receive treatment for syphilis,
but they got so much else.
medicine is as much art as it is science."

4. a row of crows on a rickety fence.
   no book learnin'.
   po' as dirt,
   never heard Monsieur Bechet
   play the clarinet.
   this experiment is not a crime,
   but a rite of sacrifice

5. no banana splits on sunday,
   no Brooks Brothers,
   no color t.v. & waterbed,
   no tickets to the county fair.
   no treatment! no treatment!
   no treatment! no treatment!

CIVIL SERVANT

ESSEX HEMPHILL

FOR NURSE EUNICE RIVERS

I could perform my job no other way:
obey instructions or be dismissed,
which would end my nursing career.
I was a Colored nurse,
special, one of few.
I didn't question the authority
the government doctors exercised over me.
Their control of life and death
and my sense of duty and responsibility
were parallel and reciprocating.
My father, Tuskegee Institute, and Dr. Dibble
had trained me to obey
the instructions of white men,
and all men.
I didn't talk back,
raise my voice in protest,
or demand the doctors save the men.
It wasn't my place to diagnose,
prescribe, or agitate.

When the doctors told me
to prevent the men
from getting treatment elsewhere,
I did. I supplied their names
to all county health officials.
They agreed to withhold treatment
even after penicillin was discovered
to be an effective cure for bad blood.

Essex Hemphill was a well-known poet who died in 1995.
Originally published in Essex Hemphill, Ceremonies *(New York: Dutton, 1992), 22–24. Copyright*
© *1992 by Essex Hemphill. Used by permission of Dutton, Inc.*

The government doctors
viewed the men
as syphilis experiments.
I troubled myself
to remember their names.
I visited their homes
between annual checkups
to listen to their hearts
and feel their pulses.
They had aches and pains
and complaints too numerous to name,
but I soothed them. I tried.
I gave them spring tonic
for their blood.
I couldn't give them medicine.
I tried to care for everyone
including the women,
the old folks, and children.
I became an adopted member
of many of the families I visited.
I ate at their tables,
sat at their sickbeds,
mourned at their funerals.
I married one of their sons.

I never thought my duty
damned the men.
They were sick with bad blood,
but I thought they were lucky.
Most Colored folks in Macon
went from cradle to grave
without ever visiting a doctor.
The ones with bad blood were envied
because they received free
medical attention, food,
and rides to the health sites
come checkup time.

As the men died, I wept
with their wives and families.
I was there to comfort them,

to offer fifty dollars
if they let the doctors
"operate"—
cut open the deceased
from scrotum sack to skull.
They were usually horrified
by my offer,
fearing disfigurement
or the courting of blasphemy.
I assured them no one would know
that their hearts and brains
had been removed.
I suggested fifty dollars
could cover burial costs
and buy unexpected food
and clothes.

I never thought my silence
a symptom of bad blood.
I never considered my care complicity.
I was a Colored nurse, a proud
graduate of Tuskegee Institute,
one of few, honored by my profession.
I had orders, important duties,
a government career.

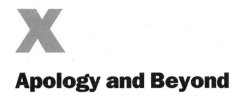

Apology and Beyond

LEGACY COMMITTEE REQUEST

Tuskegee Syphilis Study Legacy Committee[1]

In 1932, the United States Public Health Service (USPHS) initiated the Tuskegee Syphilis Study to document the natural history of syphilis. The subjects of the investigation were 399 poor black sharecroppers from Macon County, Alabama, with latent syphilis and 201 men without the disease who served as controls. The physicians conducting the Study deceived the men, telling them they were being treated for "bad blood."[2] However, they deliberately denied treatment to the men with syphilis and went to extreme lengths to ensure that they would not receive any therapy from other sources. In exchange for their participation, the men received free meals, free medical examinations, and burial insurance.[3]

On 26 July 1972 a front-page headline in the *New York Times* read, "Syphilis Victims in U.S. Study Went Untreated for 40 Years."[4] The accompanying article publicly revealed the details of the Tuskegee Syphilis Study—"the longest non-therapeutic experiment on human beings in medical history."[5] In the almost twenty-five years since its disclosure, the Study has moved from a singular historical event to a powerful metaphor. It has come to symbolize racism in medicine, ethical misconduct in human research, paternalism by physicians, and government abuse of vulnerable people.

The Tuskegee Syphilis Study continues to cast its long shadow on the contemporary relationship between African Americans and the biomedical community. Several recent articles have argued that the Tuskegee Syphilis Study has predisposed many African Americans to distrust medical and public health authorities.[6] The authors point to the Study as a significant factor in the low participation of African Americans in clinical trials and organ donation efforts and in the reluctance of many black people in seeking routine preventive care. As one AIDS educator put it, "so many African American people that I work with do not trust hospitals or any of the other community health care service providers because of that Tuskegee Experiment. It it like . . . if they did it then they will do it again."[7]

The Tuskegee Syphilis Study Legacy Committee is dedicated to preserving the

The Legacy Committee was formed in 1996 to pressure the U.S. government to make a formal apology to the survivors, their families, and the Tuskegee community.
Printed by permission of John C. Fletcher, cochair.

memory of the Study while moving beyond it, transforming the legacy into renewed efforts to bridge the chasm between the health conditions of black and white Americans. To this end, the Committee is pursuing two inseparable goals: 1) to persuade President Clinton to publicly apologize for past government wrongdoing to the Study's living survivors, their families, and to the Tuskegee community, and 2) to develop a strategy to redress the damages caused by the Study and to transform its damaging legacy.

In his recent apology for the government's role in human radiation experiments (1944–1974), President William J. Clinton claimed that "the American people . . . must be able to rely upon the United States to keep its word, to tell the truth, and to do the right thing," and that "when the government does wrong, we have a moral responsibility to admit it."[8] President Clinton is not alone in his belief that an apology for past wrongs is "doing the right thing." Recently, the Southern Baptist Church apologized to all African Americans for its stand on slavery during the Civil War and the Prime Minister of Japan similarly apologized to the people of the United States for the attack on Pearl Harbor.[9]

And yet, these apologies do not merely acknowledge wrongdoing: they act as a first step toward healing the wounds inflicted. President Clinton, for example, saw his apology as "laying the foundation stone for a new era"[10] in trying to regain the trust of the country.

It is within this context of doing the right thing, redressing past injuries, and regaining trust that the Committee adamantly believes that a Presidential apology to the victims of Tuskegee is critical to heal the devastating wounds that remain from this shameful episode in the history of medical research.

1. *A Presidential Apology for the Tuskegee Syphilis Study*
   a) *Moral and physical harms to the community of Macon County*

It is clear that the U.S. government scientists irreparably harmed hundreds of socially and economically vulnerable African-American men in Macon County, their family members, and their descendants by deliberately deceiving them and withholding from them state of the art treatment. When the Tuskegee Study began, the standard therapy for syphilis consisted of painful injections of arsenical compounds, supplemented by topical applications of mercury or bismuth ointments. Although this therapy was less effective than penicillin would later prove to be, in the 1930s every major textbook on syphilis recommended it for the treatment of the disease. After penicillin became available, the researchers withheld its use as well. Published medical reports have estimated that between 28 and 100 men died as a result of their syphilis.[11] Due to a lax study protocol, we cannot be sure that all the men had latent syphilis. It is therefore entirely possible that the infected men passed syphilis to their sexual partners and to their children in utero.[12] Thus physical harm may not be limited just to the men enrolled in the Study.

b) *No public apology has ever been made*

In the aftermath of a Health, Education and Welfare task force report, a Senate hearing, and an out of court legal settlement, the u.s. government provided economic compensation and continues to give free health benefits to the surviving subjects and their families. However, no public apology has ever been offered for the moral wrongdoing that occurred in the name of government medical research. No public official has ever stated clearly to the nation that the Tuskegee Syphilis Study was morally wrong from its inception, and no public official has ever apologized to the survivors and their families. Yet, an apology is sorely needed. The Committee believes that an apology from the President could facilitate the healing of the victims and the nation.

c) *The harmful legacy of the Study*

The historical record makes plain that African American's distrust of the medical profession predates the revelations of the Tuskegee Syphilis Study and involves a myriad of other social and political factors. Nevertheless, the Study has become a powerful symbol for the fear of exploitation in research and the deprivation of adequate medical care that is widespread in the African-American community. Recent articles argue that Tuskegee has created a climate of suspicion that taints the relationship between many African Americans and the medical profession. The Tuskegee Study is offered as the reason why few blacks participate in research trials,[13] why the need for transplant organs by African Americans widely surpasses the supply,[14] and why African Americans often avoid medical treatment.[15] It is also offered as an explanation as to why rumors about genocide persist in the African-American community, ranging from the notion that AIDS is a plot to exterminate black people to the idea that needle exchange programs fuel a drug epidemic that disproportionately affects black neighborhoods.[16] For many African Americans, the fact that the Tuskegee Study occurred at all proves that black life is not valued. The Committee believes that an apology combined with a strategy for addressing the damages of the Tuskegee legacy would begin the process of regaining the trust of people of color.

d) *The harm done to the community and the University*

Because the name of the Study points to Tuskegee Institute (now Tuskegee University) rather than the United States Public Health Service, it clouds the funding and responsibility for the Study. Although facilities and staff of the Tuskegee Institute were involved, primary direction came from the government under the auspices of the USPHS. The notoriety of the Study obscures the achievements of the Tuskegee Institute in improving the health care of African Americans. These achievements include initiating the National Negro Health Week, building the John A. Andrew Hospital, creating the John A. Andrew Clinical Society, establishing a nurse training school, and organizing a school for midwives.

The Apology: Context and Opportunity

The Committee urges President Clinton to apologize on behalf of the American government for the harms inflicted at Tuskegee. The apology should be directed to those most directly harmed: to the elderly survivors of the Study, to their families, and to the wider community of Tuskegee and its University. Also included within the apology should be all people of color whose lives reverberate with the consequences of the Study.

As the highest elected official of the United States, the President should offer the apology for the Study which was conducted under the auspices of the United States government. The significance of a presidential apology was recognized recently when the President apologized to those harmed by Cold War radiation experiments as a way to regain confidence of the American people. In the context of President Clinton's stated desire to bridge the racial divide, this apology provides the opportunity to begin to heal the racial wounds that persist in this country.

Given the ages of the living participants and the period of time since the Study was disclosed, we believe that the apology should be offered swiftly. There are only eleven survivors; a twelfth died as recently as March 3, 1996. We recommend that the government issue the apology from Tuskegee University, perhaps linked with an early meeting of the new National Bioethics Advisory Commission (NBEAC). Because the Tuskegee Study is a starting point for all modern moral reflection on research ethics, a meeting of the NBEAC at Tuskegee in conjunction with a presidential apology would be an ideal new beginning.

Transforming the Legacy

Although a public apology is necessary to heal the wounds of Tuskegee, it alone would not be sufficient to assure the nation that research like the Tuskegee Syphilis Study will not be duplicated. Despite the significance of a Presidential apology, it must not be an isolated event. Consequently, the Committee also recommends the development of a mechanism to move beyond Tuskegee and to address the effects of its legacy. The Committee strongly urges the development of a professionally staffed Center at Tuskegee University, focused on preserving the national memory of the Study and transforming its legacy.

Regret for past mistakes must be accompanied by a determination to prevent future wrongs. Until now for black Americans the legacy of the Tuskegee Syphilis Study has been a negative one—a symbol of their mistreatment within American society. The proposed Center could help transform the legacy of Tuskegee into a positive symbol for all Americans by demonstrating the importance of acknowledging past wrongs, rebuilding trust, and practicing ethical research.

The new Center's mission would be to preserve the national memory of the Syphilis Study for public education and scholarly research, and to analyze and disseminate findings on effective and ethically acceptable ways to address the profound mistrust that is the tragic and enduring legacy of this Study, especially among African Americans and other persons of color. (See Appendix 1.)

Although the Committee sees the creation of a Center as the most valuable attempt to redress the damages of Tuskegee, we envision several possible concurrent programs. These include:

1) a Minority Health Initiative, similar in scope to the newly established Women's Health Initiative;
2) training programs for health care providers to better understand the social and cultural issues of providing health care and of conducting research in communities of color;
3) a clearinghouse to help investigators conduct ethically responsible research.

The Committee recommends that funding for the Center must combine government and private funding. The announcement of a federal challenge grant would be very useful as a catalyst for future fundraising efforts.

It is undeniable that the Tuskegee Syphilis Study has adversely affected the attitudes that many African Americans hold toward the biomedical community and the United States government. But despite the long shadow that it casts, we now have an opportunity to challenge this legacy and create a more beneficial one.

Appendix 1

Possible functions for a Tuskegee research center:

a) to create and maintain a public museum in Tuskegee, Alabama, to preserve the memory of the Study and to provide a focal point for efforts to transform its negative legacy;
b) to provide a place for scholars to examine the ethical, legal, and social significance of the Study and other issues in bioethics;
c) to conduct public education on the Study and its legacy in schools, community organizations, and medical institutions;
d) to aid in the production of audiovisual aids for public education that will place the Study within its broadest social and historical context and provide suggestions for transforming its past legacy;
e) to assure the rigorous preservation of presently endangered documents and other records to further encourage studies of race, ethnicity, and medicine;
f) to offer support for medical researchers seeking ways to conduct research in diverse populations that is both scientifically sound and ethically responsible.

Appendix 2

Tuskegee Syphilis Study Legacy Committee

Ms. Myrtle Adams
  Chairman, Macon County Health Care Authority
  704 Patterson St.
  Tuskegee, AL 36088

Ms. Patricia Clay
  Administrator, Macon County Health Care Authority
  PO Drawer 180
  Tuskegee, AL 36088

Dr. James A. Ferguson
  Dean, School of Veterinary Medicine
  Patterson Hall
  Tuskegee University
  Tuskegee, AL 36088

Dr. John C. Fletcher, co-chair
  Director, Center for Biomedical Ethics
  Cornfield Professor of Religious Studies
  University of Virginia
  Box 348 HSC
  Charlottesville, VA 22908

Dr. Vanessa Northington Gamble, chair
  Associate Professor of History of Medicine and Family Medicine
  University of Wisconsin Medical School
  1300 University Ave.
  Madison, WI 53706

Dr. Lee Green
  Assistant Professor
  University of Alabama
  PO Box 870312
  Tuscaloosa, AL 35487

Ms. Barbara Harrell
  Director, Division of Minority Health
  Alabama Department of Public Health
  434 Monroe St.
  Montgomery, AL, 36130-3017

Dr. Bill Jenkins
  Epidemiologist
  Centers for Disease Control and Prevention
  1600 Clifton Road, NE, MS-E02
  Atlanta, GA 30333

Dr. James H. Jones
   Professor of History
   University of Houston
   2202 Swift Road
   Houston, TX 77030
Dr. Ralph Katz
   Professor
   Department of Behavioral Sciences and Community Health
   School of Dental Medicine
   University of Connecticut Health Center
   Farmington, CT 06030
Ms. Joan Echtenkamp Klein
   Assistant Director for Historical Collection and Services
   Health Sciences Library, Box 234
   University of Virginia Health Sciences Center
   Charlottesville, VA 22908
Dr. Susan Reverby
   Luella LaMer Professor for Women's Studies
   Wellesley College
   106 Central St.
   Wellesley, MA 02181
Dr. Reuben Warren
   Associate Director for Minority Health, CDC
   Centers for Disease Control and Prevention
   1600 Clifton Road, NE, MS-D39
   Atlanta, GA, 30333
Mr. Anthony Winn
   Program Analyst
   Minority Health Professions Foundation
   20 Executive Park Drive, #2021
   Atlanta, GA 30333

NOTES

1. The Committee was established at a meeting at Tuskegee University, January 18–19, 1996. All communications with the Committee should be addressed to the Chair of the Committee, Vanessa Gamble, M.D., PhD, History of Medicine Department, 1300 University Ave., Madison, WI 53706 (608) 262-5319. FAX: (608) 262-2317; email: vngamble@facstaff.wisc.edu. A list of the Committee members is attached. The Committee wishes to thank Judith A. Houck for her assistance in the preparation of this report.

2. The term "bad blood" encompassed several conditions including syphilis, anemia, and fatigue.

3. For a complete history see Jones, James H, *Bad Blood: The Tuskegee Syphilis Experiment*, new and expanded ed., New York: Free Press, 1993.

4. Jean Heller, "Syphilis Victims in the U.S. Study Went Untreated for 40 Years," *New York Times,* 26 July 1972: 1, 8. The story first broke the previous day in the *Washington Star.*

5. Jones, *Bad Blood,* 91.

6. See for example, Asim, Jabari, "Black paranoia far-fetched? Maybe, but understandable," *The Phoenix Gazette* February 23, 1993 Op-Ed: A13; Karkabi, Barbara, "Blacks' health problems addressed," *The Houston Chronicle* April 10, 1994 Lifestyle: 3; "Knowledge, attitudes and behavior; conspiracy theories about HIV puts individuals at risk," *AIDS Weekly,* November 13, 1995.

7. Thomas, Stephen B. and Quinn, Sandra Crouse, "The Tuskegee Syphilis Study, 1932–1972: Implications for HIV Education and AIDS Risk Programs in the Black Community," *Am J of Pub Health.* 1991; 81: 1503.

8. President William J. Clinton, "In Acceptance of Human Radiation Final Report," Washington, DC, October 3, 1995.

9. See for example, Neibuhr, Gustav, "Baptist group votes to repent stand on slaves," *New York Times* 21 June, 1995: A2 and Watanabe, Teresa and David Holley, "Japan Premier offers apology for WWII role," *Chicago Tribune* 15 August, 1995: A10.

10. Clinton, 3 October, 1995.

11. Jones, *Bad Blood,* 2.

12. Hammonds, Evelynn M, "Your silence will not protect you: Nurse Eunice Rivers and the Tuskegee Syphilis Study," in *The Black Women's Health Book: Speaking for Ourselves* ed. Evelyn C. White, 2nd ed., Seattle: Seal Press, 1994: 323–331.

13. Gamble, Vanessa, "A Legacy of Distrust: African Americans and Medical Research," *Am J of Preventive Medicine,* November/December 1993: 35–38.

14. "Fear Creates Lack of Donor Organs Among Blacks," Weekend Edition, National Public Radio, 13 March 1994.

15. See for example, Voas, Sharon, "Aging black sick, scared; past abuses, tradition keep them from clinic," *Pittsburgh Post-Gazette,* August 27, 1995: B1.

16. Bates, KG, "Is it Genocide?" *Essence,* September 1990: 76; Thomas, Stephen, and Quinn, Sandra, "Understanding the Attitudes of Black Americans," In Stryker, J. and Smith, MD, eds. *Dimensions of HIV Preventions: Needle Exchange,* Menlo Park: The Henry J. Kaiser Family Foundation; 1993: 99–128; Kirp, David and Bayer, Ronald, "Needles and Race," *Atlantic.* July 1993: 38–42.

STATEMENT OF ATTORNEY FRED GRAY

Press Conference, April 8, 1997, Shiloh Missionary Baptist Church

Statement of Fred D. Gray Attorney for the Living Participants and the Heirs of the Deceased Participants in the Tuskegee Syphilis Study

Fred D. Gray has represented the participants in the Tuskegee Syphilis Study from July, 1972 to date. This statement is being released during a press conference held at Shiloh Missionary Baptist Church, in Notasulga, Macon County, Alabama on April 8, 1997. In addition to Attorney Gray and members of his law firm, the following participants of the Study are also present: Charlie Pollard, Herman Shaw, Carter Howard, Fred Simmons and Ernest Hendon.

The First Traumatic Experience

Sixty-five years ago, beginning in 1932, the United States Government, through its public health service, committed one of the greatest frauds, injustices, and misrepresentations against 623 African-Americans who were citizens of Macon County, Alabama. The men were misled into participating in a study of untreated syphilis sponsored, financed, and supported by the federal government for over 40 years. The government induced these men to participate in a program in which the government represented that the participants were being treated for whatever their ailments were, even though they were not told the ailment. They never gave their consent to be involved in the Study, nor did they realize that they were a part of a Study until the story broke in July of 1972. There were no rules and regulations governing the Study. Available at this press conference is a copy of Chapter 17 of *Bus Ride To Justice* by Fred D. Gray, published by Black Belt Press. This chapter sets forth in detail the facts and circumstances surrounding the Study. An accurate account of the Study can also be found in *Bad Blood* by James H. Jones.

In response to the national showing of the film Miss Evers' Boys *in February 1996 and to request a formal federal apology, attorney Fred D. Gray and five of the study survivors called a press conference at the Shiloh Missionary Baptist Church on 8 April 1997.*
Reprinted by permission of Fred D. Gray Sr.

In July 1972, Fred D. Gray began to represent these participants and on July 24, 1973, filed a lawsuit which was amended on August 1, 1974.

In 1974, the lawsuit was settled, and the Government agreed to pay approximately seven million dollars to the living participants and the heirs of the deceased participants. Subsequent to the disbursement of these funds, interest on the proceeds has also been disbursed to the participants and heirs. In total, more than 6,000 persons have shared in the settlement. As a part of the settlement agreement, the government was ordered to continue its program of providing health care for the living participants and some widows of participants for the rest of their lives, and to provide free burial service for the participants at their death. The government also terminated the Study.

As a result of the publicity, Congress passed laws which prohibit similar occurrences to what occurred in the Tuskegee Syphilis Study. Safeguards are now in place to ensure that what happened to these men will never happen to any other human being.

The government's persuasion of these men to participate in the Study was the first traumatic experience that occurred in 1932. Other traumatic occurrences have happened since then with regard to these men.

The Second Traumatic Experience

On February 22, 1997, during Black History Month and on President Lincoln's birthday, Home Box Office telecast its premiere of a movie called *Miss Evers' Boys*. Allegedly, *Miss Evers' Boys* was based on the facts involving the participants in the Tuskegee Syphilis Study. The film does not accurately portray the facts of what occurred to the participants in the Tuskegee Syphilis Study. Thus, the premiere showing of *Miss Evers' Boys* and its repeated showings were another great tragedy which occurred in the lives of these men. On Monday, February 24th, four of the participants reviewed *Miss Evers' Boys* and the following are their comments and the comments of their counsel, Fred D. Gray, on some of the inaccuracies and how they feel about *Miss Evers' Boys*:

1. They were startled, amazed, and very unhappy about the way in which they were projected in the movie. They feel unanimously that the film does not accurately portray the events and circumstances of the Tuskegee Syphilis Study as they participated in it, and as they observed Miss Eunice Rivers, the nurse involved in the Study.
2. The movie opened by stating that these men were solicited to participate in a program for treatment of syphilis, and that they were treated over a period

of time until such time as the money for treatment became unavailable. The movie further stated that treatment was discontinued for the lack of funds. However, according to the movie, money became available to study untreated syphilis in the men. **The fact is, the participants in the Tuskegee Syphilis Study were never treated for syphilis from the beginning of Study until the end.**

3. The film showed a Dr. Brady, an African-American physician who was projected as the supervisor of the Study, and Miss Rivers' immediate supervisor. There was no such African-American who generally supervised Miss Rivers nor the Study. All of the supervisors were white. The persons who conceived and presented the matter to the health service for financing were all white. The doctors who actually came to Macon County and examined these individuals were all whites, and not African-Americans. The white Macon County health officer, Dr. Murry D. Smith accompanied Miss Rivers when they were recruiting participants for the Study.

4. The entire emphasis of the film tends to shift the blame from the federal government to an African-American doctor and an African-American nurse. This Study was conceived, financed, executed, and administered by the federal government. The African-American professionals who participated in it were victims as were the 623 African-American participants.

5. The film conspicuously omits the role that the State of Alabama, through its Board of Health played in the Study. The Alabama Health Department cooperated with the federal government in continuing not to treat the participants after penicillin became available, notwithstanding the fact that Alabama laws required such treatment.

6. In the film, there were four men who were projected as *Miss Evers' Boys*. They, basically, were projected as musicians and dancers, and they represented the other 619 men who participated in the Study. That is not true. The men who participated in the Study, for the most part, were hard working, reputable persons in their communities. Each of my clients, after reviewing the film, stated, Miss Rivers was always professional and courteous to them. She did not accompany them to night clubs. They did not dance, play music and entertain people at night clubs with Miss Rivers. The entire depiction of them as dancers and "shuffling sams" is a great misrepresentation, and does not accurately represent them, nor the other persons who were participants in this study.

7. From this general representation of these four men, not only will viewers of the movie think that they were representative of the other 619 men who were in the Study, but viewers would also believe that these men were

typical of African-Americans who lived in Macon County at that time and even now. It is a tremendous insult and a gross misrepresentation of projecting African-American men as being typical of those projected as the four *Miss Evers' Boys.*

8. There is nothing in the historical account and nothing that these men remember observing about Miss Rivers which would indicate that she had a love affair with one or more of the participants as it was set forth in the film. Miss Rivers did not give penicillin to one participant and withhold it from all the others.

Don't Subject the Participants of the Tuskegee Syphilis Study to a Third Traumatic Experience

Some 65 years after the Study began and over 25 years with knowledge of the Study, local and national community support of these participants has finally come by way of requesting that the federal government make an apology to these individuals for the harm, embarrassment, and injuries that it has caused them and their heirs. I am informed that several persons and organizations have requested that the government make an apology to these men. We understand that the Honorable Donna Shalala, Secretary of Health and Human Services, has discussed this matter with the President. The participants and their counsel join in the request for such an apology. To date, no official contact has been made from the federal government to the participants nor their counsel concerning an apology. The participants have some views concerning an apology.

In additional to an apology, the participants believe that they should be appropriately recognized for their contributions to the nation.

In a letter to President Clinton dated March 26, 1997, as counsel for the participants I stated:

> There are eight living participants, the youngest of whom is 87 years old. In view of the fact that these men and their heirs have suffered substantially, the remaining participants and I would consider it an honor to meet with you to discuss an appropriate manner to resolve the issue. On behalf of these men, we are ready, willing and able to share their views with you or your representatives at your convenience.

In 1932, these men were taken advantage of by being used as human guinea pigs. Their lives were placed in jeopardy as part of a Study on the effects of untreated syphilis without their knowledge and consent. Sixty-five years later, they have been entirely misrepresented in the manner they are projected in *Miss Evers' Boys.* They are now requesting that an appropriate apology be made, and they be recognized for the contributions they made to the nation.

On Monday, April 7, 1997, counsel for the participants received a telephone call from The White House. He was informed that his letter was received and was under consideration. Counsel believes that the President will act favorable upon our request.

HERMAN SHAW'S REMARKS

Friday, May 16, 1997, The White House, Washington, D.C.

Statement of Herman Shaw
Living Participant in Tuskegee Syphilis Study

On behalf of all the survivors who are here today, and those who could not attend, and on behalf of the heirs of my fellow participants who have died, I wish to thank President Clinton for inviting us to the White House. It has been over 65 years since we entered the program. We are delighted today to close this very tragic and painful chapter in our lives.

We were treated unfairly and to some extent like guinea pigs. We were not pigs. We were not dancing boys as we were projected in the movie, *Miss Evers' Boys*. We were all hard working men, not boys, and citizens of the United States. The wounds that were inflicted upon us cannot be undone.

I am saddened today to think of those who did not survive and whose families will forever live with the knowledge that their death and suffering was preventable.

Mr. President, we want to also thank our lawyer, Attorney Fred Gray, who has represented us during these 25 years, and who has helped to make this day possible.

This ceremony is important because the damage done by the Tuskegee Study is much deeper than the wounds any of us may have suffered. It speaks to our faith in government and the ability of medical science to serve as a force for good.

As I said at the press conference at Shiloh Missionary Baptist Church in Notasulga, on April 8, in addition to an apology, we want to construct in Tuskegee a PERMANENT MEMORIAL. A place where our children and grandchildren will be able to see the contributions that we, and others, made to this country. I am glad that I have helped form the Tuskegee Human Rights Multicultural Center which will be for the purpose of creating such a lasting memorial.

In my opinion, it is never too late to work to restore faith and trust. And so, a quarter of a century after the Study ended, President Clinton's decision to gather us here; to allow us to finally put this horrible nightmare behind us as a nation, is a most welcomed decision.

Mr. Herman Shaw of Tallassee, Alabama, became the key spokesman for the survivors of the study. He died in December 1999 at the age of ninety-seven.
Statement handed out at the White House, 16 May 1996.

In order for America to reach its fullest potential we must truly be one America—black, red and white together; trusting each other, caring for each other, and never allowing the kind of tragedy which happened to us in the Tuskegee Study to ever occur again.

Mr. President, words cannot express my gratitude to you for bringing us here today—for doing your best to right this tragic wrong, and resolving that America should never again allow such an event to occur. Because of your leadership I am confident that we never will.

Now, ladies and gentlemen, I have the great pleasure of doing something I always wanted to do and never thought I would have the privilege. I present to you the Honorable William Clinton, President of the United States.

PRESIDENT WILLIAM J. CLINTON'S REMARKS

Remarks by the President in Apology for Study Done in Tuskegee

The East Room

2:26 P.M. EDT

THE PRESIDENT: Ladies and gentlemen, on Sunday, Mr. Shaw will celebrate his 95th birthday. (Applause.) I would like to recognize the other survivors who are here today and their families: Mr. Charlie Pollard is here. (Applause.) Mr. Carter Howard. (Applause.) Mr. Fred Simmons. (Applause.) Mr. Simmons just took his first airplane ride, and he reckons he's about 110 years old, so I think it's time for him to take a chance or two. (Laughter.) I'm glad he did. And Mr. Frederick Moss, thank you, sir. (Applause.)

I would also like to ask three family representatives who are here—Sam Doner is represented by his daughter, Gwendolyn Cox. Thank you, Gwendolyn. (Applause.) Ernest Hendon, who is watching in Tuskegee, is represented by his brother, North Hendon. Thank you, sir, for being here. (Applause.) And George Key is represented by his grandson, Christopher Monroe. Thank you, Chris. (Applause.)

I also acknowledge the families, community leaders, teachers and students watching today by satellite from Tuskegee. The White House is the people's house; we are glad to have all of you here today. I thank Dr. David Satcher for his role in this. I thank Congresswoman Waters and Congressman Hilliard, Congressman Stokes, the entire Congressional Black Caucus. Dr. Satcher, members of the Cabinet who are here, Secretary Herman, Secretary Slater, a great friend of freedom, Fred Gray, thank you for fighting this long battle all these long years.

The eight men who are survivors of the syphilis study at Tuskegee are a living link to a time not so very long ago that many Americans would prefer not to remember, but we dare not forget. It was a time when our nation failed to live up to its ideals, when our nation broke the trust with our people that is the very foundation of our democracy. It is not only in remembering that shameful past that we can make amends and repair our nation, but it is in remembering that past that

William J. Clinton was president of the United States in 1996 when the formal federal apology was provided.
Press Release, The White House, Office of Press Secretary, 16 May 1996.

we can build a better present and a better future. And without remembering it, we cannot make amends and we cannot go forward.

So today America does remember the hundreds of men used in research without their knowledge and consent. We remember them and their family members. Men who were poor and African American, without resources and with few alternatives, they believed they had found hope when they were offered free medical care by the United States Public Health Service. They were betrayed.

Medical people are supposed to help when we need care, but even once a cure was discovered, they were denied help, and they were lied to by their government. Our government is supposed to protect the rights of its citizens; their rights were trampled upon. Forty years, hundreds of men betrayed, along with their wives and children, along with the community in Macon County, Alabama, the City of Tuskegee, the fine university there, and the larger African American community.

The United States government did something that was wrong—deeply, profoundly, morally wrong. It was an outrage to our commitment to integrity and equality for all our citizens.

To the survivors, to the wives and family members, the children and the grandchildren, I say what you know: No power on Earth can give you back the lives lost, the pain suffered, the years of internal torment and anguish. What was done cannot be undone. But we can end the silence. We can stop turning our heads away. We can look at you in the eye and finally say on behalf of the American people, what the United States government did was shameful, and I am sorry. (Applause.)

The American people are sorry—for the loss, for the years of hurt. You did nothing wrong, but you were grievously wronged. I apologize and I am sorry that this apology has been so long in coming. (Applause.)

To Macon County, to Tuskegee, to the doctors who have been wrongly associated with the events there, you have our apology, as well. To our African American citizens, I am sorry that your federal government orchestrated a study so clearly racist. That can never be allowed to happen again. It is against everything our country stands for and what we must stand against is what it was.

So let us resolve to hold forever in our hearts and minds the memory of a time not long ago in Macon County, Alabama, so that we can always see how adrift we can become when the rights of any citizens are neglected, ignored and betrayed. And let us resolve here and now to move forward together.

The legacy of the study at Tuskegee has reached far and deep, in ways that hurt our progress and divide our nation. We cannot be one America when a whole segment of our nation has no trust in America. An apology is the first step, and we take it with a commitment to rebuild that broken trust. We can begin by making sure there is never again another episode like this one. We need to do more to ensure that medical research practices are sound and ethical, and that researchers work more closely with communities.

Today I would like to announce several steps to help us achieve these goals. First, we will help to build that lasting memorial at Tuskegee. (Applause.) The school founded by Booker T. Washington, distinguished by the renowned scientist George Washington Carver and so many others who advanced the health and well-being of African Americans and all Americans, is a fitting site. The Department of Health and Human Services will award a planning grant so the school can pursue establishing a center for bioethics in research and health care. The center will serve as a museum of the study and support efforts to address its legacy and strengthen bioethics training.

Second, we commit to increase our community involvement so that we may begin restoring lost trust. The study at Tuskegee served to sow distrust of our medical institutions, especially where research is involved. Since the study was halted, abuses have been checked by making informed consent and local review mandatory in federally-funded and mandated research.

Still, 25 years later, many medical studies have little African American participation and African American organ donors are few. This impedes efforts to conduct promising research and to provide the best health care to all our people, including African Americans. So today, I'm directing the Secretary of Health and Human Services, Donna Shalala, to issue a report in 180 days about how we can best involve communities, especially minority communities, in research and health care. You must—every American group must be involved in medical research in ways that are positive. We have put the curse behind us; now we must bring the benefits to all Americans. (Applause.)

Third, we commit to strengthen researchers' training in bioethics. We are constantly working on making breakthroughs in protecting the health of our people and in vanquishing diseases. But all our people must be assured that their rights and dignity will be respected as new drugs, treatments and therapies are tested and used. So I am directing Secretary Shalala to work in partnership with higher education to prepare training materials for medical researchers. They will be available in a year. They will help researchers build on core ethical principles of respect for individuals, justice and informed consent, and advise them on how to use these principles effectively in diverse populations.

Fourth, to increase and broaden our understanding of ethical issues and clinical research, we commit to providing postgraduate fellowships to train bioethicists especially among African Americans and other minority groups. HHS will offer these fellowships beginning in September of 1998 to promising students enrolled in bioethics graduate programs.

And, finally, by executive order I am also today extending the charter of the National Bioethics Advisory Commission to October of 1999. The need for this commission is clear. We must be able to call on the thoughtful, collective wisdom of experts and community representatives to find ways to further strengthen our protections for subjects in human research.

We face a challenge in our time. Science and technology are rapidly changing our lives with the promise of making us much healthier, much more productive and more prosperous. But with these changes we must work harder to see that as we advance we don't leave behind our conscience. No ground is gained and, indeed, much is lost if we lose our moral bearings in the name of progress.

The people who ran the study at Tuskegee diminished the stature of man by abandoning the most basic ethical precepts. They forgot their pledge to heal and repair. They had the power to heal the survivors and all the others and they did not. Today, all we can do is apologize. But you have the power, for only you—Mr. Shaw, the others who are here, the family members who are with us in Tuskegee—only you have the power to forgive. Your presence here shows us that you have chosen a better path than your government did so long ago. You have not withheld the power to forgive. I hope today and tomorrow every American will remember your lesson and live by it.

Thank you, and God bless you. (Applause.)

2:41 P.M. EDT

THE ETHICS OF CLINICAL RESEARCH IN THE THIRD WORLD

MARCIA ANGELL

An essential ethical condition for a randomized clinical trial comparing two treatments for a disease is that there be no good reason for thinking one is better than the other.[1,2] Usually, investigators hope and even expect that the new treatment will be better, but there should not be solid evidence one way or the other. If there is, not only would the trial be scientifically redundant, but the investigators would be guilty of knowingly giving inferior treatment to some participants in the trial. The necessity for investigators to be in this state of equipoise[2] applies to placebo-controlled trials, as well. Only when there is no known effective treatment is it ethical to compare a potential new treatment with a placebo. When effective treatment exists, a placebo may not be used. Instead, subjects in the control group of the study must receive the best known treatment. Investigators are responsible for all subjects enrolled in a trial, not just some of them, and the goals of the research are always secondary to the well-being of the participants. Those requirements are made clear in the Declaration of Helsinki of the World Health Organization (WHO), which is widely regarded as providing the fundamental guiding principles of research involving human subjects.[3] It states, "In research on man [sic], the interest of science and society should never take precedence over considerations related to the wellbeing of the subject," and "In any medical study, every patient—including those of a control group, if any—should be assured of the best proven diagnostic and therapeutic method."

One reason ethical codes are unequivocal about investigators' primary obligation to care for the human subjects of their research is the strong temptation to subordinate the subjects' welfare to the objectives of the study. That is particularly likely when the research question is extremely important and the answer would probably improve the care of future patients substantially. In those circumstances, it is sometimes argued explicitly that obtaining a rapid, unambiguous answer to the research question is the primary ethical obligation. With the most altruistic of motives, then, researchers may find themselves slipping across a line that prohibits treating human subjects as means to an end. When that line is crossed, there is very

Dr. Marcia Angell is the editor of the New England Journal of Medicine.
Originally published in the New England Journal of Medicine, 337 (September 1997): 847–49.
Reprinted by permission of the publishing division of the Massachusetts Medical Society.

little left to protect patients from a callous disregard of their welfare for the sake of research goals. Even informed consent, important though it is, is not protection enough, because of the asymmetry in knowledge and authority between researchers and their subjects. And approval by an institutional review board, though also important, is highly variable in its responsiveness to patients' interests when they conflict with the interests of researchers.

A textbook example of unethical research is the Tuskegee Study of Untreated Syphilis.[4] In that study, which was sponsored by the U.S. Public Health Service and lasted from 1932 to 1972, 412 poor African-American men with untreated syphilis were followed and compared with 204 men free of the disease to determine the natural history of syphilis. Although there was no very good treatment available at the time the study began (heavy metals were the standard treatment), the research continued even after penicillin became widely available and was known to be highly effective against syphilis. The study was not terminated until it came to the attention of a reporter and the outrage provoked by front-page stories in the *Washington Star* and *New York Times* embarrassed the Nixon administration into calling a halt to it.[5] The ethical violations were multiple: Subjects did not provide informed consent (indeed, they were deliberately deceived); they were denied the best known treatment; and the study was continued even after highly effective treatment became available. And what were the arguments in favor of the Tuskegee study? That these poor African-American men probably would not have been treated anyway, so the investigators were merely observing what would have happened if there were no study; and that the study was important (a "never-to-be-repeated opportunity," said one physician after penicillin became available).[6] Ethical concern was even stood on its head when it was suggested that not only was the information valuable, but it was especially so for people like the subjects—an impoverished rural population with a very high rate of untreated syphilis. The only lament seemed to be that many of the subjects inadvertently received treatment by other doctors.

Some of these issues are raised by Lurie and Wolfe elsewhere in this issue of the *Journal*. They discuss the ethics of ongoing trials in the Third World of regimens to prevent the vertical transmission of human immunodeficiency virus (HIV) infection.[7] All except one of the trials employ placebo-treated control groups, despite the fact that zidovudine has already been clearly shown to cut the rate of vertical transmission greatly and is now recommended in the United States for all HIV-infected pregnant women. The justifications are reminiscent of those for the Tuskegee study: Women in the Third World would not receive antiretroviral treatment anyway, so the investigators are simply observing what would happen to the subjects' infants if there were no study. And a placebo-controlled study is the fastest, most efficient way to obtain unambiguous information that will be of greatest value in the Third World. Thus, in response to protests from Wolfe and others to the secretary of Health and Human Services, the directors of the National Institutes of Health (NIH) and the Centers for Disease Control and Prevention (CDC)—the organizations sponsoring the studies—argued, "It is an unfortunate fact that the current standard of perinatal care for the HIV-infected pregnant women in the sites of the studies does not include any HIV prophylactic intervention at all," and the inclusion of placebo controls "will result in the most rapid, accurate, and reliable answer to the question of the value of the intervention being studied compared to the local standard of care."[8]

Also in this issue of the *Journal*, Whalen et al. report the results of a clinical trial in Uganda of various regimens of prophylaxis against tuberculosis in HIV-infected adults, most of whom had positive tuberculin skin tests.[9] This study, too, employed a placebo-treated control group, and in some ways it is analogous to the studies criticized by Lurie and Wolfe. In the United States it would probably be impossible to carry out such a study, because of long-standing official recommendations that HIV-infected persons with positive tuberculin skin tests receive prophylaxis against tuberculosis. The first was issued in 1990 by the CDC's Advisory Committee for Elimination of Tuberculosis.[10] It stated that tuberculin-test-positive persons with HIV infection "should be considered candidates for preventive therapy." Three years later, the recommendation was reiterated more strongly in a joint statement by the American Thoracic Society and the CDC, in collaboration with the Infectious Diseases Society of America and the American Academy of Pediatrics.[11] According to this statement, "the identification of persons with dual infection and the administration of preventive therapy to these persons is of great importance." However, some believe that these recommendations were premature, since they were based largely on the success of prophylaxis in HIV-negative persons.[12]

Whether the study by Whalen et al. was ethical depends, in my view, entirely on the strength of the preexisting evidence. Only if there was genuine doubt about the benefits of prophylaxis would a placebo group be ethically justified. This is not the place to review the scientific evidence, some of which is discussed in the editorial of Msamanga and Fawzi elsewhere in this issue.[13] Suffice it to say that the case is debatable. Msamanga and Fawzi conclude that "future studies should not include a placebo group, since preventive therapy should be considered the standard of care." I agree. The difficult question is whether there should have been a placebo group in the first place.

Although I believe an argument can be made that a placebo-controlled trial was ethically justifiable because it was still uncertain whether prophylaxis would work, it should not be argued that it was ethical because no prophylaxis is the "local standard of care" in sub-Saharan Africa. For reasons discussed by Lurie and Wolfe, that reasoning is badly flawed.[7] As mentioned earlier, the Declaration of Helsinki requires control groups to receive the "best" current treatment, not the local one. The shift in wording between "best" and "local" may be slight, but the implications are profound. Acceptance of this ethical relativism could result in widespread exploitation of vulnerable Third World populations for research programs that could not be carried out in the sponsoring country.[14] Furthermore, it directly contradicts the Department of Health and Human Services' own regulations governing U.S.-sponsored research in foreign countries,[15] as well as joint guidelines for research in the Third World issued by WHO and the Council for International Organizations of Medical Sciences,[16] which require that human subjects receive protection at least equivalent to that in the sponsoring country. The fact that Whalen et al. offered isoniazid to the placebo group when it was found superior to placebo indicates that they were aware of their responsibility to all the subjects in the trial.

The *Journal* has taken the position that it will not publish reports of unethical research, regardless of their scientific merit.[14,17] After deliberating at length about the study by Whalen et al., the editors concluded that publication was ethically justified, although there remain differences among us. The fact that the subjects gave informed consent and the study was approved by the institutional review board at the University Hospitals of Cleveland and Case Western Reserve University and by the Ugandan National AIDS Research Subcommittee certainly supported our decision but did not allay all our misgivings. It is still important to determine whether clinical studies are consistent with preexisting, widely accepted ethical guidelines, such as the Declaration of Helsinki, and with federal regulations, since they cannot be influenced by pressures specific to a particular study.

Quite apart from the merits of the study by Whalen et al., there is a larger issue. There appears to be a general retreat from the clear principles enunciated in the Nuremberg Code and the Declaration of Helsinki as applied to research in the Third World. Why is that? Is it because the "local standard of care" is different? I don't think so. In my view, that is merely a self-serving justification after the fact. Is it because diseases and their treatments are very different in the Third World, so that information gained in the industrialized world has no relevance and we have to start from scratch? That, too, seems an unlikely explanation, although here again it is often offered as a justification. Sometimes there may be relevant differences between populations, but that cannot be assumed. Unless there are specific indications to the contrary, the safest and most reasonable position is that people everywhere are likely to respond similarly to the same treatment.

I think we have to look elsewhere for the real reasons. One of them may be a slavish adherence to the tenets of clinical trials. According to these, all trials should be randomized, double-blind, and placebo-controlled, if at all possible. That rigidity may explain the NIH's pressure on Marc Lallemant to include a placebo group in his study, as described by Lurie and Wolfe.[7] Sometimes journals are blamed for the problem, because they are thought to demand strict conformity to the standard methods. That is not true, at least not at this journal. We do not want a scientifically neat study if it is ethically flawed, but like Lurie and Wolfe we believe that in many cases it is possible, with a little ingenuity, to have both scientific and ethical rigor.

The retreat from ethical principles may also be explained by some of the exigencies of doing clinical research in an increasingly regulated and competitive environment. Research in the Third World looks relatively attractive as it becomes better funded and regulations at home become more restrictive. Despite the existence of codes requiring that human subjects receive at least the same protection abroad as at home, they are still honored partly in the breach. The fact remains that many studies are done in the Third World that simply could not be done in the countries sponsoring the work. Clinical trials have become a big business, with many of the same imperatives. To survive, it is necessary to get the work done as quickly as possible, with a minimum of obstacles. When these considerations prevail, it seems as if we have not come very far from Tuskegee after all. Those of us in the research community need to redouble our commitment to the highest ethical standards, no matter where the research is conducted, and sponsoring agencies need to enforce those standards, not undercut them.

REFERENCES

1. Angell M. Patients' preferences in randomized clinical trials. *N Engl J Med* 1984;310:1385–7.

2. Freedman B. Equipoise and the ethics of clinical research. *N Engl J Med* 1987;317:141–5.

3. Declaration of Helsinki IV, 41st World Medical Assembly, Hong Kong, September 1989. In: Annas GI, Grodin MA, eds. *The Nazi doctors and the Nuremberg Code: human rights in human experimentation.* New York: Oxford University Press, 1992:339–42.

4. Twenty years after: the legacy of the Tuskegee syphilis study. *Hastings Cent Rep* 1992: 22(6):29–40.

5. Caplan AL. When evil intrudes. *Hastings Cent Rep* 1992;22(6):29–32.

6. The development of consent requirements in research ethics. In: Faden RR, Beauchamp TL. *A history and theory of informed consent.* New York: Oxford University Press, 1986:151–99.

7. Lurie P, Wolfe SM. Unethical trials of interventions to reduce perinatal transmission of the human immunodeficiency virus in developing countries. *N Engl J Med* 1997;337:853–6.

8. The conduct of clinical trials of maternal-infant transmission of HIV supported by the United States Department of Health and Human Services in developing countries. Washington, D.C.: Department of Health and Human Services, July 1997.

9. Whalen CC, Johnson JL, Okwera A, et al. A trial of three regimens to prevent tuberculosis in Ugandan adults infected with the human immunodeficiency virus. *N Engl J Med* 1997;337:801–8.

10. The use of preventive therapy for tuberculosis infection in the United States: recommendations of the Advisory Committee for Elimination of Tuberculosis. *MMWR Morb Mortal Wkly Rep* 1990;39(RR-8):9–12.

11. Bass JB Jr, Farer LS, Hopewell PC, et al. Treatment of tuberculosis and tuberculosis infection in adults and children. *Am J Respir Crit Care Med* 1994;149:1359–74.

12. De Cock KM, Grant A, Porter JD. Preventive therapy for tuberculosis in HIV-infected persons: international recommendations, research, and practice. *Lancet* 1995;345:833–6.

13. Msamanga GI, Fawzi WW. The double burden of HIV infection and tuberculosis in sub-Saharan Africa. *N Engl J Med* 1997;337:849–51.

14. Angell M. Ethical imperialism? Ethics in international collaborative clinical research. *N Engl J Med* 1988;319:1081–3.

15. Protection of human subjects 45 CFR § 46 (1996).

16. International ethical guidelines for biomedical research involving human subjects. Geneva: Council for International Organizations of Medical Sciences, 1993.

17. Angell M. The Nazi hypothermia experiments and unethical research today. *N Engl J Med* 1990;322:1462–4.

ETHICAL COMPLEXITIES OF CONDUCTING
RESEARCH IN DEVELOPING COUNTRIES

HAROLD VARMUS & DAVID SATCHER

One of the great challenges in medical research is to conduct clinical trials in developing countries that will lead to therapies that benefit the citizens of these countries. Features of many developing countries—poverty, endemic diseases, and a low level of investment in health care systems—affect both the ease of performing trials and the selection of trials that can benefit the populations of the countries. Trials that make use of impoverished populations to test drugs for use solely in developed countries violate our most basic understanding of ethical behavior. Trials that apply scientific knowledge to interventions that can be used to benefit such populations are appropriate but present their own ethical challenges. How do we balance the ethical premises on which our work is based with the calls for public health partnerships from our colleagues in developing countries?

Some commentators have been critical of research performed in developing countries that might not be found ethically acceptable in developed countries. Specifically, questions have been raised about trials of interventions to prevent maternal-infant transmission of the human immunodeficiency virus (HIV) that have been sponsored by the National Institutes of Health (NIH) and the Centers for Disease Control and Prevention (CDC).[1,2] Although these commentators raise important issues, they have not adequately considered the purpose and complexity of such trials and the needs of the countries involved. They also allude inappropriately to the infamous Tuskegee study, which did not test an intervention. The Tuskegee study ultimately deprived people of a known, effective, affordable intervention. To claim that countries seeking help in stemming the tide of maternal-infant HIV transmission by seeking usable interventions have followed that path, trivializes the suffering of the men in the Tuskegee study and shows a serious lack of understanding of today's trials.

After the Tuskegee study was made public, in the 1970s, a national commission was established to develop principles and guidelines for the protection of research subjects. The new system of protection was described in the Belmont report.[3]

Dr. Harold Varmus was the director of the National Institutes of Health, and Dr. David Satcher is the surgeon general of the United States.
Originally published in the New England Journal of Medicine 337 (October 1997): 1003–5.
Reprinted by permission of the publishing division of the Massachusetts Medical Society.

Although largely compatible with the World Medical Association's Declaration of Helsinki,[4] the Belmont report articulated three principles: respect for persons (the recognition of the right of persons to exercise autonomy), beneficence (the minimization of risk incurred by research subjects and the maximization of benefits to them and others), and justice (the principle that therapeutic investigations should not unduly involve persons from groups unlikely to benefit from subsequent applications of the research).

There is an inherent tension among these three principles. Over the years, we have seen the focus of debate shift from concern about the burdens of participation in research (beneficence) to equitable access to clinical trials (justice). Furthermore, the right to exercise autonomy was not always fully available to women, who were excluded from participating in clinical trials perceived as jeopardizing their safety; their exclusion clearly limited their ability to benefit from the research. Similarly, persons in developing countries deserve research that addresses their needs.

How should these principles be applied to research conducted in developing countries? How can we—and they—weigh the benefits and risks? Such research must be developed in concert with the developing countries in which it will be conducted. In the case of the NIH and CDC trials, there has been strong and consistent support and involvement of the scientific and public health communities in the host countries, with local as well as United States–based scientific and ethical reviews and the same requirements for informed consent that would exist if the work were performed in the United States. But there is more to this partnership. Interventions that could be expected to be made available in the United States might be well beyond the financial resources of a developing country or exceed the capacity of its health care infrastructure. Might we support a trial in another country that would not be offered in the United States? Yes, because the burden of disease might make such a study more compelling in that country. Even if there were some risks associated with intervention, such a trial might pass the test of beneficence. Might we elect not to support a trial of an intervention that was beyond the reach of the citizens of the other country? Yes, because that trial would not pass the test of justice.

Trials supported by the NIH and the CDC, which are designed to reduce the transmission of HIV from mothers to infants in developing countries, have been held up by some observers as examples of trials that do not meet ethical standards. We disagree. The debate does not hinge on informed consent, which all the trials have obtained. It hinges instead on whether it is ethical to test interventions against a placebo control when an effective intervention is in use elsewhere in the world. A background paper sets forth our views on this matter more fully.[5] The paper is also available on the World Wide Web (at http://www.nih.gov/news/mathiv/mathiv.htm).

One such effective intervention—known as AIDS Clinical Trials Group protocol 076—was a major breakthrough in the search for a way to interrupt the transmission of HIV from mother to infant. The regimen tested in the original study, however, was quite intensive for pregnant women and the health care system. Although this regimen has been proved effective, it requires that women undergo HIV testing and receive counseling about their HIV status early in pregnancy, comply with a lengthy oral regimen and with intravenous administration of the relatively expensive antiretroviral drug zidovudine, and refrain from breast-feeding. In addition, the newborn infants must receive six weeks of oral zidovudine, and both mothers and infants must be carefully monitored for adverse effects of the drug. Unfortunately, the burden of maternal-infant transmission of HIV is greatest in countries where women present late for prenatal care, have limited access to HIV testing and counseling, typically deliver their infants in settings not conducive to intravenous drug administration, and depend on breast-feeding to protect their babies from many diseases, only one of which is HIV infection. Furthermore, zidovudine is a powerful drug, and its safety in the populations of developing countries, where the incidences of other diseases, anemia, and malnutrition are higher than in developed countries, is unknown. Therefore, even though the 076 protocol has been shown to be effective in some countries, it is unlikely that it can be successfully exported to many others.

In addition to these hurdles, the wholesale cost of zidovudine in the 076 protocol is estimated to be in excess of $800 per mother and infant, an amount far greater than most developing countries can afford to pay for standard care. For example, in Malawi, the cost of zidovudine alone for the 076 regimen for one HIV-infected woman and her child is more than 600 times the annual per capita allocation for health care.

Various representatives of the ministries of health, communities, and scientists in developing countries have joined with other scientists to call for less complex and less expensive interventions to counteract the staggering impact of maternal-infant transmission of HIV in the developing world. The World Health Organization moved promptly after the release of the results of the 076 protocol, convening a panel of researchers and public health practitioners from around the world. This panel recommended the use of the 076 regimen throughout the industrialized world, where it is feasible, but also called for studies of alternative regimens that could be used in developing countries, observing that the logistical issues and costs precluded the widespread application of the 076 regimen.[6] To this end, the World Health Organization asked UNAIDS, the Joint United Nations Programme on HIV/AIDS, to coordinate international research efforts to develop simpler, less costly interventions.

The scientific community is responding by carrying out trials of several promising regimens that developing countries recognize as candidates for widespread delivery. However, these trials are being criticized by some people because of the use of placebo controls. Why not test these new interventions against the 076 regimen? Why not test them against other interventions that might offer some benefit? These questions were carefully considered in the development of these research projects and in their scientific and ethical review.

An obvious response to the ethical objection to placebo-controlled trials in countries where there is no current intervention is that the assignment to a placebo group does not carry a risk beyond that associated with standard practice, but this response is too simple. An additional response is that a placebo-controlled study usually provides a faster answer with fewer subjects, but the same result might be achieved with more sites or more aggressive enrollment. The most compelling reason to use a placebo-controlled study is that it provides definitive answers to questions about the safety and value of an intervention in the setting in which the study is performed, and these answers are the point of the research. Without clear and firm answers to whether and, if so, how well an intervention works, it is impossible for a country to make a sound judgment about the appropriateness and financial feasibility of providing the intervention.

For example, testing two or more interventions of unknown benefit (as some people have suggested) will not necessarily reveal whether either is better than nothing. Even if one surpasses the other, it may be difficult to judge the extent of the benefit conferred, since the interventions may differ markedly in other ways— for example, cost or toxicity. A placebo-controlled study would supply that answer. Similarly, comparing an intervention of unknown benefit—especially one that is affordable in a developing country—with the only intervention with a known benefit (the 076 regimen) may provide information that is not useful for patients. If the affordable intervention is less effective than the 076 regimen—not an unlikely outcome—this information will be of little use in a country where the more effective regimen is unavailable. Equally important, it will still be unclear whether the affordable intervention is better than nothing and worth the investment of scarce health care dollars. Such studies would fail to meet the goal of determining whether a treatment that could be implemented is worth implementing.

A placebo-controlled trial is not the only way to study a new intervention, but as compared with other approaches, it offers more definitive answers and a clearer view of side effects. This is not a case of treating research subjects as a means to an end, nor does it reflect "a callous disregard of their welfare."[2] Instead, a placebo-controlled trial may be the only way to obtain an answer that is ultimately useful to people in similar circumstances. If we enroll subjects in a study that exposes them to unknown risks and is designed in a way that is unlikely to provide results that are useful to the subjects or others in the population, we have failed the test of beneficence.

Finally, the NIH- and CDC-supported trials have undergone a rigorous process of ethical review, including not only the participation of the public health and scientific communities in the developing countries where the trials are being performed but also the application of the U.S. rules for the protection of human research subjects by relevant institutional review boards in the United States and in the developing countries. Support from local governments has been obtained, and each active study has been and will continue to be reviewed by an independent data and safety monitoring board.

To restate our main points: these studies address an urgent need in the countries in which they are being conducted and have been developed with extensive in-country participation. The studies are being conducted according to widely accepted principles and guidelines in bioethics. And our decisions to support these trials rest heavily on local support and approval. In a letter to the NIH dated May 8, 1997, Edward K. Mbidde, chairman of the AIDS Research Committee of the Uganda Cancer Institute, wrote:

> These are Ugandan studies conducted by Ugandan investigators on Ugandans. Due to lack of resources we have been sponsored by organizations like yours. We are grateful that you have been able to do so. . . . There is a mix up of issues here which needs to be clarified. It is not NIH conducting the studies in Uganda but Ugandans conducting their study on their people for the good of their people.

The scientific and ethical issues concerning studies in developing countries are complex. It is a healthy sign that we are debating these issues so that we can continue to advance our knowledge and our practice. However, it is essential that the debate take place with a full understanding of the nature of the science, the interventions in question, and the local factors that impede or support research and its benefits.

REFERENCES

1. Lane P. Wolfe SM. Unethical trials of interventions to reduce perinatal transmission of the human immunodeficiency virus in developing countries. N Engl J Med 1997;337:855–6.

2. Angell M. The ethics of clinical research in the third world. N Engl J Med 1997;337:847–9.

3. National Commission for the Protection of Human Subjects of Biomedical and Behavioral Research. Belmont reports ethical principles and guidelines for the protection of human subjects of research. Washington, D.C., Government Printing Office, 1988. GPO 887–809.

4. World Medical Association Declaration of Helsinki. Adopted by the 18th World Medical Assembly, Helsinki, 1964, as revised by the 48th World Medical Assembly, Republic of South Africa, 1996.

5. The conduct of clinical trials of maternal-infant transmission of HIV supported by the United States Department of Health and Human Services in developing countries. Washington, D.C.: Department of Health and Human Services, July 1997.

6. Recommendations from the meeting on mother-to-infant transmission of HIV by use of antiretrovirals. Geneva, World Health Organization, June 23–25, 1994.

THE USES AND ABUSES OF TUSKEGEE

AMY L. FAIRCHILD & RONALD BAYER

The Tuskegee Syphilis Study has come to symbolize the most egregious abuse of authority on the part of medical researchers. Tuskegee has also come to serve as a point of reference for African Americans distrustful of those with power, emblematic of the history of a people enslaved and then subject to social, legal, and political oppression after the end of formal servitude. When Tuskegee as a symbol of research abuse and Tuskegee as an emblem of racial oppression are merged, a potent device is at hand for uncovering profound social injustice. When, however, the legacy of Tuskegee is incautiously invoked—when its legacy is abused—it can serve to make a careful consideration of complex matters involving research with socially vulnerable people all but impossible.

To understand both the uses and abuses of Tuskegee requires that we understand the oft-told—and sometimes mistold—story of what happened between 1932 and 1972. The seminal study by James Jones, *Bad Blood*, provides the indispensable reference.[1]

As part of its study of the long-term effects of syphilis begun in 1932, the U.S. Public Health Service (PHS) denied treatment to 399 African American men suffering from the tertiary effects of the disease. The PHS launched its 40-year study using a group of patients originally identified in Macon County, Alabama, as part of a demonstration project that recommended mass testing and treatment of syphilis in the South. When money for testing and treatment dried up in the midst of the depression, PHS officers saw an opportunity to prove that syphilis among African Americans was "almost a different disease from syphilis in the white."[2]

Researchers and physicians involved in Tuskegee chose not to inform the study's participants that they were infected with syphilis or educate them regarding its treatment or prevention. During the study's recruitment period, PHS officers knowingly provided inadequate treatment for syphilis as a means of securing the support of the state department of health. Although subjects were not told that they had syphilis or were receiving modified treatment for it, the act of offering any kind of treatment helped in luring subjects to the study and gaining their trust.

Amy L. Fairchild is assistant professor of public health and Ronald Bayer is professor of public health in the Program in the History of Public Health and Medicine, Joseph L. Mailman School of Public Health, Columbia University.
Originally published in Science *284 (7 May 1999): 919–21. Reprinted by permission of the American Association for the Advancement of Science and Amy L. Fairchild and Ronald Bayer.*

Once the study was under way, scientists deliberately misled the men, telling them that they were receiving treatment for "bad blood"—a generic term that referred to a variety of ailments—rather than syphilis.

Receiving broad cooperation from state and local health officers, local medical practitioners, the military, and the Tuskegee Institute, the PHS successfully thwarted all efforts the men made to receive treatment from other sources. The PHS gave only a placebo to those expecting a full course of treatment. The intent of this study of untreated syphilis—albeit one clearly undermined by the therapy the PHS administered during the enrollment period—was to observe the untreated men until death: "Everyone is agreed that the proper procedure is the continuance of the observation of the Negro men used in the study with the idea of eventually bringing them to autopsy."[3] In 1950, one of the study's originators triumphantly declared, "We now know, where we could only surmise before, that we have contributed to their ailments and shortened their lives."[4]

Penicillin dramatically altered the treatment of syphilis. The PHS's Division of Venereal Diseases—the driving force behind the Tuskegee study—began using penicillin in several of its clinics across the nation in the early 1940s.[5] Despite the promise of the new treatment, Tuskegee directors withheld penicillin from its subjects. Not only did the PHS remain committed to seeing the study through to its end, but also used penicillin as a rationale for continuing the study. Never again would the PHS find such a group of untreated individuals.[6]

Even after the study was exposed in 1972, the PHS officials involved with Tuskegee refused to admit wrongdoing. They justified the study on the grounds that they had simply observed a group of men who would not have received treatment anyway and for whom treatment—even penicillin—would not have provided benefit. In any case, argued PHS officers, the men—who believed they were receiving treatment, who were thwarted at each juncture at which they sought outside treatment, and who were threatened with losing free medical care and death benefits if they left the study—had been "free" to leave the study and receive treatment at any time.

Although Tuskegee was a study that the PHS adapted to changing circumstances, from this account it is possible to derive three critical features that characterize the nature of the consistent research abuses that occurred over the course of forty years. The study involved, first, deceptions regarding the very existence and nature of the inquiry into which individuals were lured. As such, it deprived those seeking care of the right to choose whether or not to serve as research subjects. Second, it entailed an exploitation of social vulnerability to recruit and retain research subjects. Finally, Tuskegee researchers made a willful effort to deprive subjects of access to appropriate and available medical care, which changed over time, as a way of furthering the study's goals.

Thus viewed, Tuskegee touched on issues central to research ethics and can serve as a standard against which to judge contemporary examples of research abuse.[7] But, as a historical event involving the exploitation of African Americans that entailed the examination of a racist thesis, the legacy of Tuskegee and the outrage it has spawned are suffused with race. When the story broke in 1972, there was intense but brief discussion in the medical and public-health press. Some of the problems raised by Tuskegee were, in some limited sense, resolved with the passage of the National Research Act of 1974. The act created institutional review boards (IRBS) and charged them with approving all federally funded human research. But while Tuskegee lay dormant in the popular press for the next decade, it served a critical function in the African American press, becoming a metaphor for genocide.

Within weeks of the first news reports of Tuskegee, the African American press and African American political leaders characterized the forty-year experiment as "outright genocide."[8] *Jet* magazine, for instance, created a new news section on "Genocide." Along with the rest of the African American press, it began to view a host of issues—the lack of health services; birth control, abortion, and involuntary sterilization; adoption; overexposure to X rays; research among prisoners and infants; prison riots; the U.S. Census—through the lens of Tuskegee.[9] "Tuskegee" crystallized a history of medical neglect and abuse that was a consequence of social and political disempowerment.[10]

It is not surprising, then, that Tuskegee has found potent invocations in the context of the AIDS epidemic, which has so disproportionately affected African Americans. Particularly when falsely remembered, as a tale of how poor African American men were deliberately infected with syphilis,[11] the story of Tuskegee rang true, for it resonated with suspicions of an epidemic manufactured to annihilate a people.[12] James Small, a black studies professor at City College of New York, summed up the views of many when he concluded, "Our whole relationship to whites has been that of their practicing genocidal conspiratorial behavior on us—from the whole slave encounter to the Tuskegee Study."[13]

In this paper we examine the uses and abuses of Tuskegee in three highly visible AIDS-related debates, which spanned the past decade: the clash over the provision of sterile injection equipment to intravenous drug users, the conflict over unidentified anonymous HIV seroprevalence studies, and the debate over the investigation of interventions to reduce the rate of HIV transmission from pregnant women to their offspring in Third World countries.

Needle Exchange

The provision of sterile injection equipment to intravenous drug users has been proposed as a way of interrupting the spread of HIV infection since the mid-

1980s.[14] The debate over needle exchange within the African American community unfolded against a backdrop of suspicions that the failure to provide adequate treatment to drug users represented a form of genocidal neglect—most potently captured in the legacy of Tuskegee.[15]

Needle exchange compounded a community's sense of outrage over a failure to provide effective drug treatment. Drawing on this community outrage, Congregational minister Graylan Ellis-Hagler succeeded in his forceful campaign to shut down a Boston needle-exchange program in 1986 by extending the genocide analogy: "First the white establishment push drugs in the community. They cripple the community politically and economically with drugs. They send males to jail. Then someone hands out needles to maintain the dependency."[16]

Wherever needle-exchange proposals emerged, black leadership gave voice to their dismay and fury. In New York City the dual specters of genocide and Tuskegee explicitly helped to shape the debate surrounding the nation's first controlled clinical trial of the intervention.[17] Because of political opposition to needle exchange from both law-enforcement proponents and the African American community, the city's health commissioner was compelled to present his 1988 needle-exchange effort as a small experiment designed to determine whether such a radical innovation could reduce the incidence of infection among drug users without encouraging drug use. Ironically, the very political cover that the experiment was designed to provide set the stage for the charge of "Tuskegee." As the *Amsterdam News* noted, "Given [the commissioner of health's] knowledge of the Tuskegee experiment—it would seem to us that he would want everything that he is doing to be above suspicion."[18]

Benjamin Ward, the city's African American police commissioner, alluded to the Tuskegee syphilis trials when he explained that his community felt "a particular sensitivity to doctors conducting experiments, and they too frequently seem to be conducted against blacks."[19] Hilton B. Davis, a Harlem City Council member, more pointedly characterized the program as a "genocidal campaign."[20] Rev. Reginald Williams echoed his sentiments, combing the imagery of Tuskegee and genocide: "Why," he demanded, "must we again be the guinea pigs in this genocidal mentality?"[21]

When David Dinkins, long opposed to needle exchange, assumed the office of mayor in 1990, thus becoming the city's first African American chief executive, he almost immediately ended the trial. Dinkins felt that "we need to go at fighting drugs in the first instance and I don't want to give people the paraphernalia to continue using drugs."[22] Ironically, when the city moved even further by withdrawing funds from a community program that provided bleach to drug users for needle cleansing, Dr. Mathilde Krim, the well-known head of the American Foundation for AIDS Research, drew a comparison to Tuskegee and concluded, "It will be genocide, pure and simple."[23]

By the mid-1990s, the intense African American opposition to needle exchange had all but vanished—eroded by the apparent effectiveness of such efforts and by the fragmentation of opinion among African American leaders. Nevertheless, opposition remains, and when it finds expression, Tuskegee continues to serve as a touchstone for criticism. Thus in 1997, Harlem Hospital psychiatrist and drug-treatment expert Dr. James Curtis denounced such programs, stating that they amounted to "reckless experimentation on human beings" akin to "a replay of the infamous Tuskegee experiment."[24]

Yet as Tuskegee ceased to serve as a tool for critics of needle exchange, it increasingly became a symbol for the advocates of such efforts, who denounced the failure of federal officials to fund such programs. It was in this context that a furious debate emerged when the NIH funded a clinical trial in Anchorage, Alaska, to answer the question of whether over-the-counter sale of injection equipment— a practice permitted in Alaska but prohibited in many jurisdictions with serious drug problems—was more effective than formal needle-exchange programs. In October 1996, Peter Lurie and Sidney Wolfe, physicians at Ralph Nader's Public Citizen's Health Research Group, sharply attacked the $2.4 million study. In a series of letters, they charged that the study was "deceptive" in failing to inform participants of the relative benefits of the needle exchange and that it " 'actively prevented' [those assigned to the pharmacy arm] from obtaining access to clean needles through the needle exchange."[25] Equally troubling, they noted one of the study's measures of efficacy—the incidence of hepatitis B infection—was utterly preventable through the provision of a vaccine. Lurie and Wolfe concluded, "The parallels here to the Tuskegee Syphilis Study . . . are clear. . . . [In] the Tuskegee study known effective treatment for a life-threatening disease was withheld, in this human experiment, two known effective means of prevention—hepatitis B vaccine and the provision at no cost of sterile needles and syringes—are being withheld."[26]

In an unprecedented move, Harold Varmus, head of the NIH, suspended the study pending review by an outside committee headed by Yale physician and expert on research ethics Robert Levine. The panel included James Childress, a senior figure in the field of medical ethics. Levine's panel reported back to Varmus in December, concluding that the study was no Tuskegee, primarily because the drug users in the study would, in fact, have ready access to clean syringes. Indeed, the study protocol stipulated that those assigned to the study's pharmacy arm would be instructed on how and where to buy clean needles over the counter. The panel described the critique of the study as "misunderstanding, mischaracteriza- tion, or both."[27] Significantly, the panel also endorsed the study's protocol regard- ing hepatitis B infection, asserting that it was not a typical service of needle- exchange programs and that study participants had easy access to it already.

With the study set to move forward, Arthur Caplan and George Annas, two prominent bioethicists, argued that neither the need to determine the efficacy of over-the-counter syringe sales nor the addition of NIH funds to offer hepatitis vaccines to those requesting them altered the basic ethics of the study. Caplan and Annas maintained that the study amounted to allowing researchers to "stand by and observe as their subjects develop devastating diseases that could be prevented." "This," they continued, "is the lesson learned in the notorious Tuskegee syphilis study. . . . It is not ethically acceptable to learn from the misery of the vulnerable without protecting them from known risks of serious harm." Concluded the two, "There is no excuse for not pursuing every reasonable avenue, including both drugstore sales and needle exchange programs, to get sterile needles into the hands of these people."[28]

Both iterations of the needle-exchange debate revolved around pressing questions of fairness in dealing with vulnerable populations. Both focused on the question of whether withholding (or providing) an innovative intervention could be justified given the risks and burdens of prevailing conditions in the HIV epidemic. Both challenged public-health priorities. But the charge of the Tuskegee-like abuse of research subjects was inappropriate in each instance. The failure to provide adequate treatment options for drug addiction, central to the complaint of African American opponents of needle exchange, most certainly represents tragic neglect on the part of the health-care system and an example of gross inequity. But while Tuskegee may serve as a powerful means of bringing serious, difficult questions to light, not all injustices are the equivalent of those represented by Tuskegee. Needle-exchange efforts do not represent a substitute for drug treatment. They simply attempt to prevent the acquisition of a lethal infection. Whereas in Tuskegee the PHS used the social circumstances of poor African American men to manipulate them into a study that would deprive them of treatment, proposals to provide sterile injection equipment seek to address the vulnerable situation of those exposed to HIV by offering a potentially life-saving intervention. The emphasis on the provision of clean needles rather than on treatment may, arguably, reflect a mistaken ordering of social priorities. Indeed, it may well reflect the extent to which the needs of the most vulnerable receive inadequate attention. But it does not demonstrate a disregard for the basic principles of research ethics.

Strong as is the evidence for the relative efficacy of needle exchange, the failure to establish such programs also does not constitute Tuskegee-like abuse. Every social policy failure, every demonstration of neglect, every injustice is not the equivalent of what happened in Macon County, although they may share common racist underpinnings. Even the challenged Alaska study was not comparable to Tuskegee. However one evaluates the evidence, it is clear that those who were to be enrolled would not suffer the kind of covert manipulation designed to deprive individuals of access to potentially effective care experienced by the men studied in Tuskegee. Only insofar as the original study failed to offer hepatitis B vaccination to participants did it arguably involve an ethical lapse—a lapse addressed by the

NIH despite the recommendations of its ethical review panel. But that lapse, in and of itself, did not constitute the kind of abuse represented by Tuskegee.

Blinded Seroprevalence Studies

The conflict over blinded seroprevalence studies involved charges that, as in Tuskegee, vulnerable individuals were unwitting subjects of surveillance. Further, critics charged that those responsible for the studies withheld critical information bearing on diagnosis and the need for treatment.

Beginning in 1988, health departments across the nation, with the support from the federal Centers for Disease Control and Prevention, conducted studies of HIV infection in the population by testing blood samples, stripped of all personal identifiers, that were drawn from hospital, clinic, and emergency-room patients. When subject to ethical review in the 1980s, experts deemed such screening unproblematic.[29] It involved samples of blood, not identifiable individuals. The privacy of no one could be violated. Informed consent was hence unnecessary.[30] But what made the studies—based on unconsented testing—ethically acceptable also precluded notification of infected individuals. Since there was little that could be done for people with asymptomatic HIV infection in the late 1980s, there was widespread consensus that the blinded surveys were ethically permissible and served a critical public-health need.

As early clinical intervention became the standard of care for both adults and infants with HIV, these studies came under legislative, clinical, and ethical attack. Notably, it was only those studies involving women and infants—arguably vulnerable by definition or history—that drew the critical challenge. Nettie Mayersohn, a democratic representative to the New York State Assembly who believed infected babies—most of whom were the children of poor, minority women—had a right to testing and treatment, explained that when she first learned of the CDC studies in May 1993, she was struck by the semblance to Tuskegee: "I was just so astounded. This was the Tuskegee experiment all over again."[31] Mayersohn accordingly introduced her "Baby AIDS Bill" to make newborn HIV testing and parental notification mandatory.

Mayersohn gained press attention for her cause by interesting *New York Newsday* columnist Jim Dwyer.[32] In the opening salvo of his Pulitzer Prize–winning series on newborn testing, he quoted Dr. Arthur Amman, a professor of pediatrics at the University of California and head of the Pediatric AIDS Research Foundation, who was among the first to argue the similarities between blinded surveillance and Tuskegee but who, unlike Mayersohn, opposed mandatory testing. "The maintenance of anonymous test results at a time when treatment and prevention are readily available," he observed, "will be recorded in history as analogous to the Tuskegee 'experiment.' "[33] Amman was joined by Scott Isaacman, a lawyer and staff physician with the Cook County Department of Health, who in 1993 accused epidemiologists of "ignoring the difference between human subjects and laboratory animals" and of using the logic "used by the PHS to abrogate responsibility for the Tuskegee Syphilis studies."[34]

The analogy helped to sharpen the attack on blinded surveillance even as Mayersohn, though not all her allies, sought to promote mandatory newborn testing. As she pressed the legislature to adopt a policy requiring the state to test all newborn babies for HIV and notify parents or guardians of the results, Mayersohn played on themes of Tuskegee's deception.[35] Her most powerful rhetorical challenges, however, drew on Tuskegee's shameless exploitation of the most vulnerable. Mayersohn argued that blinded surveillance was "a policy that conspires to deny medical treatment and care . . . to the most vulnerable among us."[36] She claimed it "unconscionable for us to continue treating helpless babies as useful, but expendable, statistical tools."[37] In 1996, after her mandatory-testing bill passed the state legislature, she jubilantly declared, "We will no longer allow infants to be used as statistical tools in some scientific experiment."[38]

Congressional representative Gary Ackerman, whom Mayersohn had helped elect to the New York State Senate years earlier, took up the gauntlet at the national level. In May 1995 he unveiled legislation to unblind the CDC newborn seroprevalence study.[39] H.R.1289 instructed states requiring infant HIV surveillance testing promptly to disclose that information to a child's parent or guardian. For Ackerman, it was simply unacceptable that unconsented testing continue in a context precluding notification of those needing treatment. Women, he asserted, knew that if their child were infected with a disease like syphilis or hepatitis, doctors would notify them. They had every reason to believe that would also be the case with HIV. Hence, they were the objects of deception when the CDC tested their babies and failed to disclose critical clinical findings.[40] Ackerman's bill sought to unblind the CDC survey, and in so doing sought to achieve his second goal of mandatory newborn testing. It was that second goal that remained clouded to many.

Perhaps because of its ambiguity, Ackerman's "Newborn Infant HIV Notification Act" carried the bipartisan support of more than 220 House members. Most striking, whereas the Mayersohn bill for mandatory testing in New York State was opposed by virtually all African American and Latino activists, the Ackerman bill won the critical endorsement of 31 members of the Congressional Black Caucus, some of whom withdrew their names from the legislation as debate intensified, the question of mandatory testing came to dominate, and Ackerman's alignment with Mayersohn became clear.

So soaked in the rhetoric of Tuskegee was the blinded seroprevalence debate that Ackerman did not even need to name the Alabama atrocity when he made his final bid to unblind the CDC's study on 11 May. Speaking before the House Commerce Committee, Ackerman warned, "There was one point in our society, a very dark day when people were allowed to walk around after being tested with a dread disease just so the medical establishment could . . . see what happens. . . . Let's not fall back to that kind of an era."[41] In response to the broad support behind Ackerman's bill, the CDC—opposed to mandatory testing—preempted Ackerman's proposal and announced it would suspend the newborn serosurvey, effective 12 May 1995. Ackerman, ironically, angrily alleged that the CDC was driven by the simple desire to avoid the taint of Tuskegee.[42]

Despite the fact that local, national, and international reviews of the ethics of blinded seroprevalence studies provoked no objection when they were initially launched, changing therapeutic prospects appeared to alter radically the context within which such efforts were conducted. In this new context, were the charges of "Tuskegee" appropriately applied to the newborn serosurveys? Had not public-health officials chosen to take information from socially marginalized populations without informing individuals that they were the objects of study, without notifying them of their HIV infection, and without offering them potentially effective treatments? That so many political leaders identified with the interests of the most socially vulnerable evidenced deep concerns about the blinded seroprevalence studies suggests that the answer to each of these questions was complex. That those responsible for the conduct of blinded surveys could not give assurance that the communities they identified as being at greatest risk would, in fact, receive the resources needed for HIV care and prevention only exacerbated the situation.

Nevertheless, on several critical accounts, blinded seroprevalence failed to meet basic criteria that could arguably reflect the abuses of Tuskegee. Neither the CDC nor state public-health departments engaged in blinded testing made efforts to deprive individuals of the opportunity for voluntary testing through which they could discover if they were infected. Nor was there an effort to divert women who sought diagnostic testing from treatment for themselves or their infants. Indeed, the very purpose of the studies was to identify *populations* at increased risk for HIV so that efforts to identify *individuals* in need of care could be given the greatest priority. Unlike Tuskegee, which sought to withhold treatment from men with syphilis, officials hoped to use the blinded seroprevalence studies as a prod to enhance the prospects that therapeutic interventions would be directed to those most in need.

Maternal-Fetal HIV Transmission Prevention Trials in the Third World

In the case of Third World trials to prevent maternal-fetal HIV transmission, two core elements of Tuskegee were at issue: the exploitation of impoverished, vulnerable populations and the denial of access to effective treatment.

In February 1994, the Data Safety and Monitoring Board of the U.S. National Institute of Allergies and Infectious Diseases interrupted AIDS Clinical Trial Group (ACTG) Study 076.[43] The preliminary data revealed a statistically significant and dramatic difference in vertical HIV transmission rates from mothers to their newborns between women who received the active regimen and women in the placebo group. The rate for the former was 8.3 percent, for the latter, 25.5 percent.

The regimen quickly became the standard of care in industrialized nations. There is no question but that further placebo-control trials of efforts to reduce vertical transmission in the wake of clinical trial 076 would be considered unethical in the United States or any other advanced industrial nation. No trial that would deny access to the ACTG 076 regimen, or to an intervention thought to hold the promise of being at least as effective as, if not more effective than, the prevailing standard of care, would satisfy the requirements of ethical review.

In developing countries, however, where maternal-fetal transmission represents an epidemiological disaster, the costs of the 076 regimen ($800 for the drug alone) put zidovudine therapy out of reach. In Uganda, for example, the cost of the zidovudine component of the ACTG 076 regimen represented 400 times the yearly per-capita expenditure on health care. It was, therefore, a matter of some urgency that trials begin to determine whether radically cheaper alternatives to the ACTG 076 regimen could achieve some measure of reduced maternal-fetal HIV transmission. In all, 15 placebo-controlled trials—9 funded by the CDC or NIH, 5 by other governments including Denmark, France, and South Africa, and one funded by the United Nations Program on Acquired Immune Deficiency Syndrome (UNAIDS)—were launched in developing countries. All had been subject to careful ethical review.

Nevertheless, on 18 September 1997, Dr. Marcia Angell, executive editor of the *New England Journal of Medicine*, denounced the placebo-control trials in Africa, Asia, and the Caribbean. "Zidovudine," she wrote, "has already been clearly shown to cut the rate of vertical transmission greatly and is now recommended in the United States for all HIV-infected pregnant women."[44] Citing the Declaration of Helsinki for authority, she noted that control groups had to be provided with the best current therapy, not simply that which was available locally. Failure to observe this ethical mandate "could result in widespread exploitation of vulnerable Third World populations for research programs that could not be carried out in the sponsor country." She concluded, "The justifications are reminiscent of those for the Tuskegee study: Women in the Third World would not receive antiretroviral treatment anyway, so the investigators are simply observing what would happen to the subject's infants if there were no study."

Writing later in the *Wall Street Journal*, Angell asserted: "All the rationalizations boil down to asserting that the end justifies the means—which it no more does in

Africa than it did in Alabama. It is easy to see the findings of the Tuskegee study from a safe distance of 25 years. But those so offended by the comparison of the African research with Tuskegee have yet to show how these studies differ in their fundamental failure to protect the welfare of human subjects."[45] Peter Lurie and Sidney Wolfe, who had leveled the charge of Tuskegee in Anchorage, Alaska, provided the basis for Angell's editorial.[46] They stated: "Many people will hear in these experiments echoes of the notorious Tuskegee syphilis study. . . . This time, the people of color affected are babies from Africa, Asia, and the Caribbean, many hundreds of whom will die unnecessarily in the course of this unethical, exploitative research."[47]

Despite the allure of the Tuskegee analogy in studies that denied access to the standard of care in industrialized nations, the disanalogies are striking. However problem-ridden the efforts to obtain informed consent in the Third World settings, it is clear that, unlike Tuskegee, investigators made efforts to inform the enrolled women that they would be part of a study to reduce maternal transmission of HIV and that some would receive a placebo. Additionally, no effort was made to exploit the social vulnerability of the women involved. Indeed, it was the very poverty of *the nations within which these women lived* that served as the predicate for the challenged studies. Only to the extent that women living in poor Third World countries could be said to have a realizable claim on the care available to women in industrialized nations would the conduct of a placebo trial have mirrored the deprivations of Tuskegee. But then any trial to find a cheaper and potentially less effective regimen than that which was standard in the industrialized world—whether it relied on a placebo-control design or not—would have been unethical as well. To the extent that the search for a less costly and potentially less effective intervention could be justified by the desperate need to find affordable interventions, the analogy to Tuskegee was simply misleading.

Yet to the extent that women in poor countries have a moral—as contrasted with a realizable—claim on the care available to women in industrialized nations, critics helped to underscore the profound injustice that characterizes the world distribution of medical resources. Unfortunately, the invocation of Tuskegee launched a furious methodological debate that diverted attention from an analysis of the very poverty and inequality that necessitated the challenged studies.

Conclusion

When we understand Tuskegee as emblematic of a history of racism and the experience of social, economic, and political disempowerment, its legacy does much to explain the atmosphere of mistrust that surrounds research, especially when the subjects of study are poor, vulnerable, and the potential targets of exploitation. That legacy is especially helpful in explaining the profound suspicions expressed by African Americans when the prospects of medical experimentation present themselves. Thus understood, Tuskegee heightens the importance of carefully and sensitively seeking to establish trust where it is absent or where historical experience has shattered it. As important, Tuskegee can draw our attention to the inevitable moral challenges that will emerge when research involves those who, for cultural, historical, political, or economic reasons, are socially vulnerable.

But for Tuskegee to serve as a useful analogy for illuminating research abuse, the challenged study must meet some reasonable, general criteria. It must involve deception regarding the nature and very existence of the research study; it must capitalize on social deprivation or vulnerability; and, not only must it fail to provide the best available effective therapy, but it must also contrive to keep individuals from receiving such therapy.

The past decade has demonstrated that the charge of "Tuskegee" is extremely effective in riveting public attention, but just as research demands of its practitioners that they adhere to standards of moral responsibility, challenges to research carry with them certain moral obligations. Those who would use Tuskegee to indict research efforts bear responsibility for how they deploy the legacy of that awful historical episode.

Not every disagreement about whether a particular study raises troubling ethical questions justifies the invocation of Tuskegee. Not every ethical lapse involving vulnerable populations is the equivalent of Tuskegee. Finally, not every injustice in the social context within which research occurs recreates the conditions that prevailed and were exploited in Alabama. The reckless invocation of the misdeeds of federal researchers between 1932 and 1972 risks derailing serious and sustained discussion of the unique dilemmas posed by contemporary research with vulnerable populations under conditions of social deprivation. Tuskegee is an unwieldy weapon in public discourse. It makes current research abuses, when subject to careful scrutiny, pale in comparison to the historic syphilis study, thus minimizing their gravity. Alternatively, in instances where contemporary problems in justice exceed the bounds of Tuskegee, its invocation ironically guarantees inadequate discussion. The ethical challenges raised by the problems of drug use, ensuring access to HIV testing and treatment resources for those in greatest need, and the world economic order should not require "Tuskegee" to merit our attention.

In the end, the abuse of Tuskegee has consequences not only for present discussion but also for the past. It threatens to rob Tuskegee of its unique value and meaning. It misuses the memory of the 399 African American men whose most basic rights were violated for 40 years. In so doing it diminishes the significance of their suffering.

REFERENCES

1. James H. Jones, *Bad Blood: The Tuskegee Syphilis Experiment* (New York: The Free Press, 1981, 1993).

2. Ibid., p. 6, quoting letter from Moore to Clark, 28 September 1932.

3. Ibid., p. 132, quoting letter from Vonderlehr to Wegner, 18 July 1933.

4. A. M. Brandt, "Racism and Research: The Case of the Tuskegee Syphilis Study," *Hastings Center Report* 8 (1978): 25, quoting O. C. Wegner, "Untreated Syphilis in Male Negro," unpublished transcript, 1950, p. 3. Tuskegee File, Centers for Disease Control, Atlanta, Ga.

5. Jones, *Bad Blood*, p. 178.

6. Ibid., p. 179, quoting a letter from Bauer to Doren, 27 November 1951, Tuskegee File, Centers for Disease Control, Atlanta, Ga.

7. D. L. Kirp, "Blood, Sweat, and Tears: The Tuskegee Experiment and the Era of AIDS," *Tikkun* 10, no. 3 (May 1995); and D. J. Rothman, "Were Tuskegee and Willowbrook 'Studies in Nature'?" *Hastings Center Report* (April 1982): 5–7.

8. "Genocide at Tuskegee," *New York Amsterdam News*, 26 August 1972. See also "Govt. Uses 600 Blacks as 'Human Guinea Pigs,'" *Jet*, 10 August 1972; and "Black Caucus Demands Reparations for Victims of U.S. Syphilis Study," *Jet*, 17 August 1972.

9. "Black Babies Used as Guinea Pigs in Dangerous Research," *Amsterdam News*, 31 March 1973; "'Guinea Pig' Experiments Are Conducted in Prisons," *Jet*, 24 August 1972; "Blacks as Guinea Pigs," *Amsterdam News*, 27 January 1973; F. E. Ruffin, "Birth Control, a Choice: Genocide or Survival?" *Essence*, September 1972; Al Rutledge, "Is Abortion Black Genocide?" *Essence*, September 1973; D. Alexander, "A Montgomery Tragedy: The Relf Family Refused to Be the Nameless Victims of Involuntary Sterilization," *Essence*, September 1973; "Black Psychologists to Present Genocide Petition to UN," *Amsterdam News*, 3 September 1975.

10. J. H. Jones, "The Tuskegee Legacy: AIDS and the Black Community," *Hastings Center Report* 22, no. 6 (November 1992): 38.

11. H. L. Dalton, "AIDS in Blackface," *Daedlus* (Summer 1989): 205–27.

12. S. B. Thomas and J. W. Curran, "Tuskegee: From Science to Conspiracy to Metaphor," *American Journal of the Medical Sciences* 3171 (January 1999): 1–4; and S. Thomas and S. Quinn, "The Tuskegee Syphilis Study, 1932–1972: Implications for HIV Education and AIDS Risk Reduction Programs in the Black Community," *American Journal of Public Health* 81 (1991): 1498–1505.

13. K. Grisby Bates, "Is It Genocide? Conspiracy Theory about AIDS and the Afro-American Community," *Essence*, September 1990.

14. D. Sencer, "Choosing between Two Killers," *New York Times*, 15 September 1985; World Health Organization, *AIDS among Drug Abusers* (Copenhagen: WHO Regional Office for Europe, 1987); National Academy of Sciences, Institute of Medicine, *Confronting AIDS: Directions for Public Health, Health Care and Research* (Washington, D.C.: National Academy Press, 1986).

15. D. L. Kirp and R. Bayer, "Needles and Race: Needle Exchange Programs and African Americans," *Atlantic*, July 1993.

16. Ibid.

17. See Dalton, "AIDS in Blackface," pp. 209–10; W. Anderson, "The New York Needle Trial: The Politics of Public Health in the Age of AIDS," *AJPH* 81, no. 11 (November 1991): 1506–17; and S. Thomas and S. Quinn, "The Burdens of Race and History Shaping Black American Attitudes toward Needle Exchange Policy to Prevent HIV Infection," *Journal Public Health Policy* 14 (1993): 320–47.

18. "Needlemania," *Amsterdam News*, 30 July 1988.

19. B. Lambat, "The Free Needle Program Is Under Way and Under Fire," *New York Times*, 13 November 1988.

20. M. Marriott, "Needle Exchange Angers Many Minorities," *New York Times*, 7 November 1988, quoted in Dalton, "AIDS in Blackface," p. 209.

21. Ibid., p. 210.

22. T. S. Purdum, "Dinkins to End Needle Plan for Drug Users," *New York Times*, 14 February 1990.

23. C. Woodard, "AIDS Experts: Policy on Needles 'Genocide,'" *Newsday*, 8 June 1990.

24. R. L. Maginnis, "Threading the Needle Exchange Program," *Washington Times*, 30 April 1998. See also David G. Evans, Letter to the Editor, "Needle Exchange Programs Fail to Deliver Benefits," *New York Times*, 19 October 1997.

25. Letter from P. Lurie and S. Wolfe to H. Varmus, 12 December 1996; Letter from P. Lurie and S. Wolfe to H. Varmus, 14 December 1996.

26. Letter from P. Lurie and S. Wolfe to H. Varmus, 17 October 1996.

27. Report to the Advisory Committee to the Director of the Panel to Review the Aspects of the Study "Interventions to Reduce HBV, HCV and HIV in IDUs," Bethesda, Md., 12 December 1996.

28. A. L. Caplan and G. Annas, "Study of Needle Exchanges Puts Politics Ahead of Health," *Washington Post*, 11 February 1997.

29. R. Bayer, C. Levine, and S. M. Wolf, "HIV Antibody Screening: An Ethical Framework for Evaluating Proposed Programs," *Journal of the American Medical Association* 256 (1986): 1768–74; Office for the Protection from Research Risks, *HIV Seroprevalence Survey of Childbearing Women: Testing Neonatal Dried Blood Specimens on Filter Paper for HIV Antibody* (Atlanta, Ga.: Centers for Disease Control, 1988); "Guidelines on Ethical and Legal Conditions in Anonymous Unlinked HIV Seroprevalence Research" (Ottowa, Ontario: Government of Canada Federal AIDS Centre, May 1988); and *Unlinked Anonymous Screening for the Public Health Surveillance of HIV Infections Proposed International Guidelines* (Geneva, Switzerland: World Health Organization Global Programme on AIDS, 1989).

30. R. Bayer, "The Ethics of Blinded HIV Surveillance Testing," *AJPH* 83, no. 4 (April 1993): 496–97.

31. C. SerVaas, "Nett[ie] Mayersohn and Her Baby AIDS Bill," *Saturday Evening Post*, 11 January 1998.

32. D. M. Abramson, "Passing the Test: New York's Newborn HIV Testing Policy, 1987–1997," in *Reducing the Odds: Preventing Perinatal Transmission of HIV in the United States*, ed. Michael A. Stoto, Donna A. Almario, and Marie C. McCormick (Washington, D.C.: National Academy Press, 1999), pp. 313–40.

33. J. Dwyer, "The Privacy That Can Kill," *New York Newsday*, 15 March 1995. See also N. Hentoff, "Another Tuskegee?" *Washington Post*, 20 May 1995; and Abramson, "Passing the Test."

34. S. H. Isaacman, "HIV Surveillance Testing: Taking Advantage of the Disadvantaged," *AJPH* 83 (1993): 597–98; S. H. Isaacman and L. Miller, "Neonatal HIV Seroprevalence Studies," *Journal of Legal Medicine* 14 (1993): 413–61.

35. Press releases, 22 January 1994 and 3 July 1993, Office of Assemblywoman Nettie Mayersohn, faxed to authors on 4 February 1999.

36. Statement of Assemblywoman Nettie Mayersohn, Public Hearing of the New York State AIDS Advisory Council Subcommittee on Newborn and Prenatal HIV Testing, 8 November 1993.

37. Press release, 14 April 1994, Office of Mayersohn.

38. Press release, 26 June 1996, ibid.

39. Abramson, "Passing the Test."

40. *Congressional Record* (19 September 1995): H9059.

41. Testimony of Gary Ackerman, Hearing before the Subcommittee on Health and Environment of the Committee on Commerce, House of Representatives, 104th Cong., 1st Sess., 11 May 1995, Serial No. 104-22:8.

42. Hentoff, "Another Tuskegee?" See also R. Bayer, "It's Not 'Tuskegee' Revisited: The False Furor over HIV Testing and Newborn Babies," *Washington Post*, 26 May 1995.

43. S. A. Spector, R. D. Gelber, N. McGrath, et al., "A Controlled Trial of Intravenous Immune Globulin for the Prevention of Serious Bacterial Infections in Children Receiving Zidovudine for Advanced Human Immunodeficiency Virus Infection," *New England Journal of Medicine* 331 (1994): 1181–87.

44. Marcia Angell, "The Ethics of Clinical Research in the Third World," *NEJM* 337 (1997): 847.

45. M. Angell, "Tuskegee Revisited," *Wall Street Journal*, 28 October 1997.

46. P. Lurie and S. Wolf, "Unethical Trials of Interventions to Reduce Perinatal Transmission of the Human Immunodeficiency Virus in Developing Countries," *NEJM* 337 (1997): 853–56.

47. P. Lurie et al., written communication, 22 April 1997, quoted in Ronald Bayer, "The Debate over Maternal-Fetal HIV Prevention Trials in Africa, Asia, and the Caribbean: Racist Exploitation or Exploitation of Racism?" *AJPH* 88 (April 1998): 568.

A GUIDE TO FURTHER READING

This bibliography should serve as a general guide to the various kinds of materials that are extant on the study. Listing all the references to the Tuskegee Syphilis Study would take a volume in itself. Sources for the archives that hold the major primary documents in the study are provided. Not every secondary article is included, nor are the numerous websites. Some general works on syphilis treatment in the 1930s and on the politics in Tuskegee are listed. In 1972, when the study first made national news, and again in 1997, when President Bill Clinton made the formal apology on behalf of the U.S. government, there was a flurry of media accounts in major newspapers, television and radio reports, and web pages. There are too many to list here.

Using any standard search engine (i.e., Hotbot, Alta Vista, Yahoo) and the search terms "Tuskegee syphilis" will yield numerous citations and websites. Some of these sites are course outlines, guides to further reading, and personal comments on the study, as well as materials from the Tuskegee Syphilis Study Legacy Committee, news stories on the apology, and citations to journal articles. An excellent beginning guide to the medical literature can be found through the National Library of Medicine's website, Internet Grateful Med, http://igm.nlm.nih.gov.

The asterisk indicates that the citation, or a selection from the citation, is in this volume.

Much of the organizational work on this bibliography was done by Kristel E. E. Maney. I am more than grateful for her assistance and good spirits.

ARCHIVES AND INTERVIEWS

Alabama Department of Archives and History, Montgomery, Alabama
    Alabama Department of Public Health Administrative Files of the State Health
      Officer
District Court of the United States, Middle District of Alabama, Montgomery,
    Alabama
    Charles W. Pollard et al. v. United States of America et al., Civil Action No.
      4126-N
National Archives and Records Administration, Southeast Regional National
    Archives, East Point, Georgia
    Tuskegee Syphilis Study Administrative Records, 1930–80
National Archives and Records Administration, Washington D.C.
    United States Public Health Service Division of Venereal Diseases, Record
      Group 90 (1918–36)

National Library of Medicine, National Institutes of Health, Bethesda, Maryland
  Tuskegee Study Ad Hoc Advisory Panel Papers
Thompson, Lillian A. "Eunice Rivers Laurie (interview, 10 October 1977)." In *The Black Women Oral History Project*, ed. Ruth Edmonds Hill, 7:213–42. New Providence, N.J.: K. G. Saur Verlag, 1992.
Tuskegee University Archives, Hollis Burke Frissell Library, Washingtonian Collection, Tuskegee University, Tuskegee, Alabama
  *Dibble, Helen, and Daniel Williams. "An Interview with Nurse Rivers," 1977
  Eugene Dibble Papers
  R. R. Moton Papers
  Tuskegee Syphilis Study Papers

GOVERNMENT HEARINGS AND REPORTS

Alabama Advisory Committee to the United States Commission on Civil Rights. "Alabama Commission Report." Montgomery: State of Alabama, 1973.
*"Final Report of the Tuskegee Syphilis Study Ad Hoc Advisory Panel." Washington, D.C.: U.S. Department of Health, Education and Welfare, 1973.
*"Nomination of Dr. Henry Foster for Surgeon General of the United States." Washington, D.C.: Federal Document Clearing House, Inc., 1995.
*"Quality of Health Care and Human Experimentation, 1973." Hearings before the Subcommittee on Health of the Committee on Labor and Public Welfare, Ninety-third Congress, Washington, D.C., 1973.

PUBLISHED REPORTS ON THE STUDY

Caldwell, Joseph G. "Aortic Regurgitation in the Tuskegee Study of Untreated Syphilis." *Journal of Chronic Diseases* 26 (1973): 187–94.
Clark, E. Gurney, et al. "The Oslo Study of the Natural History of Untreated Syphilis." *Journal of Chronic Diseases* 2 (September 1955): 343.
Deibert, A. V., et al. "Untreated Syphilis in the Male Negro: III. Evidence of Cardiovascular Abnormalities and Other Forms of Morbidity." *Journal of Venereal Disease Information* 27 (1946): 301–14.
*Heller, John R., and et al. "Untreated Syphilis in the Male Negro: Mortality during Twelve Years of Observation." *Journal of Venereal Disease Information* 27 (1946): 34–38.
Olansky, Sidney, et al. "Environmental Factors in the Tuskegee Study of Untreated Syphilis." *Public Health Reports* 69 (1954): 691–98.
Olansky, Sidney, et al. "Untreated Syphilis in the Male Negro: Twenty-two Years of Serological Observation in a Selected Syphilis Study Group." *A.M.A. Archives of Dermatology* 73 (1956): 519–22.
Olansky, Sidney, et al. "Untreated Syphilis in the Male Negro: X. Twenty Years of

Clinical Observation of Untreated Syphilitic and Presumably Nonsyphilitic Groups." *Journal of Chronic Diseases* 4 (1956): 177–85.

Pesare, Pasquale J., et al. "Untreated Syphilis in the Male Negro." *Journal of Venereal Disease Information* 27 (1946): 202.

Pesare, Pasquale J., et al. "Untreated Syphilis in the Male Negro: Observation of Abnormalities over Sixteen Years." *American Journal of Syphilis, Gonorrhea, and Venereal Diseases* 34 (1950): 201–13.

Peters, Jesse J., et al. "Untreated Syphilis in the Male Negro: Pathologic Findings in Syphilitic and Nonsyphilitic Patients." *Journal of Chronic Diseases* 1 (1955): 127–48.

*Rivers, Eunice, et al. "Twenty Years of Follow-Up Experience in a Long-Range Medical Study." *Public Health Reports* 68 (1953): 391–95.

Rockwell, Donald H., et al. "The Tuskegee Study of Untreated Syphilis: The Thirtieth Year of Observation." *Archives of Internal Medicine* 114 (1961): 792–98.

Schuman, Stanley H., et al. "Untreated Syphilis in the Male Negro: Background and Current Status of Patients in the Tuskegee Study." *Journal of Chronic Diseases* 2 (1955): 543–58.

Shafer, J. K., et al. "Untreated Syphilis in the Male Negro: A Prospective Study of the Effect on Life Expectancy." *Public Health Reports* 69 (1954): 691–97.

Vonderlehr, R. A., et al. "Untreated Syphilis in the Male Negro: A Comparative Study of Treated and Untreated Cases." *Venereal Disease Information* 17 (1936): 260–65, and *Journal of the American Medical Association* 107 (1936): 856–60.

MEDICAL, NURSING, AND PUBLIC-HEALTH ARTICLES

*Angell, Marcia. "The Ethics of Clinical Research in the Third World." *N. E. J. Med.* 337, no. 12 (1997): 847–49.

Brawley, O. W. "The Study of Untreated Syphilis in the Negro Male." *Int. J. Radiat. Oncol. Biol. Phys.* 40, no. 1 (1998): 5–8.

Butler, Broadus. "The Tuskegee Syphilis Study." *Journal of the National Medical Association* 65, no. 4 (1973): 345–48.

Byman, B. "Out from the Shadow of Tuskegee: Fighting Racism in Medicine." *Minn. Med.* 74, no. 8 (1991): 15–20.

*Cave, Vernal G. "Proper Uses and Abuses of the Health Care Delivery System for Minorities with Special Reference to the Tuskegee Syphilis Study." *J. Nat. Med. Assoc.* 67, no. 1 (1975): 82–84.

Cobb, W. M. "The Tuskegee Syphilis Study." *J. Natl. Med. Assoc.* 65, no. 4 (1973): 345–48.

Coughlin, S. S., G. D. Etheredge, C. Metayer, and S. A. Martin Jr. "Remember Tuskegee: Public Health Student Knowledge of the Ethical Significance of the Tuskegee Syphilis Study." *Am. J. Prev. Med.* 12, no. 4 (1996): 242–46.

Cox, J. D. "Paternalism, Informed Consent and Tuskegee." *Int. J. Radiat. Oncol. Biol. Phys.* 20, no. 1 (1998): 1–2.

Curran, William J. "Law-Medicine Notes: The Tuskegee Syphilis Study." *New England Journal of Medicine* 289, no. 14 (1973): 730–31.

*Cutler, John C., et al. "Venereal Disease Control by Health Departments in the Past: Lessons for the Present." *American Journal of Public Health* 78, no. 4 (1988): 372–76.

Dowd, S. B., and B. Wilson. "Informed Patient Consent: A Historical Perspective." *Radiol. Technol.* 67, no. 2 (1995): 119–24.

Gerrity, Patricia L. "Public Health Initiatives and the Legacy of Tuskegee: A Case Study." *Family Community Health* 17, no. 3 (1994): 15–22.

Grunfeld, G. B. "Dissimilarities between Tuskegee Study and HIV/AIDS Programs Emphasized." *Am. J. Public Health* 82, no. 8 (1992): 1176.

Guinan, M. E. "Black Communities' Belief in 'AIDS as Genocide': A Barrier to Overcome for HIV Prevention." *Ann. Epidemiol.* 3, no. 2 (1993): 193–95.

Harris, Y., P. B. Gorelick, P. Samuels, and I. Bempong. "Why African Americans May Not Be Participating in Clinical Trials." *J. Natl. Med. Assoc.* 88, no. 10 (1996): 630–34.

Hazen, H. H. *Syphilis in the Negro: A Handbook for the General Practitioner*. Vol. Supplement No. 15, Venereal Disease Information. Washington, D.C.: Federal Security Agency, U.S. Public Health Service, 1942.

Hinton, William A. *Syphilis and Its Treatment*. New York: Macmillan Company, 1936.

*Kampmeier, R. H. "The Tuskegee Study of Untreated Syphilis." *Southern Medical Journal* 65 (October 1972): 1247–51.

———. "The Final Report on the Tuskegee Syphilis Study." *Southern Medical Journal* 67, no. 11 (1974): 56–67.

Lewis, Julian Herman. *The Biology of the Negro*. Chicago: University of Chicago Press, 1942.

McCarthy, C. R. "Historical Background of Clinical Trials Involving Women and Minorities." *Acad. Med.* 69, no. 9 (1994): 695–98.

*McDonald, Charles J. "The Contribution of the Tuskegee Study to Medical Knowledge." *J. Nat. Med. Assoc.* 66, no. 1 (1974): 1–7.

*Parran, Thomas. "White Man's Burden." In *Shadow on the Land*, 160–81. New York: Reynal and Hitchcock, 1937.

*Roy, Benjamin. "The Tuskegee Syphilis Experiment: Biotechnology and the Administrative State." *J. Natl. Med. Assoc.* 87, no. 1 (1995): 56–66.

———. "The Tuskegee Syphilis Experiment: Medical Ethics, Constitutionalism, and Property in the Body." *Harvard Journal of Minority Health* 1, no. 1 (1995): 11–15.

———. "The Julius Rosenwald Fund Syphilis Seroprevalence Studies." *J. Natl. Med. Assoc.* 88, no. 5 (1996): 315–22.

*Silver, George A. "The Infamous Tuskegee Study." *Am. J. Public Health* 78, no. 11 (1988): 1500.

Talone, P. "Establishing Trust after Tuskegee." *Int. J. Radiat. Oncol. Phys.* 40, no. 1 (1998): 3–4.

*Thomas, Stephen. B., and Sandra Crouse Quinn. "The Tuskegee Syphilis Study, 1932 to 1972: Implications for HIV Education and AIDS Risk Education Programs in the Black Community." *American Journal of Public Health* 81 (1991): 1498–1506.

"Treponemes and Tuskegee." *Lancet* 1, no. 7817 (23 June 1973): 1438.

"The Tuskegee Study." *J. Okla. State Med. Assoc.* 66, no. 2 (1973): 47–51.

*Varmus, Harold, and David Satcher. "Ethical Complexities of Conducting Research in Developing Countries." *N. E. J. Med.* 337, no. 14 (1997): 1003–5.

Vessey, J. A., and S. Gennaro. "The Ghost of Tuskegee." *Nurs. Res.* 43, no. 2 (1994): 67.

White, R. M. "Grand Dragon or Windmill: Why I Opposed the Presidential Apology for the Tuskegee Study." *J. Natl. Med. Assoc.* 89, no. 11 (1997): 719–20.

Wolinsky, Howard. "Steps Still Being Taken to Undo Damage of 'America's Nuremberg.' "*Annals of Internal Medicine* 127 (15 August 1997): 143–44.

HISTORICAL, SOCIAL SCIENCE, AND BIOETHICAL ARTICLES
AND BOOKS

Aptheker, Herbert. "Racism and Human Experimentation." *Political Affairs, Theoretical Journal of the Communist Party* LIII (2 1974): 47–59.

*Benedek, T. G. "The 'Tuskegee Study' of Syphilis: An Analysis of Moral versus Methodologic Aspects." *Journal of Chronic Diseases* 31, no. 1 (1978): 35–50.

Bowie, Sibyl Kaye. "The Tuskegee Syphilis Study: A Case Study in Crisis Communication in Public Relations." Master's thesis, University of Georgia, 1986.

Brandt, Allan M. *No Magic Bullet.* New York: Oxford University Press, 1987.

*———. "Racism and Research: The Case of the Tuskegee Syphilis Study." In *Sickness and Health in America*, eds. Judith Walzer Leavitt and Ronald L. Numbers, 392–404. 3d (rev.) ed. Madison: Wisconsin Press, 1997.

*Caplan, Arthur L. "When Evil Intrudes." *The Hastings Center Report* 22, no. 6 (1992): 29–32.

Dawson, Emory. "The Protection of Human Subjects: The Tuskegee Study." *Maxwell Review* 10, no. 2 (1974): 49–56.

Dula, Annette. "African American Suspicion of the Healthcare System Is Justified: What Do We Do about It?" *Cambridge Quarterly of Healthcare Ethics* 3 (1994): 347–57.

*Edgar, Harold. "Outside the Community." *Hastings Center Report* 22, no. 6 (1992): 32–35.

*Fairchild, Amy L., and Ronald Bayer. "Uses and Abuses of Tuskegee." *Science* 284 (7 May 1999): 919–21.

Forman, James. *Sammy Younge, Jr. : The First Black College Student to Die in the Black Liberation Movement*. New York: Grove Press, 1968.

Foster, Henry W. Jr. *Make a Difference*. New York: Scribner's Sons, 1997.

Fourter, A. W., C. F. Fourtner, and C. F. Herreid. "Bad Blood: A Case Study of the Tuskegee Syphilis Project." *J. College Sci. Teach.* 23, no. 23 (1994): 277–85.

Gamble, Vanessa Northington. "A Legacy of Distrust: African Americans and Medical Research." *Am. J. Prev. Med.* 9 November-December 1993, Suppl.): 35–38.

———. "The Tuskegee Syphilis Study and Women's Health." *J. Am. Med. Women's Assoc.* 52, no. 4 (1997): 195–196.

*———. "Under the Shadow of Tuskegee: African Americans and Health Care." *AJPH* 87 (November 1997): 1773–78.

Goldner, Jesse A. "An Overview of Legal Controls on Human Experimentation and the Regulatory Implications of Taking Professor Katz Seriously." *St. Louis University Law Journal* 38 (Fall 1993): 63–134.

Gray, Fred D. *Bus Ride to Justice: Changing the System by the System, The Life Works of Fred Gray*. Montgomery, Ala.: Black Belt Press, 1995.

*———. *The Tuskegee Syphilis Study: The Real Story and Beyond*. Montgomery: Black Belt Press, 1998.

Guzman, Jessie Parkhurst. *Crusade for Civic Democracy: The Story of the Tuskegee Civic Association, 1941–1970*. New York: Vantage Press, 1984.

Hammar, Lawrence. "The Dark Side to Donovanosis: Color, Climate, Race and Racism in American South Venereology." *Journal of Medical Humanities* 18 (Spring 1997): 29–57.

*Hammonds, Evelynn M. "Your Silence Will Not Protect You: Nurse Eunice Rivers and the Tuskegee Syphilis Study." In *The Black Woman's Health Book: Speaking for Ourselves*, ed. C. Evelyn White, 323–31. 2d ed. Seattle: Seal Press, 1994.

Hiltner, Seward. "The Tuskegee Syphilis Study under Review." *The Christian Century* 90, no. 43 (1973): 1174–76.

*Hine, Darlene Clark. *Black Women in White*. Bloomington: Indiana University Press, 1989.

*Johnson, Charles S. *Shadow of the Plantation*. Chicago: The University of Chicago Press, 1934.

Jones, James H. *Bad Blood: The Tuskegee Syphilis Experiment*. New York: Free Press., 1981, Revised Edition, 1992.

———. "The Tuskegee Legacy: AIDS and the Black Community." *The Hastings Center Report* 22, no. 6 (1992): 38–40.

Katz, Jay. "The Regulation of Human Experimentation in the United States—A Personal Odyssey." *IRB: A Review of Human Subjects Research* 9 (January/February 1987): 1–6.

*King, Patricia A. "The Dangers of Difference." *Hastings Center Report* 22, no. 6 (1992): 35–37.

Kirp, David L. "Blood, Sweat, and Tears: The Tuskegee Experiment and the Era of AIDS." *Tikkun* 10, no. 3 (1995): 50–54.

Lederer, Susan. "The Tuskegee Syphilis Study in the Context of American Medical Research." *Sigerist Circle Newsletter and Bibliography* 6 (Winter 1994): 2–4.

Norrell, Robert J. *Reaping the Whirlwind: The Civil Rights Movement in Tuskegee.* New York: Vintage, 1986.

Reverby, Susan M. "History of an Apology: From Tuskegee to the White House." *Research Nurse* 3 (July/August 1997): 1–9.

*——. "Rethinking the Tuskegee Syphilis Study: Nurse Rivers, Silence and the Meaning of Treatment." *Nursing History Review* 7 (1999): 3–28.

*Rosenkrantz, Barbara. "Non-Random Events." *Yale Review* 72 (1983): 284–96.

Rothman, D. J. "Were Tuskegee and Willowbrook 'Studies in Nature'?" *Hastings Center Report* 12, no. 2 (1982): 5–7.

——. "Research Ethics at Tuskegee and Willowbrook [letter]." *Am. J. Med.* 77, no. 6 (1984): A49.

Savitt, Todd L. "The Use of Blacks for Medical Experimentation and Demonstration in the Old South." *Journal of Southern History* 48 (August 1982): 331–48.

Shick, Tom W. "Race, Class and Medicine: 'Bad Blood' in Twentieth-Century America." *Journal of Ethnic Studies* (Summer 1982): 97–105.

Smith, Joyce E. "A Black Experiment, or the Tuskegee Study." *Consciousness IV* Series No. 2 (1973) Washington, D.C.: Howard University Library.

Smith, Susan L. *"Sick and Tired of Being Sick and Tired": Black Women's Health Activism in America, 1890–1950.* Philadelphia: University of Pennsylvania Press, 1995.

*——. "Neither Victim nor Villain: Nurse Eunice Rivers, the Tuskegee Syphilis Experiment, and Public Health Work." *Journal of Women's History* 8 (Spring 1996): 95–113.

*Solomon, Martha. "The Rhetoric of Dehumanization: An Analysis of Medical Reports of the Tuskegee Syphilis Project." *Western Journal of Speech Communication* 49, no. 4 (1985): 233–47. Reprinted in *Critical Questions: Invention, Creativity, and the Criticism of Discourse and Media*, eds. William L. Nothstine, Carole Blair, and Gary A. Copeland. New York: St. Martin's Press, 1994.

Stanfield, John H. "Venereal Disease Control Demonstrations among Rural

Blacks in the American South." *Western Journal of Black Studies* 5, no. 4 (1981): 246–53.

Taper, Bernard. *Gomillion versus Lightfoot: The Tuskegee Gerrymander Case*. New York: McGraw Hill, 1962.

Winters, Myrtle V. "A Study of the Development and Organization of the Public Health Department of Macon County, Alabama." Master's thesis, Tulane University School of Social Work, 1941.

NEWSPAPER AND MAGAZINE ARTICLES

Barker, Martha G. "Civil Rights Center Dedicated in Tuskegee." *Opelika-Auburn News*, 17 May 1998, A-1.

*Heller, Jean. "Syphilis Victims in U.S. Study without Therapy for Forty Years." *New York Times*, 26 July 1972, 1, 8.

*Junod, Tom. "Deadly Medicine." *Gentlemen's Quarterly*, June 1993, 164–71, 231–34.

Levine, Martin P. "Bad Blood: The Health Commissioner, the Tuskegee Experiment, and AIDS Policy." *New York Native* 16 February 1987, 13–16.

Shelton, Deborah L. "Legacy of Tuskegee." *American Medical News* 3 June 1996, 24–30.

Spear, Ken L. "Tuskegee Launches Bioethics Center," *Montgomery Advertiser* 15 May 1999, 1A, 2A.

Stryker, Jeff. "Tuskegee's Long Arm Still Touches a Nerve." *New York Times*, 13 April 1997, 4.

Trafford, Abigail. "The Ghost of Tuskegee." *Washington Post*, 6 May 1997, A19.

Washington, Harriet A. "Human Guinea Pigs." *Emerge: Black America's New Magazine*, 6 (1 October 1994): 24.

*Yoon, Carol Kaesuk. "Families Emerge as Silent Victims of Tuskegee Syphilis Experiments." *New York Times*, 12 May 1997, A1.

VIDEOS, AUDIOCASSETTES, AND COMPACT DISCS

Bad Blood. Video. London: Diverse Production, 1992.

*Bryon, Don. *Tuskegee Experiments*. Elektra Nonesuch 79260-2. Compact disc. 1992.

Critical Thinking in Nursing: Lessons from Tuskegee. Video. New York: National League for Nursing Videos, 1993.

The Deadly Deception. Video. NOVA, WGBH Educational Foundation Films, 1993.

Living Black and White: Tuskegee, Alabama. Video. Tuscaloosa, Ala.: University of Alabama Center for Public Television, 1996.

McDonald, Leroy. *Tuskegee Subject No. 626*. Film. Dallas: Leroy McDonald, 1991.

Miss Evers' Boys. New York: HBO, 1997.

Race Prejudice and Health Care: The Lessons of the Tuskegee Syphilis Experiment.
Audiotapes. Minneapolis: Illusion Theater, 1993.

Scott-Herron, Gill. *Bridges*. Arista: AB 4147. Compact disc, 1994.

Susceptible to Kindness: "Miss Evers' Boys" and the Tuskegee Syphilis Study. Video.
Ithaca: Cornell University Media Services, 1993.

"The Tuskegee Study." Video. New York: ABC, "Prime Time Live," 6 February
1992.

"White House Apology." Video. Atlanta: CNN Live, 16 May 1997.

FICTION

Chandler, Duane. *The Trees Don't Bleed in Tuskegee: A Play in Two Acts Based on
the Tuskegee Syphilis Study*. Unpublished manuscript. Hasbrouck Heights,
N.J., 1997.

*Feldshuh, David. *Miss Evers' Boys*. New York: Dramatists Play Service, Inc., 1995.

*Hemphill, Essex. "Civil Servant." In *Ceremonies*, 22–24. New York: Plume, 1992.

INDEX

The following abbreviations are used in the index:

DPs—Demonstration projects
HSR—Human subjects research
JRF—Julius Rosenwald Fund
TSS—Tuskegee Syphilis Study
VD—Venereal disease

Abbott, William Osler, 269–71, 273–74
Ad Hoc Committee to Consider the Tuskegee
  Study, 10 (n. 6), 26, 169–71, 463–72, 477, 514
Advisory Committee for Elimination of Tuberculosis, 580
African American churches: and JRF DPs, 63;
  influence of, 67; and TSS, 102, 132, 135, 401,
  408, 409
African American health-care researchers:
  and TSS, 5, 202, 210, 365; and syphilis treatment, 243
African American health professionals: and
  diversity, xvi; and TSS, 4, 24, 225, 344–45,
  346, 348, 349, 354, 355, 360, 365, 392, 408,
  460, 569; and syphilis treatment, 24, 68–69,
  376; and PHS, 60–61; and JRF DPs, 61; in
  Macon Co., 219; as authority figures, 225;
  and JRF, 240; and AIDS, 347; and morality,
  379; and racism, 394, 435; recruitment of,
  403; and African Americans as research
  subjects, 434–35; and Tuskegee VA Hospital,
  435; and Ad Hoc Committee to Consider
  the Tuskegee Study, 468–69
African Americans: and disease patterns, xv–
  xvi; and images of TSS, 1; as metaphor, 3–4;
  and white philanthropic support, 4; and
  conspiracy theories, 5, 278, 405, 413, 515, 517;
  and physicians' role, 5, 49–51; and syphilis,
  7, 17, 42, 54, 59–61, 64, 66, 68, 80, 239, 253,
  277, 283, 306, 310, 314, 353; and health care
  delivery systems, 8, 355–56, 359, 360, 387,
  400, 412, 424, 426, 431–32, 435, 437–39,
  559, 561; and effects of TSS, 8, 600; and Darwinism, 16, 18; and syphilis treatment, 17,
  22, 23, 176, 368; and Macon Co. mortality
  rate, 41–42; and violence, 42, 43–45; and

folk knowledge of disease, 45–49, 400; and
  midwives, 51–54; and JRF demonstration
  program, 54–58, 59, 60; and education, 59,
  61, 63, 67, 240; and autopsies, 85; and AIDS,
  278, 340, 346–47, 360, 404–6, 412–16, 425–
  26, 431–32, 436, 517, 591; and TSS, 340, 365,
  390, 405, 406, 426, 435–36, 438, 440, 515–
  16, 518–19, 520, 561, 562, 589, 591; governmental neglect of, 350; and Rivers, 375, 389,
  390; and women's history, 391; and racial
  difference, 424, 425–26, 427; and black-
  controlled hospitals, 434–35; and voting
  rights litigation, 473–74; and official apology, 562, 575
—as research subjects: identification of as
  cadavers, 3, 7, 266; history of, 3, 269–72,
  432–35; view of as less than human, 28, 33
  (n. 89), 269–70; and racism, 266, 437; and
  litigation, 272–74. See also Tuskegee Syphilis Study—subjects
Aging: and TSS, 35, 209, 227; and syphilis, 43
AIDS: African Americans' participation in education and research on, 278, 360, 408, 412–
  16, 425–26, 431–32, 517; and TSS, 278, 413,
  426, 431–32, 436, 514, 559, 591; incidence of
  among African Americans, 340, 346–47,
  404–6, 591; and genocide, 405, 406, 413, 415,
  416, 436, 510, 515, 517, 518, 561; and racial difference, 425–26; control of, 495–96, 498,
  504, 505, 506; and AIDS Clinical Trials
  Group protocol 076, 586, 598
AIDS Research Consortium of Atlanta, 518
Alabama: and lawsuit, 38; and VD control,
  110, 226, 231; and autopsy laws, 268–69; and
  public health laws, 281, 410, 569; coroner
  system in, 471; and voting rights litigation,
  473–74
Alabama Health Department: and syphilis
  treatment, 26, 569, 589; and TSS, 76, 281; and
  TSS records, 327; and Rivers, 333–35, 477;
  and state appropriations to counties, 469
Alabama State Board of Health: and TSS, 37,
  106, 408, 451, 569; and lawsuit, 38; and JRF
  DPs, 75, 240

378; and Olansky, 513; and *Miss Evers' Boys*, 531, 542, 550; and lawsuit settlement, 568
Butler, Broadus N., 157, 161, 175, 181
Buxtun, Peter J.: and TSS, 7, 8, 37, 255, 276–77, 288, 399, 418, 514; correspondence of, 105, 153–54, 411; Senate hearing testimony of, 150–56; and race, 291

Caldwell, Joseph G., 37, 164–65, 169, 377, 464, 470
Campbell, Tom, 333, 334
Cancer, 42
Caplan, Arthur, 8, 593–94
Cardiovascular disease and syphilis: and race, 4, 66, 79, 86–87, 209, 217, 283, 306, 308, 325, 368, 407, 493; untreated, 19, 117, 119, 151, 168, 256, 523; in latent stage, 25, 198–99, 206, 243; and mortality rate, 42, 122; and TSS, 75, 76, 97, 100, 125, 127, 197, 203–4, 206, 208–9, 223, 255, 309, 420–21, 468, 484, 491; treatment, 89, 198, 199–200, 228–29, 465, 470; and Bruusgaard, 194, 207, 223; and Wassermann test, 306
Carver, George Washington, 576
Case Western Reserve University, 163, 300, 581
Cassell, Robert, 5
Cave, Vernal G., 8, 25, 162, 174, 181, 202
Centers for Disease Control: and TSS continuation, 8, 15, 26, 117, 411, 470, 514; and race, 26, 411; and Buxtun, 37, 255, 277, 418; and lawsuit, 38; and SDS, 111–14; and penicillin, 167; and AIDS, 404, 414; and syphilis, 419; and medical research, 439; and Foster, 444, 446, 454; and syphilis treatment, 447; and Tuskegee Institute, 450; and TSS outcome, 523; and HIV, 580, 584, 585, 587, 598; and blinded seroprevalence studies, 595, 596, 597
Central nervous system and syphilis: and spinal taps, 21, 22, 35, 100, 326, 493–94; untreated, 25, 117, 168, 208, 209, 256, 301, 523; and race, 66, 208, 217, 230, 283, 325, 368, 407, 493; and TSS, 75, 92, 203–4, 255, 307–8, 421, 483, 486; and Bruusgaard, 194, 205, 207, 216; treatment, 228, 465, 484; in latent stage, 243; and Cooperative Clinical Study, 301
Chamberlain-Kahn Act, 497
Cheever, David W., 214
Child Health Association, 239
Children: and syphilis treatment, 38; and in-

fant mortality rates, 41–42, 46, 65; and congenital syphilis, 43, 219; and JRF DPs, 62; and TSS, 78, 227, 230, 346, 457, 460, 483, 484, 487; and syphilis transmission, 167, 560; and DPs, 239; and Heller, 332; and AIDS, 346, 404, 518; and trust in health care delivery systems, 510, 519; and medical research, 518; and official apology, 575; and HIV, 585, 586, 591, 595–96, 597–99
CIA experiments, 490
Civil rights, 415, 480
Civil rights movement, 291, 355, 405, 469
Clark, E. G., 194, 203, 204
Clark, Taliaferro: and TSS, 18–19, 23, 24, 35, 75–76, 77, 97, 245, 266, 277, 283, 368, 407, 512; and African Americans, 20; and TSS subjects, 21; and syphilis treatment, 21–22; and deception of TSS subjects, 22, 408; correspondence of, 73–75, 78–83, 240, 241, 368; and morality, 279, 286; and informed consent, 281, 284; and ethics, 282–83, 287; and peer review, 285
Class: and race, 4, 11 (n. 16), 366, 390; and Rivers, 366–67, 374, 375, 379, 380, 390, 393; and syphilis, 368, 369; and TSS, 390, 392, 394; and African Americans, 391–92, 394; and HIV/AIDS, 416
Clinical trials: African American participation in, 414, 415, 425–26, 431, 559, 561; and AIDS, 414, 415, 425–26, 586, 598; and racial difference, 427; and ethics, 578, 580, 582, 584, 585; and needle exchange programs, 592, 593
Clinton, William J.: official apology of, xvi, 1, 2, 5, 9, 38, 278, 296 (n. 10), 365–66, 431, 457, 460, 574–77; and Tuskegee Institute, 478; and TSS Legacy Committee, 560; and human radiation experiments, 560, 562; and context of apology, 562
Cohen, Paul, 169, 464
Combs, S. R., 198
Commission on the Eradication of Syphilis, 68
Commonwealth Fund, 239
Communicable Disease Center, 151, 152, 155
Congressional Black Caucus, 574, 596
Control groups, and ethics, 214–15, 578, 579, 580, 585, 587, 598. *See also* Tuskegee Syphilis Study—control group
Cooperative Clinical Studies in the Treatment of Syphilis: and TSS, 91, 222–24; and PHS,

163, 299, 300, 313; and syphilis treatment, 195; and syphilitic aortitis, 198; reports of, 219, 222, 230; African American subjects of, 220–21; and untreated syphilis, 301; and central nervous system, 307

Cornely, Paul B., 355

Cumming, H. S.: and TSS, 18–19, 23, 278; and Tuskegee Institute, 75; correspondence of, 77; and VD, 239; and HSR, 285; and serological study, 302

Cutler, John C., 8, 99–101, 412, 507, 513, 519–20

Darwinism, 16

Davis, Michael M., 59, 164, 239–41, 242, 243, 245, 382 (n. 21)

Declaration of Helsinki, 37

Deibert, Austin V.: and TSS, 35, 97, 322; correspondence of, 89–92, 220, 222; and syphilis treatment, 96, 281; and cardiovascular disease, 208

Developing countries, 584–88, 598

Dibble, Eugene H., Jr.: and TSS, 23, 24, 77, 84, 86, 87–88, 330–31, 344–45, 348, 368, 369, 469; correspondence of, 75–76; and autopsies, 85; and Rivers, 335, 371, 375; and syphilis treatment, 354; and Foster, 444

Dibble, Helen, 7, 371

Draft board. See Selective Service Commission

Du Bois, W. E. B., 390

Dull, H. Bruce, 170, 464, 465, 469

DuVal, Merlin K., 116, 159, 237, 402

Edgar, Harold, 8, 476, 489

Education: of TSS subjects, xv, 21, 116, 127, 128, 225, 252, 259, 286, 402, 405, 409, 431, 478; and African Americans, 59, 61, 63, 67, 240; and informed consent, 206, 224; and VD control, 241, 242, 497, 500, 504, 505; and HIV/AIDS, 404, 406, 408, 412–16, 431; and TSS, 563

Ehrlich, Paul, 19, 194, 242, 367

Ellison, Ralph, 366, 369

Ethics: and TSS, xv, xvi, 15, 27, 28, 29, 118, 166, 171, 172, 173, 176, 213–15, 231–32, 251, 255, 278, 280–87, 303, 365, 389, 390, 492, 517, 563, 577, 579, 594, 600; rethinking of, 6; and medical research, 7, 214–15, 232, 254, 277, 279, 285, 288–89, 297 (n. 42), 419, 422, 562–63, 576, 578–88, 590–91; of informed consent, 9, 180, 268, 278, 284, 293, 490, 585; and HEW

policies, 178; and news media, 197; and HSR, 215, 245, 246–47, 268, 272, 284–89, 293–95, 419, 422–23, 559, 577; and Co-operating Clinical Group's findings, 223; and Jones, 245, 284, 289, 293, 411, 491; and TSS reports, 252, 260, 261, 262, 263, 264 (n. 3); and PHS, 292, 410, 411; professional, 293–95, 424; and penicillin, 295 (n. 7); and Rivers, 345, 378, 380, 389, 393; and Foster, 444; and institutional review boards, 491; and HIV, 579–80, 584, 585, 598, 599, 600; and needle exchange programs, 593–94; and blinded seroprevalence studies, 595, 597

Faden, Ruth R., 282, 284

Farrakhan, Louis, 514, 516

Fed (slave), 432

Federal officials: and TSS, 4, 418; and Tuskegee Institute, 4, 478; and JRF syphilis DPs, 97; and HIV/AIDS education, 414; and VD control, 497, 499, 500, 501, 503, 504

Feldshuh, David, 5, 8, 341, 393, 527–51, 568–70, 572

Fletcher, John C., 7, 465

Folk knowledge of disease, 45–49, 400

Folktales, 433–34

Food and Drug Administration (FDA), 177, 284, 491

Foster, Henry Wendell, 8, 106, 365, 443–56

FTA-ABS (fluorescent treponemal antibody absorption) test, 107, 197, 210, 312

Gamble, Vanessa Northington, 8, 278, 459, 460, 564

Gatch, Willis, 271

Gender: and race, 4, 11 (n. 16), 366, 390; and public health work, 349, 352, 358, 360; and syphilis, 368; and Rivers, 374, 375, 379, 380, 393; and TSS, 390, 394

Genocide: and TSS, 111, 278, 412, 418, 436–37, 479, 514, 515, 561, 591, 592, 593; and AIDS, 405, 406, 413, 415, 416, 436, 510, 515, 517, 518, 561; and needle exchange programs, 415, 431, 592; fears of, 435–37

Germany, 284–85, 287, 304, 305, 313

Gibson, Count, 513, 519

Gill, D. G., 74, 82, 86, 94–95

Gillespie, E. J., 104

Gjestland, T., 194, 202, 203, 205, 207, 210, 232

ethics of, 9, 27, 215, 268, 278, 284, 293, 490, 585; and Pure Food and Drug Act Amendments, 36; and Declaration of Helsinki, 37; and HEW policies, 178; and SAG, 180; and HSR, 273, 276, 284, 399, 439–40, 519, 576, 579; history of, 282–84, 296 (n. 33), 378; and legal protections, 293; and Wile, 300; limitations of, 424; and lawsuit, 475; and blinded seroprevalence studies, 595

Insanity, and syphilis, 17, 19, 151, 523

Institutional Human Investigation Committee (IHIC), 180

Institutional review boards (IRBs), 2, 294, 426, 490–91, 591

Ipsen, Johannes, Jr., 169, 463, 469

Iskrant, Albert, 281, 290

Ivy, A. C., 215

James, Reginald, 329, 376, 385 (n. 71), 394

Japan, 313, 560

Jenkins, Bill, 458, 459–60, 564

John A. Andrew Clinical Society, 561

John A. Andrew Hospital: and TSS, 23, 35, 74, 84, 88, 132, 136, 238, 283, 322, 354; and JRF, 42; and Rivers, 342, 353; building of, 561

Johns Hopkins University, 163, 300

Johnson, Charles, 241, 243–44, 246, 356

Johnson, Price, 476

Jonas, Hans, 291, 428

Jones, H. T., 86–87

Jones, James H.: and nontherapeutic experimentation, xi, 241, 348; research of, xi–xiii, 6, 236, 238, 246, 521; and race, xii, 4, 240, 283; narrative of, xii, 6, 251, 341, 406, 481, 491, 567, 589; and morality, xii, 237, 245–46, 251, 342; and images of TSS, 1; and review of *Bad Blood*, 7, 236–47; and Rivers, 8, 11 (n. 16), 341, 342, 345, 348, 371, 373, 378, 389; and public knowledge, 236, 341; and Gray, 237–38, 481; and medical arrogance, 238, 244; and PHS, 239–40; and syphilis treatment, 242–43, 281, 382 (n. 21), 385 (n. 71), 410; and TSS subjects, 244, 409, 459; and penicillin, 245, 246, 295 (n. 7); and ethics, 245, 284, 289, 293, 411, 491; and Buxtun, 255; and TSS objectives, 266; and objections to TSS, 277; and African American health professionals, 355; and physicians, 356; and historical background of TSS, 406, 407–8, 589;

and chronology of TSS, 411; and lawsuit, 412; and TSS summary, 420; and Edgar, 493; and TSS Legacy Committee, 565

Julius Rosenwald Fund: syphilis-control DPs of, 2, 22, 34, 42, 54–58, 59, 60–66, 75, 77, 97, 163, 218, 219, 239, 241, 277, 353, 399–400, 406–7, 478; and PHS, 18, 59, 60, 75, 163, 239–41, 242, 253, 266, 406; attitudes towards experiment of, 54–58, 408; report of, 74; and morality, 286; and syphilis serology, 300; and VD control, 353, 498

Julkes, Albert, Jr., 457

Kaiser, Clyde, 169, 450, 464, 466, 469, 470, 471, 472

Kampmeier, R. H., 7, 28, 198, 203

Katz, Jay: and TSS Ad Hoc Advisory Panel, 162, 174, 181; and informed consent, 175, 282, 284; and addendum to panel report, 175–77, 297 (n. 39); and National Human Investigation Board, 285

Katz, Ralph, 565

Keidel, A., 195

Kennebrew, Elizabeth M., 108, 109–11

Kennedy, Edward: and U.S. Senate Hearings before the Subcommittee on Health of the Committee on Labor and Public Welfare, 37, 136–56, 236, 251, 412, 418; and morality, 280, 288; and U.S. Senate Committee Hearings for the Nomination of Dr. Henry Foster, 443, 447–48, 453–55

Kenney, John, 304–5

Kenny, J. A., 93

King, Martin Luther, Jr., 406

Kuhn, U. S. G., III, 170, 464, 465

Ku Klux doctors, 433

Ku Klux Klan, 17, 375, 435

Lafayette-Bulwinkle Act, 499

Laurie, Eunice Rivers. *See* Rivers, Eunice

Lawsuit: settlement of, 2, 229–30, 238, 487–88, 490, 514, 561, 568; and TSS subjects, 38, 213, 229, 229–30, 237, 328, 332, 365, 412, 473, 475, 476, 478–83; and Rivers, 378–79; and Macon Co. Medical Society, 448, 452; and Gray, 473–88, 489, 568; conclusions regarding, 475; assistance with, 475–76; and Edgar, 476, 489; plaintiffs and defendants of, 476–78; allegations of, 478–79; theory of, 479–80; and discovery, 480–81; and deceased

medical research, 428. *See also* African Americans

Minority Health Initiative, 563

Miss Evers' Boys (Feldshuh), xii, 5, 8, 9, 341, 393, 527–51, 568–70, 572

Missouri v. Holland, 313

Moore, J. E.: and Oslo Study, 19–20; and Clark, 22, 286; correspondence of, 78–80; and latent syphilis, 164; and syphilis treatment, 195; and cardiovascular disease, 198; and TSS, 283, 304; and syphilis serology, 302, 304, 310; and TSS subjects, 356

Morality: and TSS, xvi, 2, 4, 8, 10 (n. 6), 27, 37, 98, 104, 105, 108, 116–18, 151, 168, 176, 210, 237, 251, 255, 287–88, 292–95, 365, 411, 422–23, 513, 519, 561, 562; and PHS, 2–3, 29, 276, 278–79, 289–92, 295, 418; and medical research, 3, 292, 423, 562, 600; and African Americans, 16, 17, 350; and penicillin, 245, 290, 373; and TSS reports, 252, 261; and nontherapeutic experimentation, 254; and historical relativism, 276, 278, 279–80, 285–87; and Heller, 278; and official apology, 278, 295 (n. 8), 560, 561; and HSR, 279, 280–81; and graded approach to moral judgment, 287–92; and Olansky, 295 (n. 8); and Rivers, 378, 379, 393; and HIV/AIDS, 415; and VD control, 505; and government responsibility, 560; and medical resources, 599

Moral relativism, 4, 245, 276

Morbidity: and untreated syphilis, 19, 151, 168, 200, 207–8, 256; and TSS, 23–24, 25, 83, 85, 87, 97, 100, 120, 151, 165, 175, 197, 401–2, 466, 483, 485, 523; and syphilis, 59, 97–98, 168; and syphilis serology, 465

Mortality: Macon Co. mortality rates, 41–42, 46, 400; and violence, 42, 43–45; and folk knowledge of disease, 45–49; and use of physicians, 49–51; and midwives, 51–54; and JRF demonstration program, 54–58; and TSS, 97, 108, 115, 120–24, 151, 165, 197, 208, 209, 224, 227, 306, 401, 465; and untreated syphilis, 151, 175, 200, 401, 402; and Cooperating Clinical Group, 224; and racism, 437

Moss, Frederick, 574

Moton, R. R.: and TSS, 18, 23, 24, 348, 354, 368, 369; correspondence of, 75–76, 77

Moveable School: and Rivers, 342, 349–50, 351,

352–53, 387; as extension program, 349–50; federal government funding for, 354; and African American health care, 360

Murfreesboro, Tenn., 239

Murray, Albert, 369

Myers, Ira L.: correspondence of, 106; and Ad Hoc Committee to Consider the Tuskegee Study, 169, 463, 468–69, 470, 471, 472; and Foster, 446, 447, 451, 452, 453, 454; and Macon Co. Medical Society, 450; and lawsuit, 477, 480

National Archives, xi, xiii, 15, 27, 237

National Association for the Advancement of Colored People (NAACP), 213, 354, 392, 476

National Bioethics Advisory Commission (NBEAC), 562, 576–77

National Commission for the Protection of Human Subjects of Biomedical and Behavioral Research, 403, 419

National Commission on AIDS, 406, 413, 414, 436

National Commission on Venereal Disease, 199

National Conference on Venereal Disease Control, 68

National Health Conference, 599

National Human Investigation Board, 179–80, 285

National Institutes of Health: and autopsies, 83; and penicillin, 195; and ethics, 276, 277, 285, 297 (n. 42); and informed consent, 284; and prior group review, 285, 289, 292; and Nuremberg Code, 289; and TSS, 292–93, 467; and clinical studies, 426–27; and HIV, 580, 584, 585, 587, 588, 598; and placebos, 581; and needle exchange programs, 593–94

National Medical Association, 68, 355, 360

National Negro Health Movement, 349, 354

National Negro Health Week, 561

National Research Act of 1974, 439, 490, 591

National Venereal Disease Act of 1938, 303

Nation of Islam, 405, 514

Native Americans, 9, 59, 354

Nazi experimentation: and ethics, xv, 285, 289, 419; as metaphor, 3; TSS compared to, 151, 152, 176, 340, 514, 516, 521

Needle exchange programs, 415, 431, 591–95

Negro Veterans Hospital. *See* Tuskegee VA Hospital

Students for a Democratic Society (SDS), 111–14

Subject Advisory Group (SAG), 180

Sulfonamides, 305

Surgeons general: and TSS, 3, 7, 164, 176; and Foster, 8, 443–56; and syphilis treatment, 176; and morality, 290; and VD control, 498. *See also specific surgeons general*

Syphilis: and bad blood, 1, 22, 54, 61, 240, 243, 337, 365; and autopsies, 2; and race, 4, 66, 79, 86–87, 168, 208, 209, 217, 230, 240, 253, 258, 283, 306, 308, 310, 325, 368, 407, 425, 493, 504; and African Americans, 7, 17, 42, 54, 59–61, 64, 66, 68, 80, 239, 253, 277, 283, 306, 310, 314, 353; and JRF, 54–58, 59, 60–62; and whites, 59–69; congenital, 64, 219, 220, 230, 400; and PHS statistics, 155–56; natural history of, 164, 196, 203–4, 205, 216, 230, 232, 256, 257–58, 283, 290, 299, 368, 407, 419, 420, 422, 425, 509, 523, 559, 579; diagnosis of, 242–43, 244, 466, 479, 486, 495; and TSS reports, 255–56, 259, 260; laws requiring tests for, 313; and VD control, 495–506. *See also* Cardiovascular disease and syphilis; Central nervous system and syphilis; Syphilis—latent stage

—latent stage: and treatment, 17, 19–20, 28, 60, 62, 220, 485, 509; and transmission risk, 20, 164, 167, 459–60; and cardiovascular disease, 25, 198–99, 206, 243; and TSS, 28, 164, 165, 166, 196, 199, 200, 205, 220, 301, 358, 421, 559, 560; and penicillin, 28, 167, 168; correspondence concerning, 77, 90; and selection of candidates, 125, 206; and Cooperative Clinical Studies in the Treatment of Syphilis, 163; cure rate for, 165; results of treatment of, 166, 168, 199, 367, 369, 370; and Bruusgaard, 207; and syphilis serology, 210; diagnosis of, 243; and Rivers, 371–72; and natural history of syphilis, 523

—serology: and deception, 24; and JRF DPs, 58, 59, 65, 240; and VD control, 68, 500; and TSS, 76, 77, 94, 97, 100, 107, 119, 125, 132, 133, 134, 135, 136, 138, 144, 172, 196, 207, 209, 219, 220, 221, 222, 223, 227, 231, 243, 299, 301, 302–6, 467; and morbidity, 170, 465; and syphilis treatment, 195, 209, 217, 300, 492; and treponemal tests, 196, 311–13; and Oslo Study, 204, 205, 207, 217; and cardiovascular disease, 209; and latent syphilis, 210; and

congenital syphilis, 230; and PHS, 251, 301–3, 305, 308, 311, 401; and biotechnology, 299; and nontreponemal tests, 299, 301–5; and untreated syphilis, 300–301; and diagnosis credibility, 305–11; and Milbank Memorial Fund, 321; and Rivers, 327; and African American churches, 409; and origin of transmission, 460; and *Miss Evers' Boys*, 530, 531

—treatment: and PHS, 2, 15, 20, 25–26, 27, 60, 65, 68, 80–82, 483; withheld from TSS subjects, 2, 15, 25–26, 27, 116, 168–69, 175–76, 198, 205, 207, 213, 225–26, 229, 231–32, 241, 251, 257, 267, 357, 370, 401, 465, 466, 469, 479, 484, 487, 560, 569, 575, 579, 590, 600; and race, 4, 20; science of, 7; obtained by TSS subjects, 7, 26, 81, 89, 107, 120, 151, 169, 196, 197, 198, 199, 209–10, 220, 222, 230, 372, 377, 378, 410, 466, 484, 486, 487, 492; and African Americans, 17, 22–23, 30 (n. 15), 425; and JRF DPs, 18, 54–56, 58, 60, 400, 406–7; risks of, 19, 28, 118, 153, 166, 167, 170, 176, 194, 196, 200, 203, 218, 227, 254, 321–22, 369, 371, 465, 468, 484, 485, 492, 500, 509, 514; discoveries concerning, 19, 116–17, 194–95, 216; offered to TSS subjects, 21–23, 31 (n. 43), 90, 165, 220, 281, 479, 512, 568–69, 589; costs of, 23, 66, 69, 75, 80–81, 194, 242, 367, 368; and noneffective medicines, 24, 166; and Macon Co., 64, 74, 194, 368; and drug supply, 80–82; and TSS, 87, 199, 368, 370, 410, 467, 469, 471, 477; control of, 89–90, 94–96, 107; and Buxtun, 153; and Cooperative Clinical Studies in the Treatment of Syphilis, 163, 222–24; challenges of, 194–95, 198, 419; history of, 194–95, 217–18, 227–28, 281, 300–301, 495, 500, 512, 560; controversies surrounding, 241–43, 244; effects of, 257, 472; meaning of, 367, 372, 379, 401, 410, 479, 484, 492; and lawsuit, 475, 483, 479, 484, 487, 560, 569, 575, 579, 590, 600; and *Miss Evers' Boys*, 527–28, 542–46. *See also* Arsenic, as syphilis treatment; Mercury, as syphilis treatment; Syphilis—untreated

—untreated: and treatment withheld from subjects, 2, 15, 21, 116–18, 168, 193, 225–26, 354, 366, 483, 509; and TSS, 2, 19, 23, 110, 164–65, 172, 175, 203, 220, 225, 233, 253, 266–67, 281, 407, 421, 466, 492, 512–13, 567, 579, 590; and Oslo Study, 2, 19–20, 151, 203, 233,

ment, 23; formation of, 27, 37, 236, 299; and informed consent, 27, 164, 166, 171, 175, 224, 280; and HSR, 27–28, 29, 171, 173, 180–81, 251, 418–19; and subject interviews, 132–35; and Buxtun, 152; charter of, 157–61; members of, 161–62; and justification of study, 162–66, 172, 418; and ethics, 166, 171, 172, 173, 251, 280, 283–84, 292; and penicillin, 167–69, 171, 172; and continuation of study, 169–71, 402

—control group: selection of, 1, 15, 24, 119, 125, 172, 220, 401, 491–92; transfer of to syphilitic group, 24, 165, 302, 359, 380 (n. 1), 492; and syphilis treatment, 95–96, 222, 226; and syphilis, 110, 222, 226; and mortality rates, 120–24, 197, 227; interviews with, 133; and morbidity, 207–8; family status of, 227; and cardiovascular disease, 229; and lawsuit, 229–30, 476, 482, 487; and syphilis serology, 230; families of, 458, 492; and untreated syphilis, 484

—Legacy Committee, 9, 278, 459, 559–66

—subjects: education of, xv, 21, 116, 127, 128, 225, 252, 259, 286, 402, 405, 409, 431, 478; tracing of, 1–2, 98, 101, 111, 119–20, 129, 410–11, 447; syphilis treatment withheld from, 2, 15, 25–26, 27, 116, 168–69, 175–76, 198, 205, 207, 213, 225–26, 229, 231–32, 241, 251, 257, 267, 357, 370, 401, 465, 466, 469, 479, 484, 487, 560, 569, 575, 579, 590, 600; syphilis treatment obtained by, 7, 26, 81, 89, 107, 120, 151, 169, 196, 197, 198, 199, 209–10, 220, 222, 230, 372, 377, 378, 410, 466, 484, 486, 487, 492; syphilis treatment offered to, 21–23, 31 (n. 43), 90, 165, 220, 281, 479, 512, 568–69, 589; deception of, 21–25, 27, 29, 175, 246, 253, 281, 286, 291, 365, 479, 491, 512, 521, 522, 523–24, 559, 560, 567, 575, 589–90, 600; selection of, 21–26, 35, 78–80, 97, 119, 125, 172, 206, 220, 222, 224, 243–44, 401, 479, 486; dehumanization of, 28, 252, 255, 258–59, 260, 266, 370, 458, 484, 522; and timeline, 34–38; cash payments to, 36, 103, 138–39, 142, 147; certificates of appreciation for, 36, 138–39, 145, 147, 150; and Centers for Disease Control, 38; compensation of, 38, 142, 146, 147, 237, 328, 332, 338, 365, 378, 402, 403, 457, 460, 468, 470–71, 487, 488, 490, 514, 561, 568; and lawsuit, 38, 213, 229, 229–30, 237, 328, 332, 365, 412, 473, 475, 476, 478–83; and

correspondence, 87–88, 102–3; and untreated syphilis, 89–91, 105, 253; responsibility to, 100, 108, 246, 600; and Rivers, 110, 134, 135, 141, 323–27, 330, 332–33, 370–71, 373, 377; and mortality rate, 120–24, 197, 227; follow-up procedures for, 126–29, 465, 470, 483, 492; interviews with, 132–35; and Senate hearing testimony, 136–49; exploitation of, 175, 286, 425; family status of, 227; and cardiovascular disease, 228–29; and TSS reports, 255–59, 260, 261; and ethics, 295 (n. 7); and syphilis serology, 302, 303; and Moveable School, 356; identification of as cadavers, 370; and informed consent, 401; families of, 457–60, 482, 483, 487, 492, 575; and continuation of study, 464; health care of, 469, 561, 568, 479, 484, 487, 560, 569, 575, 579, 590, 600; and *Miss Evers' Boys*, 527–51, 568–70, 572; and official apology, 562; memorial to, 572, 576

Tuskegee University National Center for Bioethics in Research and Health Care, 2, 9, 562–63, 576

Tuskegee VA Hospital: and African American mortality, 41; and JRF DPs, 42; and African Americans' living conditions, 64; and cardiovascular disease testing, 76; and autopsies, 86, 221; and health care delivery systems, 98; and TSS, 103, 144, 322; and Tuskegee Institute, 354; and black-controlled hospitals, 435; and TSS subjects, 468

Tyson, Freddie Lee, 458

Uganda, 580, 588, 598

United Nations Program on Acquired Immune Deficiency Syndrome, 598

United States, and lawsuit, 477, 480, 482–83, 489, 514, 568

U.S. Army, 168, 195

U.S. Department of Defense, 177, 179

U.S. Department of Health and Human Services, 576, 580, 581

U.S. Department of Health, Education and Welfare (HEW): and TSS, 15, 37, 38, 411–12; and lawsuit, 38; and policies on HSR, 177–80, 412; and penicillin availability, 237. *See also* Tuskegee Syphilis Study—Ad Hoc Advisory Panel

U.S. District Court of the Middle District of Alabama, 236, 412

U.S. Navy, 195

U.S Public Health Service (PHS): and VD
control, xi, 239, 242, 353, 368, 496, 497, 498–
500, 501, 502–3; and TSS records, xi, 328,
472; and TSS initiation, xv, 2, 15, 34, 219,
243, 254, 276, 303, 353, 479, 559; and TSS
sponsorship, 1, 110, 116, 251, 340, 348, 411–12,
489, 507, 509, 561, 579, 589; and African
Americans as research subjects, 1–2; and
syphilis treatment, 2, 15, 20, 21, 25–26, 27,
60, 65, 68, 80–82, 176–77, 301, 368, 370,
407–8, 483, 513, 590; and spinal taps, 2, 22,
24–25, 81, 485–86; inducements of, 2, 23–25,
32 (n. 58), 36, 62, 81, 116, 126, 127–29, 130,
152, 225, 252, 259, 267, 323–24, 330, 357, 401,
409, 559, 590; and morality, 2–3, 29, 276,
278–79, 287, 289–92, 295, 418; role of, 7; and
TSS goals, 18–19; and prevalence of syphilis,
21, 34, 42–43, 60; and TSS design, 21, 35; and
TSS continuation, 23, 24; subjects' trust in,
24, 61; and race, 26, 416; and scientific bureaucracy, 29; and JRF DPs, 34, 59, 60, 75,
163, 218, 239–41, 242, 253, 266, 353, 400,
406–7; and penicillin, 35, 213, 228, 392, 410,
590; and TSS reports, 35, 219, 257; and lawsuit, 38, 229, 475, 481; and correspondence,
73–75, 87–88, 102–3, 368; and TSS salaries,
76; and TSS subjects, 125, 154, 378, 418, 589,
594; and VD statistics, 155–56; and Cooperative Clinical Studies in the Treatment of
Syphilis, 163, 195; and Macon Co. Health
Department, 170, 451, 465; and HSR, 177,
276, 288, 291, 303; and Alabama law, 226,
231; and informed consent, 231; and American Social Hygiene Association, 241–42;
and physicians, 244; and syphilis serology,
251, 301–3, 305, 308, 311, 313, 401; and ethics,
292, 410, 411; and syphilis research, 299–
300; and Kenney, 304; and autopsies, 306;
and syphilis diagnosis, 310–11; and patent
agreement, 314; and Rivers, 348, 353, 370,
379; and Tuskegee Institute, 445, 561; and
Olansky, 511–12

U.S. Senate Hearings before the Subcommittee on Health of the Committee on Labor
and Public Welfare: and TSS, 2, 365; and
Kennedy, 37, 136–56, 236, 251, 412, 418; and
TSS subjects' testimony, 136–49

U.S. Supreme Court, 313, 490

United States v. Stanley, 490

University Hospital of Cleveland, 581
University of Michigan, 163, 300
University of Pennsylvania, 163, 300
University of Virginia Hospital, 63
Usilton, L. J., 90, 122, 168, 208

Values: and scientific research, 15, 29, 263–64,
287; and informed consent, 284, 287; and
HSR, 288–89, 291, 292; and VD control,
495, 496, 505
VDRL test, 197, 210, 305, 311, 312, 501
Venereal Disease Research Act of 1936, 305
Venereal Disease Research Laboratory
(VDRL), 304, 501, 503, 511, 512
Venereal diseases: control of, 8, 239, 241–42,
258, 353, 368, 410, 419, 495–506; and African
Americans, 17, 20, 42, 59, 353; and TSS, 163
Venereal disease tests, 7. *See also* Syphilis—
serology; *specific tests*
Veterans Hospital. *See* Tuskegee VA Hospital
Vines, Kenneth, 477
Violence: and mortality rates, 42, 43–45; and
sexuality, 44, 54
Volstead Act, 239
Vonderlehr, Raymond: and TSS subjects, 21–
25; and TSS, 35, 97, 207–8, 232–33, 267, 278,
283, 322, 325, 466, 486, 512; correspondence
of, 80–96, 168, 220, 225–26; and control
subjects, 222; and autopsies, 269, 421; and
morality, 279, 286; and syphilis treatment,
281; and ethics, 282, 283, 287; and informed
consent, 284; and syphilis serology, 302, 321;
and Native Americans, 354; and spinal taps,
485; and VD control, 497–98, 505–6

Walker, Eleanor N., 101, 436
Walker, Thelma P., 358
Wallace, George, 236
Walwyn, C. A., 92–93
Ward, Benjamin, 592
Washington, Booker T., 3, 348, 349, 350, 354,
369–70, 576
Washington Serology Conference, 304, 305
Wassermann test: and TSS subjects, 21, 34; and
JRF DPs, 43, 59, 60, 64, 218; and TSS, 76, 77,
78, 79, 80; and Oslo Study, 163, 194, 216, 217;
reliability of, 242–43; and syphilis serology,
300; and cardiovascular disease, 306; and
TSS control group, 484; and syphilis treat-
ment, 492

STUDIES IN SOCIAL MEDICINE

Nancy M. P. King, Gail E. Henderon, and Jane Stein, eds.
  Beyond Regulations:
  Ethics in Human Subjects Research (1999)

Laurie Zoloth
  Health Care and the Ethics of Encounter:
  A Jewish Discussion of Social Justice (1999)

Susan M. Reverby, ed.
  Tuskegee's Truths:
  Rethinking the Tuskegee Syphilis Study (2000)